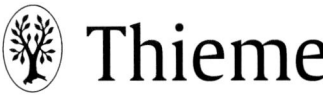

Ultrasound of the Urogenital System

Grant M Baxter, FRCR
Consultant Radiologist
Department of Radiology
Western Infirmary NHS Trust
Glasgow, UK

Paul S Sidhu, BSc, MRCP, FRCR
Consultant Radiologist
Honorary Senior Lecturer
Department of Radiology
King's College Hospital
London, UK

With contributions by
PL Allan, S Chandrasekera, D Dodds, CC Geddes,
SD Heenan, V Hughes, E Leen, J Moss, GH Muir, U Patel,
P Scott, MEK Sellars, J Traynor, MJ Weston, CJ Wilkins

450 illustrations

Thieme
Stuttgart · New York

Library of Congress Cataloging-in-Publication Data is available from the publisher.

Illustrator: Adrian Cornford

For Fig. 12.1: Markus Voll
Reproduced from Schuenke M et al. *THIEME Atlas of Anatomy–General Anatomy and Musculoskeletal System* (Stuttgart: Georg Thieme Verlag, 2005), 201

Important note: Medicine is an ever-changing science undergoing continual development. Research and clinical experience are continually expanding our knowledge, in particular our knowledge of proper treatment and drug therapy. Insofar as this book mentions any dosage or application, readers may rest assured that the authors, editors, and publishers have made every effort to ensure that such references are in accordance with **the state of knowledge at the time of production of the book.**

Nevertheless, this does not involve, imply, or express any guarantee or responsibility on the part of the publishers in respect to any dosage instructions and forms of applications stated in the book. **Every user is requested to examine carefully** the manufacturers' leaflets accompanying each drug and to check, if necessary in consultation with a physician or specialist, whether the dosage schedules mentioned therein or the contraindications stated by the manufacturers differ from the statements made in the present book. Such examination is particularly important with drugs that are either rarely used or have been newly released on the market. Every dosage schedule or every form of application used is entirely at the user's own risk and responsibility. The authors and publishers request every user to report to the publishers any discrepancies or inaccuracies noticed. If errors in this work are found after publication, errata will be posted at www.thieme.com on the product description page.

Some of the product names, patents, and registered designs referred to in this book are in fact registered trademarks or proprietary names even though specific reference to this fact is not always made in the text. Therefore, the appearance of a name without designation as proprietary is not to be construed as a representation by the publisher that it is in the public domain.

This book, including all parts thereof, is legally protected by copyright. Any use, exploitation, or commercialization outside the narrow limits set by copyright legislation, without the publisher's consent, is illegal and liable to prosecution. This applies in particular to photostat reproduction, copying, mimeographing, preparation of microfilms, and electronic data processing and storage.

© 2006 Georg Thieme Verlag,
Rüdigerstrasse 14, 70469 Stuttgart, Germany
http://www.thieme.de
Thieme New York, 333 Seventh Avenue,
New York, NY 10001, USA
http://www.thieme.com

Typesetting by primustype Hurler GmbH, Notzingen
Printed in Germany by Grammlich, Pliezhausen
10-ISBN 3-13-137441-1 (GTV)
13-ISBN 978-3-13-137441-7 (GTV)
10-ISBN 1-58890-237-4 (TNY)
13-ISBN 978-1-58890-237-5 (TNY)   1 2 3 4 5 6

Preface

We hope that you will enjoy *Ultrasound of the Urogenital System*, a comprehensive guide to the applications of ultrasound in the everyday investigation of the renal tract. Ultrasound is often used in the preliminary investigation of a problem associated with the renal tract, whether it is thought to originate within the kidney, the prostate, testes, or elsewhere in the genito-urinary tract.

With this in mind we have compiled a textbook that specifically deals with the role of ultrasound in imaging of the renal tract to include the kidneys, collecting systems, and bladder, and addresses the common pathological, medical, and surgical conditions. The prostate, testes, and penis also receive coverage since ultrasound has an increasingly important primary role in these areas. The imaging findings in each subject area are put into clinical context by two chapters giving both a medical and surgical overview, often of the same clinical problem or presentation, and clearly showing how ultrasound and the other imaging modalities play an important role in securing the diagnosis.

The failing kidney and its treatment, including transplantation, is discussed, and the many clinical and resource issues this raises for the 21st century are addressed. Genito-urinary problems are a common scenario in childhood and can continue or have implications into adulthood; thus no book on the genito-urinary tract would be complete without a chapter on the pediatric population. Although many of the chapters have been contributed by ultrasound enthusiasts, both they and the editors are conscious of the crucial role played by the other imaging modalities in patient investigation and these, too, are referred to in the book. Ultrasound contrast agents are relatively new in relation to the renal tract and to date have largely focussed on the liver. Whilst their use in the kidney, prostate, etc is in the early stages of assessment, a section has been included to discuss early results and potential future applications.

Unfortunately the results of many investigations of the genito-urinary tract will confirm clinical diagnoses of suspected carcinoma. It must be remembered that the applications of imaging also extend to treatment monitoring and assessment of response, thus the book includes a chapter on the treatment of common malignant conditions of the genito-urinary tract. Furthermore, the increasing prominence of ultrasound in interventions in this area and in imaging and treatment of renal tract trauma is included.

Clearly, the wide range of specific specialist areas covered by this textbook, albeit genito-urinary in origin, could not be addressed by one or two individuals. Therefore we have contributions from a large number of authors, all well respected in their fields. Our main aim was to produce a textbook, which, whilst not an all-encompassing tome, would be comprehensive, taking in all aspects of modern ultrasound practice. In addition we wished to produce a book of high quality images which offers the practising radiologist, sonographer, physician, and trainees insight into the contribution of ultrasound to routine clinical management, and provides them with practical, critical, and useful information which they will use throughout their working practice. We also hope this book will be read beyond the traditional imaging community since we feel it is ideal in size and detail to give a solid grounding to those renal physicians and urologists wishing to undertake their own imaging.

Grant M Baxter and Paul S Sidhu

Acknowledgments

It has indeed been an enlightening experience to see what is involved in publishing such a book, and to witness the effort, enthusiasm, and dedication required. Many of those involved, for example in illustrating, designing, typesetting, and printing this textbook, will remain unnamed. We would like to thank them collectively for their tireless effort, support, and co-operation in completing this project.

We are also aware of the time and effort invested by each contributor to produce such high quality chapters and images. We would like to thank them for this and are pleased to say that all friendships remain intact.

Finally, we wish to thank our families and friends who have supported us during this project and indeed our secretaries who manage successfully to organize the many different aspects of our work.

Contributors

Paul L Allan, BSc, MBBS, DMRD, FRCP, FRCP (Edin)
Consultant Radiologist
Royal Infirmary of Edinburgh
Part-time Senior Lecturer Radiology
University of Edinburgh
Edinburgh, UK

Grant M Baxter (see title page)

Srinath Chandrasekera, MS, FRCS, FEBU
Senior Research Fellow in Urology
Department of Urology
King's College Hospital
London, UK

David Dodds, MBChB, MRCP, FRCR
Consultant Oncologist
Beatson Oncology Unit
Western Infirmary
Glasgow, UK

Colin C Geddes, FRCP (Glas)
Consultant Nephrologist
Renal Unit
Western Infirmary
Glasgow, UK

Susan D Heenan, MB, BChir, MA, MRCP (UK), FRCR
Consultant Radiologist
Department of Radiology
St. George's Hospital and Medical School
London, UK

Vivienne Hughes, MBChB, MRCP, FRCR
Beatson Oncology Unit
Western Infirmary
Glasgow, UK

Edward Leen, MD, FRCR
Consultant Radiologist
Department of Radiology
Royal Infirmary
Glasgow, UK

Jon Moss, FRCS, FRCR
Consultant in Interventional Radiology
Department of Radiology
Gartnavel General Hospital
Glasgow, UK

Gordon H Muir, FRCS (Urol), FEBU
Consultant Urologist and Senior Lecturer
Department of Urology
King's College Hospital
London, UK

Uday Patel MB, ChB, MRCP (UK), FRCR
Consultant Radiologist
Department of Radiology
St. George's Hospital and Medical School
London, UK

Paul Scott, MRCP, FRCR
Fellow in Interventional Radiology
Department of Radiology
Gartnavel General Hospital
Glasgow, UK

Maria EK Sellars MBhB FRCR
Consultant Radiologist
Department of Radiology
King's College Hospital
London, UK

Paul S Sidhu (see title page)

Jamie Traynor, MRCP (UK)
Specialist Registrar
Renal Unit
Western Infirmary
Glasgow, UK

Michael J Weston MB, ChB, MRCP, FRCR
Consultant Radiologist
Department of Radiology
St. James' University Hospital
Leeds, UK

C Jason Wilkins, MA, MRCP, FRCR
Consultant Radiologist
Department of Radiology
King's College Hospital
London, UK

List of Abbreviations

^{51}Cr-EDTA	^{51}Cr-ethylene diamine tetraacetic acid	IMRT	intensity modulated radiation therapy
^{99}Tc-DMSA	^{99}Tc-dimercaptosuccinic acid	INR	international normalized ratio
ACDK	acquired cystic disease of the kidney	IVC	inferior vena cava
ACE	angiotensin-converting enzyme	IVU	intravenous urography
ACTH	adrenocorticotropic hormone	KDSM	keratinizing desquamative squamous metaplasia
ADI	agent detection imaging		
ADPKD	autosomal dominant polycystic kidney disease	KUB	kidneys, ureter, bladder
		LDH	lactate dehydrogenase
AFP	alpha-fetoprotein	LH	luteinizing hormone
AI	acceleration index	LHRH	luteinizing hormone-releasing hormone
ANCA	antineutrophil cytoplasmic antibody	LOC	loss of correlation
ANF	antinuclear factor	LUTS	lower urinary tract symptoms
APTT	activated partial thromboplastin time	MAG3	mercaptoacetyltriglycine
ARF	acute renal failure	MCU	micturating cystourethrography
ARPDK	autosomal recessive polycystic kidney disease	MI	mechanical index
AT	acceleration time	MPA	medroxyprogesterone acetate
ATLS	Advanced Trauma and Life Support	MRA	magnetic resonance angiography
ATN	acute tubular necrosis	MSU	midstream urine
AVF	arteriovenous fistula	MVAC	methotrexate, vinblastine, adriamycin, cisplatin
BCG	bacille Calmette–Guérin		
BEP	bleomycin, etoposide, cisplatin	PAN	polyarteritis nodosa
beta-HCG	human beta-chorionic gonadotropin	PCN	percutaneous nephrostomy
BPH	benign prostatic hyperplasia	PCNL	percutaneous nephrolithotomy
CAPD	continuous ambulatory peritoneal dialysis	PGE1	prostaglandin E1
CCI	coherent contrast imaging	PI	pulsatility index
CECT	contrast-enhanced computed tomography	PIH	pulse inversion harmonic
CIS	carcinoma in situ	pmp	per million population
CKD	chronic kidney disease	PRF	pulse repetition frequency
CPS	contrast pulse sequencing	PSA	prostate-specific antigen
CRF	chronic renal failure	PSV	peak systolic velocity
CXR	chest x-ray	PTFE	polytetrafluoroethylene
DTPA	diethylene triamine pentaacetate	PTLD	posttransplant lymphoproliferative disease
ECG	electrocardiography/electrocardiogram	PUJ	pelviuretic junction
ED	erectile dysfunction	PUJO	pelviuretic junction obstruction
EDV	end diastolic velocity	PUV	posterior urethral valve
ESR	erythrocyte sedimentation rate	RAR	renal-to-aortic ratio
ESRD	end-stage renal disease	RAS	renal artery stenosis
ESWL	extracorporeal shockwave lithotripsy	RCC	renal cell carcinoma
FAST	focussed assessment with sonography in trauma	RF	radiofrequency
		RF	retroperitoneal fibrosis
FBC	full blood count	RI	resistive index
FFP	fresh frozen plasma	ROI	regions of interest
FMD	fibromuscular dysplasia	SAE	stimulated acoustic emission
Fr	French	SCVIR	Society of Cardiovascular and Interventional Radiology
FSH	follicle-stimulating hormone		
G	gauge	SLE	systemic lupus erythematosus
GFR	glomerular filtration rate	TCC	transitional cell carcinoma
Gy	Gray	TIPSS	transjugular intrahepatic portosystemic shunt
HCG	human chorionic gonadotropin	TNM	tumor, node, metastasis
HIFU	high-intensity focussed ultrasound	TRUS	transrectal ultrasound
HIVAN	HIV-associated nephropathy	TUNA	transurethral needle ablation
HLA	human leukocyte antigen	TUR	transurethral resection
HRPC	hormone-refractory prostate cancer	TURBT	transurethral resection of bladder tumor

TURP	transurethral resection of the prostate	**VHL**	von Hippel Lindau
USCD	ultrasound cystodynomagram	**VUJ**	vesicouretic junction
VCUG	voiding cystourethrography	**VUR**	vesicouretic reflux

Table of Contents

Section 1 Nephrology   1

1 Introduction: Medical Overview 3
Introduction 3
Renal Function....................... 4
Presentation of Renal Disease 5
Natural History of Chronic Kidney Disease 8
Investigating the Patient who Presents with
Renal Disease........................ 9
Conclusion......................... 13

2 The Normal Kidney 15
Anatomical Relationships of the Kidney 15
Anatomy of the Kidney 16
Ultrasound Examination 17

3 Parenchymal Diseases of the Kidney 29
Introduction 29
Cortical Disorders..................... 30
Disorders of the Medulla/Pyramids 31
Renal Infections 33
Vascular Disorders 36
Miscellaneous Disorders 39
End-Stage Renal Disease 41

4 Chronic Renal Failure 44
Introduction 44
Diseases Associated with the Native Kidneys. ... 44
Dialysis........................... 46

5 Renal Transplantation. 54
Background........................ 54
Introduction 54
Indications and Contraindications in
Transplantation 55
Donor Supply....................... 55
Histocompatibility Testing 55
Preoperative Management 55
Surgery........................... 55
Immunosuppression 56
Imaging the Transplant Kidney............. 56
Early Complications 58
Late Complications 62
Long-Term Complications................ 66
Other Complications 66
Combined Renal and Pancreas Transplant....... 67

**6 Radiological Intervention in the Urogenital Tract
(Including Trauma and Emergencies)** 70
Principles of Ultrasound-Guided Procedures 70
Patient Preparation: General Principles 71
Nephrostomy....................... 72
Transplant Kidneys.................... 76
Drainage of Perinephric Collections 77
Ultrasound-Guided Renal Biopsy............ 78
Renal Artery Stenosis 79
Use of Ultrasound in Radiofrequency Ablation
in the Kidney....................... 80
Trauma and Emergencies................. 82

Section 2 Urology   87

7 The Urogenital Tract: Surgical Overview 89
Introduction 89
Urinary Tract Infections................. 89
Urinary Calculus Disease 90
Upper Urinary Tract Obstruction
(Hydronephrosis).................... 91
Hematuria......................... 92
Lower Urinary Tract Symptoms and Benign
Prostatic Hyperplasia.................. 93
Prostate Carcinoma 95

Focal Renal Lesions.................... 96
Urogenital Trauma 97
Penile and Scrotal Abnormalities............ 98

8 Focal Lesions of the Kidney 102
Introduction 102
Renal Cysts 102
Benign Solid Lesions 109
Malignant Tumors 111
Renal Trauma....................... 114

9 Diseases of the Collecting System and Ureters . 119
Introduction 119
Obstruction 119
Acute Obstruction. 119
Calculi 124
Congenital Abnormalities. 125
Tumors of the Collecting System and Ureters . . . 126
Miscellaneous Disorders 127

10 Diseases of the Bladder and Prostate 130
Introduction 130
Anatomy of the Bladder and Prostate. 130
Ultrasound of the Bladder and Prostate Gland . . . 133
The Abnormal Prostate and Ejaculatory
Mechanism 140
Transrectal Ultrasound-Guided Intervention 148

11 Diseases of the Testis and Epididymis 153
Introduction 153
Normal Anatomy 153
Ultrasound Examination Technique 155
Normal Ultrasound Appearances of the Testis
and Epididymis 155
Intratesticular Abnormalities 157
Extratesticular Abnormalities 168

12 Diseases of the Penis with
Functional Evaluation 181
Introduction 181
Normal Anatomy and Ultrasound Appearances . . 181
Erectile Dysfunction 182
Structural Pathology 188
Urethral Ultrasound 190

13 Oncological Management of Tumors of the
Urogenital Tract 193
Treatment of Bladder Cancer 193
Treatment of Prostate Cancer 195
Treatment of Testicular Tumors. 199
Treatment of Renal Cell Carcinoma 201

Section 3 The Urogenital Tract in the Child 205

14 Ultrasound of the Pediatric Urogenital Tract. . 207
Introduction 207
Ultrasound Imaging Techniques 207
Normal Anatomy 207
Congenital Anomalies Affecting Renal
Position and Number 208
Urinary Tract Infections 213
Cystic Renal Disease 215
Renal Tumors. 217
Renal Trauma. 218
Renal Calcification 218
Vascular Anomalies. 218
Renal Transplant. 219
Abnormalities of the Bladder and
Distal Urinary Tract. 220
Adrenal Glands. 222
Testis 223

Section 4 Other Imaging Modalities in the Urogenital Tract 231

15 Non-Ultrasound Imaging of the
Urogenital Tract. 233
Introduction 233
Problem-Solving. 239

Section 5 New Developments: Ultrasound Contrast Agents 251

16 The Native Kidney 253
Introduction: Classes of Ultrasound
Contrast Agents 253
Microbubble Behavior and Imaging Modes 254
Newer Nonlinear Imaging Modes 255
Optimization of Equipment Settings and
Practical Aspects. 255
Clinical Applications 256

17 The Transplant Kidney 264
Introduction 264
Vascular Applications 266
Potential Applications 268

Section 1

Nephrology

1 **Introduction: Medical Overview** 3
2 **The Normal Kidney** 15
3 **Parenchymal Diseases of the Kidney** 29
4 **Chronic Renal Failure** 44
5 **Renal Transplantation** 54
6 **Radiological Intervention in the Urogenital Tract (Including Trauma and Emergencies)** 70

1 Introduction: Medical Overview

C. Geddes, J. Traynor

Introduction

The field of nephrology has expanded rapidly in the last 50 years as a result of improved understanding of the pathophysiology of renal disease and the increasing success and availability of renal replacement therapy for acute and chronic renal failure.[1]

The prevalence of renal disease has increased greatly in the last few decades. This is probably a combination of a true increase in prevalence (in an aging population that has an increasing burden of co-morbid disease that can affect the kidneys), and increased recognition of the presence of renal disease. The prevalence of renal disease shows wide variability across the world that is likely to reflect differences in its true incidence and in the availability of health-care resources for detection and treatment. The United States appears to have the highest prevalence of renal disease. It has recently been estimated that 11% of the US adult population has chronic kidney disease (CKD, as defined below),[2] and the incidence of CKD requiring renal replacement therapy in the United States in 2001 was 336 per million population (pmp) per year.[3] The incidence of CKD in Europe is variable but universally much lower than the United States (Fig. 1.1).

The presence of CKD is of major importance for an individual because it is associated with a markedly increased risk of cardiovascular, infectious, and malignant complications compared with the general population.[4–7]

The incidence of acute renal disease is more difficult to ascertain but is also probably increasing. A recent comprehensive national survey in Scotland reported 297 patients pmp per year in 2002 had acute renal failure (ARF) severe enough to require dialysis treatment.[9] This compares with previous estimates in the United Kingdom of between 18 pmp per year and 187 pmp per year in publications covering the 1980s and 1990s.[10–13]

Renal replacement therapies (dialysis and kidney transplant) are expensive, and the management of renal disease places a high burden on health-care budgets compared with other specialties.

This chapter will describe the detection of renal disease and the approach to the patient with renal disease. Ultrasound scanning of the urogenital tract has a pivotal role in investigating the causes of renal disease. In selected patients it is also of value in assessing prognosis, assessing disease progression, and in treating urinary obstruction.

A basic understanding of how the normal kidney functions is important in order to appreciate the clinical manifestations of renal disease. A brief description of renal function will be followed by an overview of the presentation and investigation of adults with renal disease.

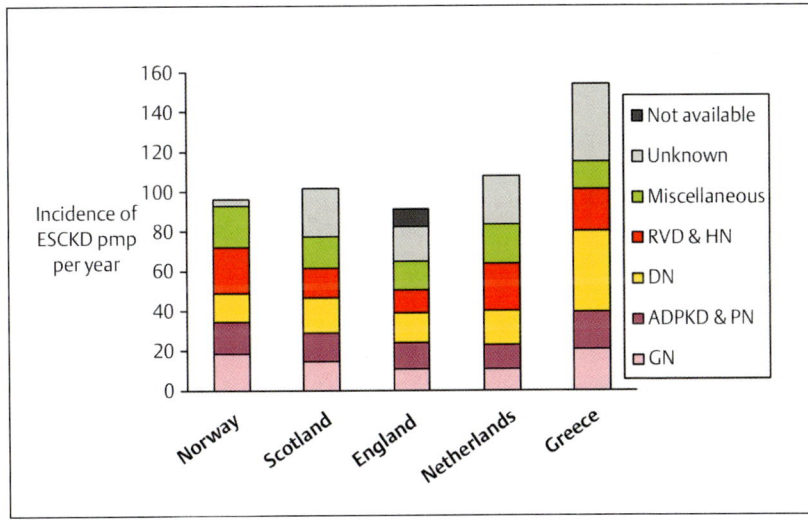

Fig. 1.1 **Variability in the incidence and cause of chronic kidney disease requiring renal replacement therapy in selected European countries for the year 2001.** Adapted from The European Renal Association (ERA-EDTA) Registry 2001 Annual Report, published June 2003[8] (RVD = renovascular disease; HN = hypertensive nephropathy; DN = diabetic nephropathy; ADPKD = autosomal dominant polycystic kidney disease; PN = chronic pyelonephritis and other interstitial diseases; GN = glomerulonephritis; ESCKD = end stage chronic kidney disease)

1 Introduction: Medical Overview

Summary points:
- The incidence of both acute and chronic kidney disease is rising
- Treatment of kidney disease places a high burden on health-care resources
- Ultrasound scanning has a pivotal role in assessing the causes and prognosis of kidney disease

Renal Function

The kidney performs several functions. The main role of the kidney is to excrete metabolic waste and control the solutes in extracellular and intracellular fluid. It also has endocrine functions and plays a major role in control of blood pressure and drug pharmacokinetics. The functions of the kidney and clinical manifestations of failure of these functions are summarized in Table 1.1.

The performance of all these kidney functions is dependent on approximately one million nephrons in each kidney (Fig. 1.2). Blood from the renal arteries is delivered to the glomerular capillaries. Ultrafiltrate enters the proximal tubule by filtration of blood through the basement membrane that lies between the endothelium of the glomerular capillary and the glomerular epithelium. The quantity and content of the ultrafiltrate is dependent on the driving pressure within the intraglomerular capillaries and the basement membrane permeability. The tubules reabsorb and secrete solute and/or water from the ultrafiltrate under the influence of numerous homeostatic factors. The tubules converge

Table 1.1 Summary of functions of the kidney and clinical consequences of impaired function

Function	Clinical consequences of impaired function
Excretion of nitrogenous waste	Elevated serum concentrations of urea & creatinine[a]
Blood-pressure control	Hypertension (or less commonly hypotension)
Sodium excretion	Extracellular fluid overload (e.g., edema) or depletion
Free water excretion	Hyponatremia or hypernatremia
Electrolyte balance	e.g., hyperkalemia
Acid–base balance	Metabolic acidosis
Erythropoietin secretion	Anemia
Vitamin D_1-hydroxylation (activation)	Hypocalcemia, hyperparathyroidism[b]
Phosphate excretion	Hyperphosphatemia, hyperparathyroidism[b]
Excretion of water-soluble medicines, e.g., digoxin, gentamicin	Medicine toxicity
Gluconeogenesis in the fasting state	Tendency to hypoglycemia
Catabolism of peptide hormones (including insulin)	Tendency to hypoglycemia

[a] Many nitrogenous waste products are excreted, but urea and creatinine are the ones most commonly measured
[b] Associated with renal bone disease and cardiovascular disease

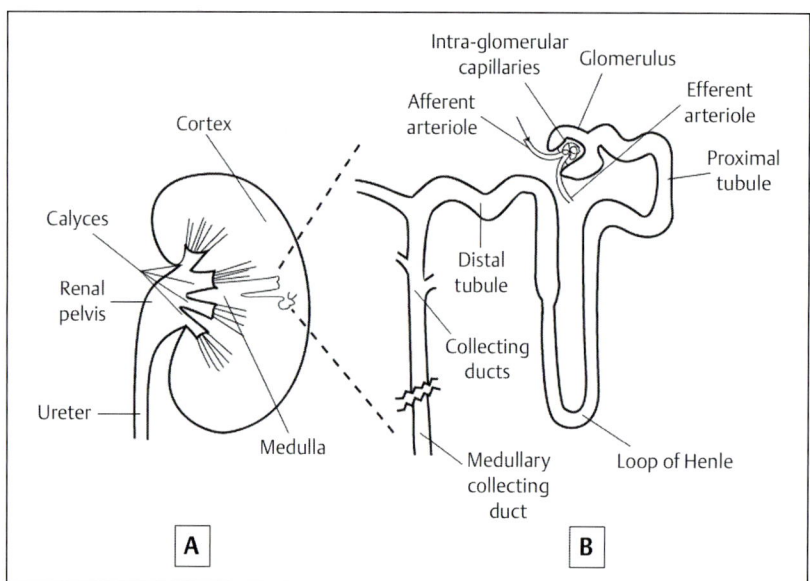

Fig. 1.2 Graphical representation of the anatomy of the whole kidney (**a**) and an expanded representation of a single nephron (**b**)

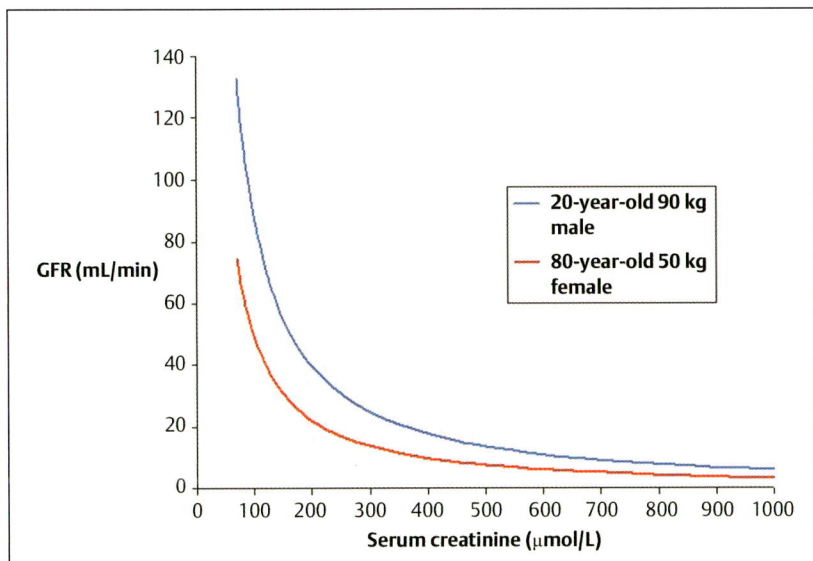

Fig. 1.3 **Relationship between serum creatinine concentration and GFR.** The relationship is dependent on muscle mass, as illustrated by the difference between the 20-year-old male and the 80-year-old female. In general a serum creatinine above the upper limit of the normal range (approximately 120 µmol/L) implies at least a 50% reduction in GFR. A rise from 100 µmol/L to 200 µmol/L reflects a greater loss of renal function than a rise from 400 µmol/L to 500 µmol/L

to form collecting ducts, calyces, and eventually the ureters, which leave each renal pelvis to drain the urine into the bladder.

Renal function is best assessed by measurement of glomerular filtration rate (GFR). This can be considered a measure of the number of functioning nephrons. As renal disease worsens the number of functioning nephrons diminishes and the GFR falls.

The most accurate measures of GFR, such as inulin clearance, are too cumbersome for routine clinical practice. For this reason measurement of creatinine clearance can be used as an estimate of GFR. Creatinine is derived from muscle metabolism. It is suitable for estimating GFR because it is produced at a constant rate, is almost entirely filtered at the glomerulus, and is not reabsorbed by the tubules. Measurement of creatinine clearance requires a 24-hour urine collection, which is often inconvenient for the patient, may lead to false results if the collection is incomplete, and precludes an immediate assessment of renal function. For these reasons measurement of serum creatinine concentration is the most commonly used test of renal function. The relationship between serum creatinine and GFR is shown in Figure 1.**3**.

It is important to appreciate that the relationship between serum creatinine and GFR is inverse but not linear. The relationship between serum creatinine and GFR is dependent on muscle mass because creatinine is derived from muscle; as shown in the graph (Fig. 1.**3**), a 20-year-old, muscular male weighing 90 kg with a serum creatinine of 200 µmol/L will have a much higher GFR than an 80-year-old female weighing 50 kg who also has a serum creatinine of 200 µmol/L.

In the setting of constant muscle mass, and in the absence of dialysis treatment, a rising serum creatinine is a reliable indicator of worsening renal function and a falling serum creatinine is a reliable indicator of improving renal function.

Presentation of Renal Disease

Renal disease may present in many ways depending on the underlying causes, the severity, and the duration of the disease. Renal disease may be primary (i.e., limited to the kidney) or secondary (i.e., occurring as part of a systemic disease affecting more than one organ).

Proteinuria and/or Hematuria

The presence of proteinuria and microscopic hematuria can easily be detected by commercially available dipstick tests. Dipstick testing of urine is performed in a number of settings. Thus proteinuria and/or hematuria may be detected at a routine insurance or employment medical, during pregnancy, or during admission to hospital for unrelated reasons. It may also be detected when investigating patients with hypertension or elevated serum creatinine.

Transient proteinuria detected by dipstick can be associated with a urinary tract infection, fever, and upright posture (orthostatic proteinuria). Persistent proteinuria with or without hematuria suggests impaired size selectivity in the glomerular basement membrane and is therefore a marker of glomerular disease. The most abundant protein in the urine in the setting of glomerular disease is albumin.

Dipstick proteinuria should be confirmed and quantified in a 24-hour urine sample or by calculating the

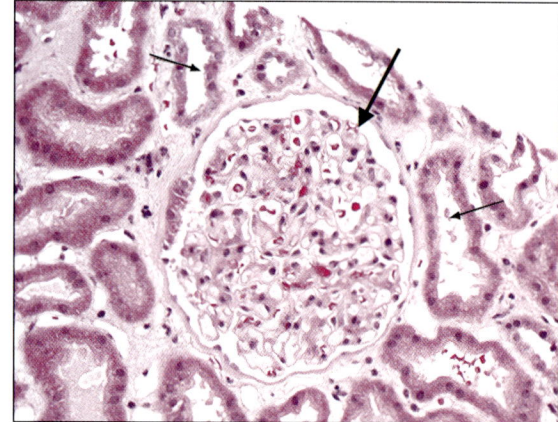

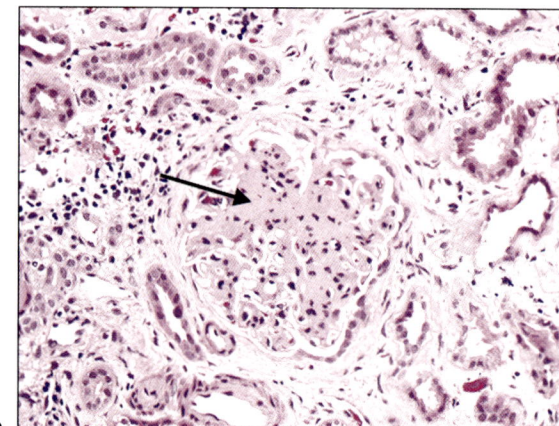

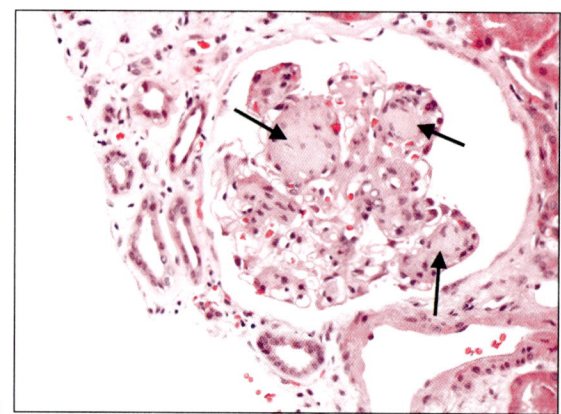

Fig. 1.4 **a** Light microscopy appearances of a cross section through a normal glomerulus (large arrow) and surrounding tubular segments (small arrow; hematoxylin and eosin stain). **b** IgA nephropathy, the most common primary glomerular disease. The main feature is expansion of the mesangium in a proportion of the glomeruli (arrow). The diagnosis is confirmed by identifying immune complexes containing IgA in the mesangium by immunofluorescence and electron microscopy. **c** Diabetic nephropathy. The commonest systemic disease with associated glomerular involvement. The main distinguishing feature is the typical nodular glomerulosclerosis (arrows). (Photomicrographs courtesy of Dr. B. Young, Pathology Dept., Western Infirmary, Glasgow, UK)

albumin:creatinine ratio on a spot urine sample. Dipstick tests for hematuria actually detect hemoglobin, so a positive test should be confirmed by microscopy to detect red cells. If red cells are not present in a patient with dipstick "hematuria" then this suggests overspill of "free" plasma hemoglobin into the urine. In this situation the presence of dipstick "hematuria" is not due to glomerular or urinary tract disease and may occur in conditions such as "march" hemoglobinuria and paroxysmal nocturnal hemoglobinuria.

The presence of proteinuria is often associated with hypertension. Depending on the severity and duration of the disease there may also be renal failure (see below). Heavy proteinuria (3 g per 24 hours) may be associated with hypoalbuminemia and peripheral edema and this triad is called the nephrotic syndrome. Identification of the nephrotic syndrome is important because the patient is at increased risk of thrombotic events, infection, and cardiovascular events.

Isolated microscopic hematuria can also be a presenting feature of glomerular disease, but other bleeding lesions throughout the length of the renal tract should always be considered (see Chapter 7).

The quantity of proteinuria, the presence of hematuria, hypertension, and renal failure, the presence of nephrotic syndrome, the presence of systemic clinical features, and the duration of proteinuria can all give clues as to the likely histological diagnosis, but there is considerable overlap between the clinical features of the many primary and secondary glomerular diseases associated with proteinuria and hematuria (Table 1.2). The commonest primary glomerulopathy in adults in the developed world is IgA nephropathy, and the commonest secondary glomerular disease is diabetic nephropathy (Fig. 1.4).

In a patient with proteinuria and hematuria the possibility of two pathologies such as glomerular disease and bladder carcinoma must always be entertained.

Renal Failure

The kidneys have a large functional reserve, but if sufficient renal parenchyma is diseased then renal failure develops. There is no simple practical definition of renal failure. Table 1.2 shows that, with the exception of elevation of serum creatinine, the clinical manifestations of failure of most of the functions of the kidney are not specific to renal failure. For this reason renal failure is usually diagnosed and monitored by measurement of serum creatinine. A pragmatic approach is to consider all patients with a serum creatinine higher than the upper limit of the "normal" range as having renal failure worthy of investigation. In the light of the

Table 1.2 Diseases to consider in the patient with chronic kidney disease*

Renal parenchymal	Prerenal	Postrenal
Primary glomerular disease e.g., IgA nephropathy, membranous nephropathy, focal segmental glomerulosclerosis, Alport syndrome	Atherosclerotic renovascular disease Hypertensive nephropathy Severe chronic left ventricular failure	Chronic reflux nephropathy/chronic pyelonephritis Chronic prostatic hypertrophy Chronic bladder atonia, e.g. spina bifida
Interstitial disease e.g., ADPKD[a] analgesic nephropathy, nephrocalcinosis, nephronopthiasis		Renal calculi
Secondary diseases e.g., diabetic nephropathy, SLE [b], amyloidosis, sarcoidosis, myeloma, systemic sclerosis, Hepatitis B, C, HIV infection		

* This table is not exhaustive but illustrates the wide range of possibilities
[a] Autosomal dominant polycystic kidney disease
[b] Systemic lupus erythematosis

earlier discussion, however, it should be appreciated that, in a patient with low muscle mass, a serum creatinine rising within the normal range may indicate important loss of renal function (Fig. 1.3).

Renal failure is usually considered as acute or chronic. Again there are no universally agreed definitions, but ARF is usually considered as occurring over a period of days or weeks and CRF occurs over several months or years.

Serum creatinine is one of the most commonly requested blood tests and, as with proteinuria or hematuria, renal failure is often detected opportunistically in patients who are attending medical services for unrelated reasons. Renal failure may also be detected in patients who are systemically unwell (in whom measurement of serum creatinine is regarded as a standard baseline investigation), have proteinuria detected on dipstick testing (see above), or develop oliguria in hospital (see Changes in Urine Volume below).

Macroscopic Hematuria

Macroscopic hematuria is usually caused by bleeding from structural lesions in the urothelial tract such as renal carcinoma, bladder carcinoma, or renal calculi. (For an overview of the causes and evaluation of macroscopic hematuria see Chapter 7.) Occasionally, intermittent macroscopic hematuria can be a manifestation of glomerular diseases such as IgA nephropathy or poststreptococcal glomerulonephritis, or can complicate autosomal dominant polycystic kidney disease (ADPKD). In the first two examples hematuria of glomerular origin can sometimes be confirmed by the presence of dysmorphic red cells on urine microscopy.

Loin Pain

Pain in the upper renal tract is usually situated in the loin/flank area and often radiates to the iliac fossa and groin. Pain in this area should raise the suspicion of renal calculi, renal infection (acute pyelonephritis), renal infarction, or unilateral ureteric obstruction. Other renal diseases are sometimes associated with chronic intermittent loin pain, especially ADPKD, IgA nephropathy, and loin pain hematuria syndrome.

Changes in Urine Volume

Urine volume is determined by both GFR and tubular reabsorption.

GFR can be maintained over a wide range of systemic blood pressure due to autoregulatory mechanisms involving the renin–angiotensin system and prostaglandins. Severe and sustained circulatory failure will lead to oliguria due to a reduced GFR.

Tubular reabsorption of filtrate is also controlled by homeostatic mechanisms. Tubular reabsorption can be inhibited by the administration of diuretics, alcohol, diabetes mellitus (due to the osmotic effects of glucose), and diabetes insipidus (impaired activity of vasopressin), all of which will result in polyuria. Diseases that impair tubular function (e.g., acute tubular necrosis, renal tract obstruction, chronic interstitial disease) may be associated with polyuria even if the GFR is reduced. This is often seen in the recovery phase of ARF and in incomplete urinary tract obstruction (see below).

In most cases of acute or chronically reduced GFR (renal failure) the tubules are also diseased. Impaired GFR and tubular function have opposing effects on urine volume and so measurement of urine volume is not usually helpful in investigating the cause of renal failure. The exception to this is sudden complete anuria in the absence of severe hypotension which is highly suggestive of complete urinary tract obstruction. It should be stressed, however, that an incomplete urinary tract obstruction will usually be associated with ongoing urine output and possible polyuria and therefore obstruction cannot be excluded on clinical grounds alone.

Changes in urine volume can be helpful in monitoring the course of ARF, as an increase in urine output is usually the first sign of recovery of renal function.

Recurrent Urinary Tract Infection

Urinary tract infection (UTI) is usually confined to the lower urinary tract. Recurrent UTI warrants investigation of the urinary tract to exclude acquired or congenital anatomical abnormalities, impaired bladder emptying, urinary obstruction, and calculi (see Chapter 7).

Renal Disease Detected by Targeted Screening

Sometimes asymptomatic patients are found to have renal disease when a relative is found to have a hereditary condition such as ADPKD, Alport syndrome, von Hippel–Lindau syndrome, or medullary cystic kidney disease. Targeted screening of relatives is important because renal disease is often asymptomatic until an advanced stage.

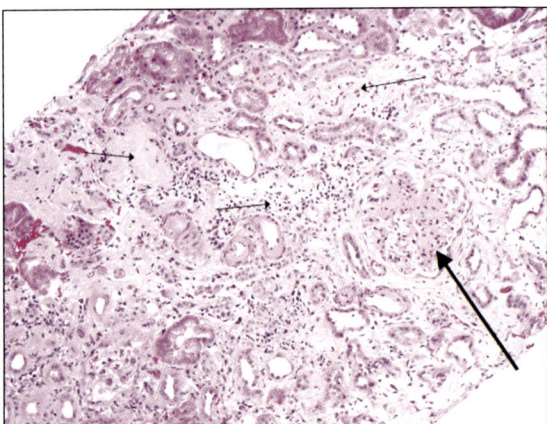

Fig. 1.5 **Histological appearances of a kidney with progressive renal failure.** Note the presence of only one glomerulus in this low power field (large arrow) and widespread replacement of tubules with extensive amorphous fibrosis and chronic inflammatory infiltrate (compared with Fig. 1.**4a**; highlighted by small arrows) The underlying diagnosis in this patient was IgA nephropathy, but these features are common to most causes of CRF. (Photomicrograph courtesy of Dr. B. Young, Pathology Dept., Western Infirmary, Glasgow, UK)

Urine Discoloration

Occasionally patients present to nephrologists with discolored urine. This is usually due to hematuria, myoglobinuria, metabolism of a variety of medicines, or rare inherited enzyme defects such as alkaptonuria.

> **Summary points:**
> - Kidney disease typically presents with proteinuria/hematuria, raised serum creatinine (renal failure), recurrent urinary tract infection, or by targeted screening for inherited diseases
> - Assessment of renal function in routine clinical practice is based on the inverse relationship between serum creatinine and GFR
> - A serum creatinine greater than the upper limit of the "normal" range usually implies renal failure and warrants further assessment
> - The distinction between acute and chronic renal failure is arbitrary. ARF occurs over days/weeks and chronic occurs over months/years

Natural History of Chronic Kidney Disease

A substantial proportion of patients with CKD will remain asymptomatic throughout their lives. Glomerular disease can often be self-limiting. Progression to CRF is an important potential consequence of CKD. It appears that progression to renal failure is secondary to a number of hemodynamic and metabolic factors that are initially protective and are independent of the nature of the underlying causes.[14] A relentless process is triggered, whereby loss of nephrons is associated with compensatory hyperfiltration in the remaining glomeruli. This causes filtration of toxic substances into the tubules, causing further nephron loss and a destructive cycle ensues (Fig. 1.**5**). Eventually, insufficient nephrons remain to maintain total GFR and renal failure develops with a progressive (often linear) deterioration in renal function.

Normal GFR is approximately 90–120 mL/min corrected for a body surface area of 1.73 m^2. Symptoms of uremia do not usually start until GFR falls below 20 mL/min and death from uremia does not usually occur until GFR is < 5 mL/min. Renal replacement therapy (dialysis or transplantation) is usually started when the GFR is 5–20 mL/min and the timing of initiation of renal replacement therapy is usually guided by patient symptoms.[15–18]

There is now increasing evidence that even minor reductions in GFR are associated with significant morbidity, including increased cardiovascular risk and malnutrition,[19,20] despite the fact that the patient is likely to have no symptoms related to the reduced GFR.

Defining Chronic Kidney Disease

The increased awareness of the prognostic importance of even a mild reduction in GFR and the availability of interventions that slow the rate of deterioration in renal function prompted the National Kidney Foundation of the United States to propose CKD as a single entity. They defined CKD as:

> "Evidence of structural or functional kidney abnormalities (abnormal urinalysis, imaging studies, or histology) that persist for at least three months, with or without a decreased GFR (as defined by a GFR of < 60 mL/min per 1.73 m^2). The most common manifestation of kidney damage is persistent albuminuria."[21]

Using a representative sample of 15 625 adults from the general population it was recently estimated that 3.3% of the US adult population has persistent albuminuria with preserved renal function (GFR > 90 mL/min), 7.5% of the population have CKD with GFR 15–89 mL/min, and 0.2% of the population have CKD with GFR < 15 mL/min (including all patients on renal replacement therapy).[22]

The definition of CKD as a single entity has been combined with increased efforts to detect kidney disease at an earlier stage, to identify patients at high risk of progression, and to design intervention strategies to prevent or slow the rate of progression. Lowering of blood pressure with regimens that include agents that inhibit the renin–angiotensin system has been shown to be highly effective at slowing the rate of deterioration in renal function for a wide range of causes.[23-25] Other interventions such as reduced dietary protein intake, immunosuppressive treatment, and intensive treatment of hyperglycemia appear to be effective in selected patients.[26-28]

Summary points:
- It is estimated that 7.5% of adults have chronic kidney disease with reduced renal function (low GFR)
- CKD has a tendency to progress to kidney failure
- Any reduction in GFR is associated with increased cardiovascular morbidity and mortality
- Increased efforts to detect CKD at an early stage will allow interventions to slow the rate of deterioration in GFR and reduce other cardiovascular risk factors

---

Investigating the Patient who Presents with Renal Disease

As described previously, dipstick testing of urine, measurement of serum creatinine, and targeted screening will identify most patients with significant kidney disease. Once detected the clinician should attempt to establish the causes, determine if reduced GFR is present (renal failure), and attempt to establish the duration of renal disease. This information will determine if any specific treatment is available, the likely response to such treatment, and provide prognostic information.

Approach to Acute Renal Failure

If a raised serum creatinine is present it is important to try to establish whether this is acute or chronic, as the differential diagnosis and urgency of investigation and treatment differ. A search for previous measures of renal function should be made. A patient with a serum creatinine of 300 μmol/L clearly has ARF if serum creatinine was 80 μmol/L two weeks before, but has CRF if serum creatinine was 300 μmol/L two weeks before and 200 μmol/L two years before that.

Previous measures of renal function are often not available or are inconclusive, but other features can be helpful. The presence of oliguria (< 0.5 mL urine per kg body weight per hour), recent onset of an acute illness, or daily deterioration in renal function are suggestive of ARF, while the presence of small kidneys (< 8 cm in adults) on ultrasound is suggestive of CRF. When considering the distinction between ARF and CRF it must be emphasized that patients with CRF often have an acute deterioration in renal function ("acute on chronic renal failure") in association with an acute systemic illness or nephrotoxic medicines.

The cause of ARF is best considered in terms of prerenal, postrenal, and renal parenchymal causes (see Table 1.**3**).

Prerenal ARF is the commonest type of ARF and impaired blood supply to the glomeruli must be considered in all cases. Prerenal causes of ARF involve impaired blood supply to the glomeruli, often associated with tubular hypoxia that can eventually lead to acute tubular necrosis (ATN). Prerenal ARF usually results in oliguria and is usually associated with minimal or no protein and blood on urine dipstick testing. Medicines that impair the vascular autoregulatory mechanisms that preserve GFR during times of impaired glomerular blood flow will exacerbate the ARF (angiotensin-converting enzyme [ACE] inhibitors, angiotensin receptor antagonists, nonsteroidal anti-inflammatory drugs [NSAIDs]). When a patient develops intravascular fluid depletion or becomes markedly hypotensive,

Table 1.3 Causes of acute renal failure

Prerenal	Postrenal	Renal parenchymal
Hypovolemic shock Septicemic shock Severe heart failure Liver failure (hepatorenal syndrome) Aortic thrombosis Polyarteritis nodosa Cholesterol emboli syndrome	Bladder outflow obstruction, e.g. prostatic carcinoma Bilateral ureteric obstruction, e.g. bladder carcinoma, invasive cervical carcinoma, retroperitoneal fibrosis Obstruction of a single functioning kidney, e.g. ureteric calculus	Acute glomerulonephritis, e.g. in association with systemic vasculitis, Goodpasture disease, poststreptococcal glomerulonephritis, hemolytic uremic syndrome Direct tubular toxicity, e.g. rhabdomyolysis, myeloma, contrast nephropathy, cisplatin Acute interstitial nephritis, e.g. allergic drug reaction, hantavirus infection Poisoning, e.g. paracetamol

these agents interfere with the normal protective vascular response, rendering the glomeruli and tubules much more vulnerable to damage from hypoperfusion and hypoxia.

Postrenal ARF implies either obstruction to bladder outflow or both ureters, unless the patient only has a single functioning kidney. Complete obstruction will cause anuria, whilst partial obstruction is often associated with polyuria because of impaired ability of the tubules to reabsorb filtrate (see Changes in Urine Volume above). Eventually this polyuria can lead to systemic extracellular fluid depletion, adding a prerenal component to the ARF and causing oliguria. The urine stasis proximal to the obstruction can often lead to UTI with systemic sepsis, leading to worsening of ARF. In this clinical situation immediate relief of the urinary tract obstruction is required to treat both the systemic sepsis and the ARF.

Acute renal parenchymal disease is a rare cause of ARF. Acute renal parenchymal disease is suspected when there is no history to suggest a prerenal cause of ARF, no evidence of systemic sepsis, and imaging reveals normal-sized, unobstructed kidneys. An acute glomerulonephritis is suspected if there is heavy proteinuria and hematuria on dipstick testing and urine microscopy reveals red cell casts. Common causes of acute renal parenchymal disease are listed in Table 1.3. Imaging does not help further with the diagnosis and renal biopsy is usually required to determine the causes when renal parenchymal disease is suspected.

When considering the causes of ARF it should be remembered that a large proportion of cases are multifactorial and that sometimes the distinctions are artificial. For example, rhabdomyolysis as a cause of ARF involves a prerenal component (related to movement of fluid from the intravascular space into the ischemic muscle) and a renal parenchymal component (related to the direct tubular toxicity of filtered myoglobin released from necrotic muscle). Similarly, small vessel vasculitis is considered as a renal parenchymal cause of ARF but in pathophysiological terms can be considered as a prerenal cause.

The vast majority of cases of ARF involve a prerenal component and the urgency of investigation and treatment should reflect the fact that prerenal failure can be seen as a marker of severity of acute systemic disease. Life-threatening hyperkalemia and respiratory failure should be addressed before more detailed assessment is performed.

The history and examination should elicit evidence of recent blood and fluid losses, evidence of and potential sites of sepsis, features of severe heart failure, ingestion of nephrotoxic medicines (including ionic contrast media), symptoms of bladder outflow obstruction, and evidence of an enlarged bladder. Repeated measures of blood pressure, pulse rate, arterial oxygen content, and body temperature help to identify circulatory failure and systemic sepsis.

Investigation to determine the causes of ARF should be directed by the history and examination but may include culture of blood and fluid from any possible source of infection, for example urine, sputum, tests of liver function and cardiac ischemia, and measurement of various factors in the blood that can help to narrow the differential diagnosis such as c-reactive protein, calcium, eosinophil count (raised in cholesterol emboli syndrome, Churg–Strauss syndrome, acute allergic interstitial nephritis), creatinine kinase (raised in rhabdomyolysis), antineutrophil cytoplasmic antibody (vasculitis), and antiglomerular basement antibody (Goodpasture disease).

Monitoring of urine volume is rarely of diagnostic value, for reasons described previously, but increasing urine volume after a period of oliguria can be a useful way of assessing response to treatment. Similarly, measurements of urine osmolality and urine sodium concentration are rarely of diagnostic value but can provide prognostic information.

Imaging to exclude urinary tract obstruction is essential in most cases, as early treatment can rapidly correct renal failure whilst prolonged obstruction can cause irreversible renal damage. Obstruction can be diagnosed by the presence of hydronephrosis; an ultrasound scan of the kidneys has the advantage over other modalities, such as CT and MR imaging, as it provides a rapid answer, is cheap, and portable. Ultrasound examination to exclude obstruction does not require the administration of ionic contrast media that are nephrotoxic and may exacerbate the ARF. If hydronephrosis is detected, CT and MR imaging are more likely to identify the cause of the obstruction than ultrasound.

Imaging to exclude obstruction should be performed as early as possible. Imaging should be regarded as a matter of urgency in a patient who has evidence of systemic sepsis of undetermined source and when there are clinical features that raise the possibility of urinary obstruction, for example known cervical carcinoma. In these cases immediate treatment of pyonephrosis by nephrostomy can be life-saving. Imaging is not necessary when clear reversible causes are present on initial assessment, therapy is instituted (e.g., intravenous fluid replacement), and there is clear evidence of a prompt response (within the first few hours of treatment) with a return to normal renal function within a few days.

Occasionally obstruction may be present without hydronephrosis. This can happen in the first few days of obstruction when the collecting system is relatively noncompliant and can also happen when the ureters and collecting systems are encased with tumor or fibrosis. In the latter situation a CT scan can identify the encasing tumor. Similarly, detection of hydronephrosis can sometimes be difficult in patients with multicystic kidneys and in this situation CT scanning and intravenous urography should be considered.

The approach described above also applies to patients with acute on chronic renal failure.

Summary points:
- The causes of ARF are best considered under the headings of "prerenal," "postrenal," and "renal parenchymal" causes
- The most frequent causes of ARF are prerenal.
- Incomplete urinary tract obstruction can cause polyuria
- Ultrasound examination to exclude urinary tract obstruction is required in cases of ARF that do not respond to initial treatment and where other clinical features point to the possibility of obstruction
- If pyonephrosis is present relief of obstruction by nephrostomy can be life-saving
- Urinary tract obstruction can occasionally be present without hydronephrosis

Approach to Patients with Chronic Kidney Disease

As described earlier, the National Kidney Foundation of the United States has suggested that CKD should be considered as a single entity, defined as evidence of structural or functional kidney abnormalities with or without a decreased GFR.[21]

The presence of persistent significant proteinuria (or albuminuria) at the level detected by dipstick tests (approximately > 300 mg protein per day, depending on how concentrated the urine is at the time of testing) is suggestive of glomerular disease and warrants further assessment. The presence of preserved renal function, as assessed by serum creatinine, suggests that either the onset of disease is relatively recent or that the disease is nonprogressive.

Identification of CKD is an opportunity to prevent, reverse, or more likely slow the rate of progression to requiring renal replacement therapy and reduce the risk of associated cardiovascular disease. Assessment of the patient with CKD is aimed at identifying the cause of CKD, assessing the severity of any impairment of each of the functions of the kidney (Table 1.1), identifying additional aggravating factors (e.g., the administration of NSAIDs), and assessing the associated cardiovascular risk factors.

Causes

There are many diseases that can cause CKD (Table 1.2) and they are best considered as renal parenchymal, prerenal, and postrenal (obstructive). Renal parenchymal diseases can be considered as primary (i.e., confined to the kidney) or secondary renal diseases (as part of a multisystem disorder). The most common causes of end-stage CKD requiring renal replacement therapy in a selection of European countries is shown in Figure 1.1.

A detailed history and examination to identify features of systemic diseases with possible renal involvement, and consumption of prescribed and proprietary medication is essential. Patients should be asked directly about a family history of inherited renal disease such as ADPKD or Alport syndrome.

The age and gender of the patient, the presence or absence of hematuria, the quantity of proteinuria, the presence of nephrotic syndrome, and urine microscopy all help to narrow the differential diagnosis, but further investigation is required to establish a firm diagnosis. Tests such as measurement of serum immunoglobulin and complement concentrations can help to narrow the differential diagnosis but are not diagnostic. Similarly, the presence of a monoclonal band on serum electrophoresis, antinuclear factor (ANF), antineutrophil cytoplasmic antibody (ANCA), or raised serum ACE concentration may all suggest renal involvement in systemic diseases such as myeloma, systemic lupus erythematosis, vasculitis, or sarcoidosis, respectively, but further investigation is required to establish the true renal diagnosis.

Imaging

Renal imaging should be performed in almost every patient with CKD. Imaging may provide a single diagnosis or may narrow the differential diagnosis. Imaging may also provide prognostic information and information to guide further investigation.

Ultrasound scanning is the most widely applied form of renal imaging, but there is also a role for the plain radiograph, intravenous urography (IVU), and nuclear imaging in selected cases. Furthermore, spiral CT and MR imaging appear increasingly valuable as they become more widely available and the speed of imaging improves.

Ultrasound is usually diagnostic for chronic obstructive uropathy, ADPKD, medullary cystic kidney disease, renal agenesis, duplex ureteric systems, and horseshoe kidney. Ultrasound can reveal morphological features that are highly suggestive of the diagnosis in conditions such as renal artery stenosis (RAS), chronic pyelonephritis, nephrocalcinosis, and von Hippel–Lindau disease.

A common finding in the investigation of patients with CKD and advanced renal failure is bilateral shrunken kidneys (< 8 cm in bipolar diameter) with cortical thinning and loss of corticomedullary differentiation. Histological appearances of these kidneys reveals extensive glomerulosclerosis, tubular atrophy, and interstitial fibrosis, and this appears to be the final common pathway for most causes of progressive CKD (Fig. 1.**5**). The finding of bilateral shrunken kidneys in a patient with CKD is therefore not diagnostic but implies further progressive renal failure is inevitable. Further invasive investigation such as renal biopsy is unlikely to provide any further useful information in these patients. Similarly, the finding of shrunken kidneys suggests that invasive treatments such as renal artery stenting for RAS or ureteric stenting for hydronephrosis are likely to be fruitless.

A diagnosis of atherosclerotic RAS should always be entertained in a middle-aged or elderly patient with CKD who is hypertensive and has evidence of atherosclerotic disease elsewhere, especially when kidney size is asymmetric. Some authors have suggested that ultrasound Doppler assessment of the renal artery is sufficiently sensitive and specific for the diagnosis of RAS.[29] Doppler ultrasound of the renal arteries appears to be highly operator-dependent and time-consuming, however. Conventional renal arteriography remains the gold standard for the diagnosis of RAS, but has the disadvantage that it is invasive and can be associated with life-threatening complications, including contrast nephropathy or cholesterol emboli syndrome. In many centers, including ours, magnetic resonance angiography (MRA) is now the investigation of choice in patients with suspected RAS.[30] MRA can also be used to calculate individual kidney GFR, as well as providing information on kidney size, cortical thickness, and renal artery patency. MRA therefore offers the prospect of providing a large amount of information from a single test.

Recent evidence suggests that a low resistive index (RI) using Doppler ultrasound is predictive of a beneficial response to revascularization in patients with RAS.[31] This finding requires further confirmation but could provide a further role for ultrasound in the assessment of patients with CKD.

Consequences of Chronically Diseased Kidneys

Chronically diseased kidneys have an increased likelihood of developing cystic change. This appears to be associated with an increased risk of developing renal carcinoma.[32,33] The kidneys can be imaged with ultrasound or CT depending on availability. The native kidneys should not be forgotten as a potential source of hematuria in patients on dialysis or patients with a renal transplant, and some authors advocate regular surveillance of the native kidneys in these patients.

Chronically diseased kidneys are also at increased risk of infection, which can lead to abscess formation within the kidney or in the surrounding tissue (perinephric abscess). Patients with ADPKD often experience acute loin pain due to hemorrhage within a cyst. This is usually self-limiting and the offending cyst can sometimes be identified on ultrasound or CT scanning. Ultrasound-guided puncture of the offending cyst can lead to an improvement in pain and should be considered if there are clinical features that suggest the cyst is infected.

Summary points:
- Identification of CKD is an opportunity to slow the rate of progression to requiring renal replacement therapy and reduce the risk of associated cardiovascular disease
- The causes of CKD are best considered as renal parenchymal, prenal and postrenal
- Renal parenchymal diseases can be considered as primary or as part of a multisystem disorder
- Imaging should be performed in most patients with CKD

- Ultrasound scanning may provide a single diagnosis or may narrow the differential
- Measurement of kidney size and resistive index can provide useful prognostic information
- Other non-invasive imaging modalities such as MR and spiral CT appear increasingly useful, especially for assessing renovascular disease
- Chronically diseased kidneys should not be forgotten as a source of hematuria or sepsis in patients on renal replacement therapy

Conclusion

Renal disease is common and consumes a large proportion of health resources in developed countries. ARF usually presents in the context of severe systemic illness, but it is important to exclude other causes such as urinary obstruction or acute renal parenchymal disease.

Increasing recognition of the cardiovascular risk associated with even mild reduction in renal function and an improved understanding of the pathophysiology of progressive renal failure has led to a focus on CKD as a single entity. Early detection and investigation of CKD to attempt to prevent or slow progression toward the need for renal replacement therapy is expected to greatly reduce morbidity and mortality.

At present ultrasound is the renal imaging modality most widely used to investigate patients with ARF and CKD. Other modalities such as CT and MR imaging offer some advantages over ultrasound in imaging renal arteries, renal masses, and identifying the cause of any urinary obstruction. Ultrasound is likely to remain the first-line renal imaging investigation for most patients with renal disease, however, because of its widespread availability and portability. The application of advanced ultrasound techniques such as measurement of RI may be of value in selected cases in the future.

References

1. EdREN. The website of the Renal Unit of the Royal Infirmary of Edinburgh. The early development of dialysis and transplantation. http://renux.dmed.ed.ac.uk/EdREN/Unitbits/historyweb/HDWorld.html . 17-1-2004.
2. Coresh J, Astor BC, Greene T, Eknoyan G, Levey AS. Prevalence of chronic kidney disease and decreased kidney function in the adult US population: Third National Health and Nutrition Examination Survey. Am J Kidney Dis 2003;41:1–12.
3. US Renal Data System. 2003 Annual Data Report. Atlas of end-stage renal disease in the United States. Bethesda, MD: National Institutes of Health, National Institute of Diabetes and Digestive and Kidney Diseases: 2003.
4. Foley RN, Parfrey PS, Sarnak MJ. Epidemiology of cardiovascular disease in chronic renal disease. J Am Soc Nephrol 1998;9:16–23.
5. Vanholder R, Van Biesen W. Incidence of infectious morbidity and mortality in dialysis patients. Blood Purif 2002;20: 477–480.
6. Vamvakas S, Bahner U, Heidland A. Cancer in end-stage renal disease: potential factors involved (editorial). Am J Nephrol 1998;18:89–95.
7. Marple JT, MacDougall M. Development of malignancy in the end-stage renal disease patient. Semin Nephrol 1993; 13:306–314.
8. ERA-EDTA Registry. ERA-EDTA Registry 2001 Annual Report. Amsterdam: Academic Medical Center: 2003.
9. Khan IH, Smith C, Metcalfe W, Simpson K, Baharani J, Martin H, Lawson L, Prescott G,Ritchie C. Scottish Executive Health Department Chief Scientist Office Executive Summaries. The epidemiology of acute renal failure in Scotland. http://www.show.scot.nhs.uk/cso/Publications/ExecSumms/OctNov03/Khan.pdf . 1-11-2003. 28-2-2004.
10. Feest TG, Round A, Hamad S. Incidence of severe acute renal failure in adults: results of a community based study. BMJ 1993;306:481–483.
11. Khan IH, Catto GRD, Edward N, MacLeod AM. Acute renal failure: factors influencing nephrology referral and outcome. Q J Med 1997;90:781–785.
12. Stevens PE, Tamimi NA, Al Hasani MK, Mikhail AI, Kearney E, Lapworth R, Prosser DI, Carmichael P. Non-specialist management of acute renal failure. QJ Med 2001;94: 533–540.
13. Robertson S, Newbigging K, Isles CG, Brammah A, Allan A, Norrie J. High incidence of renal failure requiring short term dialysis: a prospective observational study. Q J Med 2002;95:585–590.
14. Rennke H, Anderson S, Brenner BM. Structural and functional correlations in the progression of renal disease. In: Tisher C, Brenner B, eds. Renal Pathology. Philadelphia: 1989:43–66.
15. Beddhu S, Samore MH, Roberts MS, Stoddard GJ, Ramkumar N, Pappas LM, Cheung AK. Impact of timing of initiation of dialysis on mortality. J Am Soc Nephrol 2003;14: 2305–2312.
16. Traynor JP, Simpson K, Geddes CC, Deighan CJ, Fox JG. Early initiation of dialysis fails to prolong survival in patients with end-stage renal failure. J Am Soc Nephrol 2002;13: 2125–2132.
17. Korevaar JC, Jansen MA, Dekker FW, Jager KJ, Boeschoten EW, Krediet RT, Bossuyt PM. When to initiate dialysis: effect of proposed US guidelines on survival. Lancet 2001;358:1046–1050.
18. Beddhu S, Samore MH, Roberts MS, Stoddard GJ, Ramkumar N, Pappas LM, Cheung AK: Impact of timing of initiation of dialysis on mortality. J Am Soc Nephrol 2003;14: 2305–2312.
19. Mann JF, Gerstein HC, Pogue J, Bosch J, Yusuf S. Renal insufficiency as a predictor of cardiovascular outcomes and the impact of ramipril: the HOPE randomized trial. Ann Intern Med 2001;134:629–636.
20. Locatelli F, Fouque D, Heimburger O, Drueke TB, Cannata-Andia JB, Horl WH, Ritz E. Nutritional status in dialysis patients: a European consensus. Nephrol Dial Transplant 2002;17:563–572.

21. National Kidney Foundation. K/DOQI clinical practice guidelines for chronic kidney disease: Evaluation, classification and stratification. Am J Kidney Dis 2002;39(suppl. 1).
22. Coresh J, Astor BC, Greene T, Eknoyan G, Levey AS. Prevalence of chronic kidney disease and decreased kidney function in the adult US population: Third National Health and Nutrition Examination Survey. Am J Kidney Dis 2003;41:1–12.
23. Lewis EJ, Hunsicker LG, Bain RP, Rohde RD. The effect of angiotensin-converting-enzyme inhibition on diabetic nephropathy. The Collaborative Study Group [see comments] [published erratum appears in N Engl J Med 1993 Jan 13;330(2):152]. N Engl J Med 1993;329:1456–1462.
24. The GISEN Group. Randomised placebo-controlled trial of effect of ramipril on decline in glomerular filtration rate and risk of terminal renal failure in proteinuric, non-diabetic nephropathy. (Gruppo Italiano di Studi Epidemiologici in Nefrologia) [see comments]. Lancet 1997;349:1857–1863.
25. Nakao N, Yoshimura A, Morita H, Takada M, Kayano T, Ideura T. Combination treatment of angiotensin-II receptor blocker and angiotensin-converting-enzyme inhibitor in non-diabetic renal disease (COOPERATE): a randomised controlled trial. Lancet 2003;361:117–124.
26. Klahr S, Levey AS, Beck GJ, Caggiula AW, Hunsicker L, Kusek JW, Striker G. The effects of dietary protein restriction and blood-pressure control on the progression of chronic renal disease. Modification of Diet in Renal Disease Study Group [see comments]. N Engl J Med 1994;330:877–884.
27. Ballardie FW, Roberts IS. Controlled prospective trial of prednisolone and cytotoxics in progressive IgA nephropathy. J Am Soc Nephrol 2002;13:142–148.
28. UK Prospective Diabetes Study (UKPDS) Group. Intensive blood-glucose control with sulphonylureas or insulin compared with conventional treatment and risk of complications in patients with type 2 diabetes (UKPDS 33). Lancet 1998;352:837–853.
29. Radermacher J, Chavan A, Schaffer J, Stoess B, Vitzthum A, Kliem V, Rademaker J, Bleck J, Gebel MJ, Galanski M, Brunkhorst R. Detection of significant renal artery stenosis with color Doppler sonography: combining extrarenal and intrarenal approaches to minimize technical failure. Clin Nephrol 2000;53:333–343.
30. Schoenberg SO, Rieger J, Johannson LO, Dietrich O, Bock M, Prince MR, Reiser MF. Diagnosis of renal artery stenosis with magnetic resonance angiography: update 2003. Nephrol Dial Transplant 2003;18:1252–1256.
31. Radermacher J, Chavan A, Bleck J, Vitzthum A, Stoess B, Gebel MJ, Galanski M, Koch KM, Haller H. Use of Doppler ultrasonography to predict the outcome of therapy for renal-artery stenosis. N Engl J Med 2001;344:410–417.
32. Ishikawa I. Acquired cystic disease: mechanisms and manifestations. Semin Nephrol 1991;11:671–684.
33. Marple JT, MacDougall M, Chonko AM. Renal cancer complicating acquired cystic kidney disease. J Am Soc Nephrol 1994;4:1951–1956.

2 The Normal Kidney

G. M. Baxter

Anatomical Relationships of the Kidney

The normal anatomical relationships of the kidney have been appreciated for many years. They are retroperitoneal organs lying on either side of the vertebral column, traditionally the left kidney lying at a higher level than the right and being shaped as the name implies (Fig. 2.**1a**). In general the lower poles lie more laterally than the upper.

Medially they are bordered by the psoas muscle, with the aorta on the left and the inferior vena cava (IVC) on the right, and superiorly by the adrenal glands. The anterior relationships of the kidneys are many (Fig. 2.**1b**). The kidneys themselves are surrounded by perirenal fat with a further layer of renal fascia both anteriorly and posteriorly, i.e. Gerota's fascia, which separates the perirenal from the pararenal spaces. Although not visualized on ultrasound, these are much better appreciated on computed tomography (CT; Fig. 2.**2**)

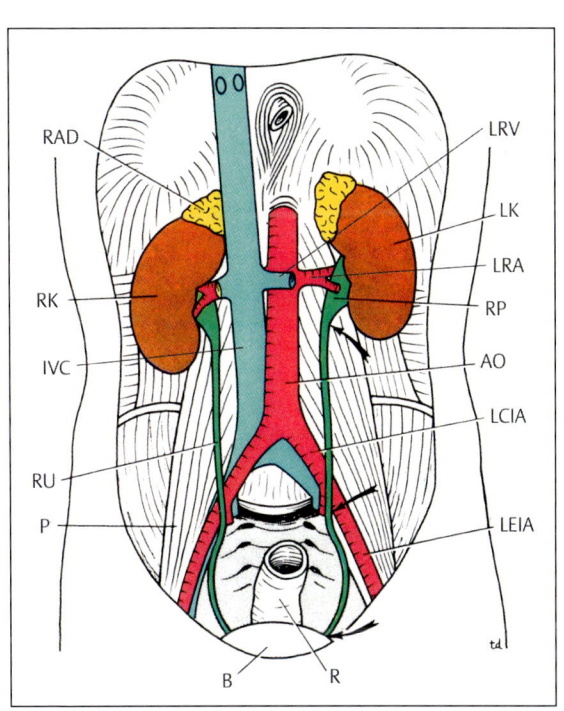

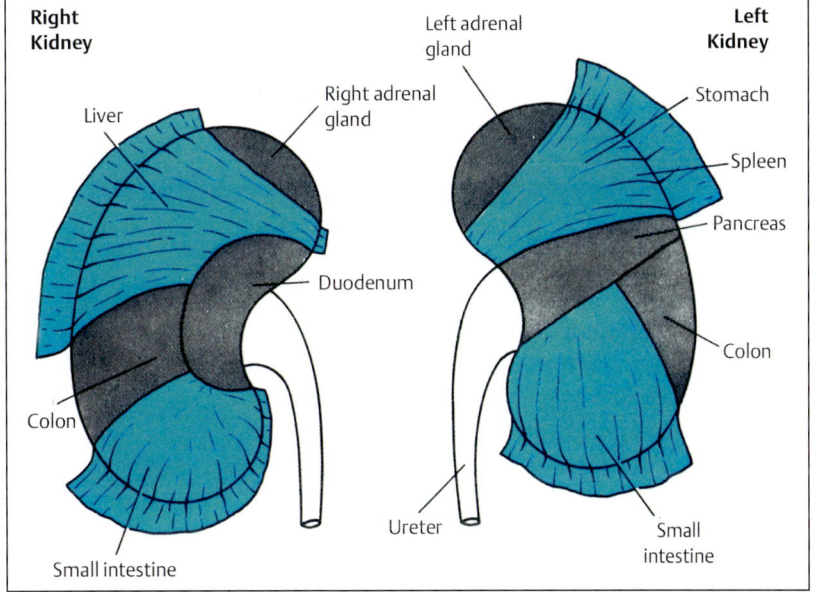

Fig. 2.**1 a Coronal depiction of the anatomy of the posterior abdominal wall and retroperitoneum**
(AO = aorta, B = bladder; IVC = inferior vena cava; LCIA = left common iliac artery; LEIA = left external iliac artery; LK = left kidney; LRA = left renal artery; LRV = left renal vein; P = psoas; R = rectum; RAD = right adrenal gland; RK = right kidney; RP = renal pelvis; RU = right ureter)
b The anterior relationships of the right and left kidney. The visceral peritoneum has been left in blue

2 The Normal Kidney

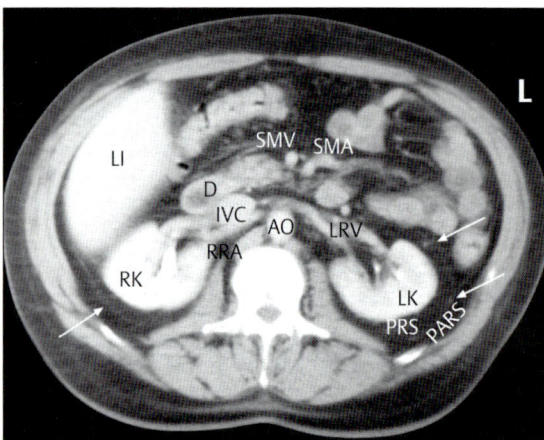

Fig. 2.**2 Axial CT scan through the renal area.** The main anatomical structures have been marked. The perirenal and pararenal spaces are separated by the anterior and posterior perirenal fascia, more commonly known as Gerota's fascia (arrows)
(AO = aorta; D = duodenum; IVC = inferior vena cava; LI = liver; LK = left kidney; LRV = left renal vein; PARS = pararenal space; PRS = perirenal space; RK = right kidney; RRA = right renal artery; SMA = superior mesenteric artery; SMV = superior mesenteric vein)

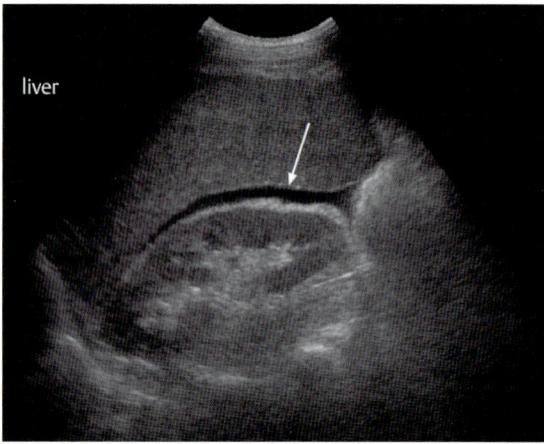

Fig. 2.**3 A small amount of ascitic fluid is seen between the liver and right kidney** (arrow). This is a key area to check for abdominal fluid

and are more easily delineated when retroperitoneal fluid or inflammation is present. On the right, the reflection of peritoneum between the inferior surface of the liver and kidney, i.e. the hepatorenal fossa or Morrison's pouch, is generally appreciated when ascitic fluid or fluid of any nature is present within the upper abdomen. This area between the right kidney and liver is often one area to specifically view when small amounts of abdominal fluid require detection (Fig. 2.**3**).

Anatomy of the Kidney

Embryologically the kidney begins within the pelvis and ascends to its normal anatomical position in the retroperitoneum of the upper abdomen. It is therefore possible that this superior migration can be prematurely interrupted at any point in the process. If the kidney is not observed in its normal anatomical position then, it should be sought within the lower abdomen or pelvis. The kidney develops from a number of "lobes" in the fetus, which normally merge, resulting in a kidney with a smooth surface. However, some may persist on the surface of the kidney, giving a slightly normal but nodular appearance known as fetal lobulation (see p. 24, Fetal Lobulation).[1]

Renal length is often quoted as being 10–12 cm, but a much wider range is normally visualized in patients with normal renal function, and any specific measurement should be related to the patient's age and build, including height and weight.[2] If renal size falls below these values, any comment on renal function without biochemical correlation should be guarded. In addition, it is important to remember that in some patients, because of the axis of the kidney, it may be difficult to measure a "true" renal length and some foreshortening may occur. Furthermore, there is both interobserver and intraobserver variation in such measurements and again this has to be taken into consideration.[3] What is certain, however, is that ultrasonic measurements are generally smaller than those traditionally used, for example with intravenous urogram (IVU), largely due to the lack of any radiographic magnification factor and the fact that ultrasound is the most accurate modality for defining renal length when compared with plain film, IVU, or renal angiography.[4]

The kidney itself is surrounded by a fibrous capsule with the renal parenchyma lying immediately beneath it. The cortex occupies the most peripheral margin, then the inner medulla, which consists of the renal pyramids arranged in an orderly fashion around the renal sinus, which largely consists of fat. Projections of cortex extending into the sinus between the pyramids are called septa or columns of Bertin.[1]

Apart from fat, the renal sinus contains the renal vessels, i.e. the artery and vein, and the renal pelvis. The tips of the pyramids project to the calyces, which point to form the collecting system and renal pelvis (Fig. 2.**4**). The renal pelvis in the majority is largely confined to the renal sinus. However, it may project out and be "extrarenal" in position. This is of no significance apart from that it may be confused with a parapelvic cyst, hydronephrosis, or even in certain circumstances a perirenal fluid collection.

The renal veins lie anterior to the arteries and divide at renal sinus level. Most kidneys are supplied by a single

Ultrasound Examination

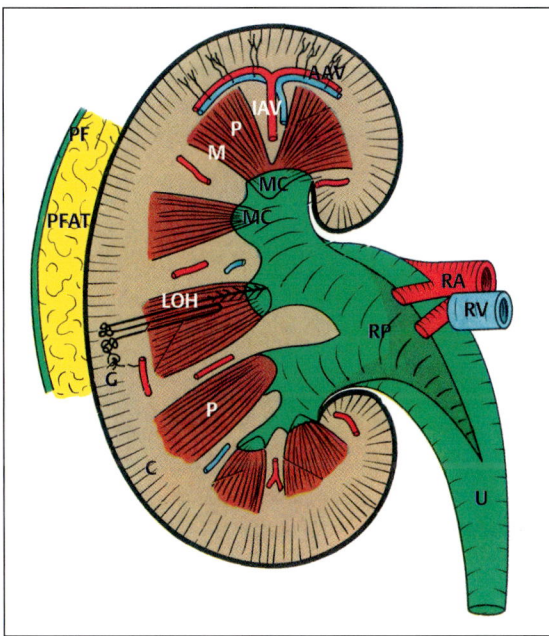
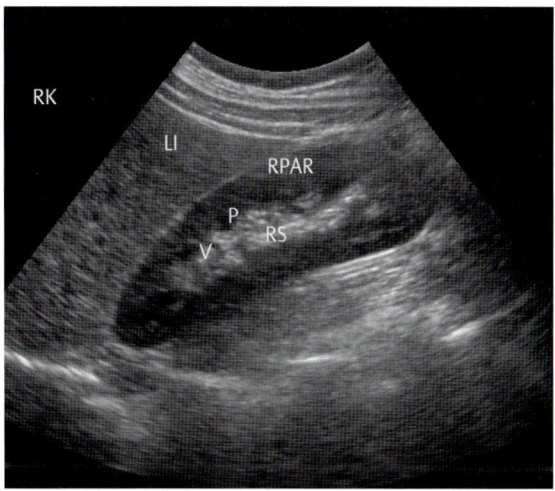
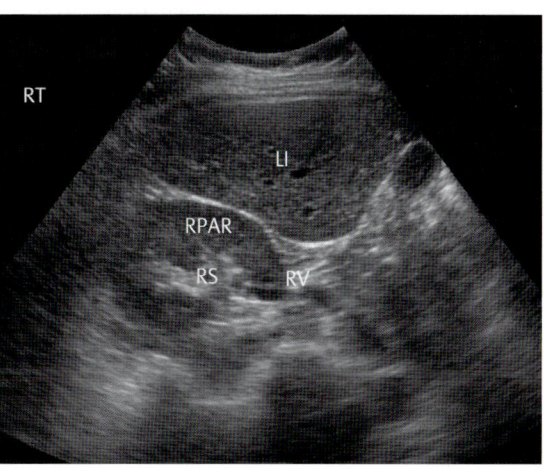

Fig. 2.4 **a** Schematic representation of the normal kidney. **b** Normal kidney, longitudinal axis. **c** Transverse axis for comparison
(AAV = arcuate artery and vein; C = cortex; G = glomerulus; IAV = interlobar artery and vein; LI = liver; LOH = Loop of Henle; M = medulla; MC = minor calyx; P = pyramid; PF = perirenal fascia; PFAT = perirenal fat; RA = renal artery; RP = renal pelvis; RPAR = renal parenchyma; RS = renal sinus; RV = renal vein; U = ureter; V = vessel)

renal vessel. However, accessory vessels are well-documented with an incidence of 20–27%.[5,6] The main renal vessel itself divides into a number of segmental branches which then subdivide into interlobar branches with, finally, small branches running around the corticomedullary junction, called the arcuate vessels.

Summary points:
- The kidneys are paired retroperitoneal organs and embryologically ascend from the pelvis to the abdomen
- The kidney develops from a number of lobes which, if they persist, may give a nodular surface known as fetal lobulation
- Renal length depends upon height, weight, age, and sex
- The renal sinus contains fat, renal pelvis, the renal artery, and the renal vein
- Most kidneys are supplied by a single artery; the incidence of accessory vessels is 20–27%

Ultrasound Examination

Technique

The patient is fasted as for an upper abdominal scan. However, it is normal in many institutions if only the kidneys are being interrogated not to specifically fast the patient, although this will clearly vary from center to center. The examination normally begins with the patient lying in the supine position; the right kidney is normally assessed first. The liver may be used as an acoustic window; the transducer is generally in a subcostal or intercostal position, depending on the patient's build. The examination can be conducted in quiet respiration or the patient may be asked to breath-hold on inspiration. Imaging is normally performed in the longitudinal and axial planes. The kidney is then re-examined with the patient in the right oblique position, i.e. the right side raised, this being particularly useful if there is difficulty visualizing either the upper or lower poles in the supine position, which may occur for a number of reasons. The left kidney is also visualized, initially with the patient supine; scanning is performed in a more posterior and lateral position than that of the right kidney. In general terms the left kidney is a little more difficult to visualize due to bowel gas in the adjacent splenic flexure and/or small bowel, and because of this it is often necessary to raise the patient into a left oblique position and even into the full left lateral decubitus position to obtain suitable and complete access. The spleen, like the liver on the right, may also be used as an acoustic window.

Prone scanning may be useful in children, but in general terms is not merited in the adult apart from when performing a traditional renal biopsy.

With regard to the gray-scale findings, a number of criteria are normally considered. These include the renal size, parenchymal thickness, and subjective correlation with the patient's age and build. In addition, the renal parenchymal echogenicity is also routinely assessed. Vasculature can also be assessed, although only superficially with gray-scale ultrasound. However, a more detailed examination can be performed with the color Doppler technique.

Apart from measuring renal length and assessing parenchymal thickness and echogenicity, it is important that the perirenal structures and organs are assessed. If a renal abnormality is present, then assessment of the entire urogenital tract, renal vein, IVC, liver, and retroperitoneum is appropriate.

Assessment Criteria

Renal Size

The left kidney is normally a little larger than the right (Table 2.**1**).[2,7] It is important when measuring renal size to measure the full length of the kidney, as previously mentioned, as it is easy to foreshorten and obtain a falsely low measurement. In general, multiple measurements give a more overall accurate measurement and routine measurements made in the supine and oblique positions help overcome any potential underestimation (Fig. 2.**5**). With good technique, measurement errors should be within 1.85 cm in the adult. However, inexperience and poor technique is likely to increase the margins of error. Renal length, however, is a good working overall assessment of the kidney and in most patients provides a fairly accurate assessment of renal size. Nevertheless, small differences in measurements should be interpreted with caution. These measurements are used commonly by the renal physician in conjunction with other criteria to help determine whether renal failure is likely to be acute or chronic. As a rule of thumb a renal length of > 10 cm is normal and < 9 cm would be regarded as abnormal, dependent on age, weight, and size of patient. A kidney < 8 cm is almost certainly a manifestation of chronic disease.

Volume measurements of the kidney can also be calculated either by measuring the area of the kidney

Table 2.**1** Normal values for renal length, including renal volume and renal length calculation for children > 1 year

Median renal length (cm)		No. of subjects
Right	Left	
10.9 (9.8–12.2)	11.2 (10.1–12.3)	665[2]
11.00 (10.2–11.8)	11.2 (10.3–12.1)	175[31]
Renal volume		
134 cm³	146 cm³	665[2]
Children > 1 year of age		
Renal length = 6.79 + 0.22 × age (cm)		203[32]

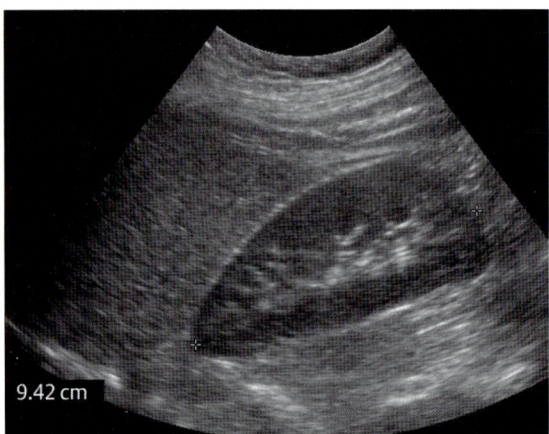
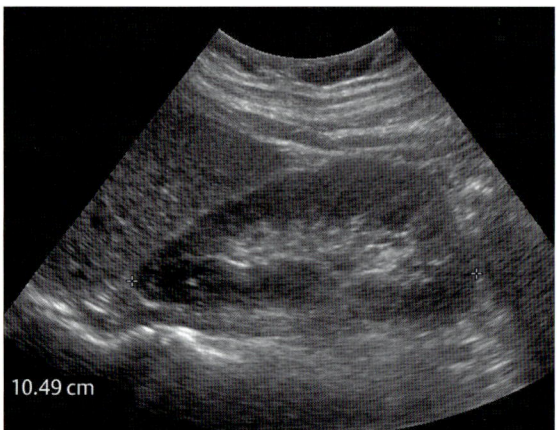

Fig. 2.**5 a** Longitudinal axis measurement of the right kidney with the patient in the supine position. The kidney measures 9.42 cm. **b** The same patient as in Fig. 2.5a but in the right oblique position. The kidney now measures 10.49 cm. It is important to turn the patient to optimize the maximum renal length for accurate measurements

in serial slices and summing (an accurate method) or by using various computerized elliptical drawings around the kidney itself. Both methods have errors, however, and as with renal length, these specific measurements, although important, may be less important than a change in value over a specific time period. A simpler and less time-consuming alternative for volume calculation is to measure the length, anterior-posterior, and transverse diameters of the kidney, and multiply all three by 0.5.

One study measuring renal length and parenchymal volume concluded that in those with normal renal function the length on the kidney was the most important measurement, whilst in end-stage renal failure the parenchymal volume was more appropriate.[8]

Parenchymal Thickness

Although cortical and parenchymal thickness can be measured, it is important to remember that this is variable and, like renal length, depends upon age[2,9] and size of the patient and exactly where the cortex or parenchyma is being measured. For completeness, the cortical thickness is the distance between the capsule of the kidney and the outer margin of the pyramid, whilst the parenchymal thickness is the distance between the capsule and the margin of the sinus echo (Fig. 2.**6**). In my opinion, the latter is easier to perform and more reproducible and is likely to be of more value if serial measurements are being performed. The size and cortical thickness of kidneys vary and, like most physiological measurements, there is a degree of overlap between normal and disease states. No normal values have been published. In general terms, both renal length and parenchymal thickness are reduced in patients with impaired renal function, although clearly in some patients length may be more affected than thickness and vice versa. It has been shown that there is a linear relationship between thickness and length of the kidney. When this was correlated with biopsy and clinical outcome, irreversible change was present in those kidneys with a parenchymal thickness of < 1.0 cm or a renal length < 9.0 cm.[10,11]

As a rule of thumb, an experienced individual will assimilate renal length and cortical thickness appearances to give a global assessment of renal size in relation to the clinical condition and biochemical values if stated.

Renal Echogenicity

The third parameter normally assessed is the cortical echogenicity and this is done by comparing it with the adjacent liver or spleen. Echogenicity varies with age, i.e., at birth the cortex is relatively hyperechoic due to

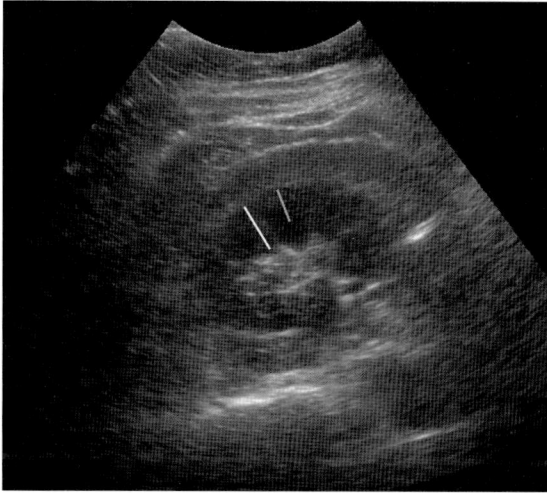

Fig. 2.**6 Axial image of the right kidney.** The cortical thickness (distance between capsule and outer margin of the pyramid) is shown in green and the parenchymal thickness (distance between the capsule and the margin of the sinus echo) in white

an increased number of glomeruli compared with the adult.[12] Furthermore, corticomedullary differentiation is increased and sinus fat is almost absent. By adulthood the cortex is less echogenic and the sinus fat hyperechoic. A further assessment is also made of the degree of corticomedullary differentiation in conjunction with the appearance of the medullary pyramids.

The normal kidney can usually be easily identified because of the contrast between the darker parenchyma and the bright sinus fat. The cortical renal reflectivity can be easily subjectively assessed by comparison with the adjacent organs, i.e. liver or spleen, assuming of course these organs are normal, which may not necessarily be the case (Fig. 2.7).

In general the cortex is less echogenic than that of the liver[13] and spleen, although the degree of contrast will vary depending on machine settings and various processing programs, which can range from high contrast to flatter, lesser degrees of contrast. What is appreciated, however, is if the renal cortex has a brighter echogenicity than the liver, this is a good indicator of renal parenchymal disease. Those kidneys that have an echogenicity equivalent to or less than that of the liver will in fact have normal renal function.[14,15] It is important to remember that despite these "working rules," patients with normal-appearing kidneys may still have disease.

The medullary pyramids are generally darker than the overlying cortex and are identified by their regular distribution around the inner margin of the parenchyma adjacent to the renal sinus. The pyramids are not seen as routinely in the native kidney as, for example, when compared with a transplant kidney, where

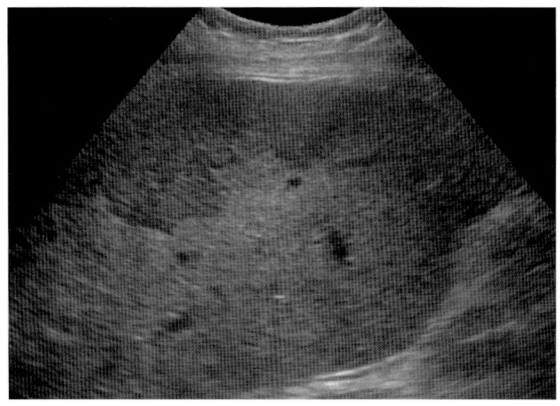
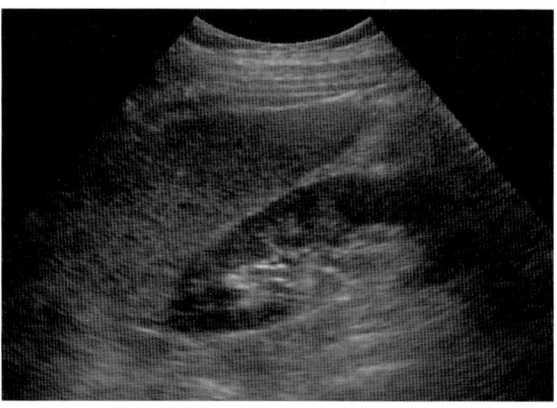

Fig. 2.**7 a** Image of a liver showing a geographical variation in echogenicity consistent with an area of normal liver and an area of fatty infiltration. **b,c** Images of the right kidney, at exactly the same settings, against different areas of the liver; in (**b**) the kidney looks much darker than in (**c**) but this variation is simply the relative contrast with the changing liver background

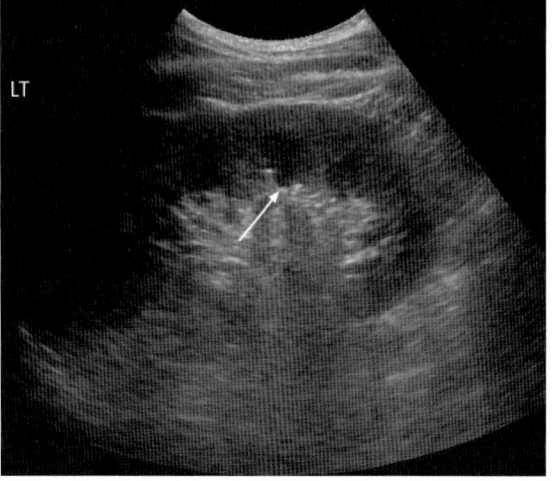
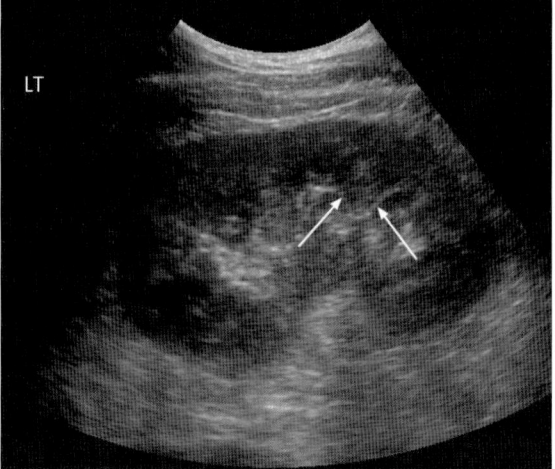

Fig. 2.**8 a** Longitudinal image of the left kidney showing some bright fine echoes around the renal pyramid (arrow). This is likely to represent interlobar arterial calcification. **b** The same kidney as in Fig. 2.**8a** showing more extensive interlobar arterial calcification (arrows). This type of fine calcification is normally related to the renal pyramids

resolution is generally excellent due to its superficial position. Small reflective foci may be seen adjacent to the pyramids and these are likely to represent the interlobular and arcuate vessels (Fig. 2.**8**). Visualization of the margins between the pyramids and cortex are normally well-defined, but in any condition resulting in inflammation and/or edema, this corticomedullary differentiation may be lost, or depending on the condition, can even be enhanced.

The renal parenchyma normally reduces with age whilst simultaneously there is generally an increase in the amount of fat within the renal sinus. This slight thinning can be normal; in general it does not result in a reduction in renal length.

> **Summary points:**
> - The kidneys should be examined with the patient in multiple positions, e.g., supine, oblique, decubitus
> - A renal length > 9.0 cm is regarded as normal
> - No normal range of parenchymal thickness measurements exist. However, a thickness of < 1.0 cm is associated with irreversible change
> - Renal echogenicity equal to or less than that of the liver is associated with normal renal function

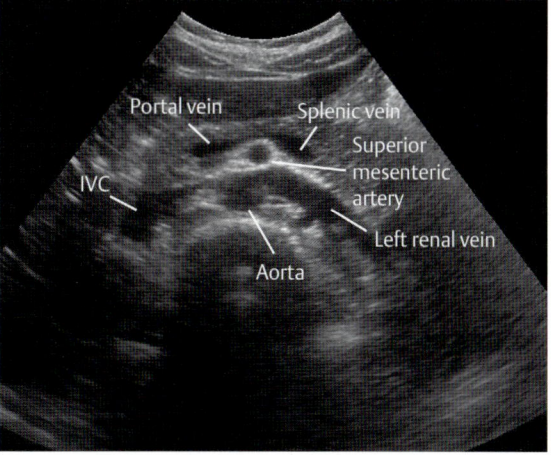

Fig. 2.**9 Transverse image of the retroperitoneum at renal level.** The vascular anatomy has been labeled. (IVC: inferior vena cava).

Renal Vasculature

Although the renal arteries and veins can be visualized on gray-scale ultrasound (Fig. 2.**9**), for quantitative information the color Doppler technique is required. Power Doppler can also be used and is generally said to improve intrarenal vascular registration from either pole due to its angle independence. However, by repositioning the patient and angulation of the probe, similar sensitivity is normally obtained with the color flow technique.

A number of techniques are normally required in the one patient to successfully visualize the renal arteries from their origin at the aorta to the renal hilum. In thin patients both vessels can be visualized from an anterior midline approach at their origin at the abdominal aorta. Although the main vessels may be seen, it is important to appreciate that no ultrasonic study to date has reliably visualized accurately the accessory arteries we know exist.[16] In addition, a number of other positions, including both oblique and decubitus positions, are normally required in an attempt to visualize both the right and left renal arteries. It is important to state, however, that Doppler examination of the entire length of the renal vessels is technically difficult and can result in failure to visualize both in as many as 40% of patients depending on patient build, habitus, bowel gas, etc. (Fig. 2.**10**).[16] The normal peak systolic velocity (PSV) in the main renal artery is < 1.5–1.8 ms^{-1} whilst the normal renal-to-aortic ratio (RAR) of the PSV values is < 3.5. Anything greater than these values is in keeping with a > 60% stenosis of the main renal artery. The sensitivity and specificity using these techniques vary significantly between institutions, making a consensus value difficult to quote.

The intrarenal vessels are easier to demonstrate and interrogate and can be visualized in the vast majority of cases.[6,17] They are first identified with color Doppler ultrasound with spectral waveforms recorded from the upper, middle, and lower parts of the kidney. This allows averaging of these values and on a rare occasion even the detection of an accessory vessel. When evaluating the vasculature for suspected renal artery stenosis (RAS), the intrarenal acceleration time (AT) and acceleration index (AI) are measured. An AT of < 0.07 seconds and an AI > 3 ms^{-2} would be regarded as normal (see Chapter 3, Parenchymal Diseases of the Kidney).

The use of microbubble contrast agents has certainly improved the visualization of both the main and intrarenal vessels. However, to date this has not resulted in an improvement in the overall sensitivity or specificity of the technique.[18]

The classical normal renovascular waveform is a low-resistance waveform, i.e., the diastolic flow is approximately one third to one half that of the PSV. This relationship is seen from the main renal artery to the interlobar and arcuate vessels (Fig. 2.**11**). In the adult, typical normal resistive index (RI) values vary between 0.55 and 0.65. Variability in the RIs, however, are appreciated in the young and in general the RI also tends to increase with age.[19] Therefore interpretation again should be cautions. As a working rule, in the majority of the adult population, an RI of 0.65–0.7 is considered as the upper limit of normal. Although an RI > 0.7 is regarded as abnormal,[20] in one study 70% of patients with parenchymal disease had an RI of < 0.7 and this bore no relationship to cortical echogenicity or serum creatinine.[21] A recent article by Splendiani, however, demonstrated that RI may be of prognostic significance, as those patients with chronic nephropathy who had a normal RI on presentation had a good outcome with stable function at three years, whilst those whose RI was elevated had progressive renal failure.[22] In acute renal failure (ARF) a progressive lowering of RI correlates well with recovery following diagnosis and medical treatment.[23] In essence, whilst 0.7 can be regarded as normal in the adult, its importance must be in conjunction with the gray-scale ultrasound and clinical

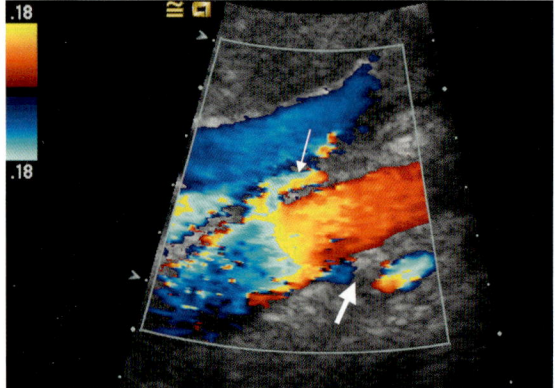

Fig. 2.**10 a** An unusually clear longitudinal image of the abdominal aorta and the origins of both the right (arrow) and left (thick arrow) renal arteries. Imaging conditions must be optimal to acquire this type of image and normally this can only be obtained in thin patients. A number of imaging planes are normally required to visualize the origins of the renal vessels, including supine and multiple obliques. **b** Spectral Doppler waveform of the right kidney with a normal PSV of 1.20 ms^{-1}. This was measured in the proximal right renal artery just posterior to the IVC with the patient in the supine position. **c** Spectral Doppler waveform of the left renal artery with a PSV of 1.00 ms^{-1} This was measured in the proximal left renal artery with the patient in a high left oblique position.

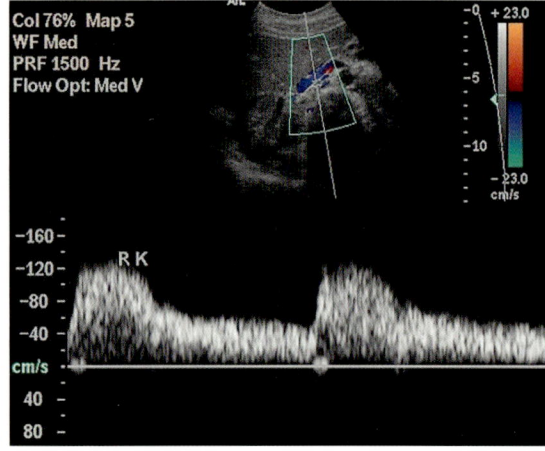
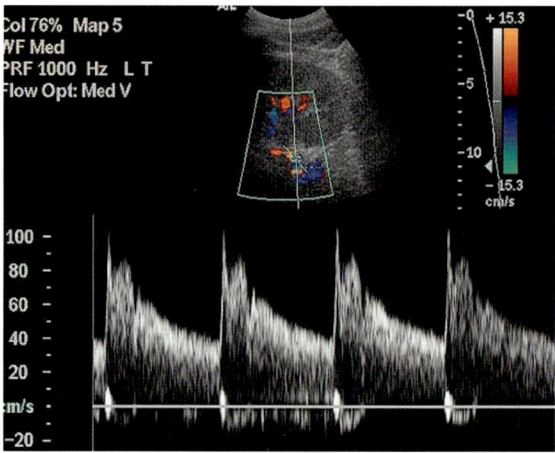

findings, although clearly it can be of use in serial studies.

Similarly, the renal veins can be visualized either anteriorly or from the flank approaches. The renal veins are generally larger than their arterial counterparts; blood within them is normally echo-free.

Very often the clinical question is simply whether the vessel is patent or occluded and this can often be resolved with the use of color flow.

Renal Collecting System

The renal sinus contains a large amount of fat and hence is bright on ultrasound. The major renal vessels pass through it. Small components of the renal sinus can extend around the papilla and septa of Bertin or even run through the upper or lower pole, seen as a thin echogenic line, i.e. the parenchymal junctional defect. An excessive amount of fat in the renal sinus is known as sinus lipomatosis, which can be diagnosed on CT or inferred at IVU by stretching of the pelvicalyceal system. Conditions that predispose to fat deposition, such as patients on steroids, may contribute. Just as an excess of fat can increase the renal sinus echo, renal sinus fat

Fig. 2.**11 Normal color flow ultrasound showing good depiction of the intrarenal vasculature with flow to the periphery of the cortex.** An interlobar vessel has been sampled and the typical low-resistance spectral Doppler waveform of the kidney is clearly demonstrated

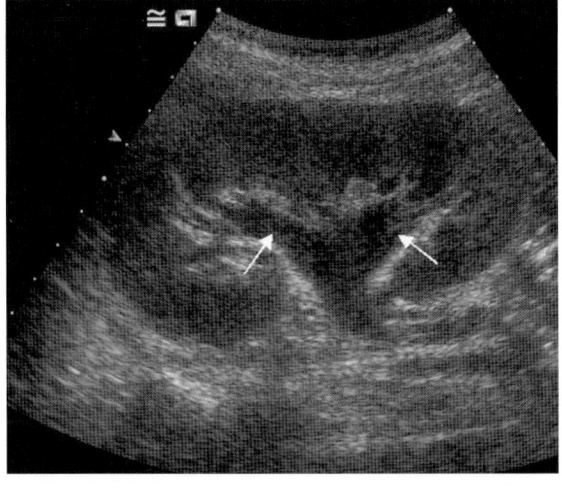
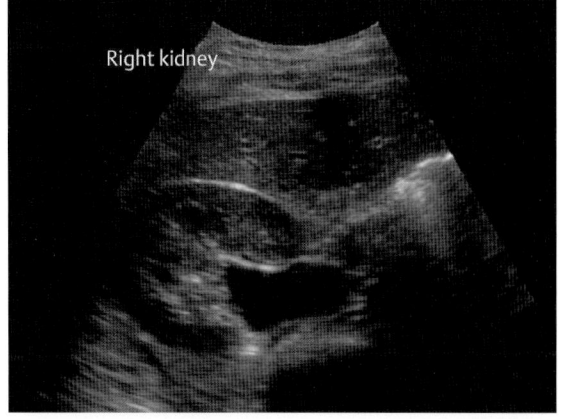
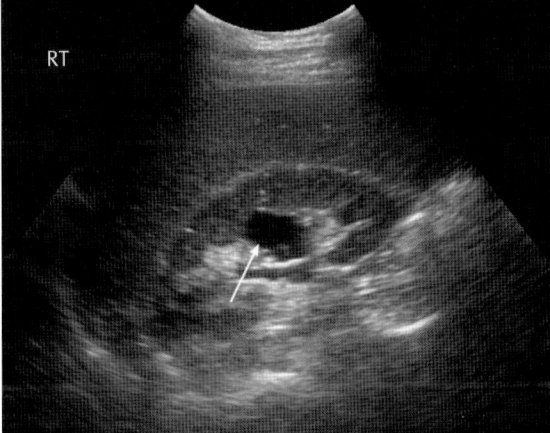
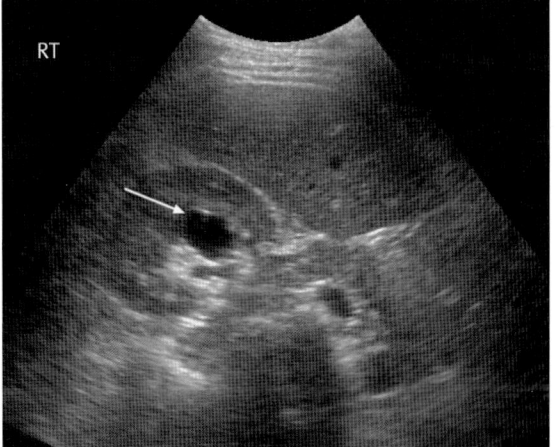

Fig. 2.12 **a** Longitudinal scan of the left kidney showing "splitting" of the renal sinus by the collecting system (arrows) in early hydronephrosis. **b** Transverse image of an extrarenal pelvis. **c** Longitudinal image of a parapelvic cyst (arrow). **d** Transverse image of the parapelvic cyst (arrow) as in Fig. 2.12c. There is no connection with the collecting system

can also be reduced, for example in cachectic patients, and very occasionally in those with tumor infiltration or edema.

Normally the collecting system cannot be distinguished within the renal sinus. However, in those patients who are undergoing a diuresis or have a full bladder, the renal pelvis and/or major calyces may be mildly prominent; with early hydronephroses this appearance is known as "splitting" of the renal sinus echoes (Fig. 2.12a). If suspected or indeed if there is a question of renal obstruction or a "full pelvis," a repeat scan following bladder emptying will restore the normal pelvic appearances in the latter. It is important to remember that not all hydronephrosis on ultrasound is obstructive and nonobstructive dilatation should also be considered. In an attempt to differentiate, an RI > 0.70 has been used to try and identify obstruction, although as this value depends upon the phase of the obstruction cycle it remains controversial.[24]

Prominence of the collecting system particularly on the right is common in pregnancy and indeed obvious dilatation can be seen in approximately two thirds of patients by 36 weeks.[25] These changes normally resolve within the first few days following delivery, although minor distension may persist for a little time. Contributing factors to this dilatation is likely to include the mechanical impression of the enlarging uterus, hormonal factors, and increased blood flow. However, debate remains as to the exact cause.

The renal pelvis, as mentioned previously, normally lies within the sinus. However, it may also lie partly or completely outside the kidney, i.e. the extrarenal pelvis (Fig. 2.12b). This should be distinguished from obstruction, parapelvic cyst, or other pararenal collections, and in this situation the axial image is often helpful (Fig. 2.12c,d), particularly if connection to the calyceal system is visualized.

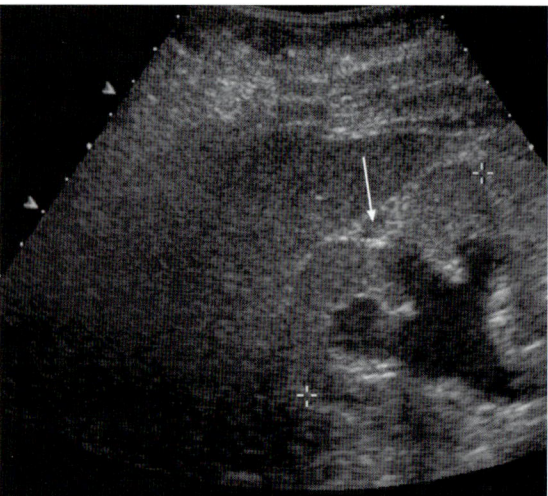

Fig. 2.**13** A small (7.2 cm) slightly echogenic kidney in a 30-year-old female patient with a history of childhood infection and urinary reflux. The collecting system is dilated and there is complete loss of cortex overlying one of the calyces (arrow). These appearances are typical of focal pyelonephritis secondary to reflux nephropathy.

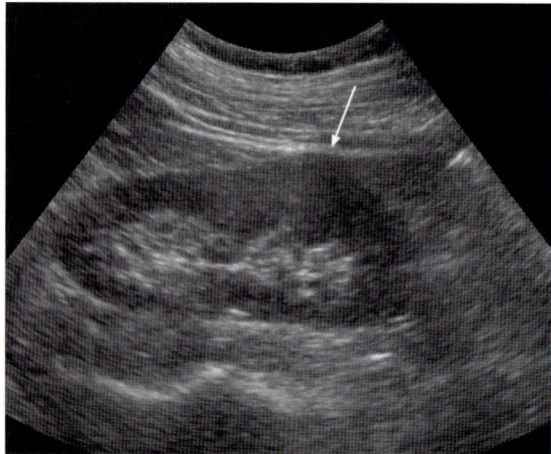

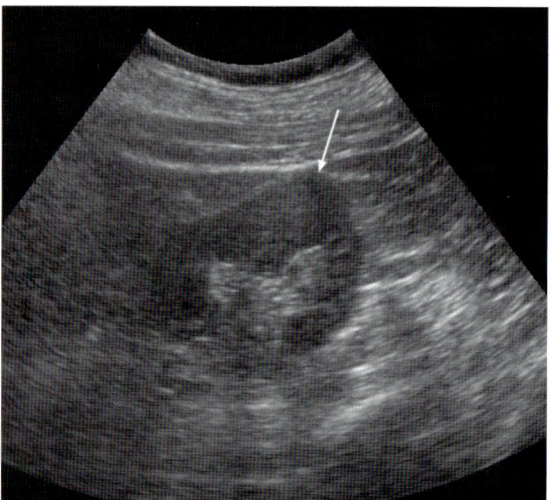

The renal sinus contains the renal vasculature, i.e. the renal artery and vein. The vascular properties are discussed above.

> **Summary points:**
> - Doppler examination of the main renal artery is technically difficult and failure rates can approach up to 40%
> - Intrarenal vessels can be sampled in almost all cases
> - The normal renovascular waveform is a low resistance waveform
> - The RI is normally < 0.7
> - Physiological hydronephrosis is seen in those who are well-hydrated, have a full bladder, and in pregnancy

Normal Variants

Fetal Lobulation

As mentioned previously, a number of lobes in the fetus fuse and form the adult kidney.[1] Normally this fusion is undetectable on ultrasound. However, on occasion one or two may remain and, as a consequence, produce a bulge in the renal outline which on occasion can be difficult to distinguish from tumor or focal hypertrophy in response to an area of cortical scarring (Fig. 2.**13**). In such cases it is possible to see that the cortical indentation lies between the pyramids rather than overlying it; this implies it is most likely to represent persistent fetal lobulation. Splenic humps and other developmental cortical bulges are due to focal areas of normal tissue, which lie adjacent to nearby organs. Although initially the appearances may suggest a mass, careful examination shows a normal cortex and thickness with maintenance of normal intrarenal architecture (Fig. 2.**14**). The normal color Doppler appearances have been said to be a helpful distinguishing feature between a true mass and a local bulge. Sometimes a repeat scan is justified, particularly when appearances are marked; occasionally CT may be used to confirm the diagnosis, i.e. to exclude a tumor.

Fig. 2.**14 a** Longitudinal and (**b**) transverse images of the left kidney showing a cortical bulge or "splenic hump" (arrow). This is a normal variant. When severe these can be confused with tumor, and either a CT scan or interval ultrasound scan is required to clarify

Septa of Bertin

This developmental variation is again related to fetal lobulation, as when these coalesce the deeper parts of the cortex become trapped and embedded into the renal sinus lying between the papilla. They do not usually distort the overlying anatomy.[1] It can on occasion be confused with tumor, although in general terms they are identical to the overlying cortex and cause no local distortion. In general, differentiation from tumors is often straightforward. Where doubt persists, CT scanning with intravenous contrast is normally helpful (Fig. 2.15).

Congenital Variants

It is not possible to cover the entire gamut of congenital variants of the urogenital tract and as such only the commoner variants directly related to the structure of the kidney will be commented upon. Other variants, for example congenital megaureter and posterior valves, will be discussed in the appropriate chapters.

Duplex Collecting System and Ureters (see Chapter 9, Diseases of the Collecting System and Ureters)

Minor variants of the upper and lower moieties of the collecting systems will not be apparent on ultrasound. Moderate to marked degrees of variation are likely to show as two separate renal sinuses split by a band of normal renal cortex, i.e. a septa of Bertin. The point of junction of both complexes is very difficult to identify with ultrasound even when the ureters are dilated. In this situation examination of the bladder is important, as a ureterocele may be identified, which is often associated with the upper moiety, the lower moiety being more associated with reflux (Fig. 2.16).[26]

Ectopic Kidneys

If the kidney is not in its normal anatomical position in the renal bed, then the possibility that it may be absent or ectopic (assuming there has been no previous surgery) should be considered. The presence of a contralateral enlarged kidney, which is otherwise normal in appearance, implies that the remaining kidney is either congenitally absent or nonfunctional, whereas a normal-sized kidney may indicate that the remaining kidney lies at a site below the normal renal bed. A careful search from the renal bed inferiorly as far down as the pelvis is justified, 80% being found below the level of the iliac crest and on the ipsilateral side.[27] Generally the ectopic kidney is similar to that of a normal kidney. However, pelvic kidneys may have an unusual orienta-

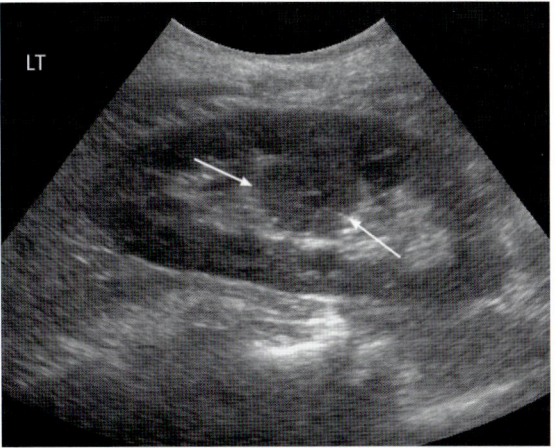
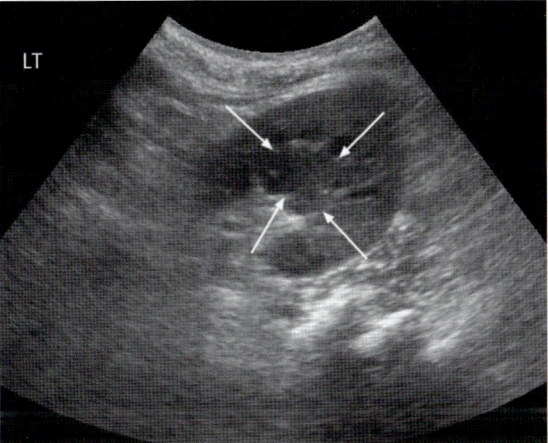

Fig. 2.15 a Longitudinal and (b) transverse images of a prominent column of Bertin (arrows). The invaginated column of tissue is identical to the overlying cortex and there is no anatomical distortion

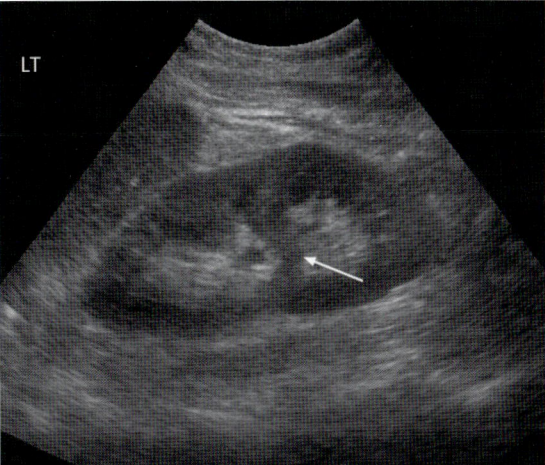

Fig. 2.16 Longitudinal image of the left kidney with a band of tissue traversing it (arrow) and splitting the renal sinus. Appearances are likely to reflect a duplex collecting system. Kidneys with duplex systems in general tend to be slightly larger than those with conventional collecting systems

2 The Normal Kidney

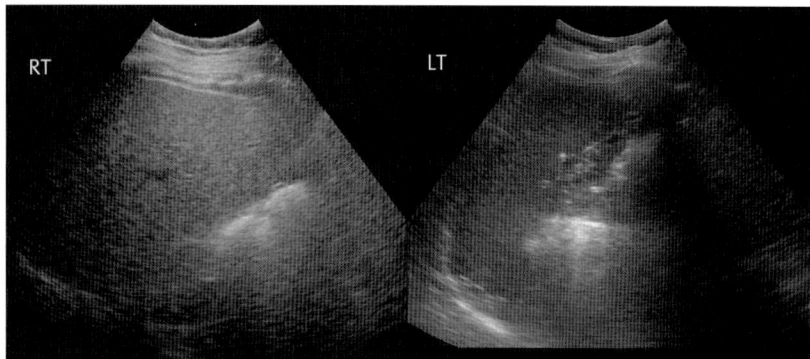

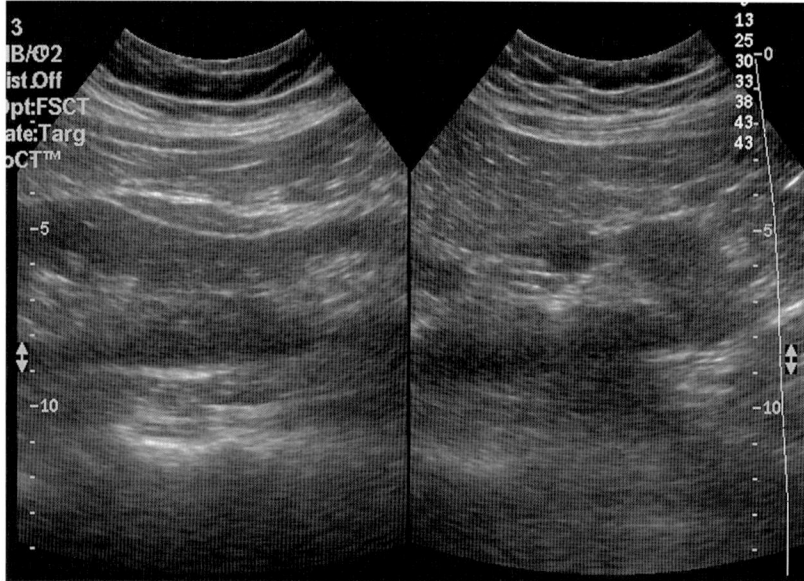

Fig. 2.17 **a** Ultrasound scan through both the right and left renal areas, showing no visible renal tissue. **b** A scan through the left lower abdomen and midline just below umbilical level showed an enlarged kidney measuring 15 cm in the lower left lumbar area (left side of image) which joins with a separate mass of renal tissue in the midline (right side of image). The appearances are those of crossed-fused ectopia

tion within the pelvis and may also show some pelvicalyceal dilatation. It may be detected as part of a clinical examination and be falsely misinterpreted, which can on occasion lead to confusion, with misinterpretation as a bowel-related colonic tumor, appendix mass/abscess,[28] or lymph node mass. This should be avoidable, however, as one renal bed will be empty and will probably be occupied by bowel. In addition, color Doppler may prove helpful in identifying the normal renal vasculature within the mass.

The ectopic kidney can, of course, cross the midline and lie under and attach inferiorly to the normally positioned kidney. This condition is known as crossfused ectopia and produces a very long kidney, generally speaking, with two separate sinus echoes (Fig. 2.17).

Horseshoe Kidneys

The incidence of horseshoe kidney based upon previous autopsy data and more recently a literature review of 12 studies is approximately 1 in 600 births.[29] Horseshoe kidneys are distinguished by a bridge of renal tissue connecting the lower poles of the kidneys. This can vary in thickness and, if of adequate thickness, can be visualized as a parenchymal band crossing the midline. Visualization of the "isthmus" depends upon many factors related to ultrasound, i.e. patient build, etc. It lies in front of the aorta and IVC and can be confused with a lymph node mass or retroperitoneal tumor. In general, however, the fact that this tissue may be renally related can be gleaned from the fact that the lower poles of the kidneys lie more medial than the upper, and that there is often a degree of mild rotation of the collecting system, which lie more anteriorly than in the normal situation (Fig. 2.18).

Hypoplasia and Atrophy

Often these two entities are difficult to differentiate, and indeed this differentiation is generally of little clinical consequence. Congenital hypoplasia is thought to occur secondary to some form of intrauterine insult, which has resulted in poor renal development. Atrophy again can be secondary to a number of renal insults. However, childhood reflux nephropathy is one of the commoner causes (Fig. 2.13). In cases where one kidney is clearly smaller and may be of reduced cortical thickness, overall function and contribution of each kidney with an isotope scan is often of help.

Agenesis

Agenesis is more common than ectopia and is more common on the left side and, as mentioned previously, in contrast to ectopia, the contralateral kidney generally shows evidence of compensatory hypertrophy. The incidence is approximately 1 in 1500.[30] Furthermore, bowel mainly occupies the empty renal bed; where ultrasound remains suggestive but nondiagnostic, an isotope scan or CT scan often clarifies the matter. The cause of agenesis is not fully appreciated, however. Some may be secondary to unilateral cystic dysplastic kidneys which have progressively atrophied over time. Clearly bilateral renal agenesis is detected in the developing fetus usually as part of the investigation of oligohydramnios and is essentially incompatible with life.

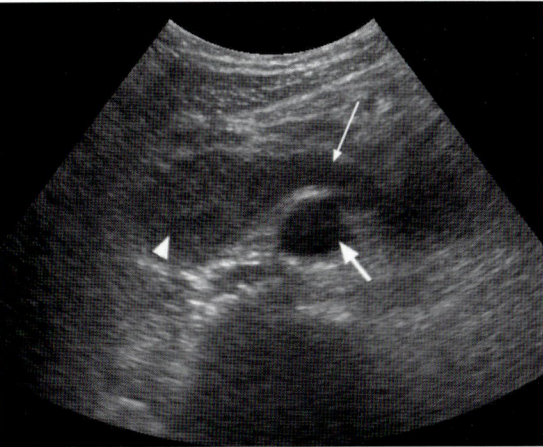

Fig. 2.**18 Transverse section through the lower abdomen showing the abdominal aorta** (thick arrow) **and a bridging piece of tissue running anterior to it** (thin arrow). This is the isthmus of a horseshoe kidney. Part of the right side of the horseshoe can be appreciated (arrowhead)

Summary points:
- Splenic humps and septa of Bertin are normal appearances of renal tissue that can on occasion be confused with tumors
- In a duplex system the upper moiety is associated with a ureterocele, whilst the lower moiety is associated with ureteric reflux
- Ectopic kidneys can occasionally be confused with colonic or appendix masses
- The incidence of horseshoe kidney is 1 in 600 births and can occasionally be confused for retroperitoneal adenopathy
- The incidence of renal agenesis is 1 in 1500; it is more common on the left

References

1. Hodson J. The lobar structure of the kidney. BJN 1972; 44:246–261.
2. Emamian SA, Nielsen MB, Pedersen JF, Ytte L. Kidney dimensions at sonography: correlation with age, sex and habitus in 665 adult volunteers. AJR 1993;160:83–86.
3. Ablett MJ, Coulthard A, Lee RE, Richardson DL, Bellas T, Owen JP, et al. How reliable are ultrasound measurements of renal length in adults? Br J Radiol 1995;68:1087–1089.
4. Ninan VT, Koshi KT, Niyamthullah MM, Jacob CK, Gopalakrishnan G, Pandey AP, et al. A comparative study of methods of estimating renal size in normal adults. Nephrol Dialy Transpl 1990;5:851–854.
5. Olin JW, Piedmonte MR, Young JR, DeAnna S, Grubb M, Childs MB. The utility of duplex ultrasound scanning of the renal arteries for diagnosing significant renal artery stenosis. Ann Int Med 1995;122:833–838.
6. Helenon O, El Rody F, Correas JM, et al. Color Doppler ultrasound of renovascular disease in native kidneys. Radiographics 1995;15:833–854.
7. Brandt TD, Neiman HL, Dragowski MJ, Bulawa W, Claykamp G. Ultrasound assessment of normal renal dimensions. J Ultrasound Med 1982;1:49–52.
8. Mazzotta L, Sarteschi LM, Carlini A, Antonelli A. Comparison of renal ultrasonographic and functional biometry in healthy patients and in patients with chronic renal failure. Arch Ital Urol Androl 2002;74:206–209.
9. Buchholz NP, Abbas F, Biyabani SR, Afzal M, Javed Q, Rizvi I, et al. Ultrasonic renal size in individuals without known renal disease. J Pak Med Ass 2000;50:12–16.
10. Roger SD, Beale AM, Cattell WR, Webb JA. What is the value of measuring renal parenchymal thickness before renal biopsy? Clin Radiol 1994;49:45–49.
11. Webb JAW. The role of ultrasonography in the diagnosis of intrinsic renal disease. Clinical Radiology 1994;49: 589–591.
12. Hricak H, Slovis TL, Callen CW, Callen PW, Romanski RN. Neonatal kidneys: sonographic anatomic correlation. Radiology 1983;147:669–702.
13. Manley JA, O'Neill WC. How echogenic is echogenic? Quantitative acoustics of the renal cortex. AJKD 2001;37: 706–711.
14. Hricak H, CruZ C, Romanski RN, Uniewski MH, Levin NW, Madrazo BL, et al. Renal parenchymal disease: sonographic histologic correlation. Radiology 1982;144:141–147.
15. Platt JF, Rubin JM, Bowerman RA, Marn CS. The inability to detect kidney disease on the basis of echogenicity. AJR 1988;151:317–319.
16. Desberg AL, Paushter DM, Lammert GK, et al. Renal artery stenosis: evaluation with color flow imaging. Radiology 1990;177:749–753.

17. Baxter GM, Aitchison F, Sheppard D, Moss JG, McLeod MJ, Harden PN, et al. Colour Doppler ultrasound in renal artery stenosis: intrarenal waveform analysis. Br J Radiol 1996;69:810–815.
18. Claudon M, Plouin PF, Baxter GM, Rhoban T, Maniez Devos D. Renal arteries in patients at risk of renal artery stenosis: Multicenter evaluation of the echo-enhancer SH U 508A at color and spectral Doppler US. Radiology 2000;214:739–746.
19. Rivolta R, Cardinale L, Lovaria A, Di Palo FQ. Variability of renal echo-Doppler measurements in healthy adults. J Nephrol 2000;13:110–115.
20. Terry JD, Rysavy JA, Frick MP. Intrarenal Doppler: characteristics of aging kidneys. J Ultrasound Med 1992;11:647–651.
21. Mostbeck GH, Kain R, Mallek R. Duplex Doppler sonography in renal parenchymal disease. Histopathologic correlation. J Ultrasound Med 1991;10:189–194.
22. Splendiani G, Parolini C, Fortunato L, Stumiolo A, Costanzi S. Resistive index in chronic nephropathies: predictive value of renal outcome. Clinical Nephrology 2002;57:45–50.
23. Quaia E, Bertolotto M. Renal parenchymal diseases: is characterisation feasible with ultrasound? Eur Radiol 2002;12:2006–2020.
24. Mostbeck GH, Zontsich T, Turetschek K. Ultrasound of the kidney: obstruction and medical diseases. Eur Radiol 2001;11:1878–1889.
25. Peake SC, Roxburgh HB, Langlois S le P. Ultrasonic assessment of the hydronephrosis of pregnancy. Radiology 1983;146:167–170.
26. Fernbach SK, Feinstein KA, Spencer K, Lindstrom CA. Ureteral duplication and its complications. Radiographics 1997;17:109–127.
27. Meyers MA, Whalen GP, Evans JA, Viamonte M. Malposition and displacement of bowel in renal agenesis and ectopia: new observations. AJR 1973;117:323–333.
28. Mokoena T, Nair R, Degiannis E. Ectopic kidney presenting as an appendix mass or abscess. South African Journal of Surgery 1996;34:142–143.
29. Weizer AZ, Silverstain AD, Auge BK, Delvecchio FC, Raj G, Albala DM, et al. Determining the incidence of horseshoe kidney from radiographic data at a single institution. J Urology 2003;170:1722–1766.
30. Mascatello V, Lebowitz RL. Malposition of the colon in left renal agenesis and ectopia. Radiology 1976;120:371–376.
31. Miletic D, Fuckar Z, Sustic A, Mozetic V, Stimac D, Zauhar G. Sonographic measurement of absolute and relative renal lengths in adults. J Clin Ultrasound 1998;26:185–189.
32. Rosenbaum DM, Korngold E, Teele RL. Sonographic assessment of renal length in normal children. AJR Am J Roentgenol 1984:142:467–469.

3 Parenchymal Diseases of the Kidney

P. L. Allan

Introduction

There are a wide variety of conditions which can diffusely affect the renal parenchyma and produce varying degrees of renal impairment. In patients with acute renal failure (ARF), the primary role of ultrasound is to exclude obstruction as a cause of the failure, which will be the case in about 5–10% of cases.[1] For the remainder, the diagnosis will depend upon a combination of the clinical situation, biochemical findings, and, in a proportion of patients, renal biopsy. Many of these disorders do not produce specific changes in the appearances of the kidneys on ultrasound, but analyzing any changes that are seen, in the light of the clinical situation, may allow a differential diagnosis to be made.

Some disorders affect mainly the cortex, others affect primarily the medulla, and some may affect the parenchyma as a whole. During the ultrasound examination, attention should be given to each of the components of the kidney.

Renal size and overall appearance: In some acute disorders, swelling and edema of the kidney may be seen, although in most cases the size of the kidneys is within normal limits. In chronic renal disease the kidneys tend to contract in size, but this is variable and there is little or no correlation with either renal function, or the cause of renal disease.[2] These small, relatively echogenic kidneys may be difficult to distinguish within the retroperitoneal fat and may only be identified through their movement on respiration (Fig. 3.1). In some patients with end-stage renal disease (ESRD), changes of acquired cystic disease of the kidney may be seen and parenchymal calcification can be seen with some disorders.

Cortex: The appearances of the cortex may be within normal limits, or show an abnormal increase or decrease in echogenicity: Normal renal echogenicity is less than that of the adjacent liver or spleen (assuming that these are normal). In some acute conditions edema and swelling of the cortex are seen. Cortical scarring may be seen (Fig. 3.2); this is distinguished from fetal lobulation as it is usually opposite a calyx or pyramid, whereas the cortical "defects" in fetal lobulation lie between pyramids. Cortical calcification can occur but it is less common than medullary, or collecting system calcification.

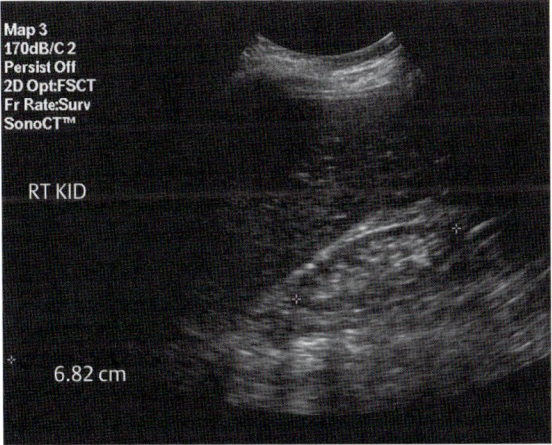

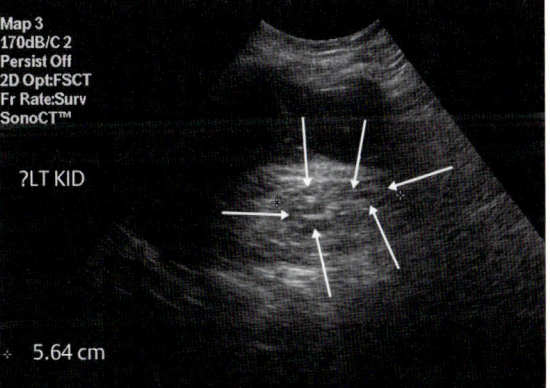

Fig. 3.1 **a** A kidney measuring 6.8 cm in length in a patient with chronic renal disease. **b** A smaller kidney that is more difficult to identify in another patient (arrows); it is easier to appreciate in real-time as it moves with respiration

Medulla/pyramids: The appearances of the pyramids can vary, depending upon a number of factors relating to the medullary tissues, or to the adjacent cortex. Normal pyramids are of lower echogenicity than the adjacent cortical tissue and are evenly spaced around the margins of the renal sinus. In acute cortical disorders the pyramids may be more visible due to greater contrast between them and the increased cortical echogenicity. In other cases there may be a decrease in corticomedullary differentiation. In patients with a primary abnormality of the medulla, the pyramids may be enlarged and hypoechoic, as sometimes seen in acute

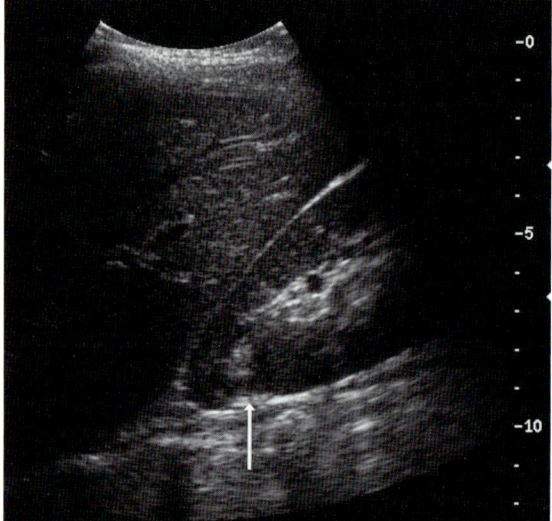
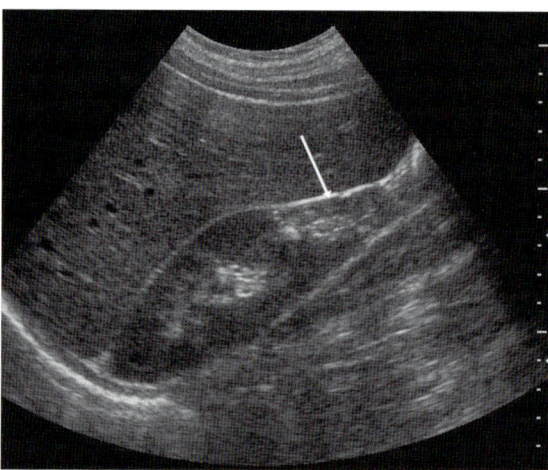

Fig. 3.**2** **a** A small scar at the upper pole of the right kidney (arrow). **b** More marked scarring at the lower pole of another right kidney (arrow)

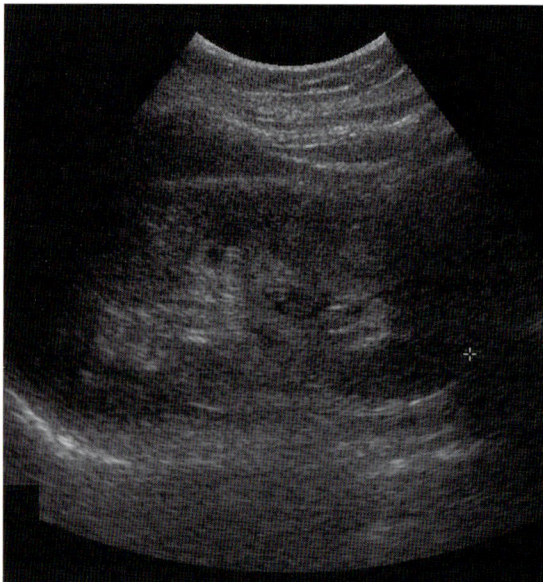

Fig. 3.**3** A diffusely echogenic kidney with loss of corticomedullary differentiation in a patient with acute glomerulonephritis

tubular necrosis (ATN), or show increased echogenicity, as in cases of nephrocalcinosis.

Renal sinus: The region of the renal sinus appears as an area of increased echogenicity in the central part of the kidney because of the fat that it contains surrounding the major vessels. It is not usually involved in diffuse parenchymal disease but may be reduced in size with severe parenchymal edema, or show a relative increase in size with parenchymal atrophy. The components of the collecting system are more prominent in cases of ureteric obstruction and calyceal prominence can be noted in cases of papillary necrosis.

Renal vessels: Color and spectral Doppler provide information on local conditions in the vessels at the point of interrogation, as well as indirect evidence on the peripheral circulation in the kidney from changes to the spectral waveform.

Cortical Disorders

Glomerulonephritis

There are several inflammatory and noninflammatory pathologies which can affect the glomerulus and interfere with its function; many have an autoimmune component. Clinically, they result in hematuria and proteinuria and a variable degree of renal impairment.

There are no specific features on ultrasound and the kidneys will appear normal in many cases. In some cases there is a variable increase in the cortical echogenicity (Fig. 3.**3**). This is nonspecific and there is no relationship with the pathological type, degree of renal impairment, or prognosis; there is some correlation between cortical echogenicity and the degree of inflammatory infiltrate or fibrosis found on histology but this is of little clinical value.[3] In acute cases the kidneys may show some enlargement and decreased corticomedullary differentiation with a tendency to shrink if chronic disease develops.

Acute Cortical Necrosis

This is a rare cause of ARF in the West but is more common in India and Eastern Asia.[4] Classically it is associated with abruptio placentae, or postpartum hemorrhage but it can also occur with shock, sepsis, snake bites, and exposure to toxins. There is microvascular thrombosis, and a diffuse intravascular coagulopathy develops resulting in cortical ischemia, except for a thin subcapsular rim of tissue supplied by capsular vessels. There is loss of the normal corticomedullary differentiation and ill-defined patchy areas of increased echogenicity within the parenchyma; the peripheral, perfused rim of parenchyma may be distinguished as an hypoechoic, subcapsular zone (Fig. 3.4).[5] Calcium may be deposited at the junction of the ischemic and peripheral zones; this may develop within a few days from the onset of renal failure.

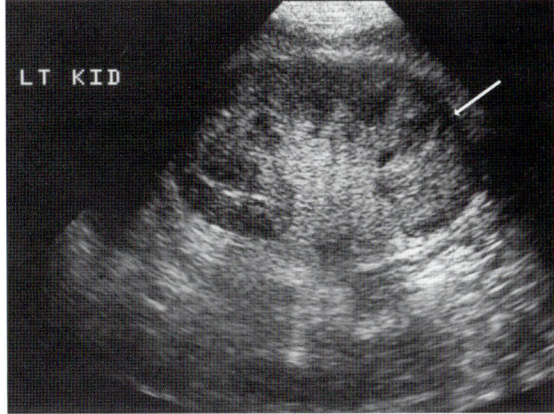

Fig. 3.4 A kidney with acute cortical necrosis showing generally increased echogenicity but with a thin rim of perfused parenchyma (arrow)

Acute Interstitial Nephritis

Acute interstitial nephritis usually results from an immunologically-induced hypersensitivity reaction to a drug or infective antigen.[6] Rarely, it is associated with sarcoid, systemic lupus erythematosus, or malignancy. Histologically, there are diffuse inflammatory infiltrates in the interstitial tissues of the kidney. Clinically, it can imitate ATN, as there is usually a degree of tubular dysfunction. On ultrasound, the kidneys may be normal or enlarged, depending on the severity of the condition; the echogenicity of the cortex may be normal or increased and the finding of a markedly echogenic parenchyma in a patient with ARF (Fig. 3.5) should raise the possibility of acute interstitial nephritis.[7]

Cortical Nephrocalcinosis

Cortical nephrocalcinosis is rare compared with medullary nephrocalcinosis. Focal calcifications can occur following trauma, infarction, or infection; they may also be associated with tumors. Diffuse cortical calcification may be seen following acute cortical necrosis, renal transplant rejection, Alport syndrome, and rarely with chronic glomerulonephritis. Following acute cortical necrosis the calcification is characteristically seen at the junction between the viable and necrotic regions; this can be seen as early as six to seven days after the onset of the disorder.[5]

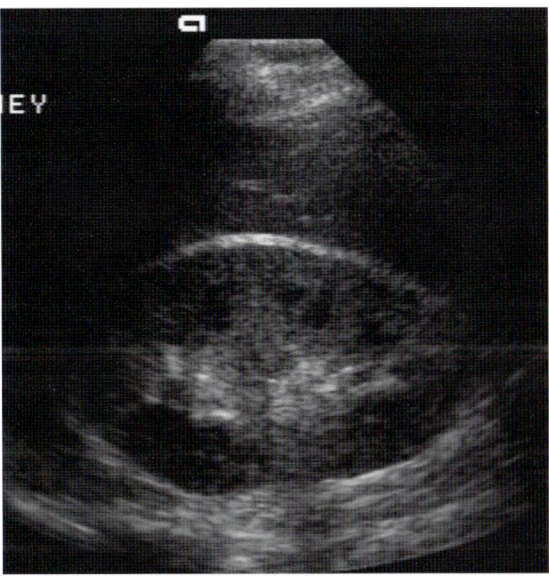

Fig. 3.5 A diffusely enlarged, echogenic kidney in a patient with acute interstitial nephritis. However, the appearances are nonspecific and are similar to those seen in several other acute disorders of the renal parenchyma

Disorders of the Medulla/Pyramids

Acute Tubular Necrosis

Acute tubular necrosis (ATN) is one of the most common causes for ARF in hospital patients.[8,9] The injury is usually due to a combination of cellular ischemia and direct tubular epithelial cell injury induced by nephrotoxins. The tubules are more vulnerable to ischemia because of their relatively high metabolic rate and the relatively poor blood supply with low oxygenation when compared with the more luxuriant flow to the cortex and glomeruli. In addition, sloughing of cells and

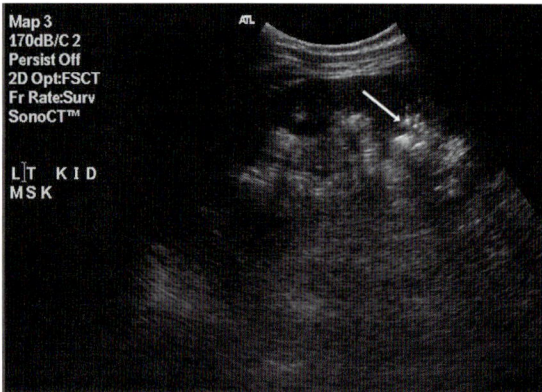

Fig. 3.6 Echogenic foci in the region of the medullary pyramids (arrow) in a patient with medullary sponge kidneys. A little patchy shadowing is visible but this is not a strong feature

debris into the tubular lumen leads to obstruction by proteinaceous casts. There are several factors which may contribute to the development of this disorder, including ischemia and hypotension, drugs and toxins, sepsis and myoglobinuria/hemoglobinuria. In any individual case, more than one factor is often involved.

The kidneys often appear normal in these patients, and the main role of ultrasound is to exclude obstruction as a cause of the renal failure. Changes which may be identified on ultrasound include diffuse swelling of the kidneys, increased prominence of the medullary pyramids due to edema, or some increase in cortical echogenicity with preservation of corticomedullary differentiation. Doppler ultrasound shows an increase in the resistive index (RI) in the intrarenal vessels,[10] with those patients who suffer persistent renal dysfunction tending to have higher values than those who recover adequate function.[11]

■ Renal Papillary Necrosis

Renal papillary necrosis is part of a spectrum of chronic tubulointerstitial nephritic disorders in which there is progressive scarring and fibrosis of tubulointerstitial structures. This is the final common pathway to ESRD for many disorders, including analgesic nephropathy, diabetes, vesicoureteric reflux (VUR), sickle cell disease, sarcoid, chronic transplant rejection, and heavy-metal poisoning. Over 50% of cases in the United Kingdom are associated with diabetes. In renal papillary necrosis, ultrasound will not show any changes until the disease is advanced and the papillae have sloughed away producing small round, or triangular cystic areas at the site of the missing papilla. Calcification of affected papillae can occur, particularly in cases of analgesic nephropathy, resulting in echogenic foci in the region of the papillae, described as a "garland pattern" around the renal sinus.[12] Sloughed papillae may result in ureteric obstruction and dilatation of the pelvicalyceal system.[13,14]

■ Medullary Sponge Kidney

The cause of medullary sponge kidney is uncertain, but it is thought that it may be a minor developmental anomaly, and links with other disorders such as Caroli disease, Marfan syndrome, and Ehlers–Danlos syndrome have been reported.[15] In medullary sponge kidney there are ectatic and cystic changes affecting the medullary collecting ducts; small calculi can form within these dilated segments. Ultrasound may show small, calcific foci in the region of the pyramids but it may just show increased echogenicity of the pyramids if the calculi are too small to show up as distinct entities (Fig. 3.6).

■ Nephrocalcinosis

There is a wide range of disorders which result in medullary nephrocalcinosis. Raised serum calcium, phosphate, or an alkaline urine can result in nephrocalcinosis. The commonest causes are primary hyperparathyroidism and renal tubular acidosis, although any disorder leading to hypercalcemia may be implicated and a list of these is given in Table 3.1.[16] Frusemide therapy is recognized as a cause of nephrocalcinosis in infants and recent reports suggest that nephrocalcinosis may also be seen in adults who are abusing frusemide to lose weight or reduce edema.[17] The calcification is predominantly medullary in location but may rarely be seen within the cortex. Ultrasound has been shown to be reliable in the detection and grading of nephrocalcinosis in children.[18] The calcified areas appear on ultrasound as regions of increased echogenicity in the medulla. Initially the calcium deposits may appear as rings around the periphery of the medullary pyramids;[19] with more marked deposition of calcium, the whole pyramid is involved (Fig. 3.7). Acoustic shadows may be absent if the calcium depositions are individually small in diameter in relation to beam width; with more marked degrees of calcification, acoustic shadowing can be variable in prominence.

Hyperechogenic medullae are not always the result of nephrocalcinosis and may be seen in patients with gout (where urate deposits and the associated interstitial nephritis are responsible) and in primary hyperaldosteronism in which chronic hypokalemia results in changes within the tubules and adjacent interstitial tissues.

Table 3.1 Causes of nephrocalcinosis[16]

Medullary		
Renal tubular acidosis		
Oxalosis*		
Papillary necrosis		
Medullary sponge kidney		
Frusemide abuse		
Bartter Syndrome		
Hypercalcemia	Primary hyperparathyroidism	Hypercalcemia of malignancy
	Sarcoid	Cushing disease
	Vitamin D excess	Milk-alkali syndrome
Cortical		
Renal cortical necrosis		
Chronic glomerulonephritis		
Transplant rejection		
Tuberculosis		
Oxalosis*		

* Oxalosis typically causes both cortical and medullary nephrocalcinosis

Summary points:
- In patients with ARF, obstruction will be responsible in 5–10%
- Ultrasonic features of glomerulonephritis are variable and are often normal
- RI maybe of prognostic significance in patients with ATN
- Renal papillary necrosis is associated with diabetes in approximately 50% of cases in the UK

Renal Infections

A spectrum of infective disorders can affect the kidneys. The commonest form is acute bacterial pyelonephritis, but infection can be associated with obstruction, calculi, reflux, diabetes, immunosuppression, catheters, or hematogenous spread. The infection can affect primarily the parenchyma, or the collecting system, or both.

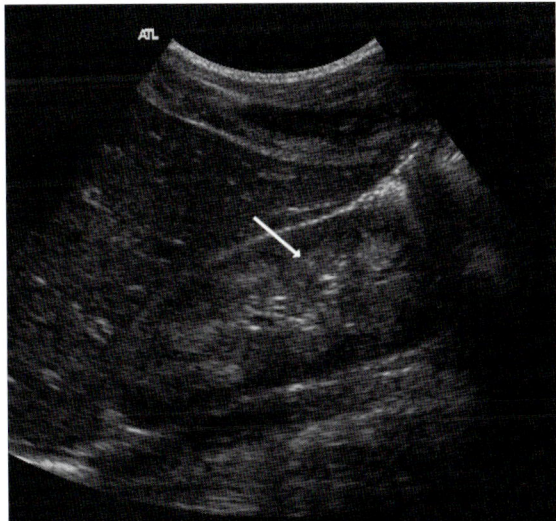

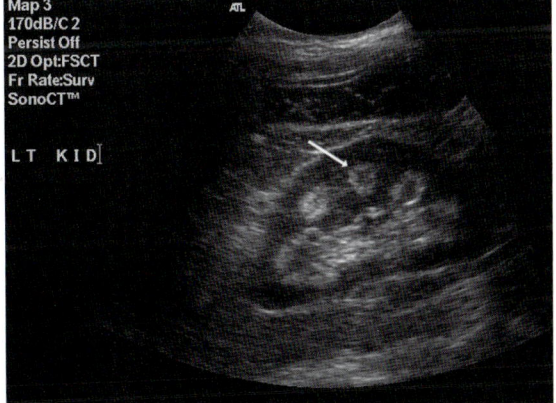

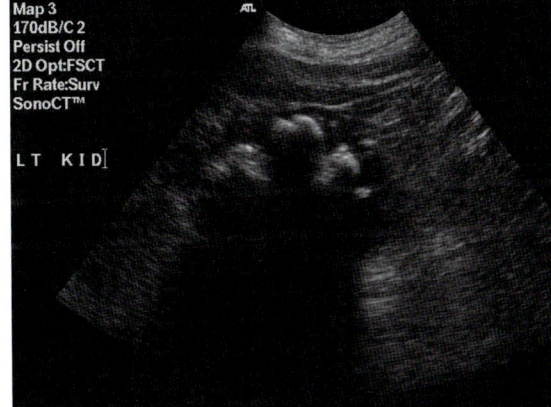

Fig. 3.7 **a** Early nephrocalcinosis identified as echogenic pyramids (arrow). **b** More marked changes showing as rings and echogenic pyramids (arrow). **c** Marked nephrocalcinosis in a patient with end-stage renal disease (ESRD)

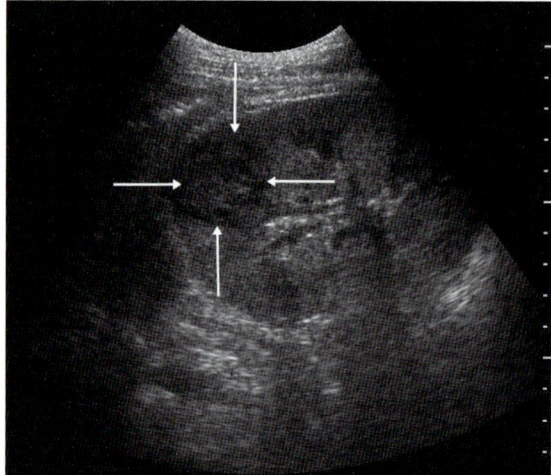

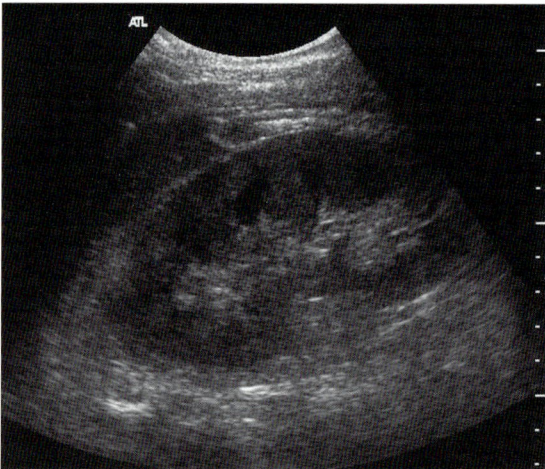

Fig. 3.8 **a** Focal lobar nephronia at the upper pole of a kidney (arrows). **b** Six weeks later this area has returned to normal

In some patients focal areas of reduced echogenicity may be identified, corresponding to marked focal inflammatory change; these may resolve with appropriate antibiotic therapy, or may go on to frank abscess formation. These focal inflammatory areas are sometimes called focal lobar nephronia, or acute focal pyelonephritis. The appearances on ultrasound are variable; the affected kidney may be generally enlarged and focal areas of increased, reduced, or mixed echoes may be seen within it (Fig. 3.8). Focal areas of low echogenicity characteristically have no evidence of acoustic enhancement distally; some mass effect can also be apparent.[22,23]

Renal Abscess

Occasionally, renal parenchymal infections will progress to abscess formation; other abscesses may result from hematogenous spread of infection, particularly with *Staphylococcus aureus*.[24] Diabetes, renal calculi, and ureteric obstruction are also predisposing factors for the development of renal abscesses.[25] Abscesses may be single or multiple, and appear on ultrasound as hypoechoic areas within which low level echoes from debris and pus may be apparent; distal acoustic enhancement is a feature because of the liquid nature of the contents. Infection can spread into the collecting system, resulting in a pyonephrosis, or into the perirenal space to produce a perirenal abscess. Distinction between an abscess and an infected renal cyst may be difficult, although the smoother walls of a cyst may be apparent around the debris-laden collection.[20]

Pyelonephritis

Acute bacterial pyelonephritis is the most common renal infective disorder, occurring more commonly in females. These infections usually respond to antibiotics, have no lasting sequelae, and patients do not usually attend for ultrasound examinations. Ultrasound is performed in patients who do not respond to therapy, have a severe infection, or who are considered to have a possible structural or functional abnormality which may predispose to infection. Even in severe infections, the kidneys may look normal on ultrasound.[20] Diffuse or focal swelling of the kidney may be seen; evidence of a predisposing factor, including calculi and/or obstruction, may be discovered. The parenchymal echo pattern may be patchy in appearance due to focal areas of edema and inflammatory infiltration, or even focal hemorrhagic necrosis.[21]

Emphysematous Pyelonephritis

Emphysematous pyelonephritis is a necrotizing renal infection characterized by gas production within the renal parenchyma, or perirenal tissues.[20] *E. coli* is the cause of the infection in 60–70% of cases and some 90% of cases of emphysematous pyelonephritis occur in diabetics, usually associated with obstruction.[26,27] Bright foci of gas may be seen in the parenchyma, perirenal tissues, or within the collecting system. Percutaneous drainage has shown promising results; this can be done using ultrasound for guidance, but computed tomography (CT) may be required if the gas obscures the anatomy of the renal area.[28]

Xanthogranulomatous Pyelonephritis

This is a rare chronic inflammatory condition which is associated with chronic obstruction and may affect part of the kidney, or the entire organ. *Proteus mirabilis* is the most common causative agent. The chronic inflammatory process is characterized by the replacement of the renal parenchyma with a diffuse or segmental cellular infiltrate of lipid-laden macrophages/foam cells (xanthoma cells); this results in the destruction of normal renal tissue, with cavitation, fibrosis, and a chronic granuloma. On ultrasound, a mass is seen in the renal bed but normal renal architecture is not apparent; hydronephrosis may be identified (Fig. 3.**9**).[29] Heterogenous areas of increased and decreased echoes are visible and calculi may be seen within the mass, although these can be difficult to see clearly due to the surrounding inflammatory, fibrotic tissue. Perinephric fluid collections may be seen in a small number of patients. Diagnosis can be difficult on ultrasound unless the possibility of xanthogranulomatous pyelonephritis is considered. Focal xanthogranulomatous changes in a kidney are usually well-circumscribed and can be difficult to differentiate from a tumor.[30,31]

Tuberculosis

Tuberculosis of the renal tract is usually the result of hematogenous spread of pulmonary tuberculosis and can affect the parenchyma, as well as the collecting system and ureters. In parenchymal disease, the bacilli favor the high cortical blood flow, oxygen saturation, and increased blood viscosity found in the efferent arterioles. If they proliferate, the infection then ruptures into the proximal tubule and the bacilli congregate in the apex of the Loop of Henle in the medulla, forming medullary granulomas and abscesses which can rupture into the collecting system, leading to ureteric strictures and bladder fibrosis.

The early stages are not apparent on ultrasound, but parenchymal abscesses, cavities, foci of calcification, and dilated calyces become visible as the disease progresses. Increasing destruction of the renal architecture is seen as the infection spreads through the kidney;[32,33] segmental or generalized dilatation of the collecting system can be seen as a result of strictures and fibrosis. Ultrasound-guided fine needle aspiration is reported to be of value in confirming the diagnosis of renal tuberculosis in patients with consistently negative urine cultures for acid-fast bacilli.[34] Eventually the kidney becomes shrunken and fibrotic. Extensive calcification may be present; this appearance is sometimes referred to as an autonephrectomy (Fig. 3.**10**).

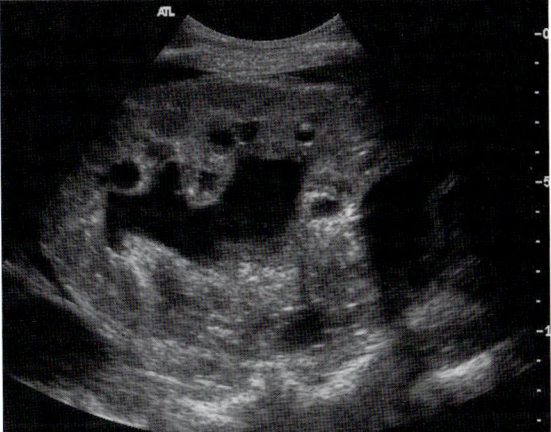
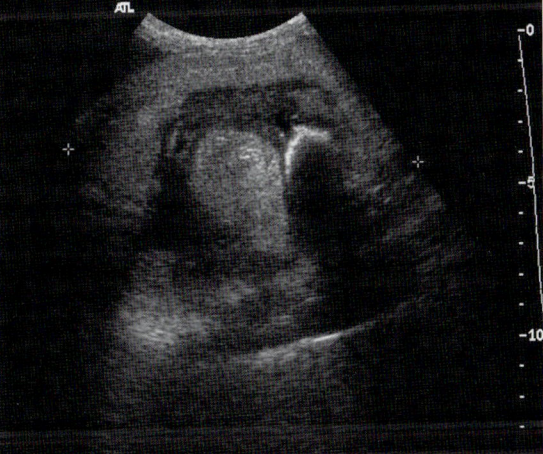

Fig. 3.**9 a** Xanthogranulomatous pyelonephritis of a kidney showing a dilated collecting system surrounded by parenchyma replaced by chronic inflammatory tissue. **b** Another case showing complete replacement of renal parenchyma by an abnormal structure; a calculus is present within this mass

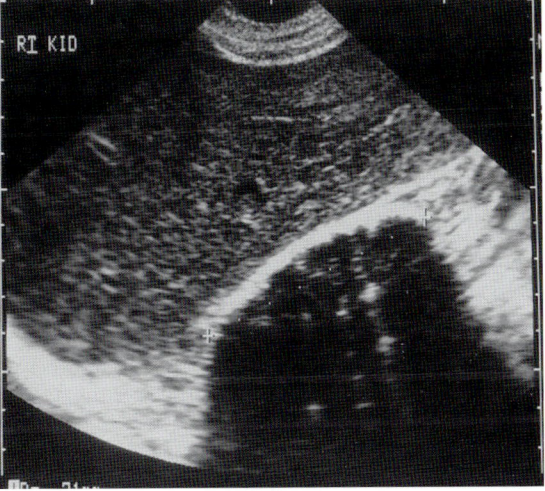

Fig. 3.**10** Autonephrectomy. A densely calcified kidney resulting from tuberculous infection

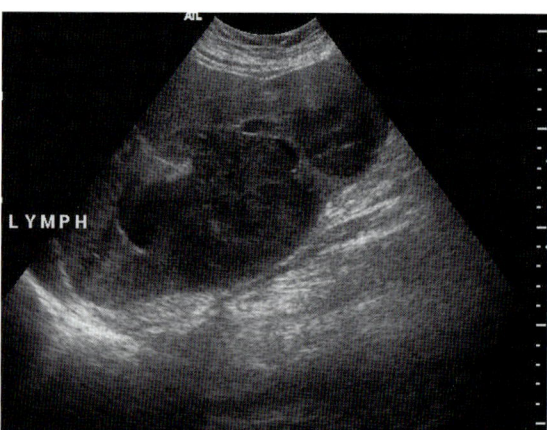

Fig. 3.11 Non-Hodgkin lymphoma affecting the kidney in a patient with AIDS

Acquired Immune Deficiency Syndrome

Patients with human immunodeficiency virus (HIV) infection who develop acquired immune deficiency syndrome (AIDS) will be more likely to suffer episodes of bacterial and fungal renal infections. They are also at increased risk of developing non-Hodgkin lymphoma, which has a predilection for extranodal sites such as the kidney (Fig. 3.11), and Kaposi sarcoma, although this has a tendency to affect the lower renal tract rather than the kidney. Amyloid may also be found in these patients.

Patients with AIDS can also develop an HIV-associated nephropathy (HIVAN). Biopsy shows focal segmental glomerulosclerosis and focal glomerulonephritis.[35] Tubular abnormalities have also been reported. Clinically, patients have proteinuria and may go on to develop uremia and renal failure.

On ultrasound, kidneys may be of normal size and appearance, or enlarged; a globular appearance was reported in half of the kidneys examined in one series[36] together with abnormal parenchymal echogenicity in up to 89% of the kidneys, decreased corticomedullary definition, and a reduction in renal sinus fat. Focal medullary and cortical calcification may be seen in patients with atypical tuberculous or fungal infections.[37] There have been reports of patients with AIDS developing hemolytic uremic syndrome and associated acute cortical necrosis, although this appears to be a rare complication.[38]

Other Infections

Fungal infections are usually seen in diabetic, cachectic, or immunosupressed patients. *Candida* infection is the most common, but *Aspergillus* and *Cryptococcus* are sometimes responsible. The infection can develop in the parenchyma with areas of destruction. Infection of the collecting system can result in the development of fungal masses within the collecting system.

Hydatid disease of the kidneys is rare. The findings are similar to those found elsewhere with a cystic lesion which contains daughter cysts, or "hydatid sand"; wall calcification may be seen.[39]

Schistosomiasis affects the bladder and ureters, producing strictures that, in turn, result in obstruction reflux, infection, and stone formation. These lead to scarring of the renal parenchyma from chronic tubulointerstitial nephritis;[40] amyloid may also be a feature of schistosomiasis and affect the renal parenchyma.

Summary points:
- The kidney is generally ultrasonically normal in patients with infection
- Xanthogranulomatous pyelonephritis may be difficult to differentiate from a renal tumor
- Tuberculosis of the renal tract is usually secondary to hematogenous spread from the lung
- Patients with AIDS can develop an HIVAN

Vascular Disorders

Renal Artery Stenosis

The two main causes of renal artery stenosis (RAS) are atheroma, which accounts for 90% of cases of RAS, and fibromuscular hyperplasia, which accounts for rather less than 10% of cases.[41] Aortic aneurysms, arteritis, and trauma can also result in narrowing of the main renal arteries, or their major branches. RAS may have a role in the development of hypertension in up to 5% of patients with hypertension, and recognition of this contributing factor is important, as renal artery angioplasty can result in cure of the hypertension, or a significant reduction in the problems associated with blood-pressure control in these cases. Ischemic nephropathy results from impairment of the renal blood flow sufficient to produce ischemia and excretory dysfunction.[41,42]

There are two components in the ultrasound assessment of RAS: Firstly, examination of the main renal arteries and their origins from the aorta; and secondly, assessment of the waveform characteristics of the intrarenal segmental and interlobar arteries.[43] Color Doppler has made it easier to identify the main renal arteries as they leave the aorta, usually just below the level of the superior mesenteric artery (Fig. 3.12). Scanning obliquely from the left side for the proximal right renal artery and the right side for the left artery may be helpful.[44] Other useful landmarks include the left renal vein as it runs toward the aorta, as the left renal artery is usually in proximity to the vein, and the inferior vena cava (IVC) for the right renal artery as the artery can be identified as it passes behind the cava. If the renal arteries cannot be identified from an anterior approach, scanning from the flank and posterolateral aspect may be of value; the liver can be used as a window on the right side (Fig. 3.**13**). Identification of both renal arteries can take considerable time and may not be achieved in every case, with the left renal artery being the more difficult to locate. Experienced operators in specialized departments report 75–80% success rate for obtaining technically adequate examinations.[45] In addition, accessory renal arteries, which occur in up to 40% of individuals in postmortem studies,[46] cannot be detected reliably.

Examination of the intrarenal vessels is more straightforward as these are located easily with color or power Doppler and a spectral display of the waveform can then be obtained.[47,48] It is best to position the sample volume initially with the patient breathing gently. The sample volume should be placed over distal segmental or interlobar arteries, as the RI tends to be a little higher in the larger vessels at the hilum.[44] Final positioning and acquisition of the waveform is then carried out during a short period of suspended respiration.

A variety of Doppler findings have been associated with a significant stenosis of the main renal arteries. These are shown in Table 3.**2**. A peak systolic velocity (PSV) > 180 cms^{-1} and a renal artery/aorta PSV ratio of > 3.5 are the most useful parameters for significant stenosis (> 60% diameter reduction) of the main renal arteries, providing an accurate angle correction can be made.[49] If visualization of the proximal main renal arteries is impossible, then an indirect assessment can be made from the waveform in the intrarenal arteries, where an acceleration time (AT) of > 0.07 s^{-1} [50] and a tardus parvus (slow and small) waveform[47] have also been shown to correlate with a significant stenosis of more than 70% diameter reduction (Fig. 3.**14**). It must be remembered that Doppler ultrasound is less accurate for lesser degrees of stenosis, so it is not reliable or useful as a screening technique for the condition. However, a positive result in selected patients indicates that further imaging techniques, such as magnetic resonance (MR) arteriography should be considered.

In distinction to renal arterial disease producing hypertension, idiopathic hypertension produces changes in the renal vessels, which over time result in hypertensive nephropathy. In patients with chronic changes it can be difficult to assess the significance of any associated stenosis and the potential value of angioplasty in improving renal function and blood-pressure control.

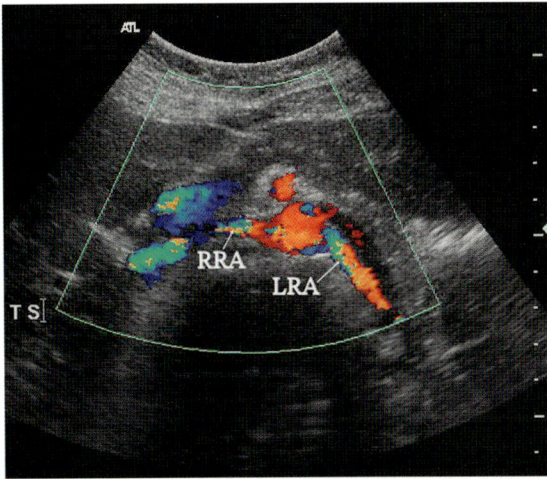

Fig. 3.**12** A transverse scan of the aorta and IVC, showing the origins of the main left and right renal arteries (RRA: right renal artery, LRA: left renal artery)

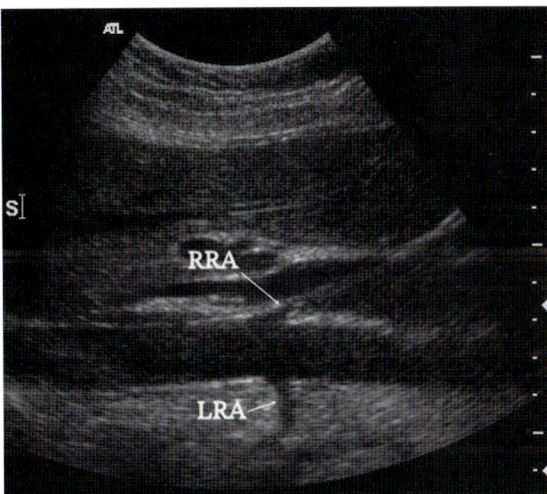

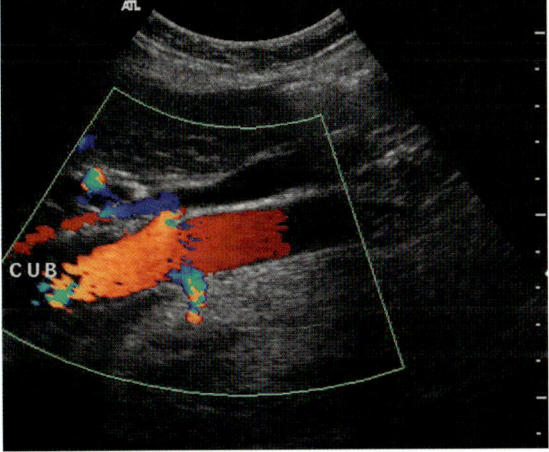

Fig. 3.**13** **a** A coronal scan through the liver showing the upper aorta and the origins of the renal arteries (arrows). **b** A color Doppler scan in the same plane

3 Parenchymal Diseases of the Kidney

Table 3.2 Indices for renal artery stenosis

Velocity in proximal renal artery	> 180 cm^{-1}
Renal artery/aorta velocity ratio (RAR)	> 3.5
Acceleration time (AT)	> 0.07 s
Acceleration index (AI)	< 3.78 ms^{-2}
Resistive index (RI)	< 0.5

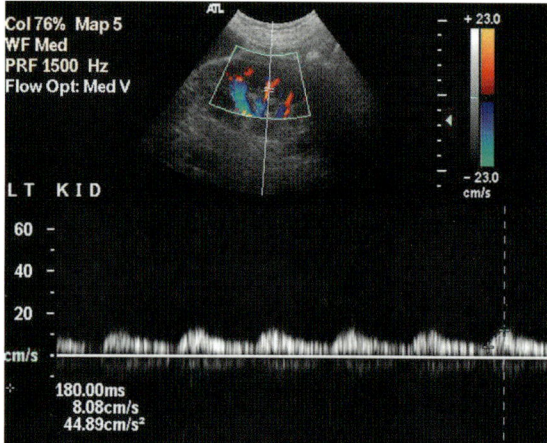

Fig. 3.**14** A color and spectral Doppler examination of the left kidney showing a tardus parvus waveform and a slow acceleration time of 0.18 s

An RI > 0.8 in the segmental renal arteries of a kidney with RAS correlates well with a poor response to angioplasty or surgery.[51]

Renal Artery Occlusion

This can result from a variety of causes, including acute hemorrhage into an atheromatous plaque, trauma, dissection of the aorta, and emboli. Chronic, unilateral occlusion may be asymptomatic, whereas an acute occlusion produces loin pain and hematuria. With complete sudden occlusion of the main renal artery, the kidney may appear normal, or slightly enlarged. Color Doppler will confirm the lack of arterial flow within the kidney. With time, the kidney atrophies. Occlusion of a segmental artery will produce segmental infarction; this can produce focal swelling of the affected segment,[52] but this may be minimal or absent and may not be recognized unless the kidney is examined carefully with color or power Doppler.

Other Arterial Abnormalities

Intrarenal arteriovenous fistulae (AVF) and aneurysms are usually the result of renal biopsy, or other renal trauma. In one series, careful examination of transplanted kidneys following biopsy showed a new AVF in 16.7% of patients.[53] Fortunately the vast majority of these closed off spontaneously: 50% within 48 hours and 75% within four weeks, with three AVF persisting for more than one year. None of the AVF required intervention. AVF characteristically show a focal tissue bruit on color Doppler at the site of the fistulous communication. Examination of the segmental artery supplying this area shows increased diastolic flow as a result of the decreased vascular resistance. The segmental vein draining the fistula shows increased velocity of flow and may show a varying degree of arterialization of flow with systolic variation. In the same series,[53] four pseudoaneurysms were detected in kidneys following biopsy; all closed spontaneously. Intrarenal aneurysms may be mistaken for cysts, unless color Doppler is applied. True aneurysms of the renal artery may occasionally develop as a result of vascular degeneration and atherosclerosis and, again, color Doppler will distinguish them from parapelvic cysts or other collections (Fig. 3.**15**).[44]

Renal Vein Thrombosis

In adults, this is associated with the nephrotic syndrome (usually the result of membranous glomerulonephritis), hypercoagulability disorders, or tumor invasion. Dehydration is more commonly associated with renal vein thrombosis in infants but it may occasionally be seen in adults, particularly in hot climates. Bilateral main renal vein thrombosis is very rare in adults and many patients will have segmental, or subsegmental venous thromboses, which cannot usually be identified on ultrasound, although they may cause a detectable decrease in diastolic flow, which can be identified through an abnormally high RI.

Renal vein thrombosis is seen more frequently in neonates; predisposing factors include dehydration, sepsis, polycythemia, umbilical vein catheters, birth asphyxia, and maternal diabetes.[54] Thrombosis commences in smaller segmental veins then propagates toward the main renal vein and IVC. In the acute phase, the thrombosed intrarenal veins appear as highly echogenic streaks.

When renal veins were ligated in a group of dogs, the affected kidney or renal segment became swollen with predominantly reduced parenchymal echogenicity and heterogeneity, together with loss of corticomedullary differentiation in the acute phase.[55] After two to three weeks the affected kidney, or segment, starts to contract and echogenicity increases as scarring and fibrosis develop.

In cases of main renal vein thrombosis, color Doppler will show an absence of flow in the vein, which may appear a little enlarged in the acute phase; less severe, intrarenal venous thrombosis cannot be visualized directly. Arterial flow is affected in a variable manner, depending upon the extent of the thrombosis and its speed of development: In acute main vein thrombosis there is a marked increase in intrarenal vascular resistance which can result in absent or reversed diastolic flow in the equivalent artery. Less extensive venous thrombosis results in decreased diastolic flow and an increase in the RI in the artery to a variable extent and care should be taken if indirect Doppler evidence is being used to confirm or exclude significant renal vein thrombosis.[56]

Renal vein occlusion can also be seen in patients with renal tumors, typically a renal cell carcinoma, which can extend into the IVC from the renal vein (Fig. 3.**16**).

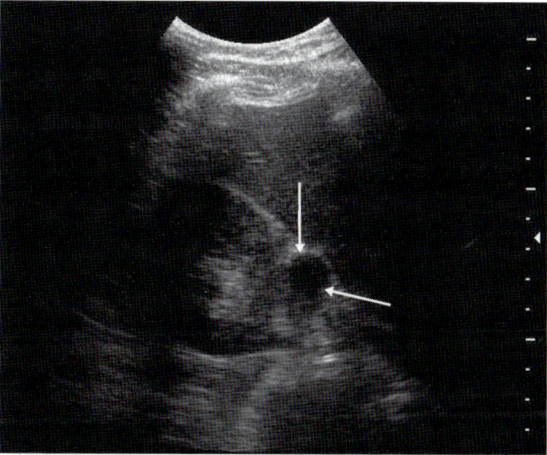

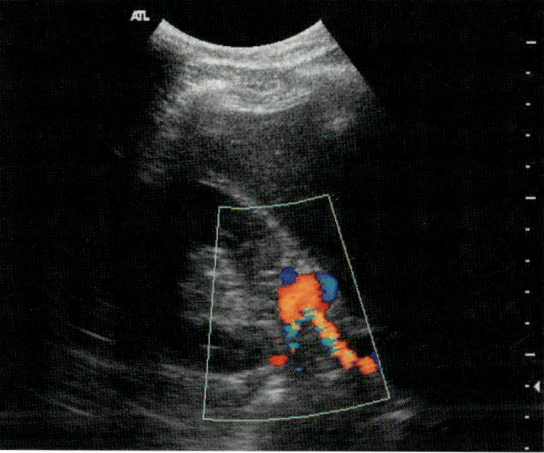

Fig. 3.**15** **a** A transverse scan of the right kidney shows a cystic area adjacent to the kidney (arrows). **b** Color Doppler shows this to be an aneurysm of the distal renal artery

> **Summary points:**
> - Accessory renal arteries cannot reliably be detected with ultrasound
> - A RI > 0.8 correlates closely with a poor outcome from angioplasty or surgery for RAS
> - In renal vein thrombosis, reduced or reverse diastolic flow may be seen in the accompanying renal artery depending upon the speed of onset and degree of occlusion

Miscellaneous Disorders

Diabetes

Diabetes is the commonest cause of ESRD in the United States and Europe. The kidneys are mainly affected by vascular disease and hypertension, but recurrent infections and neuropathic bladder changes can contribute to renal impairment. In the initial stages of renal involvement there is an increase in glomerular filtration rate (GFR) and a concomitant small increase in renal size, but as the disease progresses the kidneys generally become smaller.[57,58] Patients with established diabetic nephropathy show an increase in RI on Doppler studies when compared with individuals with normal or only mildly impaired renal function.[58,59] Renal papillary necrosis may occur in diabetics (see above) and they are also more prone to bacterial and fungal infections. Xanthogranulomatous pyelonephritis and emphysematous pyelonephritis (see above) are more common in diabetics.

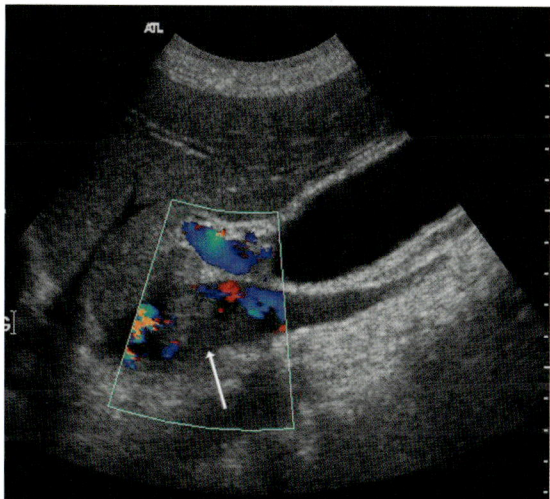

Fig. 3.**16** Sagittal view of the upper IVC behind the liver, showing a soft tissue mass within it (arrow) as a result of tumor extending from the renal vein in a patient with renal cell carcinoma

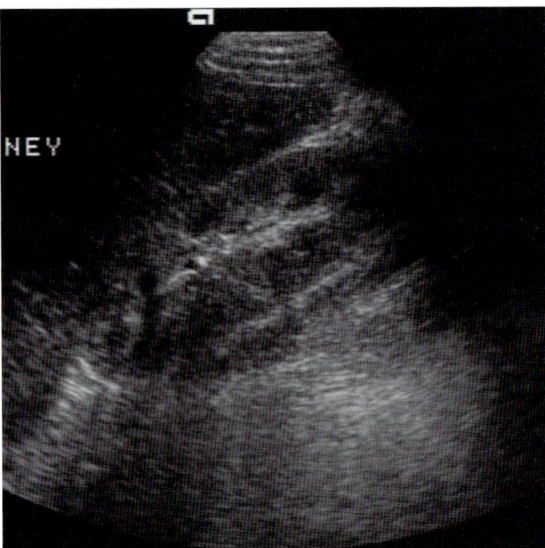

Fig. 3.17 Wegener granulomatosis affecting the right kidney. The increased echogenicity and reduction in size are, however, nonspecific

Amyloid

In amyloid, insoluble, fibrillar proteinaceous material is deposited in the kidney. Initially this is found in the glomeruli, but later, in more severe cases, it can be found elsewhere within the parenchyma. Several types of amyloid disease can be identified depending on the exact nature of the protein material and its distribution. The kidneys are often involved in systemic forms of amyloid, with 90% of primary amyloid patients showing proteinuria and 50% having a raised urea at the time of presentation; these findings also occur in myeloma-related and secondary forms of the disorder. About half of patients with secondary amyloidosis and a lower proportion with the primary form will die of renal failure.[60]

In the acute or early stages the kidneys may be enlarged and edematous, but if the disease progresses they slowly shrink in size and show increasing parenchymal echogenicity with preservation of corticomedullary differentiation.[61] In these chronically diseased kidneys there are no specific features to suggest amyloid, although the presence of an amyloid-related condition, such as rheumatoid arthritis, may suggest the diagnosis.

Connective Tissue Disorders and Vasculitides

Connective tissue disorders can affect the kidneys in a variety of ways. Systemic lupus erythematosus (SLE) affects primarily the glomeruli and tubulointerstitial disease; giant cell arteritis affects the aorta and main renal arteries, whereas polyarteritis nodosa (PAN) tends to affect the medium-sized interlobar arteries and Wegener granulomatosis (Fig. 3.**17**) or Henoch–Schonlein purpura affect the smaller arcuate or more peripheral vessels. In addition, amyloid (see above) may be associated with connective tissue disorders, or therapy for the disease may affect the kidneys. The appearances of the kidneys on ultrasound are nonspecific and do not allow distinction from other forms of progressive renal disease, renal biopsy being required for accurate diagnosis. As vasculitis affects the intrarenal vessels, there is a tendency for the RI to be elevated in connective tissue disorders; in SLE an increase in the RI is reported to correlate with the creatinine level and the presence of interstitial disease on biopsy.[62]

Sickle Cell Disease

Papillary necrosis can occur in patients with sickle cell disease as a result of damage that occurs during episodes of sickling and hemolysis. In addition, there have been reports of increased medullary echogenicity or more diffuse involvement of the parenchyma.[63] The reason for this is not yet clear, but it has been suggested that the diffuse parenchymal changes may reflect glomerular and interstitial fibrosis, whereas the medullary changes may be due to microcalcification, or even deposits of iron. As the intrarenal vessels are involved, there is an increase in the RI compared with "normals," particularly in patients with severe disease.[64]

Hepatorenal Syndrome

This can occur in either acute or chronic liver disease. There is marked vasoconstriction of the intrarenal vessels as a result of complex interactions among a multitude of neurohumoral disturbances, which leads to vasodilatation and pooling of blood in the splanchnic vessels, resulting in underfilling of the systemic arterial system and consequent compensatory vasoconstriction and a reduced GFR.[65,66] The role of ultrasound in these patients is to exclude obstruction or changes of renal parenchymal disease as a possible cause for the impaired renal function. Doppler ultrasound will show an increased RI as a result of the vasoconstriction and this can be demonstrated before azotemia develops, allowing identification of those at risk of kidney dysfunction and hepatorenal syndrome.[67,68] It has been suggested that liver transplant patients with evidence of hepatorenal syndrome prior to the operation tend to have a more stormy and protracted recovery period after transplantation.

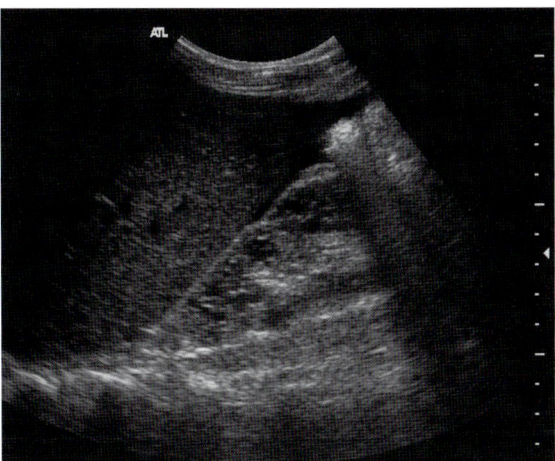

Fig. 3.18 **ACDK.** A scan of the right kidney showing multiple tiny cysts throughout the parenchyma in a patient on hemodialysis

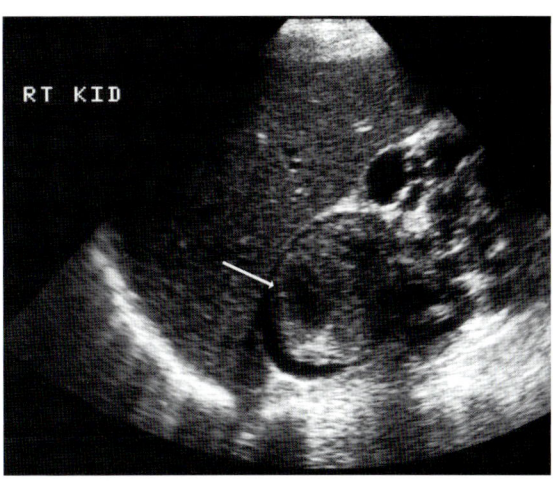

Fig. 3.19 **Carcinoma in a patient with ACDK.** A solid lesion is seen at the upper margin of this kidney (arrow) with significant disorganization of the remainder of the visible parenchyma

Hemolytic Uremic Syndrome

This is the commonest cause of ARF in children and is usually linked to infection with an enterohemorrhagic strain of *E. coli* from undercooked food. It is characterized by the simultaneous occurrence of hemolytic anemia, thrombocytopenia, and renal failure.[69] The renal failure is caused by a thrombotic microangiopathy affecting the intrarenal vessels.[70] Consequently, Doppler will show a significant increase in the RI; the clinical value of this measurement is that, in patients who show recovery of renal function, the RI starts to fall prior to biochemical improvement, thus allowing some prediction of outcome.

End-Stage Renal Disease

Failure of the kidneys and ESRD is the eventual outcome of many renal pathologies. In many cases the kidneys contract and have an echogenic parenchyma, but this is not always the case and renal size does not correlate with function.

Acquired Cystic Disease of the Kidneys

Acquired cystic disease of the kidneys (ACDK) was originally associated with patients on hemodialysis, but it is now recognized that it can occur in patients on other forms of renal replacement therapy, as well as in patients with severe chronic renal disease who have not yet progressed to dialysis.[71] Histologically there are proliferative changes leading to the formation of small adenomas and cysts (Fig. 3.18); rarely carcinoma may develop (Fig. 3.19). The ultrasound appearances depend upon the severity of the changes. There may be a few small cysts in small, or normal-sized kidneys, or more marked changes with multiple small cysts and enlargement of the kidneys. The severity of the changes are more marked in patients who have been on renal replacement therapy for longer periods.[72] A successful transplant appears to protect against the development of these changes in patients without evidence of ACDK before the operation and there is some evidence that the changes may regress in some patients following transplantation.[73,74]

> **Summary points:**
> - Diabetes is the commonest cause of ESRD in the Western world
> - RF is an important cause of death in patients with both primary and secondary amyloid
> - Sickle cell disease is a recognized cause of papillary necrosis
> - Ultrasonic appearances of ACDK are generally more severe in patients on long-term renal replacement therapy
> - Carcinoma is a rare complication of ACDK

References

1. Ritchie WW, Vick CW, Glocheski SK, Cook DE. Evaluation of azotaemic patients: diagnostic yield of initial US examination. Radiology 1988;167:245–7.
2. Webb JA. The role of ultrasonography in the diagnosis of intrinsic renal disease. Clin Radiol 1994;49:589–91.

3. Page JE, Morgan SH, Eastwood JB, Smith SA, Webb DJ, Silly SA, Chow J, Pottier A, Joseph AE. Ultrasound findings in renal parenchymal disease: comparison with histological appearances. Clin Radiol 1994;49:867–70.
4. Chugh KS, Jha V, Sakuja V, Joshi K. Acute cortical renal necrosis—a study of 113 patients. Ren Fail 1994;16:37–47.
5. Sefczek RJ, Beckman I, Lupetin AR, Dash N. Sonography of acute renal cortical necrosis. Am J Roentgenol 1984;142:553–4.
6. Kodner CM, Kudrimoti A. Diagnosis and management of acute interstitial nephritis. Am Fam Physician 2003;67:2527–34.
7. Gross HH, Hricak H, Filly RA. Ultrasonography in patients with acute renal failure. In: Resnik MI, Saunders RC, eds. Ultrasound in urology, 2nd ed. Baltimore: Williams and Wilkins: 1984:147–168.
8. Thadhani R, Pascual M, Bonventre JV. Acute renal failure. New Eng J Med 1996;334:1448–1460.
9. Esson ML, Schrier RW. Diagnosis and treatment of acute tubular necrosis. Ann Int Med 2002;137:744–52.
10. Izumi M, Sugiura T, Nakamura H, Nagatoya K, Imai E, Hori M. Differential diagnosis of prerenal azotemia from acute tubular necrosis and prediction of recovery by Doppler ultrasound. Am J Kid Dis 2000;35:713–9.
11. Platt JF, Rubin JM, Ellis JH. Acute renal failure: possible role of duplex Doppler in distinction between acute pre-renal failure and acute tubular necrosis. Radiology 1991;179:419–23.
12. Weber M, Braun B, Kohler H. Ultrasonic findings in analgesic nephropathy. Nephron 1985;39:216–22.
13. Vijayaraghavan SB, Kandasamy SV, Mylsamy A Prabhakar M. Sonographic features of necrosed renal papillae causing hydronephrosis. J Ultrasound Med 2003;22:951–6.
14. Cheung H, Chan PS, Metreweli C. Case report: echogenic necrotic renal papillae simulating calculi. Clin Radiol 1992;46:61–2.
15. Rommel D, Pirson Y. Medullary sponge kidney - part of a congenital syndrome. Nephrol Dial Transplant 2001;16:634–6.
16. Monk RD, Bushinsky DA. Nephrolithiasis and Nephrocalcinosis. In: Comprehensive Clinical Nephrology 2nd ed. Johnson RJ, Feehally J, eds. Elsevier: Mosby: 2003:731–44.
17. Kim Y-G, Kim B, Kim M-K, Chung S-J, Han H-K, Ryu J-A, Lee Y-H, Lee K-B, Lee JY, Huh W, Oh H-Y. Medullary nephrocalcinosis associated with long-term furosemide abuse in adults. Nephrol Dial Transplant 2001;16:2303–09.
18. Dick PT, Shuckett BM, Tang B, Daneman AKooh SW. Observer reliability in grading nephrocalcinosis on ultrasound examinations in children. Paediatr Radiol 1999;29:68–72.
19. al-Murrani B, Cosgrove DO, Svensson WE, Blaszczyk M. Echogenic rings - an ultrasound sign of early nehrocalcinosis. Clin Radiol 1991;44:49–51.
20. Papanicolaou N, Pfister RC. Acute renal infections. Radiol Clin Nth Am 1996;34:965–95.
21. Rigsby CM, Rosenfield AT, Glickman MG, Hodson J. Haemorrhagic focal bacterial nephritis: findings on gray scale sonography and CT. Am J Roentgenol 1986;146:1173–77.
22. Cheng CH, Tsau YK, Hsu SY, Lee TL. Effective ultrasonographic predictor for the diagnosis of acute lobar nephronia. Pediatr Infect Dis J 2004;23:11–14.
23. Farmer KD, Gellett LR, Dubbins PA. The sonographic appearances of acute focal pyelonephritis, 8 years experience. Clin Radiol 2002;57:483–7.
24. Dembry LM, Andriole VT. Renal and perirenal abscesses. Infect Dis Clin North Am 1997;11:663–80.
25. Yen DH, Hu SC, Tsai J, Kao WF, Chern CH, Wang LM, Lee CH. Renal abscess: early diagnosis and treatment. Am J Emerg Med 1999;17:192–7.
26. Michaeli J, Mogle P, Perlberg S, Heiman S, Caine M. Emphysematous Pyelonephritis. J Urol 1984;131:203–8.
27. Pontin AR, Barnes RD, Joffe J, Kahn D. Emphysematous pyelonephritis in diabetic patients. Br J Urol 1995;75:71–4.
28. Narlawar RS, Raut AA, Nagar A, Hira P, Hanchate V, Asrani A. Imaging features and guided drainage in emphysematous pyelonephritis: a study of 11 cases. Clin Radiol 2004;59:192–7.
29. Tiu CM, Chou YH, Chiou HJ, Lo CB, Yang JY, Chen KK, Hsu MH, Wang JH, Su YG, Chang CY, Yu C. Sonographic features of xanthogranulomatous pyelonephritis. J Clin Ultrasound 2001;29:279–85.
30. Ramboer K, Oyen R, Verellen S, Vermeersch S, Baert AL, Verberckmoes R. Focal xanthogranulomatous pyelonephritis mimicking a renal tumour: CT- and MR-findings and evolution under therapy. Nephrol Dial Transplant 1997;12:1028–30.
31. Kim J. Ultrasonographic features of focal xanthogranulomatous pyelonephritis. J Ultrasound Med 2004;23:409–16.
32. Premkumar K, Lattimer J, Newhouse JH. CT and sonography of advanced urinary tract tuberculosis. Am J Roentgenol 1987;148:65–9.
33. Gibson MS, Puckett ML, Shelly ME. Renal tuberculosis. Radiographics 2004;24:251–6.
34. Das KM, Vaidyanathan S, Rajwanshi A, Indudhara R. Renal tuberculosis: diagnosis with sonographically guided aspiration cytology. Am J Roentgenol 158:571–3.
35. Herman ES, Klotman PE. HIV-associated nephropathy: Epidemiology, pathogenesis and treatment. Semin Nephrol 2003;23:200–8.
36. Di Fiori JL, Rodrigue D, Kaptein EM, Ralls PW. Diagnostic sonography of HIV-associated nephropathy: new observations and clinical correlation. Am J Roentgenol 1998;171:713–6.
37. Falkoff GE, Rigsby CM, Rosenfield AT. Partial, combined cortical and medullary nephrocalcinosis: US and CT patterns in AIDS-associated MAI infection. Radiology 1987;162:343–4.
38. Hertig A, Couprie R, Haymann J-Ph, Mougenot B, Farres N, Peraldi M-N, Rondeau E, Sraer J-D. Acute cortical necrosis in acquired immunodeficiency syndrome (AIDS). Nephrol. Dial. Transplant 1997;12:585–7.
39. Vargas-Serrano B, Ferreiro-Arguelles C, Rodriguez-Romero R, Marcos del Rio N. Imaging findings in renal hydatid disease. Eur Radiol 1997;7:548–51.
40. Barsoum RS. Schistosomiasis and the kidney. Semin Nephrol 2003;23:34–41.
41. Safian RD, Textor SC. Renal artery stenosis. N Engl J Med 2001;344:431–42.
42. Zuccala A, Zucchelli P. Ischemic nephropathy: diagnosis and treatment. J Nephrol 1998;11:318–24.
43. Mitty HA, Shapiro RS, Parsons RB, Silberzweig JE. Renovascular hypertension. Radiol Clin Nth Am 1996;34:1017–36.
44. Zubarev AV. Ultrasound of renal vessels. Eur Radiol 2001;11:1902–15.
45. Lee HY, Grant EG. Sonography in renovascular hypertension. J Ultrasound Med 2002;21:431–41.
46. Pick JW Anson BJ. The renal vascular pedicle. Anatomical study of 430 body halves. J Urol 1940;44:411–34.

47. Stavros AT, Parker SH, Yakes WF, Chantelois AE, Burke BJ, Meyers PR, Schenck JJ. Segmental stenosis of the renal artery: pattern recognition of tardus and parvus abnormalities with duplex sonography. Radiology 1992;159:107-12.
48. Patriquin HB, Lafortune M, Jequier JC, O'Regan S, Garel L, Landriault J, Fontaine A, Filiatrault D. Stenosis of the renal artery: assessment of slowed systole in the downstream circulation with Doppler sonography. Radiology 1992;184:479-85.
49. Strandness DE Jr. Duplex imaging for the detection of renal artery stenosis. Am J Kidney Dis 1994;24:674-8.
50. Handa N, Fukunaga R, Etani H, Yoneda S, Kimura K, Kamada T. Efficacy of echo-Doppler examination for the evaluation of renovascular disease. Ultrasound Med Biol 1988;14:1-5.
51. Radermacher J, Chavan A, Bleck J, Vitzthum A, Stoess B, Gebel MJ, Galanski M, Koch KM, Haller H. Use of Doppler ultrasonography to predict the outcome of therapy for renal artery stenosis. N Engl J Med 2001;344:410-7.
52. Spies JB, Hricak H, Slemmer TM, Zeineh S, Alpers CE, Zayat P, Lue TF, Kerlan RK Jr, Madrazo BL, Sandler MA. Sonographic evaluation of experimental acute renal arterial occlusion in dogs. Am J Roentgenol 1984;142:341-6.
53. Brandenburg VM, Frank RD, Riehl J. Color-coded duplex sonography study of arteriovenous fistulae and pseudoaneurysms complicating percutaneous renal allograft biopsy. Clin Nephrol 2002;58:398-404.
54. Hibbert J, Howlett DC, Greenwood KL, MacDonald LM, Saunders AJ. The ultrasound appearances of neonatal renal vein thrombosis. Br J Radiol 1997; 70:1191-94.
55. Hricak H, Sandler MA, Madrazo BL, Eyler WR, Sy GS. Sonographic manifestations of acute renal vein thrombosis: an experimental study. Invest Radiol 1981;16:30-5.
56. Platt JF, Ellis JH, Rubin JM. Intrarenal arterial Doppler sonography in the detection of renal vein thrombosis of the native kidney. Am J Roentgenol 1994;162:1367-70.
57. Soldo D, Brkljacic B, Bozikov V, Drinkovic I, Hauser M. Diabetic nephropathy. Comparison of conventional and duplex Doppler ultrasonographic findings. Acta Radiol 1997;38:296-302.
58. Derchi LE, Martinoli C, Saffioti S, Pontremoli R, De Micheli A, Bordone C. Ultrasonographic imaging and Doppler analysis of renal changes in non-insulin-dependent diabetes mellitus. Acad Radiol 1994;1:100-5.
59. Platt JF, Rubin JM, Ellis JH. Diabetic nephropathy: evaluation with renal duplex Doppler US. Radiology 1994;190:343-6.
60. Kim SH, Han JK, Lee KH, Won HJ, Kim KW, Kim JS, Park CH, Choi BI. Abdominal amyloidosis: spectrum of radiological findings. Clin Radiol 2003;58:610-20.
61. Ekelund L. Radiological findings in renal amyloidosis. Am J Roentgenol 1977;129:851-3.
62. Platt JF, Rubin JM, Ellis JH. Lupus nephritis: predictive value of conventional and Doppler US and comparison with serologic and biopsy parameters. Radiology 1997;203:82-6.
63. Walker TM, Serjeant GR. Increased renal reflectivity in sickle cell disease: prevalence and characteristics. Clin Radiol 1995;50:566-9.
64. Aikimbaev KS, Oguz M, Guvenc B, Baslamisli F, Kocak R. Spectral pulsed Doppler sonography of renal vascular resistance in sickle cell disease: clinical implications. Br J Radiol 1996;69:1125-9.
65. Cardenas A, Arroyo V. Hepatorenal syndrome. Ann Hepatol 2003;2:23-9.
66. Gines P, Guevara M, Arroyo V, Rodes J. Hepatorenal syndrome. Lancet 2003;362:1819-27.
67. Platt JF, Ellis JH, Rubin JM, Merion RM, Lucey MR. Renal duplex Doppler sonography: a non-invasive predictor of kidney dysfunction and hepatorenal failure in liver disease. Hepatology 1994;20:362-9.
68. Celebi H, Donder E, Celiker H. Renal blood flow detection with Doppler ultrasonography in patients with hepatic cirrhosis. Arch Int Med 1997;10:564-6.
69. Sens YA, Miorin LA, Silva HG, Malheiros DM, Fiho DM, Jabur P. Acute renal failure due to haemolytic uremic syndrome in adult patients. Ren Fail 1997;19:279-282.
70. Remuzzi G, Ruggenenti P. The haemolytic uremic syndrome. Kidney Int 1995;8:11-19.
71. Levine E. Acquired cystic kidney disease. Radiol Clin North Am 1996;34:947-64.
72. Thomson BJ, Jenkins DA, Allan PL, Elton RA, Winney RW. Aquired cystic disease of the kidney in patients with end stage renal failure: a study of prevalence and aetiology. Nephrol Dial Transplant 1986;1:38-43.
73. Ishikawa I, Yuri T, Kitada H, Shinoda A. Regression of acquired cystic disease of the kidney after successful renal transplantation. Am J Nephrol 1983;3:310-4.
74. Vaziri ND, Darwish R, Martin DC, Hostetler J. Acquired renal cystic disease in renal transplant recipients. Nephron 1984;37:203-5.

4 Chronic Renal Failure

M. J. Weston

Introduction

Many of the diseases discussed in the Chapter 3 (Parenchymal Diseases of the Kidney) can progress to complete renal failure. Nephrons are destroyed or lose their function. The kidneys of patients with polycystic kidney disease have a recognizable appearance with large kidneys comprised of innumerable cysts of varying sizes. Other conditions have less recognizable features once terminal uremia becomes established. A study of 67 patients with uremia during the period before dialysis was started showed that the two leading causes of uremia were chronic glomerulonephritis and diabetic nephropathy.[1] Normal kidney size and high reflectivity on ultrasound were common among the diabetic nephropathy group, whereas chronic glomerulonephritis patients had kidneys that were small and highly reflective (Fig. 4.1). There have been numerous claims for the ability of ultrasound to characterize renal parenchymal disease. However, despite ultrasound trends favoring one diagnosis or another, there is still the need for renal biopsy to reach a definite diagnosis.[2] Doppler ultrasound of the renal interlobar arteries demonstrates that the resistive index (RI) has a value in determining prognosis of renal failure. A progressive lowering of the renal RI during follow-up of acute renal failure is correlated with recovery of renal function.[2] Likewise, in chronic nephropathies a high renal RI at initial presentation predicts that there will be progressive renal failure.[3]

Small, high-reflective kidneys may be difficult to locate with ultrasound, particularly on the left, as the adjacent perirenal fat can appear very similar (Fig. 4.1b). The movement of a kidney with respiration may be the only feature that allows detection.

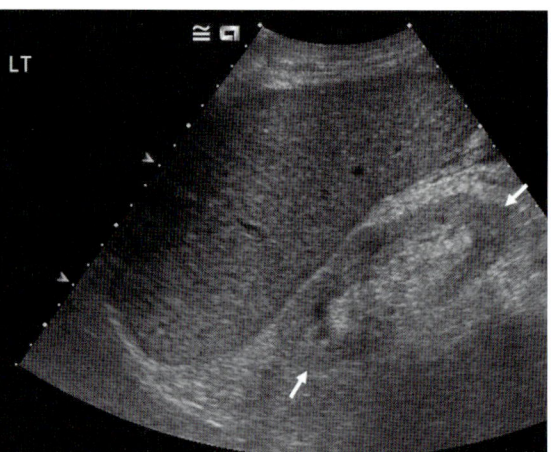

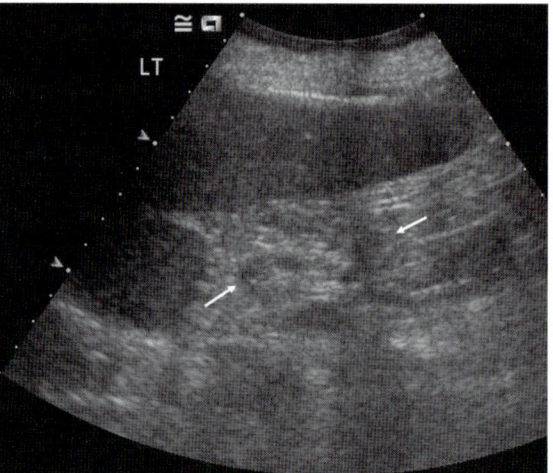

Fig. 4.1 **a** A left kidney in chronic renal failure (CRF) due to diabetic nephropathy (between arrows), demonstrating high reflectivity and normal size. **b** A small high-reflective left kidney in CRF due to chronic glomerulonephritis (between arrows), which is difficult to visualize on ultrasound

Diseases Associated with the Native Kidneys

Acquired Cystic Disease of the Kidneys

Proliferative changes in the native kidneys of patients with end-stage renal failure lead to the formation of small cysts and adenomas in up to 60% of cases. This usually occurs once the patients are on dialysis and is equally common whether hemodialysis or peritoneal dialysis is used.[4] There is a preponderance of males affected; there is also a tendency for the rate of increase in the size of kidneys due to acquired cystic disease (ACDK) to be greatest in young males.[5] This increase in size can even mimic the appearances of adult polycystic disease.[6] The frequency of ACDK increases with the duration of dialysis.[7] Once transplantation of a functioning kidney occurs, a degree of protection against the development of acquired cystic disease occurs; existing changes may even regress. Lack of regression of a focal area of cystic change in a patient following transplantation, when the rest of the cysts are regressing, is suspicious for the development of a cystic renal cell carcinoma (RCC).[8]

Ultrasound shows the presence of small cysts in the kidneys (Fig. 4.2). These cysts may number only a few but can be very numerous. If enough cysts are present, the kidneys become enlarged.[5] Small cysts may be indistinguishable from small solid lesions. This is not important. However, the development of larger or enlarging solid masses is of concern for malignant change.

Hemorrhage

ACDK is associated with an increased risk of bleeding either into the kidney or into the perinephric space. In a study of 30 dialysis patients over seven years, 17% developed large hemorrhagic cysts and 13% developed large perinephric hematoma.[9] These episodes of hemorrhage may be large enough to be life-threatening; three out of eight patients in another series died as a direct result of hemorrhage.[10] As expected the episodes of hemorrhage are more likely to occur in patients on anticoagulant therapy.

Malignant Transformation

There is an increased risk of RCC in patients with ACDK which is over and above any risk from the underlying condition or any immunosuppressive therapy.[11] The high prevalence of RCC in patients with ACDK (3.4%) makes screening of the native kidneys before transplantation sensible,[12] though there is not universal agreement that annual screening of dialysis patients is worthwhile.[13] There is also an increase in the rate of urothelial carcinoma of the upper renal tracts, particularly those with toxic nephropathies such as analgesic nephropathy, but this is unrelated to ACDK.[14] Furthermore, there is an increase in gastrointestinal malignancies in dialysis patients. In one study, a combination of fecal occult blood testing, endoscopy, and ultrasound revealed 10 malignant tumors in 178 patients starting dialysis and 34 patients on maintenance dialysis.[15] Not surprisingly, the authors advocate regular gastrointestinal screening for dialysis patients, though importantly this is based on a Japanese population with a higher prevalence of gastrointestinal disease than in Europe.

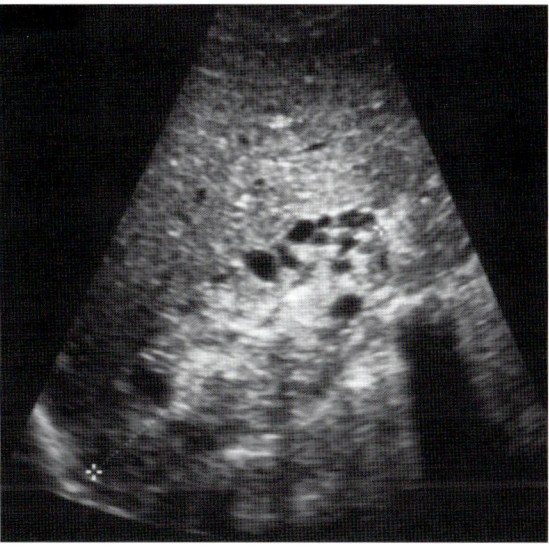

Fig. 4.2 A kidney (between cursors) in CRF, demonstrating high reflectivity and multiple small cysts

Secondary Hyperparathyroidism

Secondary hyperparathyroidism is one of the most important complications in chronic dialysis patients. Not only is it a state of increased parathyroid hormone secretion but also one of parathyroid gland hyperplasia. Ultrasound plays an essential role in the identification of enlarged parathyroid glands and the guidance of percutaneous ethanol injection for treatment.[16,17] The parathyroid glands are variable in position but are most commonly found at the upper and lower poles of the two lobes of the thyroid. The enlarged parathyroid glands characteristically are ovoid, low-reflective masses on ultrasound; they exhibit increased vascularity on color Doppler (Fig. 4.3). The vascularity decreases with appropriate treatment of the renal osteodystrophy.

Other Complications

It is estimated that 5–13% of all dialysis patients will develop renal calculi.[18] The total volume of urine production in dialysis patients is variable, but even so most patients who develop calculi will spontaneously pass the calculi. Watchful waiting is advised. However, if active treatment is needed then standard treatment with lithotripsy or ureteroscopy carries no greater complication rate than in nondialysis patients. Bilateral nephrectomy for severe, recurring stone disease is advisable in patients who are candidates for renal transplantation. There is an increased cardiovascular mortality rate in dialysis patients. It is possible, using a mea-

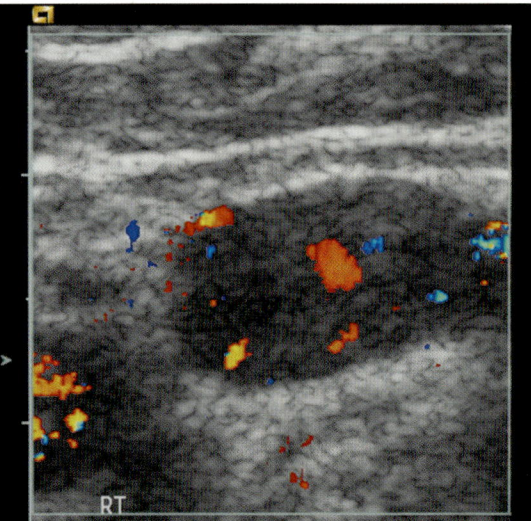

Fig. 4.3 An oval low-reflective vascular abnormality lying at the lower aspect of the left lobe of the thyroid, in keeping with parathyroid hyperplasia in a patient with CRF

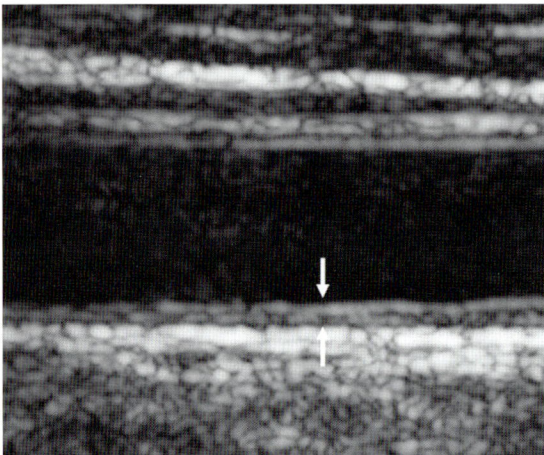

Fig. 4.4 A longitudinal view of the distal common carotid artery in a patient with chronic renal failure, demonstrating an intimamedial thickness of 1.2 mm (between arrows), suggesting an increased risk of cardiovascular disease

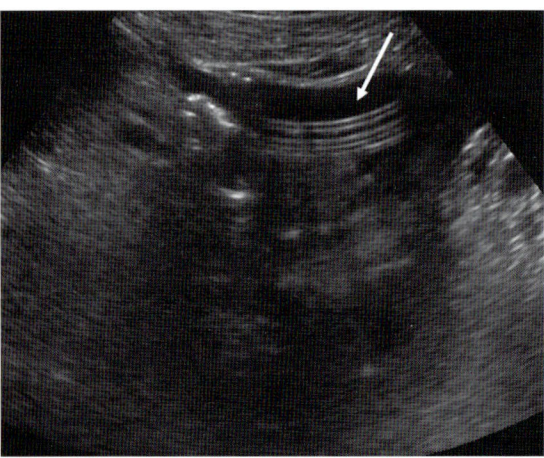

surement of the carotid intimamedial thickness to stratify the risk; those with the increased intimamedial thickness have the greatest probability of death from a cardiovascular cause (Fig. 4.4).[19]

> **Summary points:**
> - Ultrasound cannot reliably predict the underlying cause of chronic renal failure, though there are pointers
> - Once on dialysis, native kidneys may undergo cystic change
> - There is an increased risk of malignant transformation
> - Regression of cystic change may occur after transplantation

Dialysis

Continuous Ambulatory Peritoneal Dialysis

A long-term indwelling peritoneal catheter is used for the instillation of dialysis fluid into the peritoneal cavity. Then, after an interval to allow passage of waste products across the peritoneum, the fluid is drained back out. Ultrasound has a role in guiding access to the peritoneum and in assessing the complications of continuous ambulatory peritoneal dialysis (CAPD).

Exit-Site Infection and Tunnel Infection

Infection of the peritoneal dialysis catheter in its abdominal wall tunnel or at its exit through the skin is a common cause of loss of the catheter. Exit-site infections are defined as purulent discharges at the skin exit and are mostly due to *Staphylococcus aureus*; localized erythema around the catheter may be a less serious form of the infection.[20] Ultrasound is required for the diagnosis of tunnel infections and is indicated in those who have exit-site infections and those who have symptoms of peritonitis. Ultrasound features are of a low-reflective "cuff" of fluid surrounding the catheter (Fig. 4.5).[21] The presence of this pericatheter fluid predicts those that are at risk for catheter loss.[22] Measurement of the width of the pericatheter fluid may also allow prediction of which patients are responding to antibiotic treatment. One study demonstrated that patients who responded and did not require catheter removal had a decrease in the fluid width from 7 mm to 3.75 mm at two weeks.[23]

◁ Fig. 4.5 A fluid collection (arrow) is present surrounding a CAPD line

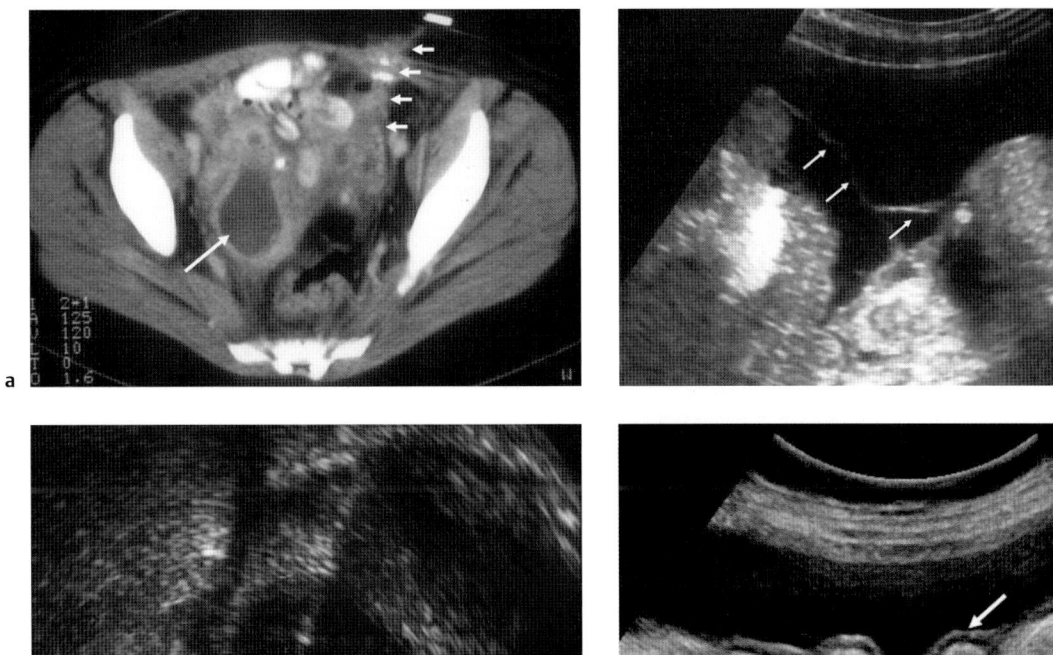

Fig. 4.6 **a** A computed tomography (CT) image of a pelvic collection (long arrow) that developed as a complication of CAPD infection (short arrows). Access for percutaneous drainage is limited by surrounding bowel and other pelvic structures. **b** Transvaginal ultrasound-guided drainage (arrow) of the collection shown on the CT image. The transvaginal route will allow drainage of fluid collections that would otherwise be inaccessible by the percutaneous route

Fig. 4.7 **a** Intraperitoneal fluid demonstrating fine stranding (arrows) in a patient on CAPD. **b** A thickened layer of peritoneum seen lying as a continuous line over the surface of several bowel loops indicative of sclerosing peritonitis (arrow)

Peritonitis

Infective peritonitis is part of the continuum of catheter-related sepsis. Infection may cause loculation of the peritoneal cavity and the development of abscesses (in approximately 1% of episodes of peritonitis).[24] Ultrasound is useful in the guidance of percutaneous drainage of these collections. The transvaginal or transrectal ultrasound-guided route may drain otherwise inaccessible collections deep in the pelvis (Fig. 4.6). Instillation of tetracycline into the emptied cavity will reduce recurrence of infection. Prolonged peritoneal dialysis and repeated episodes of infection may lead to thickening of the peritoneum, adhesion formation, and loss of free movement of bowel. The thickness of the peritoneum can be measured with ultrasound at the sternum–umbilical line distal to the xiphoid process; charts of normal thickness of the peritoneum have been developed.[25] Hemodialysis patients should show a normal peritoneal thickness.

Sclerosing peritonitis is a rare but serious complication of CAPD, which encompasses a generalized thickening of the peritoneum, encapsulating small bowel, and causing thickening of the mesentery and omentum. Sclerosing peritonitis not only leads to loculation of the dialysis fluid but also to a decrease in the permeability of the peritoneum so that dialysis filtration ceases to occur. The main risk factor is the length of time a patient has been treated with CAPD. Ultrasound features are increased small bowel peristalsis, tethering of the bowel to the posterior abdominal wall, stranding within the peritoneal fluid and "membrane" formation (Fig. 4.7). The "membrane" may show a typical trilaminar appearance. These features are all best appreciated if the ultrasound examination is performed with dialysis fluid within the peritoneal cavity.[26,27]

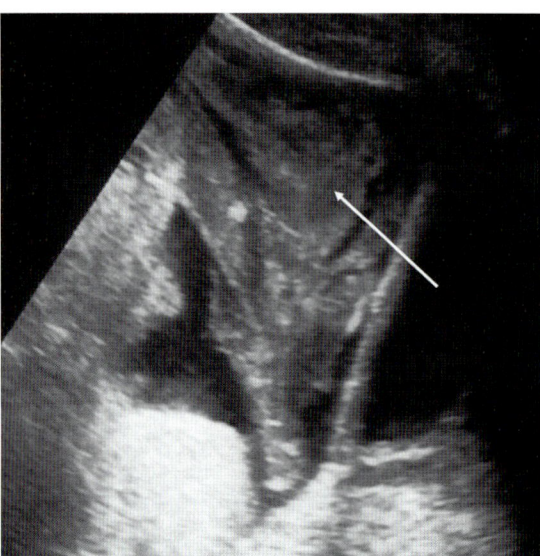

Fig. 4.8 Hemoperitoneum occurring as a complication of CAPD. The blood is shown by the presence of fine, diffuse echoes within the fluid (arrow).

> **Summary points:**
> CAPD complications include:
> - Catheter tunnel infections
> - Peritonitis
>   - Infective
>   - Sclerosing peritonitis
> - Hemoperitoneum
> - Poor fluid balance
> - Pancreatitis

Other Observations

Fluid volume and hydration status of a patient on CAPD may be assessed by measuring the diameter of the inferior vena cava (IVC) corrected for the size of the patient. Measurements < 8 mm/m² indicate underhydration; measurements > 11.5 mm/m² indicate overhydration.[28]

Gallbladder-wall thickening in ascites has been attributed to hypoalbuminemia, a common observation in patients with chronic liver disease. Studies of CAPD patients with hypoalbuminemia have failed, however, to show any increase in the gallbladder-wall thickness.[29]

Pancreatitis should be considered as a differential diagnosis for CAPD patients presenting with abdominal symptoms, particularly if they do not have any signs of infection or positive microbiology cultures. CAPD patients have an increased incidence of pancreatitis; serum amylase levels and ultrasound are unreliable in the diagnosis.[30]

Recurrent episodes of hemoperitoneum (Fig. 4.8) may be related to catheter problems and infective episodes. However, in women of reproductive age on CAPD, it may be due to hemorrhagic ovarian cyst formation and subsequent rupture. The oral contraceptive pill can suppress this complication.[31]

Hemodialysis

Hemodialysis treatment requires venous access. In long-term patients, this is best managed with the formation of an arteriovenous fistula (AVF). This allows repeated needling of the draining vein and high blood flow to facilitate rapid dialysis. Some patients require catheter-directed hemodialysis, because either they are in the acute phase of renal failure or an AVF has not yet been surgically constructed or has failed. Ultrasound guidance is recommended for all venous catheter placements; it also allows veins that might ordinarily be inaccessible to be punctured safely.[32] Furthermore, color Doppler ultrasound allows interrogation of blood-flow dynamics; finding retrograde flow in a vein about to be punctured indicates that there is a more central venous occlusion rendering the chosen site of access inappropriate.[33]

There are three main types of AVF: i) Direct anastomosis between adjacent artery and vein (typically radiocephalic or brachiocephalic); ii) Straight interposition grafts, usually with an autologous vein graft, between two distant vessels (examples are radiobasilic and brachioaxillary grafts); and iii) Loop polytetrafluoroethylene (PTFE) synthetic grafts (these may be brachiobasilic or femorofemoral). The quality of the patient's arterial and venous vessels dictates the type of AVF that is formed. Ultrasound has an important role in assessing the arteries and veins before AVF formation and is of value in looking for stenosis and other complications of established fistulae.

The nondominant arm is preferred for AVF formation. Preoperative assessment with ultrasound requires the inflow artery to be checked for atheromatous stenosis and the proposed draining vein to be checked for compressibility, size, and distensibility.[34] If the cephalic vein is being evaluated as a potential AVF outflow vein, then a minimum vein diameter of 2 mm or more predicts good fistula maturation. Whereas, a minimum cephalic vein diameter < 2 mm predicts less than 20% of fistulas will become functional.[35] Those patients who have the site of AVF planned with ultrasound have a 94% functional rate compared with only 75% functional rate for those planned with standard physical examination alone.[36] Furthermore, ultrasound planning increases the proportion of patients who are able to have fistulas rather than grafts: Fistulas may have a higher primary access failure rate than grafts but grafts have a higher subsequent long-term failure rate.[37] Grafts also require a threefold higher intervention rate to maintain their patency than fistulas do. Therefore, routine use of upper extremity Doppler ultrasound identifies many patients with veins that are suitable for use and determines arteries with optimal inflow for successful AVF formation.[38]

AVF need three weeks of maturation time to allow subsidence of edema, wound healing, dilation of the draining vein, and arterialization of the vein wall to occur, prior to commencing dialysis. Ultrasound of new AVF at two to four months can predict longer-term fistula maturity and function (Fig. 4.**9**); adequacy of fistula function is doubled if the draining vein diameter is > 4 mm, and a volume flow of 500 mL/min or greater predicts better function.[39]

Complications of Arteriovenous Fistula

Acute thrombosis: This is the commonest early complication and is usually caused by technical flaws in the surgical formation of the AVF. Acute thrombosis is clinically detected by an absent pulse or fistula "thrill." Ultrasound very readily confirms the absence of flow (Fig. 4.**10**).

Late thrombosis: This is caused either by progression of atheromatous arterial inflow disease or by stenosis of the outflow vein. The latter is commonly due to neo-intimal hyperplasia at the anastomosis or at needling sites. There is some controversy as to whether ultra-

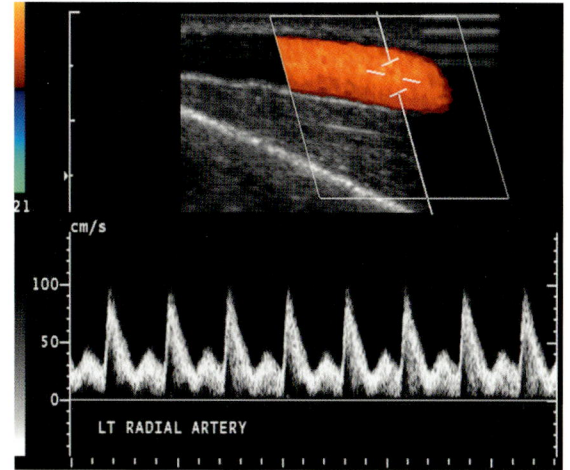
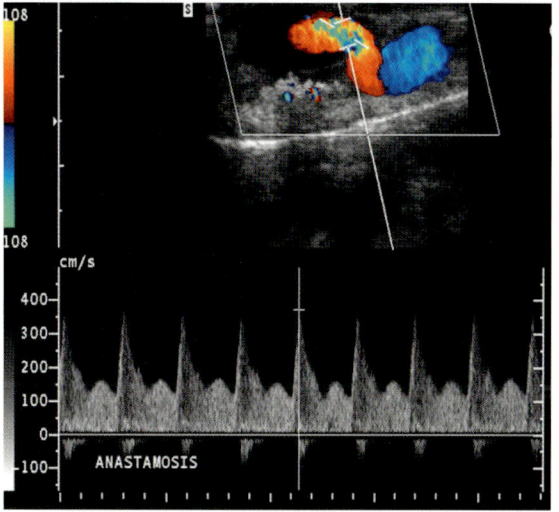

Fig. 4.**9 a** Color and spectral Doppler ultrasound of the radial artery supplying an AVF, demonstrating a monophasic waveform pattern, with forward flow in diastole. **b** The measured vascular velocity at the point of fistulation is often very high, which makes assessment of a stenosis at this point on velocity criteria alone problematic.

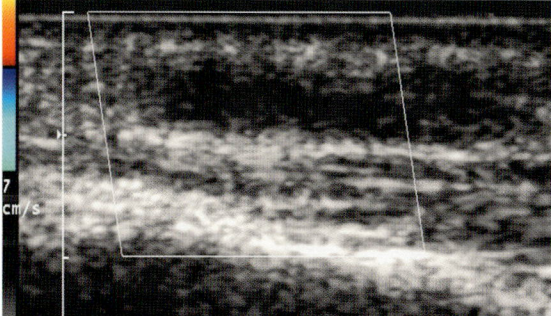
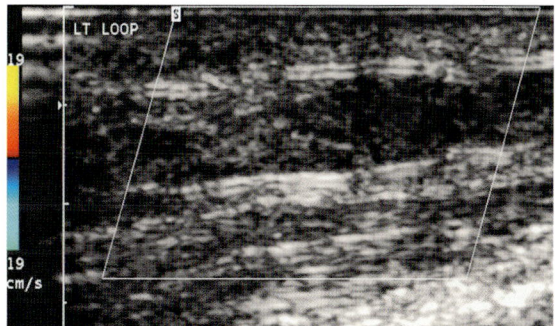

Fig. 4.**10 a** Color Doppler ultrasound image of the draining vein from an AVF demonstrates no color Doppler flow and is occluded. **b** Color Doppler ultrasound image of the arterial limb of a loop graft demonstrates no color Doppler flow and is occluded.

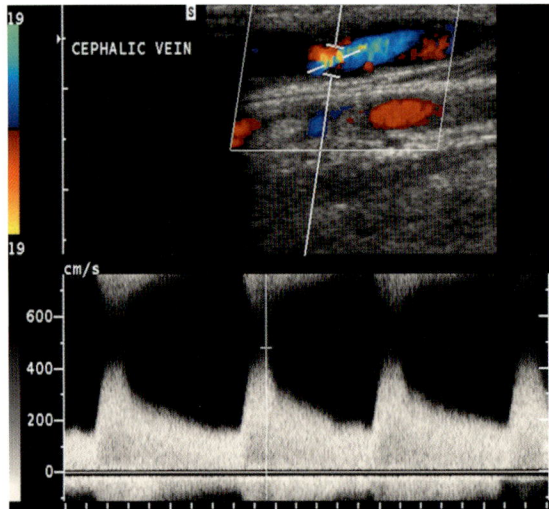

Fig. 4.11 Color and spectral Doppler ultrasound image of a focal high-velocity "jet" in the draining vein, indicative of a venous stenosis. There should be at least a doubling of velocity measurements between adjacent segments before a significant stenosis is diagnosed.

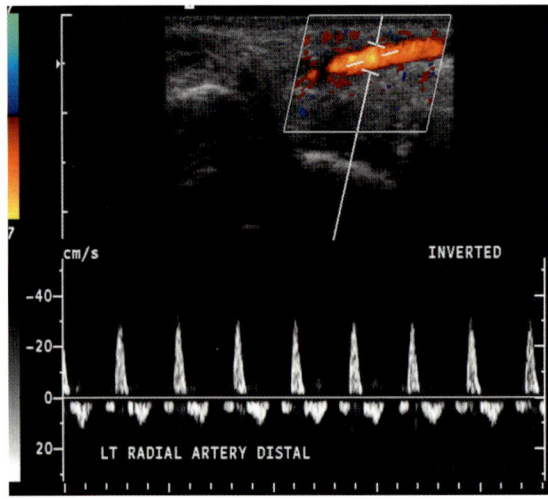

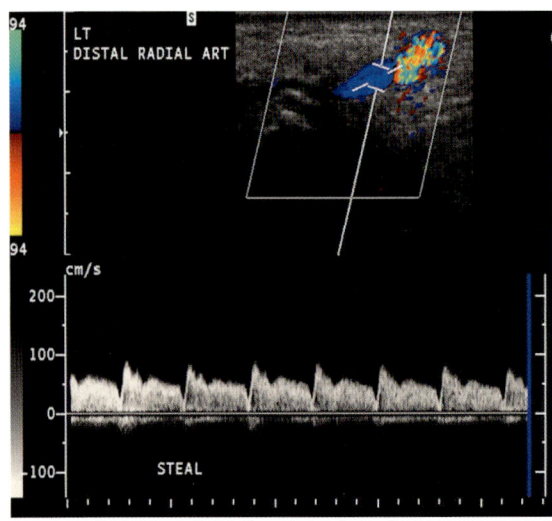

sound should be used as a routine screening tool or only in response to clinical signs of fistula malfunction. It is accepted that many clinically silent stenoses may be detected by ultrasound in an otherwise well-functioning AVF.[40] What is less clear is whether intervention to correct a silent stenosis improves overall fistula survival.[41]

There is more support for the use of ultrasound in assessing a fistula that is demonstrating clinical evidence of malfunction. Those fistulas with unequivocal clinical features of malfunction can proceed straight to catheter angiography, whereas those fistulas with only intermediate clinical evidence of fistula malfunction should have ultrasound examination. One third of this latter group are likely to show no ultrasound evidence of stenosis and so can avoid angiography.[42]

Ultrasound criteria for fistula stenosis are varied. Flow in the feeding artery and through the AVF is characteristically of continuous, low-impedance monophasic flow. A doubling of peak systolic velocity (PSV) from before a stenosis to within a stenosis is a sign of a 50% diameter stenosis. PSV > 400 cm/s suggest dysfunction, as do low-flow states of < 50 cm/s (Fig. 4.11). Volume flow is a less reproducible measure, but flow states of < 400 mL/min predict the presence of a stenosis.[43] Volume flow measurements can be improved using the ultrasound dilution technique.[44]

The steal syndrome: If the AVF is too large, it will redirect excessive blood flow—called the steal syndrome—leading to distal limb and hand ischemia in 3–7% of patients. The flow in the artery distal to the AVF should be away from the fistula and toward the hand; it should also have a multiphasic spectral Doppler waveform. Reversal of this flow and a monophasic spectral Doppler waveform indicate the presence of a steal syndrome (Fig. 4.12). An AVF may also steal excessive blood flow from proximal arterial branches. Subclavian steal, with episodes of vertebrobasilar insufficiency, has been recorded in a patient with a brachiocephalic AVF. Flow in the vertebral artery was reversed.[45,46]

Venous hypertension: This is caused by a central venous occlusion or stenosis and results in a high-pressure venous system and retrograde venous flow. Venous hypertension occurs most commonly in those

◁ Fig. 4.12 **a** Color and spectral Doppler ultrasound of flow in a radial artery distal to an AVF; normal antegrade triphasic flow in the artery toward the wrist. **b** Color and spectral Doppler ultrasound of flow in a radial artery distal to an AVF; flow reversed away from the wrist and toward the fistula. This is a "steal phenomenon" and the patient may experience symptoms of hand ischemia.

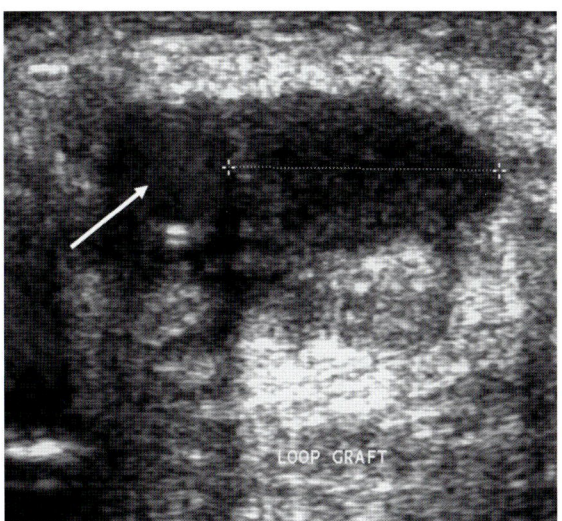
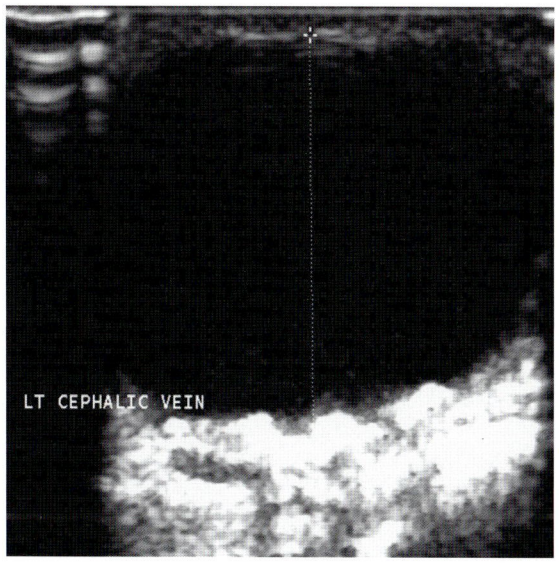
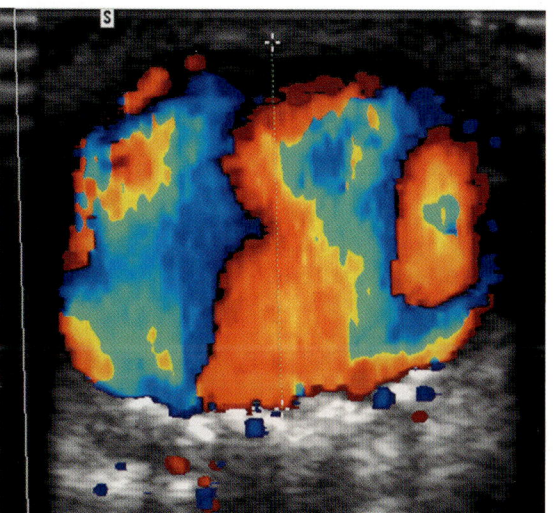

Fig. 4.**13** **a** Cross-sectional ultrasound image at the level of a small hematoma/collection (between cursors) next to an AV loop graft (arrow). **b** Cross-sectional ultrasound image of a draining vein from an AVF that has become dilated (between cursors). **c** Cross-sectional color Doppler ultrasound image of the draining vein, confirming aneurysmal dilatation (between cursors) secondary to repeated needling.

patients who have had a large-bore, central venous catheter placed in the past.

Aneurysm Formation: Venous aneurysms are usually caused by repeated needle puncture (Fig. 4.**13**). They are usually left untreated, provided the overlying skin remains intact. Sensible needle placement avoids further complications. Dilation of the inflow artery occurs with time and some patients develop true arterial aneurysms (two out of 29 in one series).[47] False aneurysms (without a surrounding vessel wall) do occur in the inflow artery but are usually secondary to malplacement of the needle. False aneurysms may be treated with ultrasound-guided thrombin injection.[48]

Summary points:
Ultrasound has a role in:
- Planning the site of AVF
- Assessing fistula maturation
- Diagnosing complications
  - Stenosis
  - Thrombosis
  - Steal phenomenon
  - Aneurysm formation

References

1. Hellstrom M, Svensson MH, Bengtsson U. Clinical and radiological renal characteristics of patients with terminal uraemia. Scand J Urol Nephrol 2002;36:455–463.
2. Quaia E, Bertolotto M. Renal parenchymal diseases: is characterization feasible with ultrasound? Eur Radiol 2002;12: 2006–2020.
3. Splendiani G, Parolini C, Fortunato L, Sturniolo A, Costanzi S. Resistive index in chronic nephropathies: predictive value of renal outcome. Clin Nephrol 2002;57:45–50.
4. Frifelt JJ, Larsen C, Elle B, Dyreborg U. Multicystic transformation of the kidneys in dialysis patients. Scand J Urol Nephrol 1989;23:51–54.
5. Ishikawa I, Saito Y, Asaka M et al. Twenty-year follow-up of acquired renal cystic disease. Clin Nephrol 2003;59: 153–159.
6. Gagnon RF, Kintzen GM, Kaye M. Acquired cystic kidney disease: rapid progression from small to enlarged kidneys simulating adult polycystic kidney disease. Clin Nephrol 2000;53:307–311.
7. Heinz-Peer G, Schoder M, Rand T, Mayer G, Mostbeck GH. Prevalence of acquired cystic disease and tumors in native kidneys of renal transplant recipients: a prospective US study. Radiology 1995;195:667–671.
8. Ishikawa I, Saito A, Chikazawa Y et al. Cystic renal cell carcinoma, suspected because of lack of regression of renal cysts after renal transplantation in a dialysis patient with acquired renal cystic disease. Clin Exp Nephrol 2003;7:81–84.
9. Levine E, Slusher SL, Grantham JJ, Wetzel LH. Natural history of acquired renal cystic disease in dialysis patients: a prospective longitudinal CT study. AJR Am J Roentgenol 1991;156:501–506.
10. Bensalah K, Martinez F, Ourahma S, Bitker MO, Richard F, Barrou B. Spontaneous rupture of non-tumoral kidneys in patients with end stage renal failure: risks and management. Eur Urol 2003;44:111–114.
11. Kliem V, Kolditz M, Behrend M et al. Risk of renal cell carcinoma after kidney transplantation. Clin Transplant 1997;11:255–258.
12. Gulanikar AC, Daily PP, Kilambi NK, Hamrick-Turner JE, Butkus DE. Prospective pretransplant ultrasound screening in 206 patients for acquired renal cysts and renal cell carcinoma. Transplantation 1998;66:1669–1672.
13. Levine E. Acquired cystic kidney disease. Radiol Clin North Am 1996;34:947–964.
14. Stewart JH, Buccianti G, Agodoa L et al. Cancers of the kidney and urinary tract in patients on dialysis for end-stage renal disease: analysis of data from the United States, Europe, and Australia and New Zealand. J Am Soc Nephrol 2003;14:197–207.
15. Ito T, Tanaka I, Kadoya T et al. Screening for gastroenterological malignancies in new and maintenance dialysis patients. J Gastroenterol 1999;34:35–40.
16. Tanaka R, Kakuta T, Fujisaki T et al. Long-term (3 years) prognosis of parathyroid function in chronic dialysis patients after percutaneous ethanol injection therapy guided by colour Doppler ultrasonography. Nephrol Dial Transplant 2003;18(Suppl 3):58–61.
17. Pavlovic D, Brzac HT. Prevention and treatment of secondary hyperparathyroidism: still a challenge for the nephrologist? Nephrol Dial Transplant 2003;18(Suppl 5): 45–46.
18. Viterbo R, Mydlo JH. Incidence and management of dialysis patients with renal calculi. Urol Int 2002;69:306–308.
19. Benedetto FA, Mallamaci F, Tripepi G, Zoccali C. Prognostic value of ultrasonographic measurements of carotid intima media thickness in dialysis patients. J Am Soc Nephrol 2001;12:2458–2464.
20. Piraino B. Peritoneal infections. Adv Ren Replace Ther 2000;7:280–288.
21. Holley JL, Foulks CJ, Moss AH, Willard D. Ultrasound as a tool in the diagnosis and management of exit-site infections in patients undergoing continuous ambulatory peritoneal dialysis. Am J Kidney Dis 1989;14:211–216.
22. Plum J, Sudkamp S, Grabensee B. Results of ultrasound-assisted diagnosis of tunnel infections in continuous ambulatory peritoneal dialysis. Am J Kidney Dis 1994;23: 99–104.
23. Vychytil A, Lorenz M, Schneider B, Horl WH, Haag-Weber M. New criteria for management of catheter infections in peritoneal dialysis patients using ultrasonography. J Am Soc Nephrol 1998;9:290–296.
24. Boroujerdi-Rad H, Juergensen P, Mansourian V, Kliger AS, Finkelstein FO. Abdominal abscesses complicating peritonitis in continuous ambulatory peritoneal dialysis patients. Am J Kidney Dis 1994;23:717–721.
25. Faller U, Stegen P, Klaus G, Mehls O, Troger J. Sonographic determination of the thickness of peritoneum in healthy children and paediatric patients on CAPD. Nephrol Dial Transplant 1998;13:3172–3177.
26. Hollman AS, McMillan MA, Briggs JD, Junor BJ, Morley P. Ultrasound changes in sclerosing peritonitis following continuous ambulatory peritoneal dialysis. Clin Radiol 1991;43:176–179.
27. Campbell S, Clarke P, Hawley C, Wigan M, Kerlin P, Butler J, Wall D. Sclerosing peritonitis: identification of diagnostic, clinical and radiological features. Am J Kidney Dis 1994;24:819–825.
28. Oe B, de Fijter CW, Geers TB, Vos PF, Donker AJ, de Vries PM. Diameter of inferior caval vein and impedance analysis for assessment of hydration status in peritoneal dialysis. Artif Organs 2000;24:575–577.
29. Kaftori JK, Pery M, Green J, Gaitini D. Thickness of the gallbladder wall in patients with hypoalbuminemia: a sonographic study of patients on peritoneal dialysis. AJR Am J Roentgenol 1987;148:1117–1118.
30. Caruana RJ, Wolfman NT, Karstaedt N, Wilson DJ. Pancreatitis: an important cause of abdominal symptoms in patients on peritoneal dialysis. Am J Kidney Dis 1986;7: 135–140.
31. Fraley DS, Johnston JR, Bruns FJ, Adler S, Segel DP. Rupture of ovarian cyst: massive hemoperitoneum in continuous ambulatory peritoneal dialysis patients: diagnosis and treatment. Am J Kidney Dis 1988;12:69–71.
32. Lau TN, Kinney TB. Direct US-guided puncture of the innominate veins for central venous access. J Vasc Interv Radiol 2001;12:641–645.
33. Conkbayir I, Men S, Yanik B, Hekimoglu B. Color Doppler sonographic finding of retrograde jugular venous flow as a sign of innominate vein occlusion. J Clin Ultrasound 2002;30:392–398.
34. Parmley MC, Broughan TA, Jennings WC. Vascular ultrasonography prior to dialysis access surgery. Am J Surg 2002;184:568–572.
35. Mendes RR, Farber MA, Marston WA, Dinwiddie LC, Keagy BA, Burnham SJ. Prediction of wrist arteriovenous fistula

35. maturation with preoperative vein mapping with ultrasonography. J Vasc Surg 2002;36:460–463.
36. Mihmanli I, Besirli K, Kurugoglu S et al. Cephalic vein and hemodialysis fistula: surgeon's observation versus color Doppler ultrasonographic findings. J Ultrasound Med 2001;20:217–222.
37. Allon M, Lockhart ME, Lilly RZ et al. Effect of preoperative sonographic mapping on vascular access outcomes in hemodialysis patients. Kidney Int 2001;60:2013–2020.
38. Malovrh M. The role of sonography in the planning of arteriovenous fistula for hemodialysis. Semin Dial 2003; 16:299–303.
39. Robbin ML, Chamberlain NE, Lockhart ME et al. Hemodialysis arteriovenous fistula maturity: US evaluation. Radiology 2002;225:59–64.
40. Malik J, Slavikova M, Malikova H, Maskova J. Many clinically silent access stenoses can be identified by ultrasonography. J Nephrol 2002;15:661–665.
41. Work J. Does vascular access monitoring work? Adv Ren Replace Ther 2002;9:85–90.
42. Dumars MC, Thompson WE, Bluth EI, Lindberg JS, Yoselevitz M, Merritt CR. Management of suspected hemodialysis graft dysfunction: usefulness of diagnostic US. Radiology 2002;222:103–107.
43. Schwarz C, Mitterbauer C, Boczula M et al. Flow monitoring: performance characteristics of ultrasound dilution versus color Doppler ultrasound compared with fistulography. Am J Kidney Dis 2003;42:539–545.
44. Tessitore N, Bedogna V, Gammaro L et al. Diagnostic accuracy of ultrasound dilution access blood flow measurement in detecting stenosis and predicting thrombosis in native forearm arteriovenous fistulae for hemodialysis. Am J Kidney Dis 2003;42:331–341.
45. Schenk WG III. Subclavian steal syndrome from high-output brachiocephalic arteriovenous fistula: a previously undescribed complication of dialysis access. J Vasc Surg 2001; 33:883–885.
46. Aschwanden M, Hess P, Labs KH, Dickenmann M, Jaeger KA. Dialysis access-associated steal syndrome: the interoperative use of duplex ultrasound scan. J Vasc Surg 2003; 37:211–213.
47. Eugster T, Wigger P, Bolter S, Bock A, Hodel K, Stierli P. Brachial artery dilatation after arteriovenous fistulae in patients after renal transplantation: a 10-year follow-up with ultrasound scan. J Vasc Surg 2003;37:564–567.
48. Ghersin E, Karram T, Gaitini D et al. Percutaneous ultrasonographically guided thrombin injection of iatrogenic pseudoaneurysms in unusual sites. J Ultrasound Med 2003;22:809–816.

5 Renal Transplantation

G.M. Baxter

Background

The road to what we now regard as the routine and successful procedure of renal transplantation has not been smooth and indeed dates back to the earliest days of Carrel's experimental attempts at transplantation at the beginning of the 20th century, which resulted in the Nobel Prize of 1912.[1] During the nonimmunosuppressed attempts at transplantation in the 1950s and then the more successful and encouraging outcomes of the twin-to-twin transplants[2] later that decade, there were so many severe setbacks and pitfalls that many groups at the time wondered whether further work in this area was justified. However, a better understanding of tissue rejection, the introduction of steroid and azathioprine in 1963,[3] and then more specifically the use of cyclosporin A by Calne et al. in the 1970s,[4] opened the door to progress.

Further improvements in surgical technique, new and more effective antirejection therapy which over the years has become less toxic, the routine use of ultrasound in the 1970s and Doppler a decade later, and the rapid development of interventional radiological techniques all combined in a very synergistic manner to make this a routine technique with the successful clinical outcome we now take for granted. It is fair to say, however, that without the fortitude and dedication of these early pioneers, it is unlikely that this status would have been achieved and indeed much of the work that will be described in this chapter owes a great debt of gratitude to those early pioneering and informative years.

Introduction

The number of patients with end-stage renal disease (ESRD) continues to rise slowly and it is estimated that it will not plateau until before the middle of the 21st century. This largely reflects a combination of an aging population and a significant improvement in long-term prognosis in this patient group, particularly in those patients with co-morbidity diseases and in particular diabetes mellitus.[5] The implication, therefore, for public health resources, in this group, is unremitting in terms of diagnosis, treatment, and long-term surveillance, and it is clear that this combination of factors is likely to constitute a serious health-resource issue.[6]

Treatment options for ESRD varies and includes hemodialysis and peritoneal dialysis; there is no doubt, however, that the treatment option of choice is renal transplantation (Fig. 5.1). Limitations of the latter option, however, are well-appreciated and well-recognized by the general public, as many public health campaigns highlight the continuing shortage of suitable donor kidneys.[7] Thankfully better donor–recipient matching,[8] use of more potent immunosuppressive regimens[9] in combination with improved surgical techniques have all resulted in an improvement in outcome, the one- and five-year graft survival rates in Europe in the mid-1990s being 77–82% and 57–64%, respectively.[10] Further improvements in these figures can be expected through earlier recognition and treatment of a variety of transplant insults and complications, and indeed current fig-

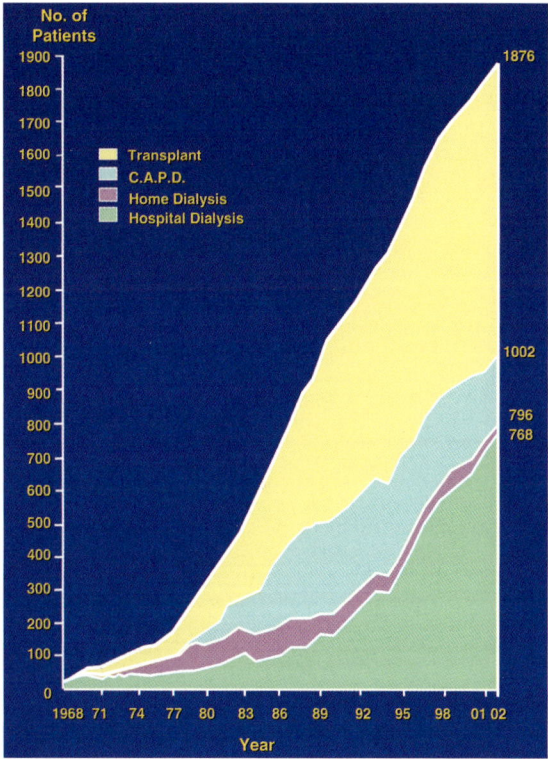

Fig. 5.1 Graph of the various forms of treatment of chronic renal failure in the West of Scotland, 1968–2002

ures show a one-year graft survival of 90% and a five-year survival of 70%, with slightly higher values for living donor kidneys, and slightly lower for second and subsequent transplants. (For current updated information see www.uktransplant.org.)

It is universally agreed that transplantation is without doubt the treatment of choice. For a number of patients with chronic renal failure, a successful renal transplant will provide a glomerular filtration rate (GFR) of 50–60 mL/min, which although only half of the normal adult value, is sufficient to return the majority of patients to a normal and independent life pattern. Such an improvement in lifestyle and quality of life is difficult, and some would say impossible to measure or cost. However, what is clear is that in the potentially harsh world of health economics, the cost-benefit of a successful and functioning transplant far outweighs that of failure, and this is one reason why many resources are focussed and targeted on the pretransplantation, peritransplantation, and posttransplantation period to ensure as high a success rate as is possible. The average normal life expectancy of a transplant kidney is 7–10 years, increasing to 15–20 years when a live donor organ is used. Although many different imaging techniques are employed in dealing with the transplant patient, there is absolutely no doubt that ultrasound is central and crucial, and that it is very useful in both the early postoperative period as a noninvasive indicator of transplant dysfunction and also in the long-term follow-up of many of these patients. This chapter will highlight the value and application of this imaging technique.

Indications and Contraindications in Transplantation

There are few contraindications to renal transplantation, and this treatment option should be considered for all patients with ESRF that is of a severity to require dialysis. Those unfit for transplantation are generally those who are unfit for anesthesia or surgery, for example severe cardiac or respiratory disease, or severe arteriopathy. In addition, the known potential problems of immunosuppression in the context of pre-existing infection and malignancy should be considered, as should the risk of disease recurrence, which is particularly associated in patients with oxalosis or active vasculitis.

Donor Supply

The main sources of organ transplantation are generally either brain-dead, ventilated organ donors or live, related donors. Although the majority of transplants in developed countries are cadaveric in origin and more live, related operations are performed in developing countries, there is no doubt that due to the current shortage of available organs there is a small but notable increase in live donor transplants now being recorded in developed countries. Indeed, both live, related and live, unrelated donor transplantation is now possible and has a very similar outcome and prognosis. Some technical differences exist in terms of surgical technique and recipient outcome between cadaveric and live, related donor transplants. However, the overall management of the recipient can be regarded as similar.

Histocompatibility Testing

In order to reduce the risk of rejection as far as possible, in particular hyperacute rejection, the detection of donor-specific antibodies in the lymphocyte cross-match test is a contraindication to transplantation.

The risk of subsequent episodes of acute rejection is partially dependent upon the degree of human leukocyte antigen (HLA) matching between donor and recipient. The genes determining the HLAs are located on chromosome 6.[11,12] The importance of HLA matching is reflected in the improved graft survival of a fully HLA-matched graft (T1/2, 17.3 years) compared with an incomplete, HLA-mismatched graft (T1/2, 7.8 years).[13,14]

Preoperative Management

The transplant procedure should be performed, certainly within 24 hours of organ retrieval and at worst 48 hours. During this period the recipient will have been chosen, appropriately prepared for theatre, i.e. screened for infection, cardiorespiratory reserve assessed, and additional dialysis given if fluid/metabolite imbalance requires correction.

A live, related donor, who can either be a family member or close friend, is screened with a combination of clinical history, examination, and HLA status assessment. Other tests vary from center to center and include a 24-hour creatinine clearance, serology, liver function tests, and a choice of intravenous urogram, dimercaptosuccinic acid (DMSA) scan, renal arteriography, and computed tomography (CT) and/or magnetic resonance (MR) imaging to assess renal function.

Surgery

Traditionally the transplant renal vessels are anastomosed to the external iliac artery and vein in the case of a cadaveric transplant and to the internal iliac vessels in a live, related transplant. In those receiving a third

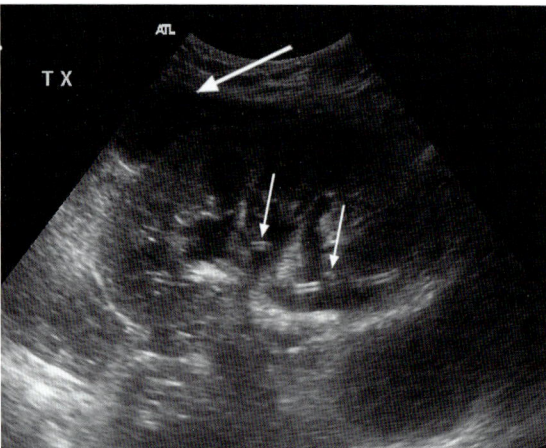

Fig. 5.2 Normal functioning transplant kidney in the early postoperative period. The ureteric stent (arrows) can easily be seen curled up within the renal pelvis and running down the proximal ureter, which is only slightly distended. A small peritransplant collection (thick arrow) is noted. This was a benign postoperative collection which did not require any intervention

transplant, an intraperitoneal approach to the iliac vasculature can be used if required. The vesicoureteric anastomosis is performed by joining a shortened donor ureter with the dome of the bladder. As a consequence of this procedure the lower end of the ureter, particularly if the ureter is left too long, may be prone to ischemic insult and may result in stricture formation, which can on occasion be functionally significant. At many centers a perioperative ureteric stent is placed; this is normally removed at three months (Fig. 5.2).

Postoperative complications vary from center to center but include bleeding (< 1%), major vascular occlusion of an artery or vein (1–2%), wound infection (1.6–6.3%), and a number of urologically-related complications, including anastomotic leak, obstruction, and hematuria (1.3–7%).[15–18]

Immunosuppression

The aim of immunosuppression is clearly to prevent rejection without inducing infectious complications or serious drug toxicity. A number of options are now available. A conventional regime may have included a combination of cyclosporine (cyclosporin A), azathioprine, and steroids (prednisolone). However, newer agents, including tacrolimus,[19] mycophenolate,[20] and sirolimus (rapamycin), are also often used. Antibody therapies, i.e. anti-interleukin 2, are effective and less toxic than the older, more traditional humoral agents, including OKT3 and antithymic globulin, and are often used in high-risk patients. Clearly, with an increased number of options, immunosuppressive regimes will vary from center to center.

The treatment of established acute rejection is normally with high-dose oral or intravenous steroids and in resistant cases immunodepletion with antibody therapy or tacrolimus. Unfortunately, there is no effective treatment for hyperacute or chronic rejection.

> **Summary points:**
> - The one- and five-year graft survivals are currently 90% and 70%
> - A combination of an aging population and increased requirements constitutes a major public health and ethical issue
> - There are few contraindications to transplantation
> - Disease recurrence posttransplantation is high in patients with oxalosis or active vasculitis
> - Immunologically well-matched kidneys have a favorable outcome

Imaging the Transplant Kidney

The transplant kidney can normally be visualized in either iliac fossa, largely lying a number of centimeters below the skin surface and therefore easily accessible. Orientation of the transplant can be variable depending on the surgical technique; however, perpendicular images can normally be obtained. As for all ultrasonic techniques, resolution depends on a well-appreciated number of factors, including patient build, depth of transplant beneath the skin surface, and the presence or absence of postoperative edema. In general a 4-MHz probe gives a good overall assessment of the kidney, perirenal, or transplant collections and also allows interrogation of the transplant vasculature, including the more deeply situated iliac vessels. A higher frequency probe (e.g., 7 MHz) does give excellent near-field resolution and therefore good anatomical detail of the transplant kidney, but in all but the thinnest of patients will probably not allow visualization of the deeper situated vascular structures.

Morphologically there is no difference between the transplant and native kidneys, which are identical, in that there is a well-defined renal parenchyma peripherally with a bright echogenic fat containing renal sinus centrally. Due to the improved resolution of the transplant kidney, the renal pyramids are more commonly visualized and are hypoechoic relative to the overlying parenchyma and are regularly spaced with no communication between them, this being a useful differentiating feature from calyceal dilatation (Fig. 5.3). It is not uncommon to observe mild hydronephrosis in the early postoperative period in the "normal" transplant kidney and this largely reflects postoperative edema with some ureteric compression at the vesicoureteric anastomosis. Although this may resolve with time, this may not always be the case. However, assuming renal function to be normal, a minor degree of dilatation is generally documented to act as a baseline on which subsequent examinations can be evaluated.

It is important not to confuse the transplant vessels, i.e. the artery and vein at the renal hilum, with a dilated or prominent renal pelvis, and these should be easily differentiated with the use of color or power Doppler. The bladder should be routinely imaged when possible and should be echo-free. The presence of intravesical turbid echoes may indicate either hemorrhage or infection, depending on the clinical situation.

Color Doppler ultrasound is extremely helpful as it provides an instantaneous assessment of the intrarenal vasculature and therefore a global impression of overall transplant perfusion and helps identify the transplant artery and vein and the iliac vessels. Although the color flow information in itself is purely qualitative, in many circumstances this information is both helpful and reassuring. As with all Doppler techniques, however, spectral Doppler analysis is required for quantification (Fig. 5.**4a,b**). The technique of color flow Doppler in the transplant has much in common with that used elsewhere, i.e. the vessel is first identified with color, the spectral gate placed over the vessel, and a Doppler tracing obtained. The spectral Doppler renal waveform is characteristically a low-resistance waveform, i.e. it has a "ski-slope" appearance, with diastolic flow normally contributing at least up to a third of the peak systolic value. Any reduction in diastolic flow may represent a pathological process. In order for color Doppler ultrasound to be used effectively in the early transplant period, serial studies are required until renal function is clinically satisfactory.

A number of Doppler indices including the pulsatility index (PI), resistive index (RI), and the systolic-to-diastolic and diastolic-to-systolic ratios can all be used, although the commonly utilized indices are the PI and RI. There is no perceived advantage to using one over the other.

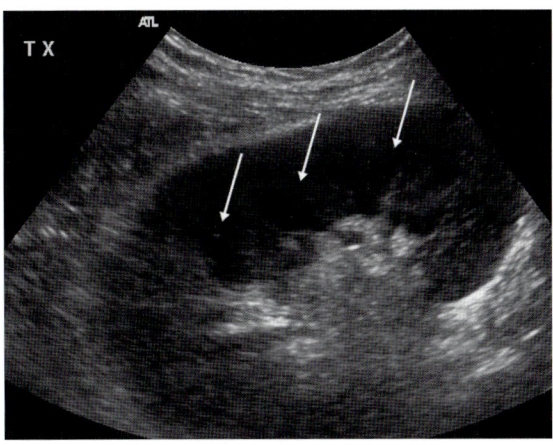

Fig. 5.**3** Normal transplant kidney. The renal pyramids (arrows) are regularly spaced and hypoechoic relative to the parenchyma. They do not communicate and are readily differentiated from calyceal dilatation

The main transplant artery can be very difficult to visualize due to its tortuosity (Fig. 5.**4c**), and possibly partly because of this, a wide range of peak systolic values have been quoted for this vessel. At our center a cut-off value of 2.5 ms^{-1} is used,[21–23] i.e. any value below this is regarded as normal, whereas above it is taken to represent a significant transplant artery stenosis. Examination of this vessel may be a time-consuming and exacting procedure due to the twists and turns previously described and the requirement of precise angle correction, and therefore accurate velocity readings cannot be overemphasized (Fig. 5.**4d**).

No specific values exist for the transplant renal vein. However, often the prime consideration, at least in the early transplant period, is simply whether flow is absent or present. It is of paramount importance that both the iliac artery and vein are identified in order to distinguish them from the renal vessels and indeed to exclude a more proximal lesion in the iliac vessel, for example the iliac artery, which may contribute or indeed be the sole cause of adverse renal function.

Pulsatility index (PI):

$$\frac{\text{peak systolic velocity} - \text{end diastolic velocity}}{\text{time-averaged mean velocity}}$$

Resistive index (RI):

$$\frac{\text{peak systolic velocity} - \text{end diastolic velocity}}{\text{peak systolic velocity}}$$

Summary points:
- A 4 MHz ultrasound probe gives the best overall assessment of the transplant kidney
- Mild hydronephrosis is "normal" in the early postoperative transplant period
- Serial color Doppler ultrasound measurements are required to monitor transplant dysfunction
- The PI and RI are the most commonly used Doppler indices; there is no advantage of one over the other
- Both the transplant and iliac vessels should be identified to avoid confusion
- The peak systolic velocity (PSV) in the transplant artery is normally < 2.5 ms^{-1}

Early Complications

Early complications are numerous and varied, and include parenchymal insults, i.e. acute tubular necrosis (ATN), acute rejection, or both, vascular occlusion, obstruction, hemorrhage, urinary leak, collections, infections, and drug toxicity related to antirejection therapy itself. Often many of these complications may be differentiated on a combination of clinical history, bacteriology, and ultrasound. When all is said and done, often the main differential diagnosis is between acute rejection and ATN and this can be very difficult clinically as symptoms are generally absent. As both entities require a different approach to treatment, early and accurate diagnosis is essential. Despite many attempts to the contrary it has not been possible to differentiate between these entities with color Doppler imaging and a histological diagnosis is still required.[24-27] Despite this limitation, ultrasound is still useful in its dual role of not only assessing and monitoring transplant dysfunction but also in assessing response to therapy.

Acute Tubular Necrosis

Acute tubular necrosis (ATN) is common in the early transplant period and up to 30% of patients may require dialysis in the early stages. Delayed graft function is rare in the live, related donor situation. ATN is principally related to both donor and donor kidney, particularly the warm ischemic time. In those patients with established ATN requiring dialysis, recovery usually occurs within one to two weeks of transplantation, although in rare cases it can be delayed for significantly longer periods of time of up to three months.

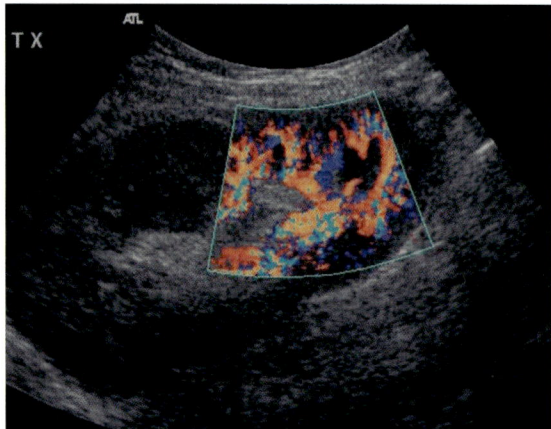

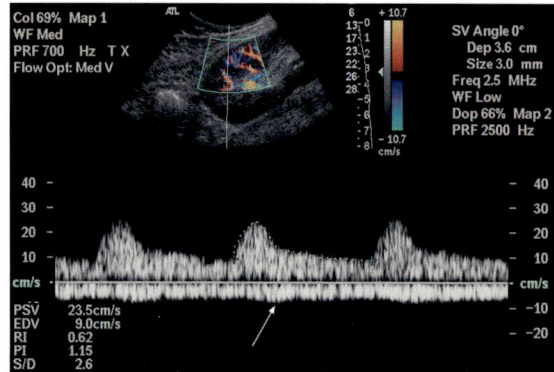

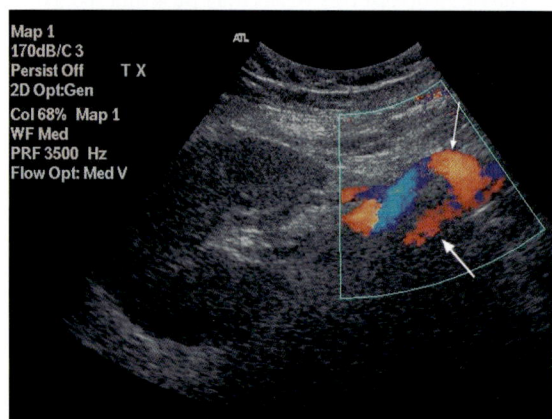

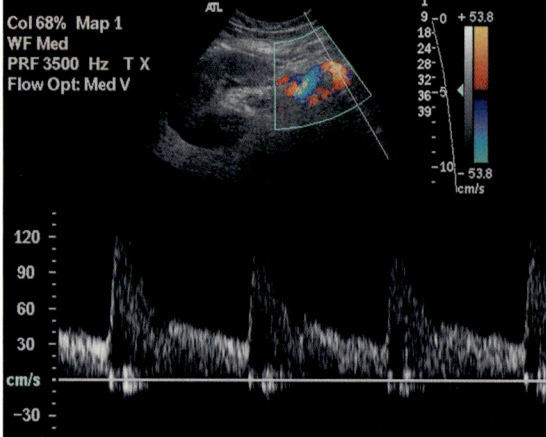

Fig. 5.4 **a** Normal color Doppler scan of the transplant kidney. The intrarenal vessels are well-visualized and extend to the periphery of the cortex. The arterial (red) and venous (blue) branches can be easily distinguished. **b** Normal spectral Doppler waveform from an interlobar artery. Having selected and drawn around an appropriate arterial waveform, the machine has automatically calculated both the PI and RI. Venous flow is noted beneath the baseline (arrow) **c** Normal color Doppler scan of the origin of the transplant renal artery (thin arrow) at its origin from the external iliac artery (thick arrow). **d** Spectral Doppler waveform of the transplant renal artery just distal to its origin. The normal renal artery waveform is well demonstrated and has a peak systolic velocity (PSV) of 1.20 ms^{-1}

Acute Rejection

Diagnosis of acute rejection is by biopsy, which in the experienced hand is safe, with the complication of hemorrhage, requiring blood transfusion, and pain relief, requiring analgesia, of less than 5%.[28] Significant complications (SMI) remain below 5% despite needle size. However, the recommended technique is using an automated core biopsy system under direct ultrasonic guidance.[29–31] Needle sizes vary from 14–18-gauge (G). However, at our institution 16 G is normally employed. Acute rejection can affect up to 40% of patients and peaks at one to three weeks posttransplantation. Assuming it is recognized early, it is normally treated with high-dose steroids or antibody therapy. Patients are normally asymptomatic although if severe, rejection can be accompanied by a flulike illness consisting of pyrexia and graft tenderness. It should always be considered in patients with deteriorating renal function and, as for ATN, the diagnosis is often very difficult, particularly in those with nonfunctioning grafts. Unfortunately, its presence has an adverse long-term prognostic indication.[32]

Delayed Function

Although the B-mode appearances of acute rejection have been well-documented,[33] these are now largely of a historical interest and should essentially no longer be observed, particularly in the postoperative transplant period, as they occur late, well after the onset of acute rejection, and are so arbitrary and inconsistent that they are of limited value. Such ultrasonic features include a reduction in corticomedullary differentiation, reduction in renal sinus echoes, increased and reduced renal parenchymal echoes, increased cortical reflectivity, and so forth. It is worthy of note, however, that observations of increased renal length[34] and cross-sectional area[35] have been reported in patients with acute rejection. Although ATN can also cause a minimal increase in renal length, it is much less marked when compared with acute rejection. As yet, however, none of these measurements have been adopted for clinical use.

With regard to Doppler ultrasound, numerous studies have been performed to assess the potential value of the technique in differentiating acute rejection from ATN, as a view to a noninvasive alternative to renal transplant biopsy. Many of the initial results were both confusing and contradictory, and this reflected a number of well-recognized factors, including inhomogeneous study populations, inadequately defined end points, and differing diagnostic criteria. In retrospect the expectation of being able to differentiate two different pathological entities with Doppler ultrasound was

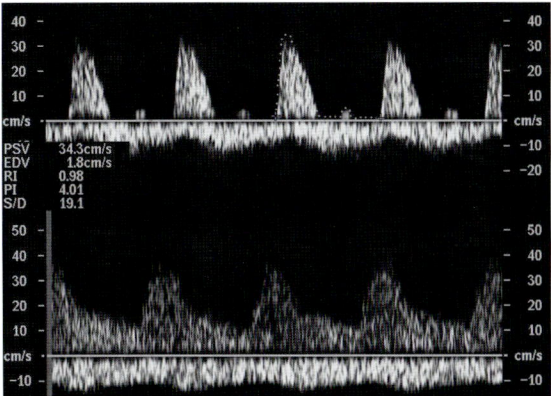

Fig. 5.5 **a** Spectral Doppler waveform from a kidney in the first week of transplantation with delayed function. On spectral analysis there was essentially complete absence of flow in diastole with a only a small focus remaining. The PI was markedly elevated at 4.01. This prompted renal biopsy which showed acute rejection. Appropriate antirejection treatment was started; the scan a few days later (**b**) showed restoration of normal diastolic flow highly suggestive of a favorable response to treatment

probably optimistic.[36,37] Nevertheless, this technique continues to have a clinical role in monitoring such patients with delayed function.[38]

The role of color Doppler, therefore, in the early postoperative period is to provide an overall qualitative impression of renal perfusion and on subsequent specific vessel interrogation, quantitative serial spectral measurements. Scanning is performed three times per week in our institution until function is established. Differentiation of pathological entities (i.e., ATN from acute rejection) is not possible despite early claims. However, serial PI or RI measurements in conjunction with the clinical and biochemical findings are a useful guide for the clinician as to whether to proceed or refrain from biopsy. A PI < 1.5 or an RI < 0.7 is normal, whereas a PI > 1.8 or an RI > 0.7 should be regarded as pathological. It is fair to say that although both ATN and acute rejection can elevate both ratios, the higher the ratio, the greater the likelihood of acute rejection. Complete absence of diastolic flow or indeed flow reversal is due to acute rejection in the majority of cases. Once a diagnosis has histologically been established, response to treatment regimes can be documented with serial spectral measurements (Fig. 5.**5**). Power Doppler can be used in addition or even as a replacement for the color Doppler technique. However, there is no evidence to date that has shown any improved benefit of doing so[39] and indeed, in my opinion, the loss of directional information is in many circumstances disadvantageous.

Other indices, including acceleration time, has shown interesting results in the early transplant period with a short acceleration time on day one being asso-

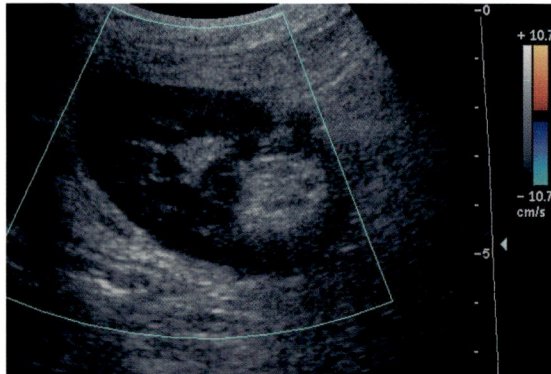

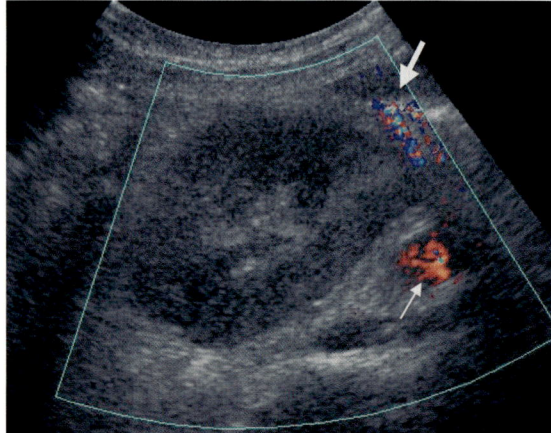

Fig. 5.**6 a** Color Doppler scan of the transplant kidney. The pulse repetition frequency (PRF) or color velocity scale is set low for increased sensitivity. Despite this there is complete absence of intrarenal flow. **b** Flow, however, can be visualized on this transverse image in the iliac artery (arrow), which lies deeper than the transplant kidney. Some flash artifact can be visualized as the color sensitivity has been increased above normal levels (thick arrow). The appearances are those of renal artery occlusion

ciated with a longer duration of delayed function and an acceleration time of < 90 ms on day five[40] with a high risk of rejection. These results, however, do remain to be substantiated and conventional RI or PI measurements remain the mainstay for Doppler monitoring.

Interestingly, with regard to outcome of the renal graft it has recently been demonstrated that an RI of ≥ 0.80 measured at least three months following transplantation is associated with subsequent poor graft performance and death.[41] This work has still to be substantiated.

Thrombosis

Arterial Thrombosis

Arterial thrombosis is rare. It occurs in the early transplant period, is often clinically silent, and may be discovered incidentally either at isotope renography or routine Doppler imaging scan in a patient with presumed delayed function. Predisposing factors include multiple renal vessels, pediatric donor kidneys, and atherosclerosis in either the donor or recipient. In general terms the process is irreversible and results in graft infarction and nephrectomy. Should the graft, however, contain multiple vessels, it is possible for one vessel to thrombose, resulting in focal segmental infarction and renal function to remain stable and satisfactory in the long term.

The ultrasound appearances are striking. There is complete absence of flow in both the kidney and the main transplant artery on color flow and spectral analysis. In this situation it is extremely important to confirm that the ultrasound machine sensitivity has been properly adjusted; a search for flow in alternative vessels at similar depth or deeper will confirm this (Fig. 5.**6**). Occasionally a spectral waveform can still be seen in the main artery; if indeed this is the case, it is normally very abnormal, with absent diastolic flow and a significantly reduced amplitude and velocity. Assuming the color features are as described, this should not alter the suspected diagnosis.

It is important to remember that absent intrarenal flow may also be seen in some patients with hyperacute rejection or renal vein thrombosis. In both these scenarios, however, color flow will be visualized in the main transplant artery with reversed diastolic flow on spectral Doppler analysis.[42] On occasion, trauma can cause an acute arterial occlusion secondary to intimal dissection; this is generally after the early transplant period and clinical history is normally highly suggestive.

Venous Thrombosis

Venous thrombosis is more common than arterial occlusion and causes acute pain and swelling of the graft, normally in association with an abrupt cessation of renal function and urine output. Typically patients are normally between the third and eight postoperative day; if the patient has delayed graft function then pain and tenderness will predominate.[43] Withholding cyclosporin and tacrolimus in the early postoperative period and the use of subcutaneous heparin or aspirin are thought to help avoid this complication. However, none of these options have been proven in clinical trials. A high index of suspicion is required, as early diagnosis and intervention may help salvage the transplant kid-

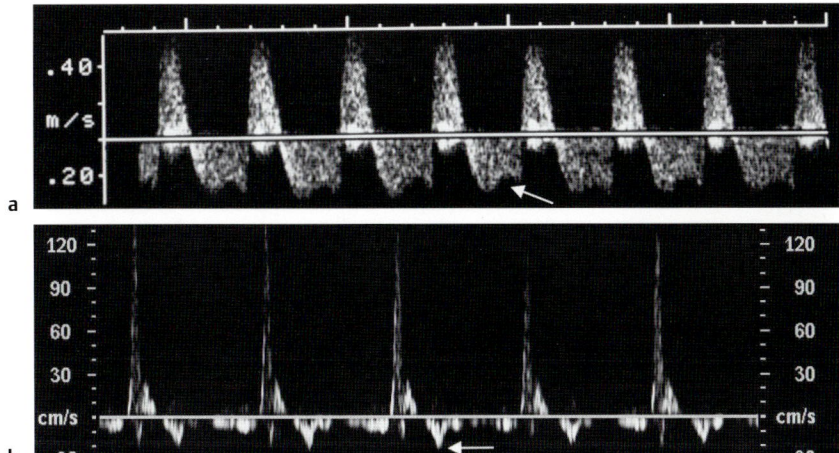

Fig. 5.7 Spectral Doppler waveforms from two different patients both of whom had graft tenderness and absent urine output in the early postoperative period. Both show reverse diastolic flow (arrows), the upper waveform (**a**) sampled from an intrarenal artery and (**b**) from the main renal artery. In both cases there was, in addition, no detectable venous flow in either the kidney or transplant vein and the features were all in keeping with renal vein thrombosis. A graft nephrectomy was performed in both cases

ney, although sadly nephrectomy is still performed in the majority of cases. Ultrasonic diagnostic criteria include a dilated transplant vein with visible echogenic thrombus, thrombus within the intrarenal system, absent flow in the transplant vein on color flow, and reverse diastolic flow in the main intrarenal arterial vessels and transplant artery on spectral Doppler analysis (Fig. 5.7).[44,45]

Low-amplitude parvus tardus–type waveform has been observed in the intrarenal vessels in this condition in patients who have incomplete renal vein occlusion and residual intravenous flow. As only a limited number of cases have been described, it is not clear whether this alters outcome or whether it remains as universally poor.[46]

Obstruction

Early obstruction within three days of transplantation normally reflects either ureteric and/or vesical blood clot and can be relieved by simple measures such as bladder irrigation. Obstruction thereafter may represent a distal ureteric stenosis, external compression of the ureter, for example by a lymphocele, abscess, or hematoma. If warranted, such collections can be drained percutaneously, either as a temporary or permanent procedure. In patients with suspected ureteric stenosis, a nephrostomy followed by contrast nephrostogram is normally performed. Depending on a number of circumstances, either reoperation or percutaneous stenting and monitoring of renal function are normally the treatment options.

Although hydronephrosis can be easily documented with ultrasound, it is important that this appearance is interpreted in conjunction with the biochemical data. Hydronephrosis should also be considered as a cause of an elevated PI or RI in the early transplant period.

Hemorrhage

Hemorrhage can occur either from the transplant kidney or the wound site. It is normally easily detected with ultrasound and is self-limiting. Intervention may be required to identify any bleeding point and subsequent hematoma. Overall, catastrophic hemorrhage is rare and is generally a consequence of either rupture or anastomotic breakdown. This is most likely when there is an associated deep wound infection or postbiopsy hemorrhage.

Urinary Leak

Urinary leak may occur in up to 6% of renal transplant patients[47] and is due to disruption or breakdown of the vesicoureteric anastomosis or necrosis of the distal ureter. Symptoms may include increasing abdominal pain, reduction in urine output, and occasionally urine leakage from the wound site. Ultrasound may demonstrate a new collection (Fig. 5.8), whereas a cystogram may show a bladder leak. Occasionally an isotope study may be helpful. Treatment is traditionally surgical repair, although a temporizing nephrostomy may be useful in certain clinical scenarios.

Posttransplantation Collections

A number of these may occur in the posttransplantation period and include abscess, hematoma, lymphocele, and urinoma. Ultrasound can identify all but cannot differentiate between these four entities. The presence of solid echoes may be seen more frequently in some than in others, but normally clinical findings in conjunction with the ultrasound appearances allow the likely nature of the collection to be recognized. If doubt

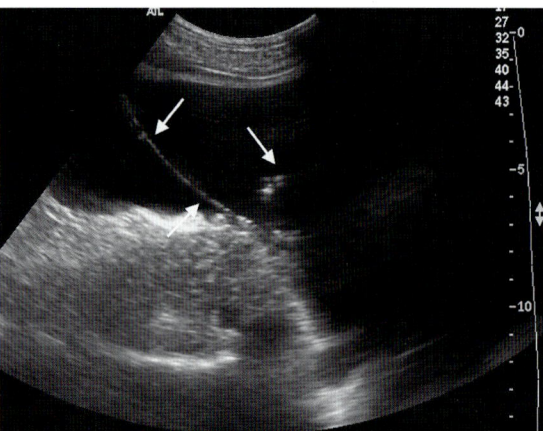

Fig. 5.8 Longitudinal scan of a large cystic collection just superior and anterior to the bladder. An 8F pigtail catheter was inserted and can be easily identified (arrows) within the collection. Analysis of the drainage fluid showed this to be urine, confirming the collection was a urinoma

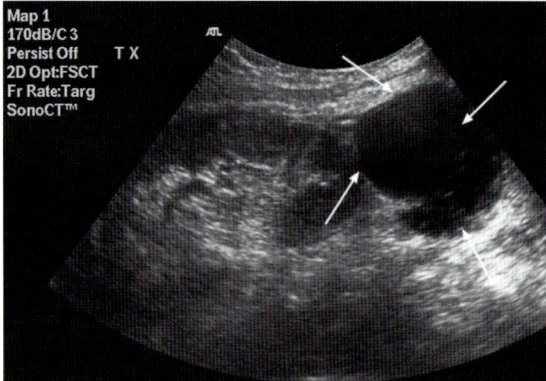

Fig. 5.9 A 4-year-old well-functioning transplant kidney. A peritransplant collection (arrows) had been noticed on multiple routine scans and was unchanged over a number of years. This was partially septated and presumed to be a lymphocele. The patient was asymptomatic and therefore no treatment was indicated

persists, however, and a definitive diagnosis is required, then this normally requires aspiration with or without formal drainage.

The most common collection is a lymphocele with an incidence of 0.6–18% (Fig. 5.9). Although various sclerosants have been instilled at an attempt at cure in the past, with mixed success, the recognized treatment is now laparoscopic marsupialization, which is both safe and effective.[48,49]

Cyclosporine and Tarcolimus Toxicity

Both agents are calcineurin inhibitors, their use representing a major advance in organ transplantation. Unfortunately, however, both are nephrotoxic and produce a reversible renovascular constriction acutely and an interstitial fibrosis chronically.[50] As a consequence, this may delay recovery from ATN and indeed may induce irreversible damage to the transplant kidney itself. Furthermore, the diagnosis of nephrotoxicity in the setting of a nonfunctioning graft is notoriously difficult and many avoid the use of such drugs if possible. Serum drug levels and renal biopsy are traditional but imperfect methods of diagnosis and ultrasound in general terms is unhelpful as these agents do not produce any significant change in diastolic flow,[51] although occasionally a reduction in flow has been recorded.

Infection

Transplant patients are subject to a number of infections in the early postoperative period, including those of the chest, wound, and urinary tract. Wound infections are likely to be due to *Staphylococcus*, whereas urinary catheters and reflux predispose to urinary tract infection (UTI). The latter may cause a deterioration in renal function, which on occasion is indistinguishable from acute rejection, and it is not unknown for pyelonephritis to be diagnosed on transplant biopsy for suspected acute rejection. Ultrasound has little or no role in the diagnosis of infection, although it is important to remember that infection can adversely affect the PI or RI ratio.

Summary points:
- 10–30% of patients require dialysis for ATN following transplantation
- Up to 40% of patients develop acute rejection following transplantation
- Color Doppler is necessary for graft monitoring; a PI < 1.5 or RI < 0.7 is normal
- Vascular occlusions, ureteric obstruction, collections, and infection can all elevate the PI and RI
- Arterial and venous occlusions carry a poor prognosis and often result in transplant nephrectomy
- Most transplant collections are benign; drainage is only performed when appropriate
- Cyclosporin toxicity has no effect on Doppler indices

Late Complications

As previously mentioned, ischemia can affect the lower aspect of the transplant ureter with secondary stricture formation, hydronephrosis, and deterioration in function. This is related to the surgical technique, which sheds the lower two thirds of the vascular supply to

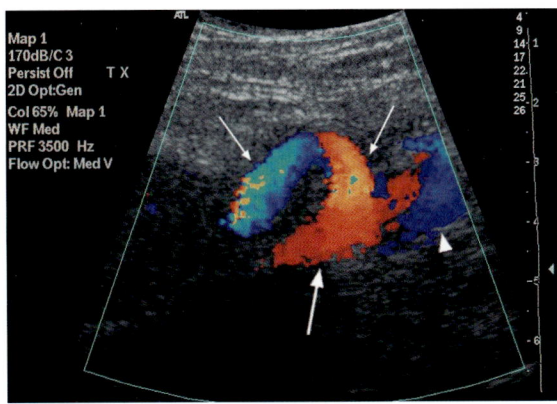 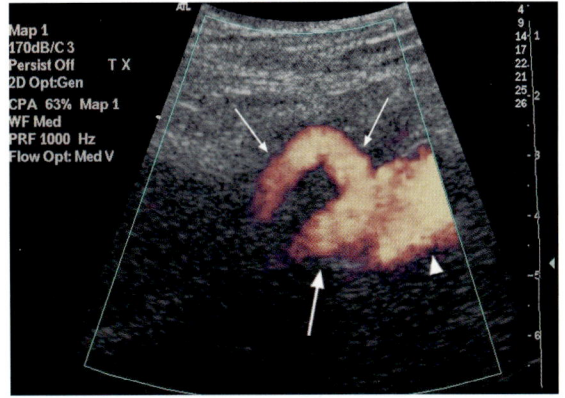

Fig. 5.**10 a** Color Doppler scan of the transplant artery (arrows) at its origin from the external iliac artery (thick arrow). The change in direction of flow within the transplant artery is easily appreciated. The external iliac vein (arrowhead) is also clearly visualized and differentiated due to the color-coding. **b** Power Doppler scan of the same area as in Fig. 5.**10a** with exactly the same labeling for comparison. There is no sense of flow direction and vessel identification is harder as a consequence

the ureter, the main supply in the transplant being the transplant renal artery itself. An overlong ureter, therefore, is at risk of an ischemic-related stenosis at its lower end. This complication may progress insidiously with a deterioration in overall renal function as a late event. Routine ultrasonic screening is therefore performed to detect this process as early as possible before permanent, severe renal damage results.

Transplant Artery Stenosis

Transplant artery stenosis occurs in up to 10% of patients.[52] Clinical suspicion is aroused in patients who have hypertension that is resistant to traditional therapy, deterioration in renal function, a combination of both, or a reduction in renal function following angiotensin-converting enzyme (ACE) inhibitor therapy. Predisposing factors include renal donor arteriosclerosis and small pediatric renal donors to adult patients. Opinions vary as to the best diagnostic test and advocates exist for isotope renography, angiography, MR imaging, and ultrasonography.[53–55] As in most situations the eventual choice will depend on local expertise and the availability of technology. We currently use color Doppler ultrasound as a first-line imaging test and if this confirms the stenosis, then angiography is performed with a view to percutaneous angioplasty and/or stenting, after appropriate clinical discussion.

Color Doppler ultrasound of the transplant renal artery is notoriously difficult due to the numerous twists and turns that the vessel may make on its route from the iliac artery to the renal hilum. This therefore requires accurate angle correction for precise spectral Doppler quantification and an awareness that it may be difficult to distinguish a focal stenosis from renal artery tortuosity. This is a potential pitfall of the technique, as the latter may also alter local hemodynamics and peak systolic velocity (PSV) readings. Although power Doppler elegantly demonstrates the twists and turns slightly better than conventional color Doppler flow, a stenosis can be masked using the power Doppler technique and therefore color Doppler is the preferred option (Fig. 5.**10**).

Any examination of the transplant renal artery must include the proximal iliac artery, as a stenosis in this area may also contribute to a reduction in renal function (Fig. 5.**11**).[56] It is fair to say, however, that the majority of lesions occur at or close to the surgical anastomosis and produce an area of aliasing on color flow imaging (Fig. 5.**12a**) which is indicative of high velocity. A PSV > 2.5 ms^{-1} within the transplant artery is diagnostic of a transplant artery stenosis (Fig. 5.**12b**).[54] We have found this value to be accurate in our center. However, other workers have found 2.0 ms^{-1} and 3.0 ms^{-1} to be better discriminators.[57,58] Clearly the exact level may depend upon many factors and it is important to use whichever is appropriate locally.

Secondary findings, including downstream turbulence, spectral broadening, and flow reversal, are all seen distal to the primary stenotic site and add both weight and confidence to the primary diagnostic findings. Due to its superficial position and relative ease of examination, the transplant artery can almost invariably be identified in all patients and therefore reliance on secondary downstream effects, including the parvus tardus effect within the intrarenal vasculature (Fig. 5.**12c**) as an aid to diagnosis, is less important than in the native kidney.[54] Intrarenal branch stenoses are also known to occur and are difficult to diagnosis not only with ultrasound but also with angiography.

It is difficult to know which patients to treat with angioplasty and/or stenting, and which simply to observe and treat conservatively. Any intervention must be clinically justified, as many of these patients remain clinically stable or even improve over time. Indeed it has also been shown that the majority of these lesions are stable and nonprogressive.[59]

Color Doppler ultrasound not only has a role in the detection of disease but also in the monitoring of such patients and in the detection of disease recurrence in those patients previously treated with angioplasty and/or stenting. Both the intrarenal RI and PSV in the transplant artery have been shown to be effective in the detection of recurrence.[60] However, at our center the preferred measurement is the latter.

Arteriovenous Fistulae

Arteriovenous fistulae (AVFs) can result from previous transplant biopsy and have an incidence of approximately 1–2%. Most are generally of little clinical significance and resolve spontaneously, as reflected in one study recording an incidence of 10% following biopsy with all but one resolving on follow-up scans,[61] whilst in another the incidence was 16.7% with 75% closing within one month and 25% (three patients) persisting longer than one year.[62] Those that remain and persist normally give rise to a spectacular and pathopneumonic color flow appearance. AVFs have been considered as a cause of both hypertension and impaired renal function. However, none of these scenarios is common. In practice these lesions are often simply observed and radiological intervention only considered if a fistula is actively bleeding or significantly increasing in size, producing a "steal syndrome" from the kidney, as in both these scenarios the benefits of embolization would be considered to outweigh those of inactivity.

Ultrasonic appearances of an AVF include a focal pool of color flow containing both arterial and venous components on spectral Doppler analysis. This can often be differentiated from "high flow" in other parts of the

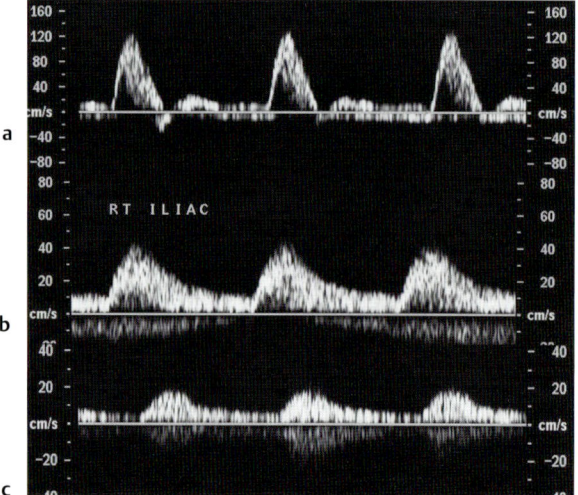

Fig. 5.**11** It is important to examine the iliac artery proximal to the origin of the transplant kidney, as iliac disease (stenosis or occlusion) can influence the transplant artery waveforms. Furthermore, it may cause a reduction in renal function. This scenario is well-demonstrated in the spectral Doppler waveforms (**a**), (**b**), and (**c**). A normal Doppler trace (a) has been shown for reference. In (**b**) a low-amplitude monophasic waveform was noted throughout the iliac artery, transplant artery, and intrarenal vessels (**c**), this all being secondary to proximal iliac disease

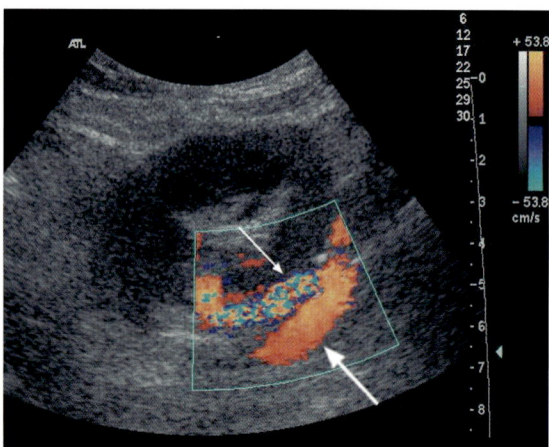

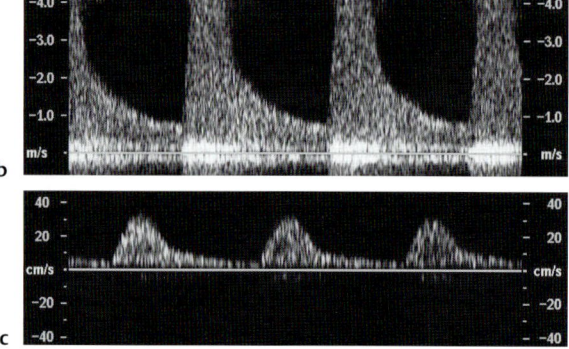

Fig. 5.**12 a** Color Doppler image at the origin of the transplant renal artery, demonstrating an area of aliasing (arrow) within the proximal transplant artery, with normal laminar flow within the iliac artery (thick arrow). The aliasing was focal, isolated, and the color velocity scale was set high. The appearances are therefore those of a transplant artery stenosis. **b** The spectral Doppler waveform through this area of aliasing in the transplant artery showed a markedly elevated PSV of 4.00 ms^{-1} and spectral broadening, all features of an RAS. **c** The spectral Doppler waveform from an intrarenal vessel in the same patient shows the parvus tardus effect, indicative of a more proximal stenosing lesion

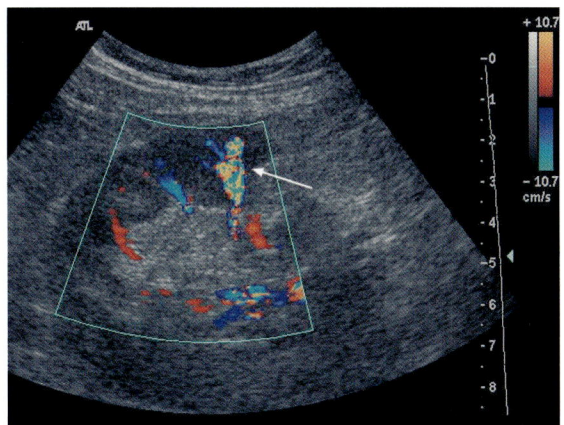
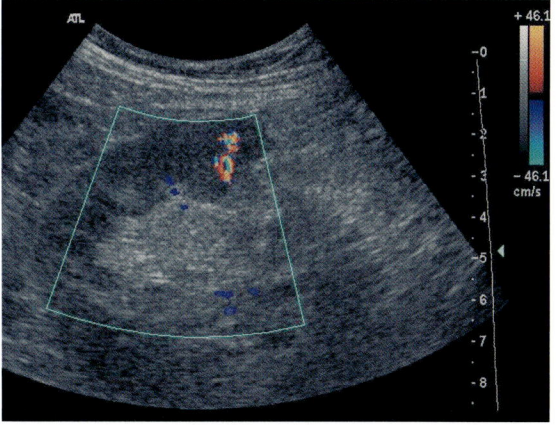

Fig. 5.**13 a** Color flow image of a 13-year-old transplant kidney demonstrates a focal pool of high flow (arrow); the velocity scale is set at a low level and a paucity of normal vessels can be visualized. The appearances are highly suggestive of an AVF.

b Same patient as in Fig. 5.**13a**. However, this time the velocity scale has been significantly increased. The normal vessels are no longer visualized and only the pathological high flow of the AVF persists. These appearances are diagnostic of an AVF

transplant kidney by increasing the pulse repetition frequency (PRF) to a level that results in nonvisualization of normal intrarenal vasculature with only the pathological flow within the fistula being observed. This simple maneuver in itself is almost diagnostic (Fig. 5.**13**). In addition to the above, spectral analysis of the arterial waveform shows increased systolic and diastolic flow within the affected area and as a result the PI or RI will remain normal or be slightly reduced in comparison with that of the surrounding vessels.[63] Venous flow can be normal or turbulent, and a large draining vein may also be visualized.

Cyclosporine and Tacrolimus Toxicity

Cyclosporine and Tacrolimus toxicity has been previously discussed and the toxic effects of both of these drugs upon renal function is well-recognized. As such it may lead to a progressive deterioration in function which can be difficult to differentiate from chronic rejection and often a therapeutic trial of dose reduction or conversion to an alternative immunosuppressive agent may be required. Following this maneuver a small but significant number of patients will respond positively.

Rejection

Acute Rejection

Acute rejection is an unusual late complication. If present then noncompliance with drug therapy should be considered. Diagnosis and treatment are as previously discussed.

Chronic Rejection

Chronic rejection is a gradual deterioration in graft function beginning at least three months following transplantation in association with the biopsy appearances of fibrous intimal thickening, interstitial fibrosis, and tubular atrophy. Previous episodes of acute rejection are the most consistent predisposing factors. No effective treatment exists, and as such all efforts are concentrated toward preventing episodes of acute rejection as a method of reducing chronic rejection. Ultrasonic features have been previously described and include increased transplant echogenicity and a reduction in the normal number of intrarenal vessels. These signs, however, are of minimal prognostic significance and the role of ultrasound is limited in diagnosis (Fig. 5.**14**).

Urinary Tract Infection

Asymptomatic bacteriuria is common and has a good prognosis. Symptomatic infections are also common and can cause pyuria, pyelonephritis (Fig. 5.**15**), and a temporary reduction in renal function. Repeated infections may lead to an underlying structural abnormality, such as calculi (Fig. 5.**16**), obstruction, or reflux. Chronic, repeated infections may occasionally lead to malacoplakia.

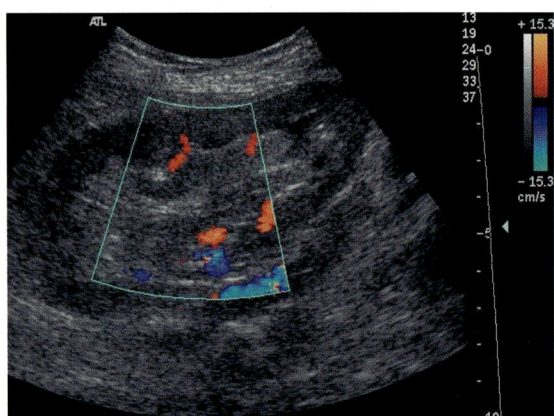
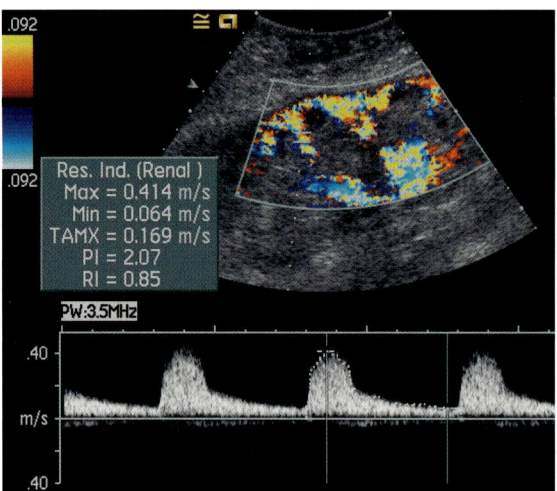

Fig. 5.14 **a** Color flow image of a 15-year-old transplant kidney with a paucity of intrarenal vessels. Renal function was good. **b** Color flow image of a 13-year-old transplant kidney. Renal perfusion is clearly better with good demonstration of small vessels to the periphery of the cortex. Renal function was similar to the patient in Fig. 5.14a

> **Summary points:**
> - The lower end of the transplant ureter is at risk of an ischemia-related stricture
> - Transplant artery stenosis occurs in up to 10% of patients
> - The PSV in the transplant renal artery is the best measurement for the detection of RAS. Cut-off values vary between 2.0 and 3.0 ms^{-1}. In our institution the cut-off value is 2.5 ms^{-1}
> - AVFs have an incidence of 1–2%. The vast majority are benign but ultrasonically interesting. Vascular steal is uncommon
> - Chronic rejection is a diagnosis of exclusion for which there is no effective treatment
> - Long-term risk factors are related to cardiovascular disease, infection, and the risk of malignancy

Fig. 5.15 Longitudinal image of a 15-year-old transplant kidney in a patient with multiple recent and recurrent UTIs. This demonstrated a focal hypoechoic area within the kidney (arrows). Flow was noted on color Doppler within it. The appearances were suspicious of tumor and the lesion was biopsied. Histology showed an area of focal pyelonephritis

Long-Term Complications

Many forms of glomerulonephritis may cause recurrent disease in the transplant kidney, although early recurrence in graft failure is rare. Recurrent disease is more commonly encountered in long-term recipients with diabetes mellitus, amyloidosis, and cystinosis. In those patients with oxalosis and active vasculitis, disease recurrence and renal damage are more common in the earlier stages following transplantation.[64] Ultrasound has no specific role apart from excluding the treatable causes of reduced renal function, which have been previously discussed.

Other Complications

Increased morbidity and mortality following renal transplantation is normally due either to cardiovascular disease, malignancy, or infections secondary to immunosuppression. Cardiovascular risk factors include hypertension, left ventricular hypertrophy, and altered liver profile. As yet, no specific targeting of these areas has provided any survival improvement.

In contrast, the incidence of infection has been significantly reduced with improvements in immunosuppression, by improved targeting of these agents, and an increased awareness of the types of infection that may occur.

The most common malignancies following transplantation are skin-related, cervical cancer, and non-Hodgkin lymphoma (Fig. 5.17). It is therefore obvious that careful supervision of the transplant population is required and it is hoped that earlier diagnosis may result in improved prognosis for each of these disorders.[65]

Combined Renal and Pancreas Transplant[66]

A detailed description of combined organ transplantation is beyond the scope of this book. In essence, however, as for the kidney, patient selection is crucial and depends upon a multidisciplinary pretransplant evaluation team. A successful outcome will restore blood glucose levels to normal, improve neuropathy in most patients, and prevent the recurrence of diabetic nephropathy in the new kidney. It may prevent the secondary complications of diabetes, but the effect on established lesions is not clear.

The standard surgical technique is that endocrine drainage of the pancreas is to the systemic venous system, i.e. the iliac vein and the exocrine drainage to the bladder. This is gradually being replaced by endocrine drainage to the portal system and enteric drainage of the exocrine. The transplanted kidney is dealt with by the standard surgical techniques.

Vascular complications are the most common and occur in 12% of cases, 5% being arterial and 7% venous. Other complications include rejection, infection, and allograft pancreatitis.

The overall survival of a combined pancreatic and renal transplant is 83.6%, 72.9% and 65.5% at one, three and five years, respectively.[67]

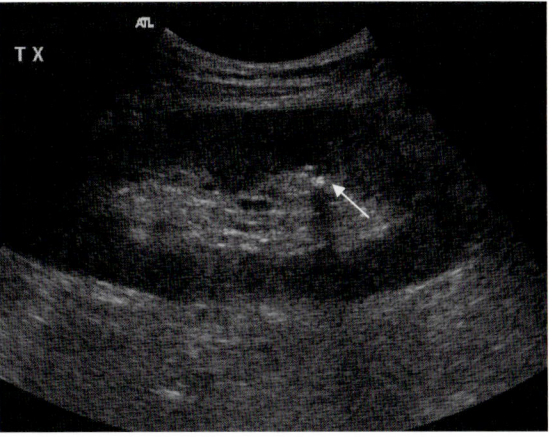

Fig. 5.16 A group of three small calculi, one with distal acoustic shadowing (arrow) is seen at the lower pole of the transplant kidney

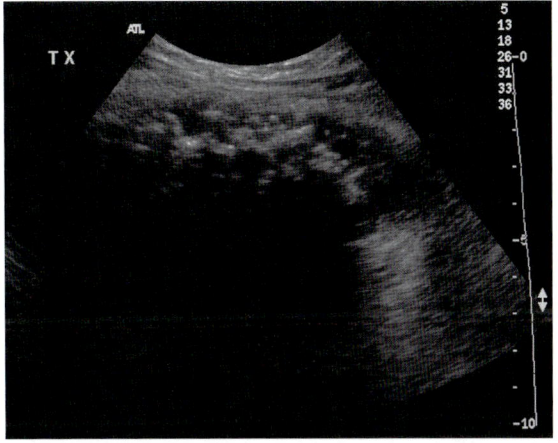

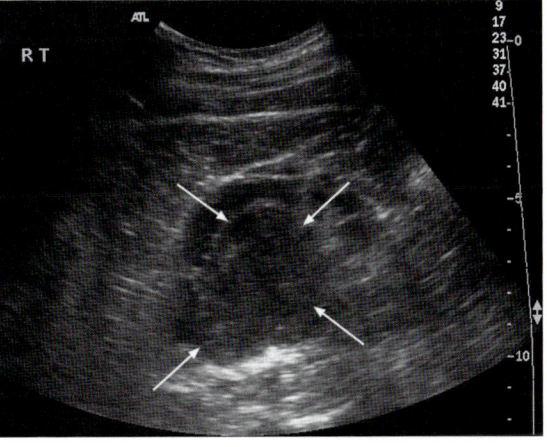

Fig. 5.17 **a** A chronic nonfunctioning transplant kidney with extensive internal calcification and distal acoustic shadowing akin to autonephrectomy. **b** Same patient as in Fig. 5.17a. The patient presented with hematuria. It is not only important to check the transplant kidney(s) in this situation but also the native kidneys. A scan of the right kidney showed a renal tumor (arrows) accounting for his symptomatology

References

1. Hamilton D. Alexis Carrel and the early days of tissue transplantation. Transplant Rev 1987;2:1–15.
2. Murray JE, Merrill JP, Harrison JH. Kidney Transplantation between seven pairs of identical twins. Ann Surg 1958; 148:343–59.
3. Starzl TE. Experience in Renal Transplantation. Philadelphia: Saunders: 1964.
4. Calne RY, White DJG, Thiru S, Evans DB, McMaster P, Dunn DC, et al. Cyclosporin A in patients receiving renal allografts from cadaveric donors. Lancet 1978;ii:323–7.
5. Charra B, Calemerd E, Ruffet M, et al. Survival as an index of the adequacy of dialysis. Kidney Int 1992;41:1286–91.
6. Valderrabano F, Jones EHP, Mallick NP. Report on the management of renal failure in Europe XXIV, 1993. Nephrol Dial Transplant 1995;10:Suppl 51:1–25.
7. Gore SM, Cable DJ, Holland AJ. Organ donation from intensive care units in England and Wales – two-year con-

fidential audit of deaths in intensive care. Br Med J 304: 349–55.
8. Takemoto S, Terasaki PI, Cecka JM, Chong YW, Gjertson DW. Survival of nationally shared HLA-matched kidney transplants from cadaveric donors. New Engl J Med 1992; 327:834–9.
9. The Canadian Multicentre Transplant Study Group. A randomised clinical trial of cyclosporin in cadaveric renal transplantation: analysis at three years. N Engl J Med 1986; 314:1219–20.
10. Berthoux FC, Jones EHP, Mehls O, Valderrabano F. Transplantation report: Report on Management of Renal Failure in Europe, XXV, 1994. Nephrol Dial Transplant 1996;11: 37–40.
11. Robinson MT, Kindt TJ. Major histocompatibility complex antigens and genes in fudamental immunology. W Paul, ed. New York: Raven Press: 1989:489–539.
12. Krensky AM. Transplant immunobiology in paediatric nephrology, 3rd ed. Baltimore: Williams & Wilkins: 1993: 1373–1389.
13. Jamison RL, Wilkinson R. The pretransplant selection and evaluation of donor and recipient. Nephrology 1997;Chapman & Hall,1072–1082.
14. Opelz G. Correlation of HLA matching with kidney graft survival in patients with or without cyclosporine treatment. Transplant 1985;40:240–3.
15. Robles J, Errasti P, Abad J, et al. Surgical complications in renal transplantation: determinant factors. Transplant Proceedings 1995;27:2258–2259.
16. Lai M, Huang C, Chu S, et al. Surgical complications in renal transplantation. Transplant Proceedings 1994;26:2 165–2166.
17. Gruber S, Chavers B, Payne W, et al. Allograft renal vascular thrombosis—lack of increase with cyclosporin immunnosuppression. Transplantation 1989;47:475–478.
18. Hakim N, Benedetti E, Pirenne J, et al. Complication of uterovesical anastomosis in kidney transplant patients: the Minnesota experience. Clinical Transplantation 1994; 8:504–507.
19. Vincenti F, Laskow DA, Neylan JF, Mendez R, Matas AJ. One-year follow-up of an open label trial of FK506 for primary kidney transplantation. Transplant 1996;61:1576–81.
20. European Mycophenolate Mofetil Cooperative Study Group. Placebo controlled study of mycophenolate mofetil combined with cyclosporin and corticosteroids for prevention of acute rejection. Lancet 1995;345:1321–5.
21. Duda SH, Erley CM, Wakat JP, et al. Posttransplant renal artery stenosis - outpatient intraarterial DSA versus color aided duplex Doppler sonography. Eur J Radiol 1993;16: 95–101.
22. Snider JF, Hunter DW, Moradian GP, Castaneda-Zuniga WR, Letourneau JG. Transplant renal artery stenosis: evaluation with duplex sonography. Radiology 1989;172:1027–1030.
23. Taylor KJW, Morse SS, Rigsby CM, Bia M, Schiff M. Vascular complications in renal allografts: detection with duplex Doppler US. Radiology 1987;162:31–38.
24. Genkins SM, Sanfilippo FP, Carroll BA. Duplex Doppler sonography of renal transplants: lack of sensitivity and specificity in establishing pathologic diagnosis. AJR Am J Roentgenol 1989;152:535–539.
25. Kelzc F, Pozniak MA, Pirsch JD, Oberly TD. Pyramidal appearance and resistive index: insensitive and nonspecific indicators of acute renal transplant rejection. AJR Am J Roentgenol 1990;155:531–535.
26. Rifkin MD, Needleman L, Pasto ME, et al. Evaluation of renal transplant rejection by duplex Doppler examination: value of the resistive index. AJR Am J Roentgenol 1987;148:759–762.
27. Rigsby CM, Taylor KJW, Weltin G, et al. Renal allografts in acute rejection: evaluation using duplex sonography. Radiology 1986;158:375–378.
28. Wilczek HE. Percutaneous needle biopsy of the renal allograft. Transplant 1990;50:790–7.
29. Tang S, Li JH, Lui SL, Chan TM, Cheng IK, Lai KN. Free-hand, ultrasound-guided percutaneous renal biopsy: experience form a single operator. Eur J Radiol 2002;41:65–69.
30. Freda A, Van Dijk LC, Van Oostaijen JA, Pattynama PM. Complication rate and diagnostic yield of 515 consecutive ultrasound-guided biopsies of renal allografts and native kidneys using a 14-guage Biopty gun. Eur Radiol 2003;13: 527–530.
31. Chan R, Common AA, Marcuzzi D. Ultrasound guided renal biopsy: experience using an automated core biopsy. Can Asso Radiol J 2000;51:107–113.
32. Pirsch JD, Ploeg RJ, Gange S, et al. Determinants of graft survival after renal transplantation. Transplant 1996; 61:1581–5.
33. Cochlin DLL, Wake A, Salaman JR, Griffin PJA. Ultrasound changes in the transplant kidney. Clin Radiol 1988;39: 373–376.
34. Pozniak MA, Kelcz F, D'Alessandro A, Oberley T, Stratta R. Sonography of renal transplants in dogs: the effect of acute tubular necrosis, cyclosporin nephrotoxicity and acute rejection on resistive index and renal length. AJR Am J Roentgenol 1992;158:791–797.
35. Parvin SD, Rees Y, Veitch PS, et al. Objective measurement by ultrasound to distinguish cyclosporin A toxicity from rejection. Br J Surg 1986;73:1009–1011.
36. Trillaud H, Merville P, Tran Le Linh P, Palussiere J, Potaux L, Grenier N. Color Doppler sonography in early renal transplantation follow-up: resistive index measurements versus power Doppler sonography. AJR Am J Roentgenol 1998; 171:1611–1615.
37. Krishnan H, Cochlin D, Moore R, Griffen P, Salaman JR. A comparison of duplex Doppler sonography and intrarenal manometry in the diagnosis of acute renal transplant rejection. Clin Transpl 1993;7:175–178.
38. Jakobsen JA, Brabrand K, Egge TS, Hartmann A. Doppler examination of the allografted kidney. Acta Radiologica 2003;44:3–12.
39. Chow L, Sommer FG, Huang J, Li KC. Power Doppler imaging and resistive index measurement in the evaluation of acute renal transplant rejection. J Clin Ultrasound 2001;29:483–490.
40. Merkus JWS, Hoitsma AJ, van Asten WNJC, Koene RA, Scotnicki SH. Doppler spectrum analysis to diagnose rejection during post transplant acute renal failure. Transplantation 1994;58:570–576.
41. Radermacher J, Mengel M, Ellis S, Stuht S, Hiss M, Schwarz A, et al. The renal arterial resistive index and renal allograft survival. N Engl J Med 2003;349:115–124.
42. Kaveggia LP, Perella RR, Grant EG, et al. Duplex doppler sonography in renal allografts: the significance of reversed flow in diastole. AJR Am J Roentgenol 1990;155:295–298.
43. Penny MJ, Nankivell BJ, Disney APS, Blyth K, Chapman JR. Renal graft thrombosis: A survey of 134 consecutive cases. Transplant 1994;58:565–9.

44. Baxter GM, Morley P, Dall B. Acute renal vein thrombosis in renal allografts: new Doppler ultrasonic findings. Clin Radiol 1991;43:125–127.
45. Reuther G, Wanjura D, Bauer H. Acute renal vein thrombosis in renal allografts: detection with duplex Doppler ultrasound. Radiology 1989;170:557–558.
46. MacLennan AC, Baxter GM, Harden P, Rowe PA. Renal transplant vein occlusion: an early diagnostic sign? Clin Radiol 1995;50:251–253.
47. Nargund VH, Cranston D. Urological complications after renal transplantation. Transplant Rev 1996;10:24–33.
48. Duepree HJ, Fornara P, Lewejohann JC, Hoyer J, Bruch HP, Schiedeck TH. Laparoscopic treatment of lymphoceles in patients after renal transplantation. Clin Transplant 2001;15:375–379.
49. Risaliti A, Corno V, Donini A, Cautero N, Baccarani U, Pasqualucci A, et al. Laparoscopic treatment of symptomatic lymphoceles after kidney transplantation. Surg Endoscop 2000;14:293–295.
50. Myers BD, Sibley R, Newton L, et al. The long-term course of cyclosporin associated chronic nephropathy. Kidney Int 1988;33:590–600.
51. Heine GH, Girndt M, Sester U, Kohler H. No rise in renal Doppler resistance indices at peak serum levels of cyclosporin A in stable kidney transplant patients. Nephrol Dialy Transplant 2003;18:1639–1643.
52. Gray DWR. Graft renal artery stenosis in the transplanted kidney. Transplant Rev 1994;8:15–21.
53. Erley CM, Duda SH, Wakat JP, et al. Non-invasive procedures for diagnosis of renovascular hypertension in renal transplant recipients and prospective analysis. Transplantation 1992;54:863–7.
54. Baxter GM, Ireland H, Moss JG, et al. Colour Doppler ultrasound in renal transplant artery stenosis: which doppler index? Clin Radiol 1995;50:618–22.
55. Gedroyc WM, Negus R, al Kautoubi A, et al. Magnetic resonance angiography of renal transplants. Lancet 1992;339:789–91.
56. Voiculescu A, Hollenbeck M, Plum J, Hetzel GR, Modder U, Pfeiffer T, et al. Iliac artery stenosis proximal to a kidney transplant: clinical findings, duplex sonographic criteria, treatment and outcome. Tranplantation 2003;76: 332–339.
57. deMorais RH, Muglia VF, Mamere AE, Garcia Pisi T, Saber LT, Muglia VA, et al. Duplex Doppler sonography of transplant renal artery stenosis. J Clin Ultrasound 2003;31:135–141.
58. Patel U, Khaw KT, Hughes NC. Doppler ultrasound for detection of renal transplant artery stenosis – threshold peak systolic velocity needs to be higher in a low risk or surveillance population. Clin Radiol 2003;58:772–777.
59. Butorovic-Ponikvar J. Renal transplant artery stenosis. Nephrol Dialy Transplant 2003;18:74–77.
60. Ruggenenti P, Mosconi L, Bruno S, Remuzzi A, Sangalli F, Lepre MS, et al. Post transplant renal artery stenosis: the hemodynamic response to revascularisation. Kid Internat 2001;60:309–318.
61. Merkus JWS, Zeebregts CJAM, Hoitsma AJ, van asten WNJC, Koene RAP, Skotnicki SH. High Incidence of arteriovenous fistula after biopsy of kidney allografts. Br J Surg 993;80: 310–312.
62. Brandenburg VM, Frank RD, Riehl J. Color coded duplex sonography of arteriovenous fisulae and pseudoaneurysms complicating percutaneous renal allograft biopsy. Clin Nephrol 2002;58:398–404.
63. Renowden SA, Blethyn J, Cochlin DLL. Duplex and color flow sonography in the diagnosis of post biopsy arteriovenous fistulae in the transplant kidney. Clin Radiol 1992; 45: 33–237.
64. Matthew TH. Recurrent disease after transplantation. Transplant Rev 1991;5:31–45.
65. Penn I. Cancer is a complication of severe immunosuppression. Surg Gynaecol Obstet 1986;162:603–10.
66. Khanna A, Patel NH, Song Z, Jindal RM. Pancreas Transplantation. In: Sidhu PS, Baxter GM. Ultrasound of abdominal transplantation. Stuttgart: Thieme International: 2002: 125–130.
67. www.insulin-free.org./article/inp.htm

6 Radiological Intervention in the Urogenital Tract (Including Trauma and Emergencies)

P. M. Scott, J. G. Moss

Principles of Ultrasound-Guided Procedures

Probe Selection and Preparation

Generally a 3–5 MHz curvilinear or sector probe will be used in renal intervention. Higher frequencies of 5–7.5 MHz are normally reserved for superficial structures such as the transplant kidney. The sector probe provides some advantages: The probe has a smaller footprint and thus allows slightly more flexibility in initial needle positioning on the skin surface.

The probe should be cleaned and then placed in one of the proprietary sterile probe covers with some gel. The gel within the cover need not be sterile. Care should be taken to achieve good apposition of probe cover to probe head. Any bubbles within the jelly under the cover should be "smoothed" off the probe head, as they degrade image quality. Sterile jelly is used between patient and sterile probe cover.

The skin is cleaned and draped. A bleb of local anaesthetic is raised at the preferred point of needle entry, which is chosen after initial scanning. It is important to eliminate any bubbles in the anaesthetic, as injecting these in the soft tissues may completely obscure subsequent attempts to guide the needle.

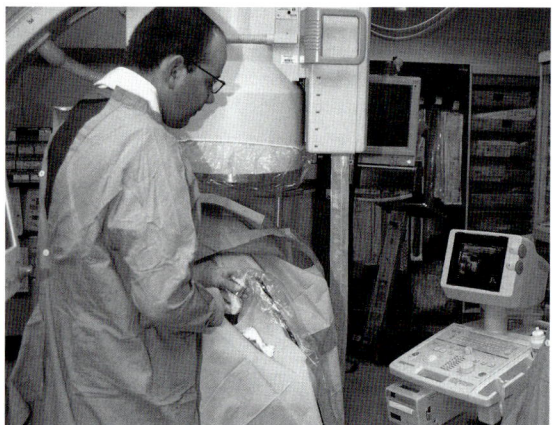

Fig. 6.1 **Ultrasound-guided internal jugular vein puncture.** The machine is placed opposite the operator in the direct line of sight, allowing the operator to see the machine without turning his or her head. This is an important general principle in ultrasound-guided procedures

Machine Placement

If possible, the ultrasound machine should be placed with the screen directly opposite the operator; often this means on the opposite side of the table. Constant straining of the neck to see an incorrectly positioned monitor makes the procedure much more difficult (Fig. 6.1).

Needle Guidance

The first principle in ultrasonic needle guidance is the need to be able to visualize the target clearly. If this is not possible, alternative image-guidance will be necessary. Generally the operator will obtain a good grayscale image of the target with the dominant hand initially. The transducer can then be transferred to the other hand and the needle then guided with the dominant hand.

Only once the target is well-visualized can needle introduction commence. Usually the local anaesthetic needle will be guided initially. The *most* crucial aspect of the technique relates to orienting the needle in *precisely* the same plane as the long axis of the ultrasound probe. Any deviation will result in loss of visualization of the needle (Fig. 6.2).

Troubleshooting

If the needle is "lost" after initial advancement, some specific maneuvers can occasionally help. Very gentle "fore and aft" movement of the transducer in the plane of the needle can sometimes bring it back into view. Occasionally very gentle angulation can also help. The target must, however, remain in view after these probe adjustments. A gentle vibration of the needle hub up and down can help by agitating tissue just around the needle, allowing minute adjustments of the probe to bring the needle fully into plane. Often the echogenic bright tip of the needle is the best-seen section.

When these adjustments fail to bring a needle back into view it is best to recommence with a fresh "line-up" rather than risk inadvertent malpositioning.

Some operators prefer to use one of the proprietary needle-guide systems available. These affix directly to the head of the ultrasound probe. Once in place, with the probe on the skin surface, the machine software marks the track the needle will take directly onto the screen, usually via a dotted line. Thus with the target visualized the probe can be manipulated until the target lies directly in the needle path. The needle then only needs to be advanced as far as the desired target.

Finally, echogenic needles are available. These are coated with a variety of substrates, which allow increased visualization, usually polymer coatings, that cause adherence of air bubbles thus increasing needle conspicuity.

Summary points:
- A 3–5 MHz curvilinear or sector probe is most frequently used
- Preparation is vital: ideally place the machine screen opposite you
- Good visualization of the target and pathway is essential
- The needle must be "in-plane" with the ultrasound probe
- If you are struggling, despite adjustment, stop. Remove the needle and try again

Patient Preparation: General Principles

Consent

Informed consent prior to the procedure is vital. Every effort should be made to obtain consent away from the procedure room when there is time for a proper explanation of the procedure and its attendant risks.

Antibiotic Prophylaxis

The majority of interventional radiologists use broad-spectrum prophylactic antibiotics prior to urogenital intervention.[1]

In nephrostomy there is certainly evidence that patients benefit from prophylaxis, with high-risk patients (urinary stones, positive urine culture, or urinary stoma) benefiting the most.[2] Use of prophylaxis is also warranted in the drainage of infected abdominal collections, although generally these patients will already be receiving intravenous antibiotics. In radiofrequency ablation antibiotics have not been routinely used.[3–5]

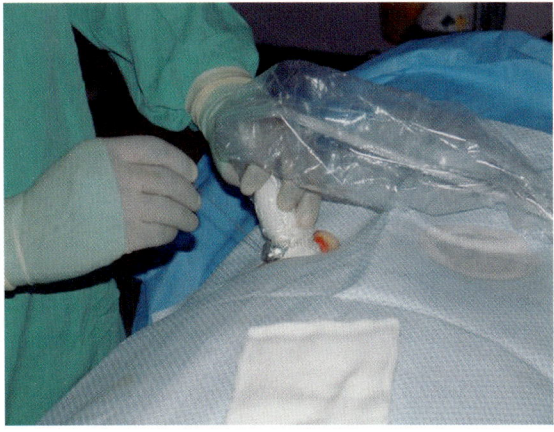

Fig. 6.2 **Several important points regarding ultrasound needle guidance.** Firstly, the area has been cleaned, covered with sterile drapes, and the skin infiltrated with local anaesthetic. Importantly, the needle is aligned such that it bisects the long axis of the probe. This is crucial for needle visualization

The choice of antibiotic is usually a broad-spectrum cephalosporin, although culture of drainage fluid will supply more specific information. In those patients with a penicillin allergy, discussion with the local bacteriology service may be helpful in choosing an alternative antibiotic to cover the procedure.

Coagulopathy

A routine full blood count and coagulation screen is not required. However, it should be carried out in some groups, specifically in patients with renal or hepatic impairment, those on anticoagulants, and those with a known coagulopathy. Acceptable limits are considered to be a prothrombin time of < 1.5 times the laboratory control (also known as the international normalized ratio [INR]) and an activated partial thromboplastin time (APTT) of < 1.5 times the control. Finally, the platelet count should be > 50×10^9 per liter.

Fresh frozen plasma (FFP) can be used to correct a raised prothrombin time if the INR is > 1.5. Usually four units are given intravenously if the INR is between 1.5 and 3.0, with the last unit running during the procedure. Alternatively, intravenous vitamin K can be used in less urgent cases.

If the patient is on intravenous heparin, this should be withheld for three hours and the APTT measured. Heparin has a half-life of 60 minutes. Platelets should be administered again during the procedure for low counts of < 50×10^9 per liter.

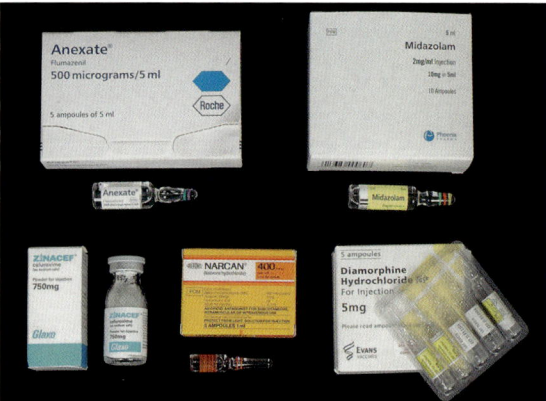

Fig. 6.3 **Commonly-used pharmacotherapy in urogenital intervention.** In the top row the short-acting benzodiazepine midazolam is seen on the right, with its reversal agent flumazenil. In the lower row, diamorphine, on the right, lies next to the opiod antagonist naloxone. Finally, the most commonly used third-generation cephalosporin antibiotic, cefuroxime, is shown bottom left

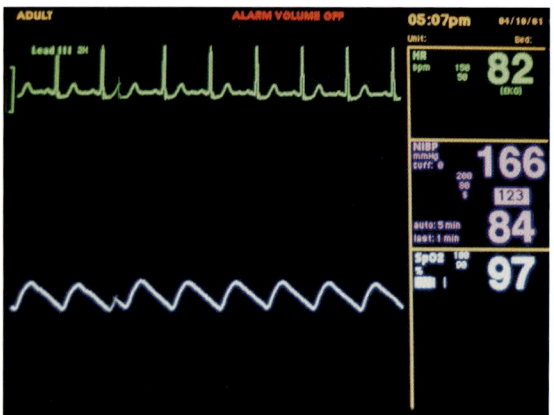

Fig. 6.4 **Patients should receive careful monitoring.** This is particularly important when any form of conscious sedation is used. Minimum acceptable monitoring should include ECG (upper trace in image), pulse oximetry (lower trace), and regular blood pressure measurements

Elevated Blood Pressure

A blood pressure above that acceptable for angiography (180 mmHg) should be avoided. In practice these are often controlled simply by using analgesia and sedation.

Sedation and Analgesia

Most practitioners use a combination of short-acting opiod analgesia and benzodiazepine. Common candidates include fentanyl or diamorphine and midazolam. Commonly combinations of 50–100 μg of fentanyl or 1–5 mg diamorphine and 1–10 mg of midazolam are used. These drugs act synergistically and can produce hypoxemia and apnoea.[6] Their action is also potentiated in renal failure, so cautious use with small incremental boluses is advisable (Fig. 6.3).

In addition, the patient must be adequately monitored with pulse oximetry, electrocardiography (ECG), and regular blood-pressure measurements. A nurse or operating department assistant must be available for this dedicated purpose.[7] In addition, the reversal agents for opiod (naloxone) and the reversal agent for benzodiazepines (flumazenil) should be available (Fig. 6.4).

Skin Preparation

Finally, the area should be cleaned with povodine iodine solution and sterile drapes applied. The skin should be anaesthetized and anaesthetic infiltrated into the intended subcutaneous track. Usually 10–15 mL of 1% lignocaine is sufficient. The maximum recommended dose is 3 mg/kg, up to a maximum of 200 mg.[8]

Nephrostomy

Percutaneous nephrostomy (PCN) is now a long-established and often-performed procedure, having been first described in 1955 by Goodwin et al.[9]

The following section will describe current indications for nephrostomy, relevant anatomy, a description of the standard technique with variations, follow-up care of patients, and a brief review of complications and their management.

Indications

There are three main categories of indication for nephrostomy:
- Ureteric obstruction
- Urinary leak
- To allow percutaneous nephrolithotomy (PCNL)

Nephrostomy is rarely required as an emergency procedure. The single definite indication for an urgent nephrostomy is the presence of infection within an obstructed kidney. In this scenario, irreversible renal damage can occur within six hours. Hyperkalemia (> 6.0 mmlo/L) is also an indication for a relatively urgent nephrostomy. However, there are medical maneuvers which can reduce the level of hyperkalemia temporarily. Indeed, it is desirable to have the serum potassium level normalized before proceeding, as hyperkalemia during the procedure can produce cardiac dysrhythmias.

Nephrostomy is an invasive procedure. In a survey of 303 patients undergoing nephrostomy, Farrell et al.[10] described a 30-day mortality rate of 3.1% and overall complication rate of 6.5%.

Given these potential complications, most practitioners would agree that percutaneous drainage should only be attempted for obstruction if retrograde stent placement is not feasible.[11]

Malignant obstruction is a common indication for nephrostomy, comprising up to 61% of patients in the series of Farrell et al.[10] Average survival following nephrostomy with or without stenting in this cohort was found to be five months.[12]

With these difficulties in mind it is important that referrals for percutaneous drainage due to malignant obstruction are appropriate. These facts should also have been discussed with the patient and patient's relatives. In general it is better to avoid placement in the first instance for unsuitable candidates. Specifically placement of a nephrostomy in those with end-stage malignancy may be inappropriate and should not be performed without consultation with the senior referring clinician first.[13]

Technique

Anatomy

The main anatomical feature guiding PCN relates to renal blood supply. The large renal vessels lie centrally and therefore a central puncture should be avoided.

The main renal arteries divide at the renal hilum into ventral and dorsal branches. The territory subtended between these main divisions is sometimes referred to as the Brödel bloodless line and lies at the junction of anterior two thirds with the posterior third of the kidney.[14] The posterior calyces are oriented in the same plane as this relatively avascular region and are therefore the preferred point of entry into the renal collecting system. Given the orientation of the kidney, this means that in a patient lying prone the posterior calyces lie roughly at an angle of 20–25° dorsal to the coronal plane (Fig. 6.**5**).

In general a puncture of a lower pole calyx, below the 12th rib, is the safest. This subcostal approach avoids the risk of transgression of the pleural space. If simple nephrostomy or stenting is the intended endpoint of the procedure, this approach is ideal.[14]

PCNL access will sometimes require access from above the 12th rib and this is associated with an increased risk of transgression of the pleural space.

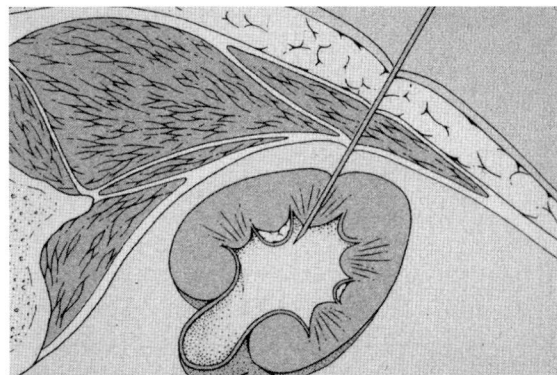

Fig. 6.**5 Needle passage into the renal collecting system.** As mentioned, an angle of 25° relative to horizontal (coronal plane) is ideal to allow puncture of a posterior calyx. In practice this is usually the angle which best allows visualization of the kidney during ultrasound scanning

Guidance

Different practitioners use different techniques to gain access to the renal collecting system. Access can be gained using solely ultrasound or fluoroscopy. The vast majority of practitioners will choose to use a combination of ultrasound and fluoroscopic guidance during the procedure, and indeed the Society of Cardiovascular and Interventional Radiology (SCVIR) guidelines specify that a high-resolution fluoroscopy unit should be available.[15] Computed tomography (CT) guidance is usually reserved for technically difficult procedures and is rarely required.

The use of ultrasound with fluoroscopy rather than fluoroscopy alone has several advantages:
- The ability to visualize overlying liver, spleen, and colon, thus avoiding inadvertent puncture
- The ability to guide the needle under real-time imaging
- Obviates the need to give iodinated contrast material prior to the procedure and reduces the overall ionizing radiation burden

The advantages of ultrasound were confirmed in a study in 1981 in which the use of a combination approach compared to fluoroscopy reduced the number of needle passes (1.4 vs. 4.1)[16] required to perform the procedure.

The technique of PCN will vary according to whether the renal collecting system is dilated or not. The *initial* approach will vary depending on this factor.

The Nondilated System

Direct calyceal puncture is extremely difficult in this group of patients. Puncture of the renal pelvis under direct ultrasound control can be performed with a 22-gauge Chiba (Neff Set, Cook, Europe) or Accustick nee-

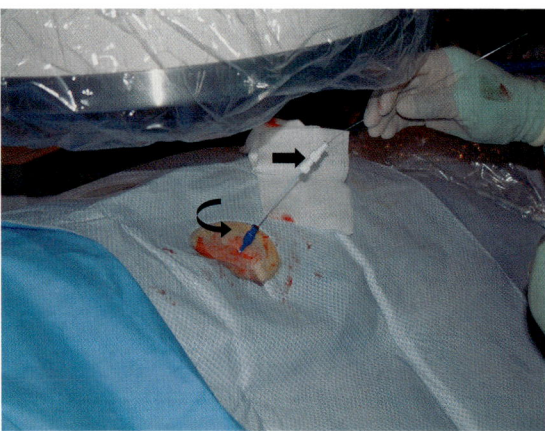

Fig. 6.6 **Using an 0.018" system for the definitive puncture, a transitional dilator system needs to be used to allow subsequent conversion to 0.035" diameter wires.** This is achieved using a three part dilator. The 6.5 Fr outer sheath is seen at the skin surface (curved arrow), its tip lying within the renal collecting system. The inner metal stiffener and plastic dilator are seen being drawn back over the 0.018" wire (straight arrow). Once removed an 0.035" wire can be introduced

dle (Accustick II Introducer System, Boston Scientific/Medi-Tech, France). After aspiration of a small amount of urine for culture, the system can be opacified and distended with dilute ionic contrast and carbon dioxide (CO_2).

The CO_2 will float on top of the urine in the prone patient, preferentially filling the posterior calyces, thus allowing calyceal puncture under fluoroscopic control. Iodinated contrast mixes only slowly with urine and often poorly outlines or fails completely to show the posterior calyces. CO_2 is preferred to room air, in case of inadvertent vascular injection.

The Dilated System

In this more common scenario a posterior calyx can be punctured under direct ultrasound control, urine aspirated for culture, and the system opacified, and then the procedure continued under subsequent fluoroscopic guidance.

Definitive access to the posterior calyx in either scenario can be achieved using either a Kellet-type 19-gauge needle, a 22-guage Chiba or Accustick needle.

Using an 19-Gauge Needle (Kellett-Type Needle)

Once the needle is in the calyx, the trochar is withdrawn. A 0.035" diameter wire can then be passed through the outer plastic dilator and coiled in the collecting system. Usually an intermediate stiffness wire is used, for example, a Coons (Cook, Europe) wire. At this point the track is dilated to 8 French (Fr) and a locking pigtail inserted, coiled, and locked in place.

Using a 22-Gauge Needle

Some operators prefer to perform the definitive puncture with a 22-gauge Chiba needle. Once within the calyx, a platinum-tipped 0.018" wire can be coiled within the collecting system. A three-part coaxial "dilator" is then placed over the 0.018" wire. The inner metal stiffener and cannula are removed.

The outer section in this system has a lumen wide enough to accept both the 0.018" wire and a 0.035" wire. A 0.035" wire is coiled in the collecting system along with the 0.018" wire. The outer cannula is carefully removed over both wires, to avoid dislodging the wires. The 0.018" wire is either removed or clipped to one side as a safety wire. This latter option is useful in difficult punctures in order to limit renal trauma. The nephrostomy insertion then proceeds as above with track dilatation and nephrostomy tube insertion over the 0.035" wire. The 0.035" wire is the last item removed (Fig. 6.**6**).

There is no clear evidence to suggest one technique is better than the other. One study comparing the two showed a reduction in the number of needle passes in the 22-gauge (1.7 vs. 2.4) group but no difference in hematuria rates or success rates.[17]

Locking the drainage catheter, once inserted, provides improved security. The clinical team must know how to unlock it and not to use force if the drain will not withdraw on gentle traction when the time comes for removal.

Further fixation with proprietary drain fixation devices such as the Drain-Fix device (Maersk Medical, UK) or Molner disk is essential. Finally, the drainage catheter is best placed within a proprietary stoma-type drainage system (Convatec, UK), rather than directly attached to a bag. This avoids the scenario of inadvertent tube dislodgment due to a heavy drainage bag providing traction at one end allied to natural patient movement overnight (Fig. 6.**7**).

Primary Antegrade Ureteric Stenting

Ureteric stenting is often performed as a two-stage procedure. This may allow the edema following nephrostomy in an obstructed ureter to subside, making subsequent stenting easier. With modern catheter and guidewire technology, many patients can be successfully stented at the time of nephrostomy. This approach was successful in 80% of ureteric obstructions in a recent study.[18] Emergency patients were not included in this study.

Insertion of an antegrade ureteric stent requires manipulation of a wire down the ureter into the bladder. Often a hydrophilic wire of sufficient stiffness will be required. Generally a stiff-angled hydrophilic wire

(Radiofocus, Guidewire M, Terumo Corporation, Tokyo) is manipulated together with a Biliary Manipulation Catheter (Torcon Blue Catheter, Cook, Europe) The angled tips of both wire and catheter allow steerage. Generally, even tight stenoses can be crossed by "helicoptering" the wire and gently advancing the tip until it passes through any stenoses. The use of a torque device to grip the wire is often necessary to gain enough purchase on the slippery hydrophilic wire. Opacification of the ureter can be helpful.

Once the Biliary Manipulation Catheter is confidently in the bladder, the hydrophilic wire is exchanged for a sufficiently stiff wire, for example an Amplatz extra or superstiff wire (Amplatz extrastiff/superstiff guidewire, Boston Scientific, Medi-Tech, France).

A peel-away sheath is required at this point to safeguard access to the kidney and reduce friction. The sheath chosen should be 1 Fr larger than the intended stent size. Usually this means 9 Fr. The tip of the peel-away is placed within the collecting system.

Many of the stents come with a thread passed through the proximal draining side holes to allow positioning of the stent if the stent is advanced too far. It is important to prevent the thread wrapping around either itself or the proximal end of the stent. Failure to do this can make retrieving the thread difficult (Fig. 6.8).

In addition to the thread, the stents have a central stiffener and a "pusher" to allow insertion of the proximal stent into the collecting system.

The insertion proceeds thus:
- The stent is inserted until the distal end lies within the bladder
- The guidewire and stiffener are withdrawn to allow the distal pigtail to form in the bladder
- The wire and stiffener are further withdrawn to allow the proximal pigtail to start forming in the renal pelvis
- Keeping the pusher apposed to the end of the stent, the wire and stiffener are withdrawn to allow the pig to fully form. Gentle forward pressure on the pusher can aid in helping to fully form this (Fig. 6.9)

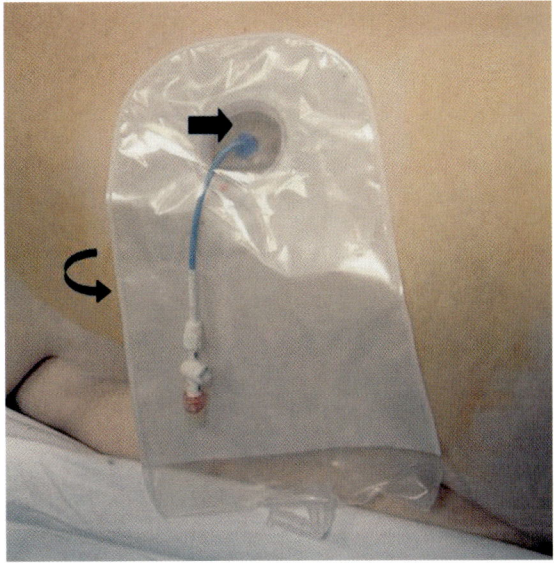

Fig. 6.7 **Stoma bag with nephrostomy.** The nephrostomy is retained with a Molner disk (straight arrow) sutured to the skin. The nephrostomy drains into a standard "stoma" bag that is not attached to the nephrostomy but to the skin (curved arrow). This minimizes the risk of inadvertent nephrostomy removal

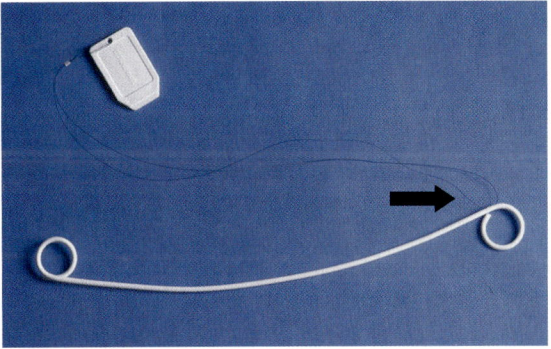

Fig. 6.8 **Ureteric stent with retraction suture.** The majority of stents come with a "thread" (arrow) through the upper pigtail to allow retraction during placement. These need to be untangled on insertion to facilitate easy removal at the end of the procedure

In extremely tight strictures an angioplasty balloon may be used to allow sufficient space for passage of the stent (Fig. 6.10).

Ideally, if a stent can be placed without causing significant hematuria, then a covering nephrostomy will not be needed. This approach should be aimed for if possible in appropriate cases. Heavy hematuria will preclude this approach.

The use of a standard 22-cm, 8-Fr double pigtail stent in most patients (ureteral stent system, Boston Scientific/Medi-Tech, France) is satisfactory. More accurate length sizing can be achieved with a bent wire technique if it is felt this is necessary. With this technique, a guidewire is passed with its tip at the point where you wish the distal end of the stent to lie. The wire is bent at the skin surface. The wire is then withdrawn until the tip lies where you wish the proximal end of the stent to lie, and bent again at the skin surface. The distance between the two kinks can be measured with a ruler to allow accurate sizing. This is rarely, if ever, required.

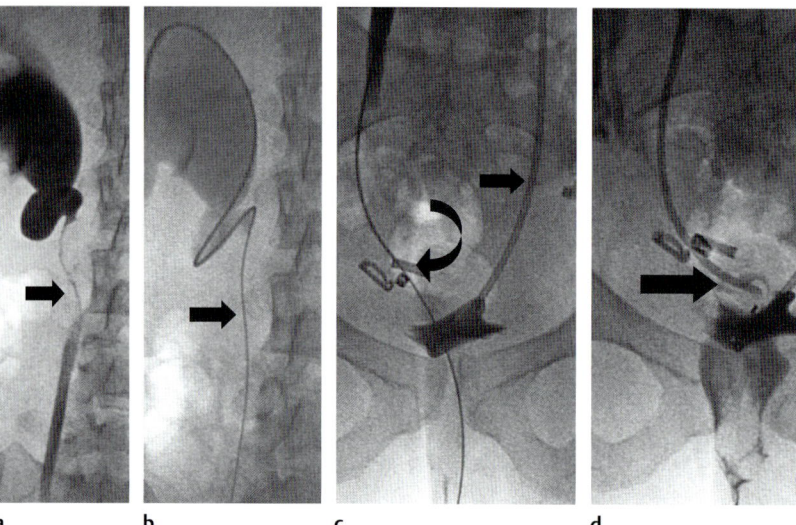

Fig. 6.9 **Stages of a ureteric stent insertion. a** Proximal ureteric stricture (straight arrow). **b** Hydrophilic wire manipulated past stricture (straight arrow). **c** Wire passed down into and through bladder, after snaring. Note left-sided stent already in situ (straight arrow) and sterilization clips (curved arrow). **d** Distal stent curled in bladder (straight arrow) after removal of wire and stiffener

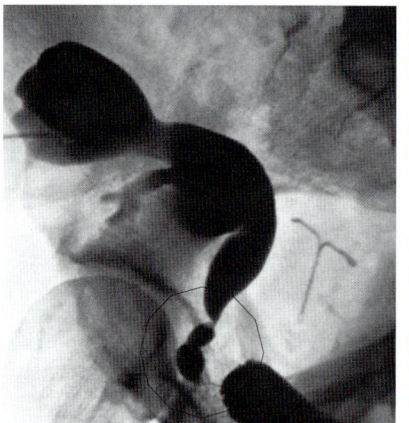
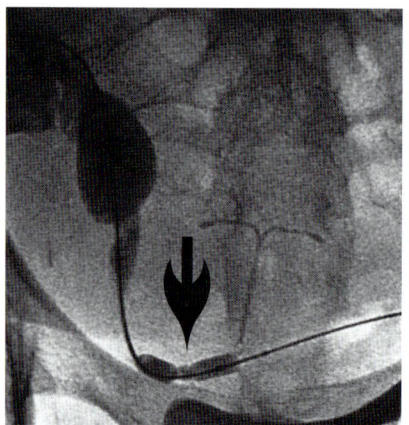

Fig. 6.**10 Tight twin transplant ureteric stricture (circled).** An angioplasty balloon (arrow) to open the strictures enough to allow subsequent passage of a ureteric stent. (From: Moss JG, Edwards R. Interventional Radiology and the Transplant Kidney. In: Ultrasound of Abdominal Transplantation. Stuttgart. New York: Thieme:2002:57. Reprinted by permission)

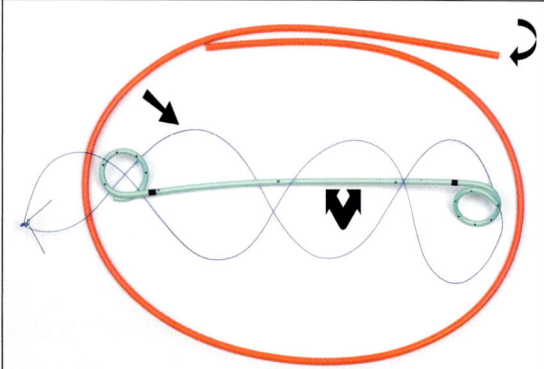

Fig. 6.**11 Shorter transplant stent (bifurcated arrow) with ethilon suture** (straight arrow) **and pusher** (curved arrow). (From: Moss JG, Edwards R. Interventional Radiology and the Transplant Kidney. In: Ultrasound of Abdominal Transplantation. Stuttgart. New York: Thieme:2002:58. Reprinted by permission)

Transplant Kidneys

A few specific features pertinent to transplant kidneys should be mentioned. In particular the operator should be aware of the very high value of the transplant kidney to the renal patient. The patient must be aware of the risks to the transplant kidney, as well as the benefits, of any procedures. A team approach involving transplant surgeon, nephrologist, and interventional radiologist is best suited in the decision-making process.

It is important in the transplant to choose an appropriate calyx for puncture in apposition to help minimize the radiation dose to the operator's hand, avoiding scar tissue, and to facilitate easy stent insertion if this is required. Direct renal pelvis puncture should be avoided.

Specific transplant stents are available and should be used. They are shorter and generally of a slightly smaller caliber. Again, primary stenting is desirable if possible. These transplant stents come without attached threads. This can be added by using a length of ethilon suture as shown (Fig. 6.**11**).

Follow-up

Immediate follow-up of patients who have had a nephrostomy should include a period of close observation for 8–12 hours. The drainage bag should also be inspected regularly to detect heavy hematuria or frank bleeding, as well as to avoid early tube blockage. It is worth providing the ward with a printed form with instructions on observation frequency, instructions on how and when to flush the catheter, an explanation of the locking mechanism, and a contact number in the radiology department.

Those patients with a significant infection burden prior to the procedure are best managed in an intermediate/high-dependency nursing unit, as subsequent decompensation can be rapid. Communication directly with the nursing and medical staff is useful in the management of problems.

Long-term nephrostomy should be avoided if at all possible. If a ureteric stent is impossible to place or continually malfunctions, a subcutaneous extra-anatomical stent should be considered.

Complications

The SCVIR has developed and published a set of quality guidelines regarding complications from nephrostomy; these include threshold rates above which your technique should be re-examined.[15]
- 98–99% technical success
- Hemorrhage in < 4% of cases
- Hemorrhage requiring embolization < 1% of cases
- Pleural transgression/nontarget organ puncture 0.1%

Tackling hemorrhage following nephrostomy can require a variety of techniques depending on the clinical scenario. Bleeding from the tract can often be stopped by insertion of a tube at least 2 Fr sizes larger.[19] Hemorrhage caused by segmental artery injury sometimes requires angiography and selective embolization.

Nephrostomy catheter dislodgment and blockage are both complications that can occur following tube insertion. Primary stenting when possible will remove these problems.

If a nephrostomy is dislodged, often a hydrophilic guidewire can be manipulated along the track into the collecting system. The chance of success diminishes with short initial dwell times.

Blocked nephrostomy tubes can be managed by sliding a peel-away sheath over the catheter into the collecting system and then exchanging for a fresh pigtail.

> **Summary points:**
> - Is the nephrostomy necessary?
> - Has a urologist seen the patient? Is a retrograde approach really impossible?
> - Very few nephrostomies need to be performed out of hours
> - Make sure you have the necessary support staff and equipment
> - Remember preassessment and postprocedure care are vital

Drainage of Perinephric Collections

In the transplant kidney a number of different fluid collections can accumulate, including:
- Hematoma
- Seroma
- Lymphocele
- Urinary collections
- Infected collections

Small hematomas, seromas, and lymphoceles are common postoperatively and generally do not require drainage unless they compromise graft function or cause significant symptoms. Most often these collections can be managed expectantly with serial ultrasound and clinical follow-up.

Enlarging collections which cause obstruction or infected collections will require drainage. Either Seldinger or "single-stab" drains can be used. Due to the close proximity to the kidney many operators will feel safer using the Seldinger approach.

A sufficiently large bore drain is required in viscous collections, usually 12–16 Fr and sometimes more than one drain if the collection is septated.

Special mention should be made of urine leaks. These most commonly occur due to anastomotic breakdown. Early leaks will generally be accompanied by pain, swelling, or fluid leak through the scar. Confirmation can be performed via isotope scanning, which will show isotope outside the collecting system or ureter. Lymphoceles too can be difficult to manage. If persistent, they can require instillation of ethanol into the cavity or surgical marsupialization.

In the native kidney, percutaneous drainage is usually reserved for infected perinephric or intrarenal collections. Confirmation using contrast-enhanced computed tomography (CECT) is useful.

The dimensions of these collections is important, with some evidence suggesting that collections of < 3–5 cm can be managed with intensive antibiotic therapy alone.[20] Ultimately, the clinical status of the patient will help determine which approach to take. The previously detailed points regarding drain size and approach are relevant.

Follow-up

Aftercare is important. Immediate follow-up is as for a nephrostomy. In addition, the drain should be flushed with 5 mL of saline every six hours following insertion. This will maintain side-hole patency. A contrast study should also be performed prior to removal to exclude fistulous connections and to confirm shrinkage of the cavity space. Prior to removal a repeat ultrasound to confirm resolution should be performed. If there is any doubt, the drain should be clamped and ultrasound performed after 24 hours before removal.

> **Summary points:**
> - Asymptomatic perinephric collections are common posttransplantation
> - A "wait-and-see" approach can be taken with most collections
> - In renal transplants urine leaks generally require surgical repair
> - Nephrostomy as a temporizing measure can be useful
> - Lymphoceles may be difficult to manage percutaneously
> - Small renal abscesses in native kidneys can be managed conservatively in some patients

Ultrasound-Guided Renal Biopsy

Renal biopsy is utilized in two main clinical scenarios: In the presence of a solid renal mass and in diffuse renal disease to allow characterization.

The general principles of ultrasound needle guidance apply. The use of color Doppler can avoid potentially catastrophic biopsy of vascular abnormalities.

In general, two classes of biopsy needle are available: hand-driven and automated. A hand-driven 14-gauge trucut needle was previously often used in diffuse renal disease. However, in the last decade automated cutting needles have replaced these and are now the norm. These automatic needles have several advantages, specifically, less crush artifact of the biopsy specimen, less time spent in kidney tissue, and less risk of laceration. They are also easier to train individuals to use.[21] Most parenchymal biopsies are now acceptably performed with a 16-gauge needle at many centers.

Preparation is as previously described in the Sections Principles of Ultrasound Guided Procedures and Patient Preparation. Traditionally the patient is positioned prone with a pillow under the midriff. Sedation can often be avoided. If using a needle-guide system, then an oblique position can be used equally effectively. Mention should be made of the abnormal platelet function in renal failure. If the patient has significant renal failure, an assessment of platelet function can be made via the bleeding time and abnormalities corrected via infusion of cryoprecipitate or desmopressin.

Specific contraindications include polycystic kidneys, active renal infection, and coagulopathy.

Problems arise with automated needles in the transplant kidney. Most automated needles once positioned have an additional "throw" of 1–2 cm. In the superficial transplant this can make positioning the needle difficult on occasion. In this scenario, one of the proprietary "nonadvancing" systems can be used.

Renal Mass Biopsy

The occurrence of indeterminate renal masses discovered as incidental findings is likely to increase as the use of abdominal cross-sectional imaging becomes more prevalent. In clearly malignant masses or simple cysts a biopsy is not necessary. In those with borderline imaging features an accurate biopsy can be useful in allowing appropriate management. This approach is particularly useful in frail patients, in whom unnecessary surgery carries a significant risk.

Those with other primary malignancies who will benefit from radiation or chemotherapy for metastases to the kidney rather than surgery for a renal primary are another group in whom the argument for image-guided biopsy is compelling.

How accurate and how safe is image-guided biopsy? Wood et al. biopsied 79 renal masses with no major complications.[22] Caoili et al. carried out biopsies using only ultrasound in 26 patients with renal mass lesions.[23] They used an 18-gauge system with the outer coaxial sheath guided to the periphery of the mass, with a 100% specificity and sensitivity, for malignancy.

In biopsy of suspected lymphoma, a 14–16-gauge needle should be used to allow a sufficiently large diagnostic sample.

Diffuse Renal Disease Biopsy

Most biopsies for diffuse renal disease are performed by renal physicians.

Song et al. studied the use of 18-gauge vs. 14-gauge cutting needles.[24] The smaller 18-gauge needle generated an equally high quality of specimen. Major hemorrhagic complications occurred in around 3% of cases with no significant difference between the two. Tang et al. confirmed this concordance in complication rate between the two needle sizes.[25] Many centers use a 16-gauge needle (Fig. 6.**12**).

The lower pole is preferred in the native kidney due to its superficial location and distance from the renal pelvis and main vessels. In general two cortical cores are required to generate sufficient tissue for light immunofluorescence and electron microscopy. Ideally the specimen should be checked by microscopy to confirm sufficient tissue is present.[21]

Follow-up

Careful follow-up for at least eight hours is required.

> **Summary points:**
> - Coaxial systems allow multiple renal biopsies through a single track
> - Biopsy of indeterminate renal mass lesions is safe and accurate
> - In diffuse disease an 18-gauge cutting needle is large enough
> - Cortical tissue is the target in diffuse disease and generally two cores will be required to obtain enough tissue

Renal Artery Stenosis

Ultrasound in the diagnosis of renal artery stenosis (RAS) is outperformed by magnetic resonance imaging (MRI) and CECT.[26] Consequently this section on RAS will be brief.

In the native kidney atherosclerotic RAS and fibromuscular dysplasia (FMD) are the two main causes. In the transplant, the cause is often multifactorial and can occur in up to 30% of patients, although on average the incidence is 10–15%.

Indications for treatment in atherosclerotic RAS include poorly-controlled hypertension, worsening renal function, and flash pulmonary edema.

The development of stent technology has led to most atherosclerotic stenoses in the native kidney being treated via primary stenting. Although primary stenting is associated with a better technical outcome than balloon angioplasty, the clinical outcomes are not dissimilar. FMD responds well to angioplasty alone.

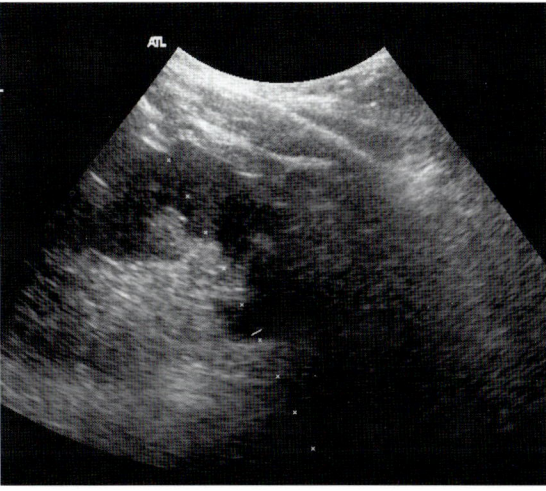

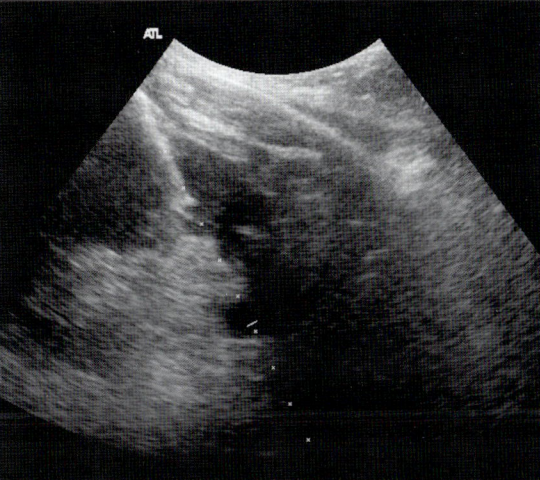

Fig. 6.**12 a** Ultrasound scan of a renal biopsy for suspected renal parenchymal disease using a needle guide. The tip of the needle is seen to lie on the surface of the kidney. The 16-gauge biopsy needle is fired (**b**) and the needle is seen to traverse the parenchyma

Technical Considerations

A detailed explanation is beyond the scope of this chapter. Several brief points can be made regarding stent deployment. Most operators use balloon-mounted stents, allowing more accurate placement, in ostial stenoses. A guiding catheter allows protected passage from the groin (or arm) to the renal ostium.

Many of the commercially available balloon-mounted stents now come in an 0.018" delivery system allowing placement in tight lesions. Rapid-exchange "monorail" systems are also useful, allowing the use of shorter guidewires (Fig. 6.**13**).

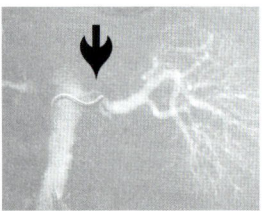 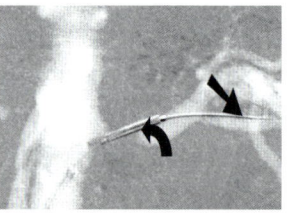 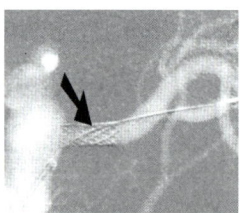

a b c

Fig. 6.13 **Deployment of a balloon-mounted renal stent.** CO_2 was used as contrast to avoid any possibility of iodinated contrast-induced nephropathy. **a** Initial image shows a tight left RAS. A Sos-Omni catheter is seen located in the ostium of the renal artery (arrow). **b** A balloon-mounted stent (curved arrow) has been passed across the stenosis on an 0.018" wire (straight arrow). **c** The balloon-mounted stent is fully open (straight arrow) and the renal artery now widely patent

Results

As mentioned above, technical success in stenting is good. Typically abolition of the stenosis occurs in 90% or more of cases.[28] Clinically the results are less definitive. Decisions regarding the need for treatment should be made in conjunction with the appropriate nephrology and surgical teams.

> **Summary points:**
> - MRI is more accurate than ultrasound in RAS
> - Renal artery angioplasty ± stenting is useful in atherosclerotic RAS

Use of Ultrasound in Radiofrequency Ablation in the Kidney

Walther et al. piloted radiofrequency (RF) ablation in the kidney in 2000. Their study evaluated the safety of the technique on a series of four patients suffering from Von Hippel–Lindau syndrome or papillary renal cell carcinoma.[29] Suspected neoplastic lesions were evaluated with intraoperative ultrasound before being treated with RF energy.

Renal function was preserved and no complications were encountered. With these results the way was opened and a number of centers began treating renal cell carcinoma with RF ablation.

Several follow-up studies[3–5] have now been produced, specifically those of Gervais et al., Mayo-Smith et al. and Farrell et al.[3–5] These groups have performed a combined number of over 100 renal tumor ablations with up to 3.5 years follow-up.

Patient Selection

As yet there is no firm data regarding which patients should be treated with percutaneous ablation and who should undergo nephron-sparing surgery. A rough consensus in the literature is beginning to emerge, however, and lesions considered would generally be < 5 cm in diameter.

These include those patients with suspected renal carcinoma who have contraindications to surgery, or have refused surgery. Some investigators have also included patients with prior nephrectomy and those with VHL requiring multiple treatments. In addition, a life expectancy longer than one year is desirable given the relatively slow growth, especially of smaller renal cell carcinomas.

Clinical Preparation and Assessment

Most of the patients can be treated as outpatients as evidenced by the three recent papers. Preassessment is necessary to identify coagulopathy and other relevant pathology. An overnight bed should be available should complications arise. Antibiotics have been safely avoided in all three large studies.

Sedation and intraprocedural monitoring as previously described are used. Some operators will use general anesthesia.

Technical Considerations

A full coverage of the subject is available in two review articles.[30,31]

RF ablation works by depositing energy within a targeted focus. The mechanism of heat generation in RF ablation relates to radiowave energy at a needle electrode trying to reach a ground point. Resistance in the tissue around this generates heat. The ground point can be either a series of pads, usually on the patient's thighs (unipolar electrode), or a proximal point of the electrode (so-called bipolar electrode).

Regardless of the technique used to deliver heat to the target, several generalizations can be made.

Cellular homeostasis is maintained up to around 40 °C. From 42–45 °C cells become more susceptible to additional insults or therapy, for example chemotherapy or radiation. At 46 °C for 60 minutes, irreversible cytotoxicity occurs, and times shorten with incremental increases in temperature. Thus four to six minutes at 50–52 °C is satisfactory and almost instant cell death occurs from 60–100 °C. Above 105 °C tissue charring occurs which can result in a surrounding "eschar," together with tissue boiling and gas production, both of which limit further effective energy deposition. Effective temperatures thus range from 50–100 °C (Fig. 6.14).

The main limiting factor in thermal ablation is the maximum treatable volume.

The design of ablation machines and needles has evolved gradually to allow treatment of increased volumes. Increased energy deposition has been facilitated by the development of umbrella electrodes and others with multiple tines. Internal cooling of electrodes allows a greater volume of tissue to be treated by preventing that portion of the lesion adjacent to the electrode from boiling. Pulsing in RF ablation achieves similar effects by alternating bursts of high and low energy pulses, allowing greater deposition of mean energy (Fig. 6.15).

Reduction of heat loss by utilizing the natural anatomy of renal tumors is a useful strategy. Most renal tumors are exophytic and as a result surrounded by an insulating layer of perinephric fat. These lesions benefit from this "oven" effect described by Livraghi et al. in 1999.[32]

Strategies are also available to reduce heat loss by convection. In vivo, blood flow causes a marked heat-sink effect. In the liver, strategies aimed at reducing portal vein blood flow have been performed surgically and angiographically. This is facilitated by the dual hepatic blood supply. More realistically, in the kidney this knowledge can be used to select vulnerable intraparenchymal and exophytic lesions, which are not cooled by a high flow central blood supply.

Target temperatures vary with manufacturer and operator. Some investigators aim for 50 °C[5] and others up to 105 °C.[4] Impedance can also be used to guide duration of therapy, with a low-impedance pattern suggesting incomplete ablation.[3]

Anatomical Considerations

An increasing size of renal tumor correlates with an increased likelihood of requirement for multiple ablations.[5] If a large tumor has a component in the renal sinus, treatment is more likely to fail.[4]

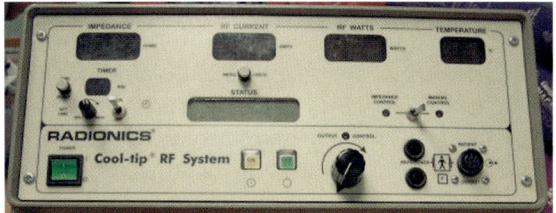

Fig. 6.**14** An RF energy generator

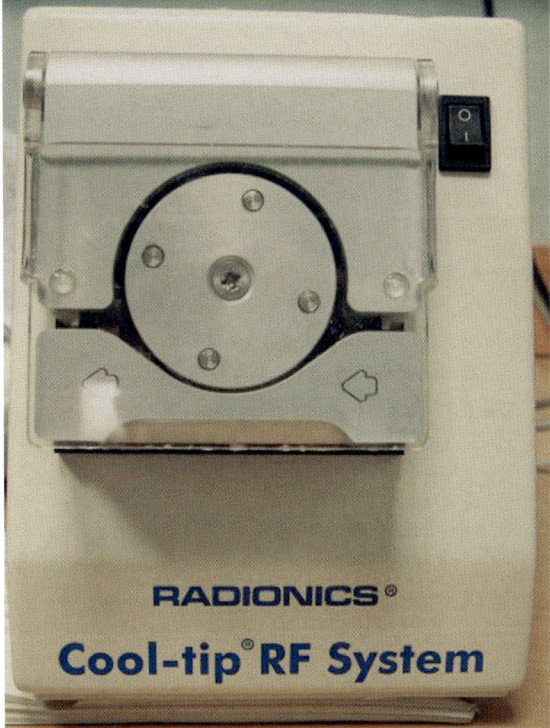

Fig. 6.**15 Pump to allow coolant circulation through ablation needle tip.** This is one of several strategies to allow ablation of larger volumes

Approach through the psoas in three patients in the Farrell et al.[3] study was associated with neuropathic pain in branches of the lumbar plexus (formed in the psoas muscle from the anterior rami of four upper lumbar nerves) and now heating the psoas muscle is avoided.[3]

Gervais encountered a single ureteric stricture when treating a lower-pole tumor[4] and care should be exercised in cases such as these.

Procedural Image Guidance

Groups have used a variety of ultrasound, CT, and MRI and combinations thereof to guide treatment. Investigators claim a variety of technical and practical advantages for each modality.

With regard to ultrasound, advantages include portability, low cost, almost universal availability, general familiarization with technique, and the ability to view real-time images during needle electrode placement. Disadvantages specific to renal neoplastic ablation include difficulty clearly delineating adjacent gas-filled structures (i.e., ascending and descending colon) and problems with visualization of the lesion if needle-tip gas production occurs. The choice of modality will often depend on operator preference.

Postprocedural Imaging

Follow-up is almost exclusively performed via CECT or if creatinine levels are raised, MR with intravenous gadolinium. Most centers use one-, three-, and 6-monthly follow-up scans and define success as lack of or minimal (< 10 HU) enhancement.

Complications

Out of 86 patients treated in the three studies mentioned above, 11 developed complications. There were three perinephric hematomas, which required no treatment. One patient developed a single skin metastasis at the site of percutaneous needle entry. This was resected. Two patients developed gross hematuria, both requiring urinary catheterisation. Finally, the three psoas complications and ureteric stricture mentioned above also occurred.

Success

A high rate of radiographic success was achieved. Mayo-Smith managed to ablate 31 out of 32 tumors. One patient refused a second treatment. Farrell's group had complete ablation at the time of writing, but all of the tumors were exophytic. Gervais had similar experience with exophytic tumors. Large tumors with sinus components faired poorly, with initial success only five out of 11 treatments.

Conclusions

RF ablation shows promise and is very attractive given the ability to treat patients on a day-case basis. Despite some limited long-term follow-up, at present, robust longitudinal data regarding tumor recurrence and patient outcome is as yet unavailable. Direct comparison with nephron-sparing surgery and alternative ablative technologies is also unavailable and controversy also exists regarding the outcome of small neoplasms in elderly patients. Thus despite very encouraging preliminary results the technique remains as yet unproven.

> **Summary points:**
> - RF ablation is a new technique for the treatment of renal tumors
> - As yet it is reserved mainly for those with contraindications to surgery or other specific indications
> - Early data shows promising results
> - A variety of different commercial RF ablation kits are available
> - Long-term data and comparison between RF ablation and surgery are, as yet, unavailable

Trauma and Emergencies

Renal Tract Trauma[33]

Trauma to the urinary tract can be either conventional or iatrogenic. In the West iatrogenic injury is by far the most common and is related to procedures such as renal biopsy, nephrostomy (Fig. 6.**16**)/nephrolithotomy,

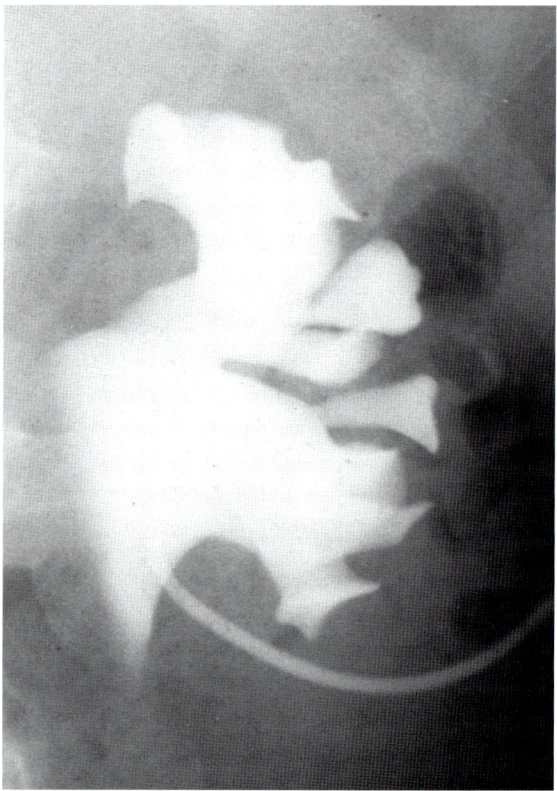

Fig. 6.**16 Nephrostogram showing a direct pelvic puncture.** This should be avoided as it risks major vessel damage

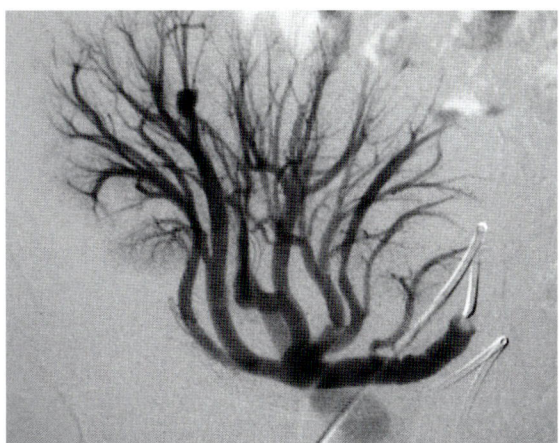
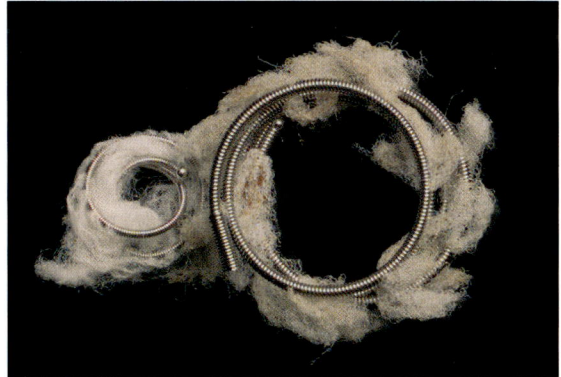
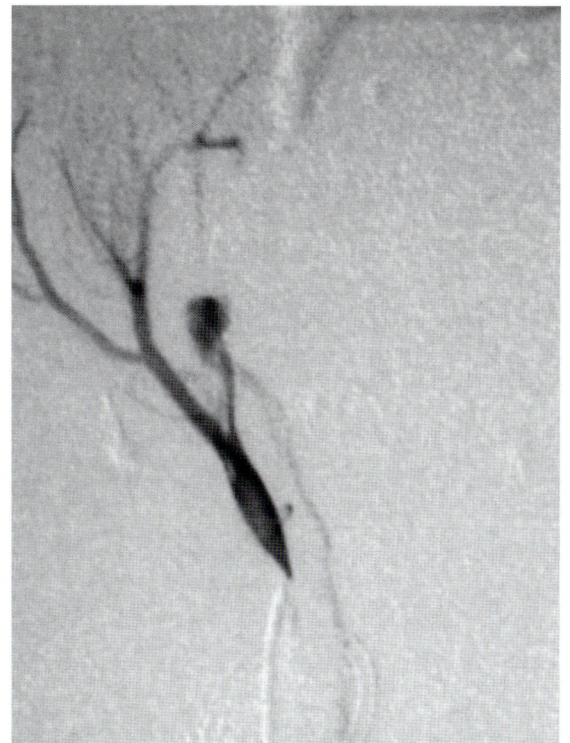
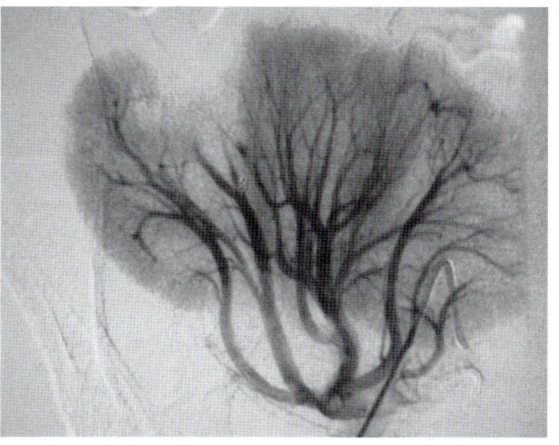

Fig. 6.17 **a** Angiogram of a renal transplant with an AVF. **b** A superselective study shows a coaxial catheter in situ through which the coils are delivered. Following coil placement (**c**) the final angiogram demonstrates successful closure of the fistula, but a small renal infarct has occurred (**d**)

instrumentation of the urinary tract, and ureteric injury during abdominal surgery. Although many of these injuries are self-limiting, others will require prompt intervention, which is increasingly done by a minimally invasive approach. The same rules apply to conventional trauma, although the approach will depend on the presence or absence of other injuries.

Renal Vascular Injuries

- Arteriovenous and arteriocalyceal fistulae
- Major pedicle disruption
- Main renal artery perforation

The vast majority of these injuries complicate renal biopsy and occur in up to 10% of cases. They are commonly seen on Doppler ultrasound, which offers an excellent method for surveillance. Provided the patient is not bleeding, suffering renal compromise, or intractable hypertension, the vast majority of arteriovenous fistulae (AVFs) can be treated conservatively and will close spontaneously. The remainder should be occluded by coil embolisation.[34] The technique using small-caliber coaxial systems has improved over the years, although it should be remembered that loss of a small amount of renal tissue is an inevitable consequence of embolization (Fig. 6.17). Open or closed conventional vascular injuries such as a sharp penetrating wound are treated in the same way. Major vascular pedicle

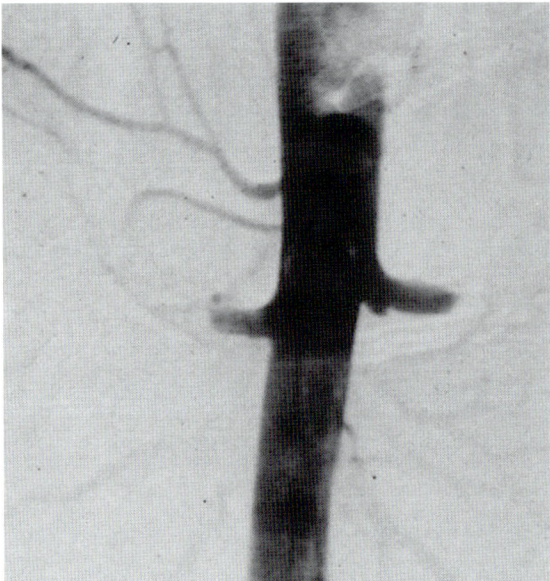

Fig. 6.**18 Aortogram of a patient who suffered major trauma.** Both renal arteries have been avulsed. (Kindly supplied by Dr. J. Tibballs, Royal Free Hospital, London, UK)

injury (Fig. 6.**18**) is a serious injury which requires open surgery and the kidney is all too often irremediably ischemic and lost.

Occasionally the main renal artery is ruptured during a renal angioplasty or stenting procedure. Although a major complication, and previously requiring salvage surgery, the vast majority can nowadays be rescued using an endovascular approach: either prolonged balloon tamponade or placement of a stent-graft (Fig. 6.**19**).

Pelvicalyceal and Ureteric Injuries

Again iatrogenic mechanisms predominate here, with an increase in the use of endourological techniques to deal with calculus disease in particular. In general the pelvicalyceal system and ureters when disrupted will almost always heal naturally, provided any obstruction is relieved and infection or disease such as cancer can be dealt with. All that is often required is a temporary nephrostomy plus possible percutaneous drainage of a urinoma. Ureteric trauma management will depend on the nature and mechanism of injury. Clearly a ligated ureter will almost always require a surgical solution, although we have occasionally embolized the main renal artery in patients unfit for surgery. Although this will infarct the kidney, it can be useful in critically ill elderly patients with advanced disease provided the other kidney is functioning.

A disrupted ureter can often be stented and this may require a combined approach from the urethra retro-

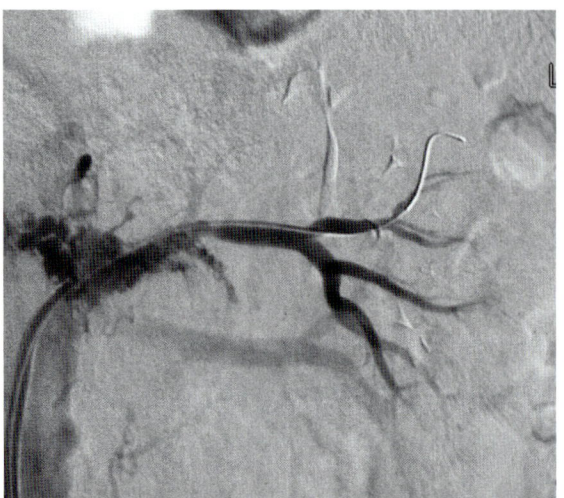

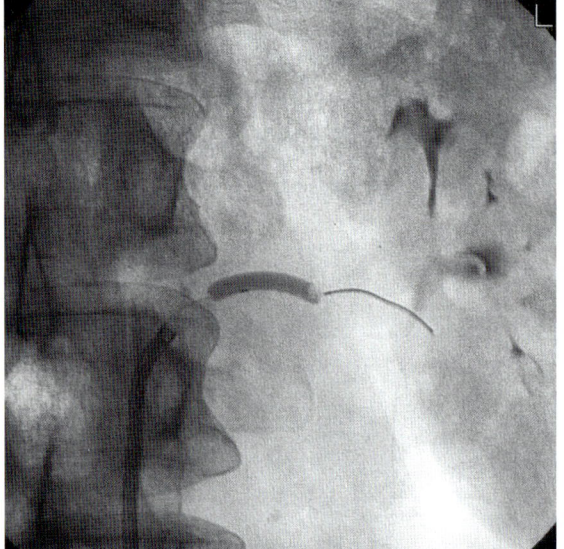

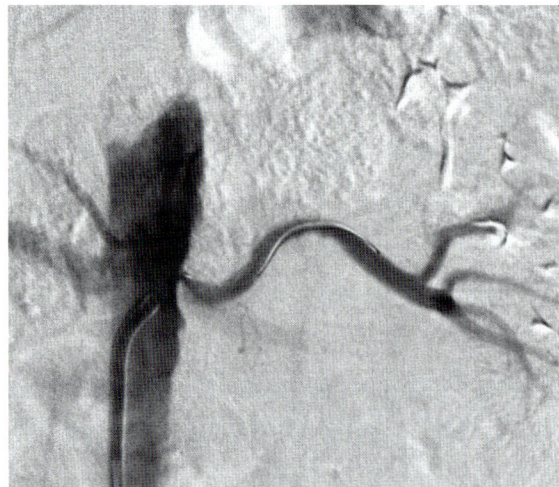

Fig. 6.**19 Patient undergoing a left renal angioplasty. a** Following balloon dilatation there is rupture of the main renal artery. Immediate balloon tamponade for 10 minutes (**b**) sealed the perforation and the kidney was preserved. No surgery was required (**c**)

gradely and the kidney antegradely. Another option with a distally disrupted or ligated ureter is a ureteroneocystostomy where a sharp guide wire or trans-jugular intrahepatic porto systemic shund (TIPSS) needle set is used from an antegrade approach and simply forced into a distended contrast-filled bladder (Fig. 6.**20**). Once a guidewire is in the bladder a stent can then be placed. This technique should not replace a surgical reconstruction but is useful in those with co-morbidity.

Finally, an extra-anatomical stent should not be forgotten as an option in dealing with major ureteric damage. Again it should not replace surgical correction if that is possible, but it has a place in the severely ill co-morbid patient.

Ureteric and Bladder Injuries

Ureteric and bladder injuries are complex and beyond the remit of this chapter. Most are due to pelvic fractures or blunt perineal trauma. Although it used to be said that the traumatized urethra should not be instrumented, this can now be done very atraumatically using angiographic skills and equipment under fluoroscopic guidance. Again a dual approach may be necessary using a suprapubic catheter and establishing a through and through wire prior to placement of a urethral urinary catheter to act as a splint.

Priapism

A priapism is a medical emergency and if not dealt with promptly leads to irreversible damage and fibrosis in the corpora. The cause can be venous or arterial in origin. If arterial in nature and when conventional pharmacological methods fail, there is a role for arterial embolization of the penile arteries. In the presence of trauma an offending arterial connection to the corpora can often be embolized.

Other Urogenital Emergencies

Occasionally other conditions will present as emergencies in the urogenital tract. Hemorrhage from an underlying cancer, particularly of the kidney, is very amenable to embolization. Chemotherapy-induced hemorrhagic cystitis again can be ameliorated by bilateral vesical artery embolization.

In conclusion, interventional radiological techniques have become firmly established in the treatment of many urogenital emergency situations. The techniques are still probably underused and should always be considered first before more invasive efforts are made.

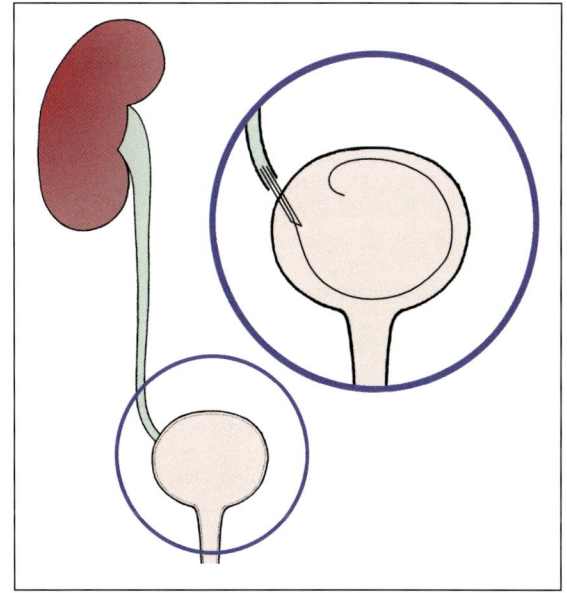

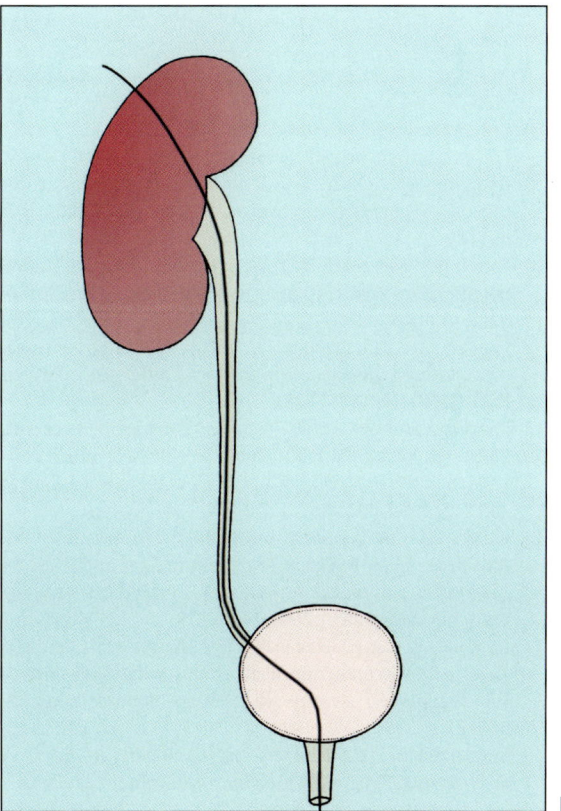

Fig. 6.**20 Technique of ureteroneocystostomy. a** A long-sheathed needle is placed antegradely across the occluded ureter into the prefilled bladder. **b** Once across, a guidewire is placed, followed by a plastic stent.

References

1. Dravid VS, Gupta A, Zegel HG, Morales AV, Rabinowitz B, Freiman DB. Investigation of antibiotic prophylaxis usage for vascular and nonvascular interventional procedures. J Vasc Interv Radiol 1998;9:401–6.
2. Gray RR, So CB, McLoughlin RF, Pugash RA, Saliken JC, Macklin NI. Outpatient percutaneous nephrostomy. Radiology 1996;198:85–8.
3. Farrell MA, Charboneau WJ, DiMarco DS et al. Imaging-guided radiofrequency ablation of solid renal tumors. Am J Roentgenol 2003;180:1509–13.
4. Gervais DA, McGovern FJ, Arellano RS, McDougal WS, Mueller PR. Renal cell carcinoma: clinical experience and technical success with radiofrequency ablation of 42 tumors. Radiology 2003;226:417–24.
5. Mayo-Smith WW, Dupuy DE, Parikh PM, Pezzullo JA, Cronan JJ. Imaging-guided percutaneous radiofrequency ablation of solid renal masses: techniques and outcomes of 38 treatment sessions in 32 consecutive patients. Am J Roentgenol 2003;180:1503–8.
6. Bailey PL, Moll JWB, Pace NL, East KA, Stanley KH. Respiratory effects of midazolam and fentanyl: potent interaction producing hypoxemia and apnea. Anesthesiology 1998;69:813.
7. NCEPOD. NCEPOD Interventional Vascular Radiology. 2000.
8. British Medical Association. Royal Pharmaceutical Society of Great Britain. British National Formulary. 2004.
9. Goodwin, WE, Casey, WC, Wolf, W. Percutaneous trocar (needle) nephrostomy in hydronephrosis. JAMA 1955;157:891–894.
10. Farrell TA, Hicks ME. A review of radiologically guided percutaneous nephrostomies in 303 patients. J Vasc Interv Radiol 1997;8:769–74.
11. Banner, MP, Ramchandani P, Pollack HM. Interventional procedures in the upper urinary tract. Cardiovasc Intervent Radiol 1991;14(5):267–284.
12. Shekkariz B, Shekkariz H, Upadhay J, Banerjee M, Becker H, Pontes JE, Wood DP, Jr. Outcome of palliative urinary diversion in the treatment of advanced malignancies. Cancer 1999;85:998–1003.
13. Kellett MJ. Interventional uroradiology. In: Grainger RG, Allison D, Adam A, Dixon AK, eds. Grainger and Allison's Diagnostic Radiology. A Textbook of Medical Imaging. Churchill Livingstone: 2001:1693–715.
14. Dyer RB, Regan JD, Kavanagh PV, Khatod EG, Chen MY, Zagoria RJ. Percutaneous nephrostomy with extensions of the technique: step-by-step. RadioGraphics 2002;22:503–25.
15. Ramchandani P, Cardella JF, Grassi CJ, Roberts AC, Sacks D, Schwartzberg MS, et al. Quality improvement guidelines for percutaneous nephrostomy. J Vasc Interv Radiol 2003;14:277–281.
16. Zegel HG, Pollack HM, Banner M, Goldberg BB, Arger PH, Mulhern C. et al. Percutaneous nephrostomy: comparison of sonographic and fluoroscopic guidance. Am J Roentgenol 1981;137:925–7.
17. Clark TWI, Clark MD, Abraham RJ, Fleming BK. Is routine micropuncture access necessary for percutaneous nephrostomy? A randomized trial. Can Assoc Radiol J 2002;53:87–91.
18. Watson GMT, Patel, U. Primary ureteric stenting: prospective experience and cost-efffectiveness analysis in 50 ureters. Clin Radiol 2001;56:568–74.
19. Millward SF. Percutaneous nephrostomy: a practical approach. J Vasc Interv Radiol 2000;11:955–64.
20. Dalla Palma L, Pozzi-Mucelli F, Ene V. Medical treatment of renal and perirenal abscesses: CT evaluation. Clin Radiol 1999;54:792–7.
21. Assessment of the patient with renal disease. In: Davison AM, Stewart Cameron J, Grünfeld J-P, Kerr DNS, ER, Winearls CQ, eds. Oxford Textbook of Nephrology. Oxford: Oxford University Press: 1997.
22. Wood BJ, Khan MA, McGovern F, Harisinghani M, Hahn PF, Mueller PR. Image-guided biopsy of renal masses: indications, accuracy and impact on clinical management. J Urol 1999;161:1470–4.
23. Caoili EM, Bude RO, Higgins EJ, Hoff DL, Nghiem HV. Evaluation of sonographically guided percutaneous core biopsy of renal masses. Am J Roentgenol 2002;179:373–8.
24. Song JH, Cronan JJ. Percutaneous biopsy in diffuse renal disease: comparison of 18- and 14-gauge automated biopsy devices. J Vasc Interv Radiol 1998;9:651–5.
25. Tang S, Li JHC, Lui SL, Chan TM, Cheng IKP, Lai KN. Freehand, ultrasound-guided percutaneous renal biopsy: experience from a single operator. Eur J Radiol 2002;41:65–9.
26. Vasbinder GB, Nelemans PJ, Kessels AGH, Kroon AA, de Leeuw PW, van Engelshoven JMA. Diagnostic Tests for renal artery stenosis in patients suspected of having renovascular hypertension: a meta-analysis. Ann Intern Med 2001;135:401–11.
27. Lee HY, Grant EG. Sonography in renovascular hypertension. J Ultrasound Med 2002;21:431–41.
28. Dorros G, Prince C, Mathiak D. Stenting of a renal artery stenosis achieves better relief of the obstructive lesion than baloon angioplasty. Cathet Cardiovasc Diagn 1993;29:191–8.
29. Walther MM, Shawker TH, Libutti SK, Lubensky I, Choyke PL, Venzon D, et al. A phase 2 study of radiofrequency interstitial tissue ablation of localised renal tumours. J Urol 2000;163:1427.
30. Goldberg SN, Gazelle GS, Mueller PR. Thermal ablation therapy for focal malignancy: a unified approach to underlying principles, techniques, and diagnostic imaging guidance. Am J Roentgenol 2000;174:323–31.
31. Goldberg SN, Dupuy DE. Image-guided radiofrequency tumor ablation: challenges and opportunities - Part I. J Vasc Interv Radiol 2001;12:1021–32.
32. Livraghi T, Goldberg SN, Lazzaroni S, Meloni F, Solbiati L, Gazelle GS. Small hepatocellular carcinoma: treatment with radiofrequency ablation versus ethanol injection. Radiology 1999;210:655–61.
33. Lang EK. Role of interventional radiology in emergency medicine. Emerg Radiol 1997;4(2):82–90.
34. Vignali C, Lonzi S, Bargellini I, et al. Vascular injuries after percutaneous renal procedures: treatment by transcatheter embolisation. Eur Radiol 2004;14(4): 723–729.

Section 2

Urology

7 The Urogenital Tract: Surgical Overview   89
8 Focal Lesions of the Kidney   102
9 Diseases of the Collecting System and Ureters   119
10 Diseases of the Bladder and Prostate   130
11 Diseases of the Testis and Epididymis   153
12 Diseases of the Penis, with Functional Evaluation   181
13 Oncological Management of Tumors of the Urogenital Tract   193

7 The Urogenital Tract: Surgical Overview

S. Chandrasekara, G. H. Muir

Introduction

The current chapter predominantly outlines the role of ultrasound, as well as other imaging modalities, in different urological clinical settings, emphasizing the urological surgeon's perception of the status of imaging in diagnosis and management.

Urinary Tract Infections

Urinary tract infections (UTIs) are a common urological problem, with the importance lying in the identification of those at risk of developing severe sequelae whilst avoiding investigation in patients with uncomplicated infections. Therefore it is useful to broadly divide UTIs into "uncomplicated" and "complicated," which dictates the extent of evaluation and the duration of treatment and also acts as an indicator of potential treatment failure (Table 7.**1**). UTIs are classified according to the dominant clinical symptom: Urethritis, cystitis, prostatitis, or pyelonephritis.[1] Clinical signs alone will not differentiate the site of the infection into an upper or lower urinary tract infection.[2] A UTI in a male patient is regarded as complicated, as in the young and the elderly male it is often associated with structural or outflow-related abnormalities. A UTI in a male patient between age 15 and 50 is uncommon.[1]

Uncomplicated Urinary Tract Infection

In females an uncomplicated UTI may be cystitis, urethritis, or pyelonephritis, with cystitis the most common. The UTI may be entirely asymptomatic or associated with symptoms of urgency, hesitancy, and pain. Common bacterial pathogens include *E. coli* (70–95%), *Staphylococcus saprophyticus*, *Proteus*, and *Klebsiella*. The probability of a UTI in a female patient is high, namely 20–35% between age 20 and 40, 10–20% of which may acquire recurrent uncomplicated infections.[1] Those patients with pyelonephritis in addition to cystitis have classical symptoms of fever, loin pain, and renal angle tenderness, but the absence of upper tract symptoms does not exclude pyelonephritis.

Table 7.1 **Factors that suggest a complicated urinary tract infection**

- Male gender
- Elderly
- Pregnancy
- Recent urinary tract infection
- Nosocomial infection
- Indwelling urinary catheter
- Recent antibiotic therapy
- Symptoms for more than seven days
- Functional or anatomical anomaly of the urinary tract
- Diabetes mellitus
- Immunosuppression

Complicated Urinary Tract Infection

Investigation beyond a posttreatment urine analysis is unnecessary for uncomplicated UTI. With acute, uncomplicated pyelonephritis, a white cell count, C-reactive protein, and blood cultures for bacteriology are necessary. An abdominal radiograph and ultrasound should be performed in both uncomplicated and complicated UTI. The plain radiograph may identify radio-opaque calculi or in rare instances demonstrate gas in the renal parenchyma, which is indicative of emphysematous pyelonephritis, or obliteration of the psoas muscle outline, a nonspecific sign of a perirenal abscess formation. An ultrasound examination is useful in excluding the presence of an abscess or pelvicalyceal obstruction. However, in some patients the upper urinary tract may be dilated in the absence of obstruction, attributed to "bacterial virulence factors."

Routine use of an intravenous urography (IVU) in uncomplicated UTI is not recommended as over 75% of patients will have a normal study.[3] However, if there is no clinical improvement within 72 hours of antibiotic therapy, further imaging is indicated. Computed tomography (CT) is the best option in such situations, as it offers greater anatomical detail of the renal parenchyma and the perirenal areas.

Emphysematous pyelonephritis is a rare, acute narcotizing condition caused by any "gas-forming" organism.[4] Diabetes mellitus, immunosuppression, urolithiasis, and renal tract obstruction are common predisposing conditions. These patients are often severely ill and may fail to respond to antibiotic therapy. Ultrasound and CT imaging are the most useful methods of

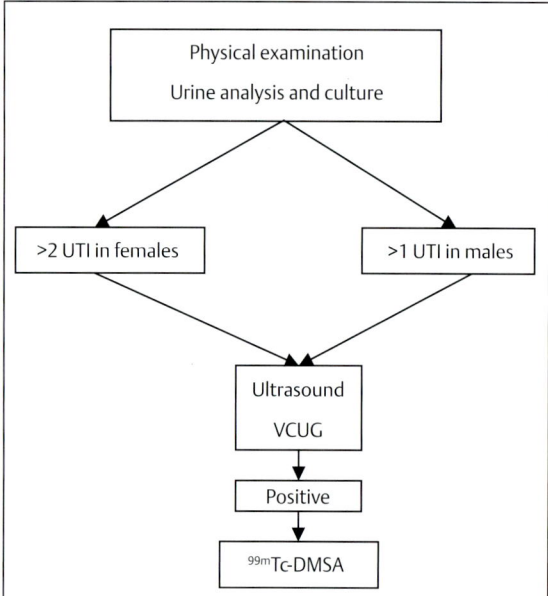

Fig. 7.1 **Investigation of a child with a urinary tract infection (UTI)**
(VCUG = voiding cystourethrography; ^{99m}Tc-DMSA = ^{99m}Tc-dimercaptosuccinic acid)

assessment, with CT imaging offering accurate anatomical detail, including areas of gas formation. Any perinephric infected fluid collection may be percutaneously drained under ultrasound guidance. There is a reported mortality rate of 50–60% in emphysematous pyelonephritis, with nephrectomy the only viable option for cure.[4]

Urinary Tract Infection in Children

UTIs are the commonest bacterial infection in children. Clinical presentation in the pediatric age group may be variable and would include failure to thrive, episodes of fever, vomiting, and dehydration.[1] Investigations are usually undertaken following the first episode of infection in male patients and following the second episode in female patients. The main objective of evaluating these patients is to exclude an underlying structural or functional anomaly that may be corrected. A diagnostic algorithm for the management of UTIs has been formulated by the European Association of Urology (Fig. 7.1).[1]

Ultrasound is the preferred imaging modality in the pediatric age group; there is the benefit of absence of ionizing radiation and adverse effects related to the use of iodinated contrast media. Ultrasound has been shown to be as accurate as IVU in detecting significant renal anomalies.[5,6]

In neonates and in children between age two and 18 years with a UTI, approximately 30% will have vesicoureteric reflux (VUR).[5] Male patients with VUR are likely to be diagnosed in infancy, whereas in female patients the diagnosis is delayed until between age two and eight years. Although VUR will resolve spontaneously in the majority of patients, UTI associated with reflux facilitates ascending infection, resulting in possible renal parenchyma cortical damage and resultant scarring. The recommended investigation for VUR in children less than age one year is a voiding cystourethrography using low-dose fluoroscopy. Indirect cystography, using either ^{99m}Tc-mercaptoacetyltriglycine (^{99m}Tc-MAG3) or ^{99m}Tc-diethylenetriamine pentaacetic acid (^{99m}Tc-DTPA) renography with reflux studies is a suitable option for older children.[1] Reflux may also be assessed using microbubble ultrasound contrast media, avoiding the use of ionizing radiation.[7] A ^{99m}Tc-dimercaptosuccinic acid (^{99m}Tc-DMSA) radioisotope scan is performed to identify renal scarring in those patients with VUR, as ultrasound is not as sensitive in the detection of renal parenchyma abnormalities.[1] The presence of renal scarring due to VUR is a relative indication for corrective surgery. This may, however, not necessarily prevent recurrence of lower UTIs. The role of IVU is limited to those who require greater anatomical detail of the upper renal tract.

Summary points:
- Divided into "uncomplicated" and "complicated" which dictates extent of evaluation and duration of treatment
- Classified into urethritis, cystitis, prostatitis, or pyelonephritis
- UTI in a male patient is regarded as complicated
- Probability of a UTI in a female patient is high

Urinary Calculus Disease

The average life-time risk of renal calculus disease is 5–10%.[8] Ureteric colic is a frequent cause of emergency urological referral, with the patient presenting with characteristic radiating loin pain, vomiting, a low-grade fever, and microscopic hematuria. The differential diagnosis is wide and includes biliary colic (on the right), peptic ulcer disease, pancreatitis, and abdominal aortic aneurysm. Urinary calculi are the commonest cause of renal colic, although sloughed renal papillae, a blood clot, and fungal debris are occasionally implicated. Investigations for renal colic that follow clinical diagnosis include analysis of urine (for red cells, leukocytes, nitrites, pH and cystene), urine culture, serum creatinine, calcium, albumin, urate, and a white cell count.[9] Appropriate imaging will immediately confirm the diagnosis and help to decide on management. The choice of imaging includes a plain abdominal radiograph combined with an ultrasound examination, IVU, or an unenhanced CT examination.

CT is likely to be the best single imaging investigation for ureteric calculi, as both radiolucent and radiopaque calculi are visualized. However, in a number of countries, including the United Kingdom, the investigation of choice in renal colic remains an IVU, a situation that is likely to change to CT imaging in the future. IVU offers accurate assessment of the calculus size, site, and the degree of renal obstruction. The absence of hydronephrosis on ultrasound does not reliably rule out renal obstruction. Over 80% of calculi < 4 mm in diameter will pass spontaneously, but this is less likely with larger calculi.[10] Patients with persistent pain, UTI, risk of pyonephrosis, renal failure, single kidney, or bilateral obstruction need urgent decompression irrespective of calculi size.

Nonobstructing calculi in the kidney may be detected incidentally, or be imaged as a consequence of investigations for pain, UTI, or hematuria. Ultrasound and CT imaging may be useful in the evaluation of radiolucent calculi. ^{99m}Tc-DMSA scintigraphy is an optional investigation used to assess the differential renal function, especially in the presence of a large "stag-horn" calculus. A complete set of investigations for calculus disease, which comprises serum creatinine, uric acid, calcium, phosphate, and a 24-hour urine assessment, is recommended for patients at high risk of forming further calculi (indicated by a positive family history or previous episodes of calculus disease). Treatment options for renal calculi include extracorporal shock-wave lithotripsy (ESWL), percutaneous nephrolithotomy (PCNL), and endoscopic surgery; open surgery is now almost never necessary for calculus disease.[9]

Bladder calculi may be formed de novo in the bladder or migrate from the upper urinary tract. Bladder calculi are now rare, with primary bladder calculi occurring most often as a consequence of structural bladder abnormalities such as diverticula or voiding dysfunction.[9] Patients usually present with lower urinary tract symptoms (LUTS), suprapubic pain, or associated complications such as UTI, hematuria, or urinary retention. A plain abdominal radiograph often reveals the bladder calculi; an ultrasound is helpful in assessing any underlying abnormality such as residual urine and diverticula. Male patients should also have urine flow rate measured, as bladder outflow obstruction is a common cause of bladder calculi formation. Management includes removal of the calculi (usually by cystoscopy) and treating the underlying cause.

> **Summary points:**
> - Ureteric colic is a frequent cause of emergency urological referral
> - CT is the best single imaging investigation for ureteric calculi
> - Persistent pain, pyonephrosis, renal failure, single kidney or bilateral renal obstruction needs urgent decompression
> - Bladder calculi are rare, occurring as a consequence of structural bladder abnormalities

Upper Urinary Tract Obstruction (Hydronephrosis)

Upper urinary tract obstruction may result from a variety of causes (Table 7.2). The presentation and natural history may vary according to the degree of obstruction. Acute upper urinary tract obstruction is often due to calculi with sloughed papillae, blood clots, renal pelvis debris, and retroperitoneal abnormalities also implicated. Chronic upper urinary tract obstruction may be further divided into equivocal (doubtful) or unequivocal. Those with equivocal obstruction may have IVU and/or ultrasound appearance of hydronephrosis or clinical symptoms such as diuresis-induced loin pain, but fail to demonstrate evidence of obstruction on ^{99m}Tc-MAG3 renography.[11] The main clinical concern with both acute and chronic upper urinary tract obstruction is the risk of any resulting renal injury causing loss of renal function.

In children pelviureteric junction (PUJ) obstruction is the commonest cause of upper tract obstruction.[11] Congenital PUJ obstruction may be visualized on ultrasound as early as the second trimester of pregnancy with antenatal imaging. Not all of the PUJ obstructions present on the antenatal ultrasound examination will persist after

Table 7.2 **Causes of hydronephrosis**

- Pelviureteric junction (PUJ) obstruction
- Congenital megaureter
- Ureterocele
- Vesicoureteric junction (VUJ) obstruction
- Ureteric stricture
- Ureteric tumor
- Pregnancy
- Tuberculosis
- Bilhaziasis
- Ureteric duplication
- Retroperitoneal pathology
  - Retrocaval ureter
  - Abdominal aortic aneurysm
  - Retroperitoneal fibrosis
- Bowel/other malignancy extending into the retroperitoneum

Table 7.3 Correlation between anteroposterior diameter of the renal pelvis and the requirement for pyeloplasty

Anteroposterior diameter of therenal pelvis (mm)	Risk of requirement for pyeloplasty (%)
< 15	2
15–20	7
20–30	29
30–40	61
40–50	67
> 50	100

birth.[11] A follow-up ultrasound examination will identify those with a persisting PUJ obstruction and allow institution of the correct management. Older children with upper urinary tract obstruction may present incidentally with pain, infection, a palpable renal mass, renal impairment, hematuria, and hypertension.[11] Dhillon et al. have demonstrated the risk of surgical correction according to the degree of hydronephrosis measured as the anteroposterior diameter of the renal pelvis (Table 7.3).[11,12] The indications for surgical correction may be further refined when combined with differential renal function ascertained with ^{99m}Tc-MAG3 renography.[11] In neonates, ^{99m}Tc-MAG3 renography may be inaccurate due to renal immaturity, with ^{99m}Tc-MAG3 renography best performed at age six weeks.[11] IVU in this setting may not add any further information and is therefore not routinely recommended.

Surgical correction is recommended when the divided renal function is < 40% and the anterior–posterior diameter of the PUJ is > 30 mm on the affected side.[11] An Anderson–Hynes pyeloplasty is the standard surgical procedure for PUJ obstruction. When there remains uncertainty, for example when the divided renal function is > 40% and the anterior–posterior diameter of the PUJ is < 30 mm, a conservative approach is usually adopted; the majority of these patients improve or remain stable.

The management of a poorly or nonfunctioning kidney (divided renal function < 15%) is more controversial; recommendations vary from an initial nephrostomy to monitor any functional improvement to immediate nephrectomy.[11] A clinical decision must be based on serial functional assessment with ^{99m}Tc-MAG3 renography. When bilateral PUJ obstruction is present, it is important to exclude voiding dysfunction as a cause. Radioisotope scans are unreliable in patients with bilateral PUJ obstruction.

In adults, unilateral hydronephrosis may be a result of an undetected, congenital PUJ obstruction. However, it is important to exclude other acquired causes, as 5% of transitional cell carcinomas (TCCs) occur in the upper urinary tract and may present as urinary tract obstruction. IVU is performed more frequently in adults than in children with upper urinary tract obstruction along with other investigations such as urine cytology, retrograde pyelography, and CT or magnetic resonance (MR) imaging of the retroperitoneum.

Bilateral upper urinary tract obstruction in the elderly male patient occurs most frequently due to high-pressure chronic retention as a result of bladder outflow obstruction. Locally advanced bladder, prostate, or gynecological tumors will occasionally cause bilateral ureteric invasion, resulting in upper urinary tract obstruction with the patients usually presenting with acute renal failure. Percutaneous nephrostomy insertion under radiological guidance is the initial management, although it is best practice to insert either a double-J stent or a metallic stent across the obstruction as soon as possible.

Summary points:
- Due to calculi, sloughed papillae, blood clots, renal pelvis debris, and retro-peritoneal abnormalities
- Acute and chronic upper urinary tract obstruction may result in loss of renal function
- Percutaneous nephrostomy insertion is possible, although it is best practice to insert a double-J stent across the obstruction as first line management
- In children PUJ obstruction is common

Hematuria

The presentation of hematuria may vary from microscopic hematuria detected on urine analysis, visible blood in the urine, to blood clots causing urinary retention. The importance of careful assessment in these patients cannot be underestimated; underlying urinary tract pathology occurs frequently. Urinary tract malignancy is found four times more often in patients with macroscopic than those with microscopic hematuria; studies have suggested a 5% and 22% incidence of bladder carcinoma with microscopic and macroscopic hematuria, respectively.[13–15]

There are a number of causes for hematuria which include both medical and surgical diseases. Glomerulonephritis, UTIs, and childhood tumors are the main differential diagnoses in the pediatric age group. Urinary stones, trauma, atypical glomerulonephritis, UTI, and IgA nephropathy should be considered in young adults, whereas over age 40 urinary tract malignancy is the main concern. Complications of benign prostatic hypertrophy, such as UTI and bladder calculi, are also a common cause in older men.

Clinical assessment of patients with any form of hematuria includes a focused history and examination,

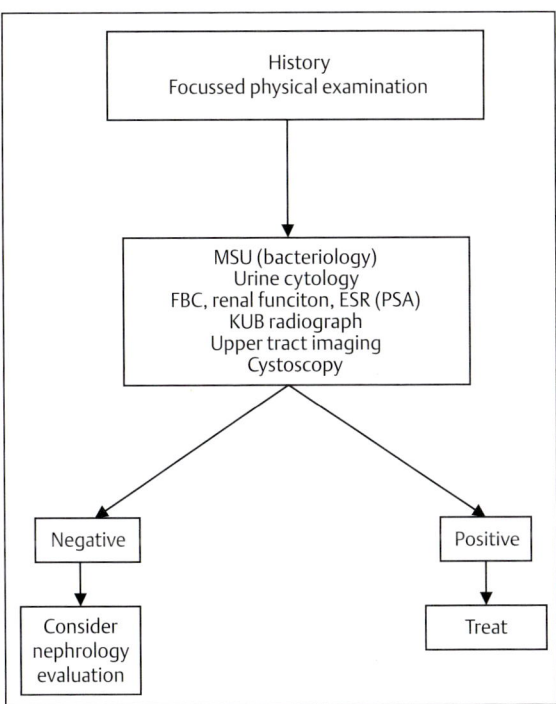

Fig. 7.2 **Investigation of hematuria**
(MSU = midstream urine; FBC = full blood count; ESR = erythrocyte sedimentation rate; PSA = prostate-specific antigen; KUB= kidneys, ureter, bladder)

urine testing, cystoscopy, and urinary tract imaging (Fig. 7.2). There remains some dispute as to the benefits of investigating microscopic hematuria in younger patients to the same extent as macroscopic hematuria in all age groups; the risk of cancer in young patients with microscopic hematuria is low.[14,16] However, a study has suggested significant disease in 18.5% of patients with microscopic hematuria, which implies that a thorough evaluation is always indicated.[14]

From the clinician's point of view, the most appropriate technique for imaging the upper renal tracts remains debatable. Ultrasound is the favored option as it is as accurate as an IVU for hydronephrosis and superior at imaging bladder tumors.[1,16] When further imaging is indicated, CT has the advantage of tumor staging and detecting nonurological causes of hematuria.[13] The most reliable method of assessing the lower urinary tract is cystoscopy.[17] If a bladder tumor is demonstrated on cystoscopy, a transurethral resection (TUR) of the tumor for histological confirmation and staging may be performed. The presence of hydronephrosis, secondary to a tumor at the ureteric orifice, is frequently a sign of muscle-invasive disease.[17] Over 90% of bladder tumors are TCCs, of which over 70% are superficial in nature.[17] The risk of recurrence varies from 50–70% according to tumor grade.[17,18] Superficial TCC may progress to invasive disease; carcinoma in situ and poorly differentiated (Grade 3) tumors pose by far the highest risk. Intravesical therapy, with either mitomycin C or epirubicin, may reduce the frequency of recurrent disease, whereas intravesical bacille Calmette–Guérin (BCG) reduces the overall recurrence rate, as well as the risk of tumor progression.[19] Patients are monitored with regular cystoscopy to detect and treat any tumor recurrence. When muscle-invasive disease is present, staging with CT or MR imaging is performed. A radionucleotide bone scan should be requested with advanced disease. Treatment options for invasive bladder carcinoma include radical cystectomy or radiotherapy, with platinum-based chemotherapy being used in advanced disease.

Summary points:
- Causes for hematuria include both medical and surgical diseases
- Urinary tract malignancy is 4x more common in macroscopic than in microscopic hematuria
- There is dispute as to the benefits of investigating microscopic hematuria in younger patients
- Assessment of any form of hematuria includes a focused history and examination, urine testing, cystoscopy, and urinary tract imaging

Lower Urinary Tract Symptoms and Benign Prostatic Hyperplasia

Lower urinary tract symptoms (LUTS), affecting up to 30% of males over age 65, are a heterogeneous group of symptoms related to the bladder and bladder outflow, further divided into storage (filling) or voiding (obstructive) symptoms (Table 7.**4**). There are numerous causes for LUTS (Table 7.**5**), of which benign prostatic hyperplasia (BPH) is the commonest. The aim of assessing patients with BPH/LUTS is to establish the diagnosis, identify the cause, and manage treatment appropriately (Fig. 7.**3**). Patients with troublesome symptoms have a

Table 7.4 **Lower urinary tract symptoms (LUTS)**

Storage (filling)
• Frequency
• Urgency
• Urge incontinence
• Nocturia
• Strangurie
Voiding (obstructive)
• Hesitancy
• Poor stream
• Postmicturition dribble
• Intermittent flow
• Feeling of incomplete emptying

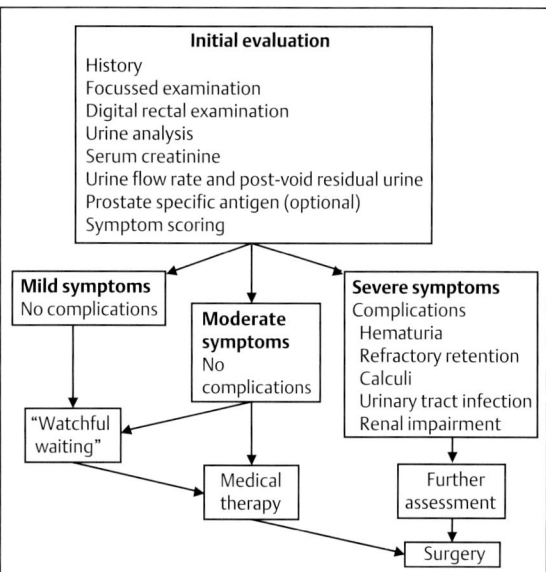

Fig. 7.3 Algorithm for management of benign prostatic hypertrophy

Table 7.5 Common causes of lower urinary tract symptoms (LUTS)

- Bladder outflow obstruction (BPH)
- Prostate carcinoma
- Urethral stricture
- Detrusor sphincter dyssnergia
- Urinary tract infections
- Nonbacterial cystitis
- Overactive bladder
- Bladder carcinoma (including carcinoma in situ)
- Bladder calculi
- Interstitial cystitis
- Age-related

Table 7.6 Indications for upper renal tract imaging with benign prostatic hypertrophy

- Renal impairment
- History of urolithiasis*
- Previous urinary tract surgery
- History of urothelial tumor*
- Hematuria
- Urinary retention

* May benefit from an IVU or CT as well

substantial improvement in quality of life following successful treatment.

The need for routine imaging of the upper urinary tract in patients with uncomplicated BPH is contentious. In a series of ultrasound examinations performed in elderly men, hydronephrosis was demonstrated in 2.5%, all the patients with hydronephrosis had a raised serum creatinine, and the number of incidental renal masses documented did not differ from that of the general population.[20] Routine imaging of the upper tracts in uncomplicated BPH is unlikely to be beneficial unless there are symptoms or clinical signs of renal disease; a postvoiding residual urine volume measurement combined with uroflowmetry should be adequate.[21] Nevertheless, in clinical practice upper tract imaging is often requested by the clinical referrers, perhaps only to reassure both the physician and the patient.

The postvoid residual urine in a normal person should be minimal, with postvoid residual urine of up to 50 mL being acceptable. Increasing amounts of postvoid residual urine become significant when associated with complications such as UTI or calculus formation. When a patient is able to void but retains > 300 mL, a state of chronic urinary retention is diagnosed.[21] Any high-pressure chronic urinary retention posses the risk of upper tract obstruction.

The indications for ultrasound imaging of the upper renal tract in BPH are detailed in Table 7.**6**.

Urodynamics (pressure-flow studies) is the most useful indicator of bladder outflow obstruction.[22] By placing a pressure transducer catheter both in the bladder and rectum during bladder filling, an accurate measurement of detrusor muscle function may be obtained.[22] A correlation between bladder-wall thickness (an indirect marker of detrusor muscle hypertrophy) and urinary outflow obstruction demonstrated on urodynamics has been suggested.[23] A bladder wall of thickness > 4 mm at 150 mL bladder capacity is suggested to be indicative of urinary outflow obstruction but is not a reliable measurement in the presence of bladder tumors or active infection. Although an attractive technique, there are difficulties with reproducing the results obtained by the original study group.[24]

Transrectal ultrasound (TRUS) is more accurate than digital rectal examination or cystourethroscopy in the assessment of prostate volume; it is an optional investigation when the prostate volume has an impact on the mode of therapy chosen. Any further imaging for LUTS can only be recommended on an individual basis, as these additional investigations, such as cystourethroscopy, abdominal radiograph, and urodynamics, are not part of the routine work-up of an uncomplicated patient.

Management and treatment of BPH is variable. "Watchful waiting" is an option for those with minimal symptoms and no associated complications. The mainstay of medical management is to treat with alpha-receptor blockers, which relax the prostatic stromal smooth muscles, and with 5-reductase inhibitors, which mainly reduce prostatic volume.[25] Larger prostates (> 40 g) are suitable for treatment with 5-reductase inhibitors. There is an inclination for some clinicians to manage mild symptoms of BPH with herbal and plant extracts (phytotherapy).[26] With increasing symptoms attributable to LUTS or other complications of BPH, surgery is appropriate. Transurethral resection of the prostate gland (TURP) is established surgical practice.[27] Larger volume prostate glands (> 100 g) are often treated with open prostatectomy, primarily as there remains concern over bleeding and inappropriate fluid absorption.[27] Photoselective vaporization of the prostate gland, via the transurethral route, using the "KTP YAG" laser (Green Light PV) or holmium laser enucleation techniques are emerging as attractive surgical alternatives even for very large prostate glands.[28]

> **Summary points:**
> - 30% of males over the age of 65 years are affected
> - Related to bladder outflow divided into storage (filling) or voiding (obstructive) symptoms
> - Benign prostatic hyperplasia is the most common cause of LUTS
> - Post-void residual urine of up to 50mL is acceptable but should normally be minimal
> - Patients have a substantial improvement in quality of life following successful treatment

Prostate Carcinoma

Prostate carcinoma is a problem of aging.[29] The lifetime risk of developing prostate cancer is 30% for microscopic disease and 10% for clinically significant disease.[30] The clinical presentation of prostate carcinoma to an extent overlaps with BPH, causing diagnostic difficulties. In the more advanced stages of prostate carcinoma, clinical presentation may be with local pain, hematuria, hemospermia, bone pain, pathological fractures, and manifestations of visceral metastases.[29] The main diagnostic tools for prostate carcinoma work-up include digital rectal examination, prostate-specific antigen (PSA) measurement, and TRUS-guided prostate biopsy.[29] In the majority of patients, prostate carcinoma develops in the peripheral zone of the prostate gland and may be palpable on digital rectal examination, but a normal digital rectal examination does not exclude the diagnosis of prostate carcinoma. The positive predictive value of PSA for prostate carcinoma detection is quoted as follows: In levels between 4 and 10 ng/mL the positive predictive value is 20–35% and for levels > 10 ng/mL it is between 50 and 80%.[29] An abnormal digital rectal exam will further increase the positive predictive value.[29]

On TRUS, the appearances of prostate carcinoma are variable; it is classically described as a low-reflective area in the peripheral zone, but may be of high or mixed reflectivity and even isoreflective to the normal prostate.[29,30] Although a TRUS biopsy may improve diagnostic accuracy and detect 50% more tumors than with physical examination alone,[31] there are no studies to support the use of TRUS biopsy as a screening tool. If there is a clinical suspicion of prostate carcinoma, systematic transrectal biopsies are obtained under ultrasound control. If the first set of biopsies are negative and there remains a high level of clinical suspicion for the presence of prostatic carcinoma, a second set of biopsies may yield a positive result in a further 20%.[31,32] Seminal vesicle biopsy may be used in selected patients for disease staging.[29]

Following diagnosis of prostate carcinoma, the stage of the disease has a major impact on the selection of appropriate treatment and prognosis.[29] TRUS is inadequate for local staging, whereas CT and MR imaging, although widely used, may not reliably predict extracapsular spread.[33,34] Accuracy of MR imaging may be improved with an endorectal coil and gadolinium contrast enhancement.[29,33] The use of microbubble ultrasound contrast agents in the evaluation of prostate carcinoma shows promise.[18,35] PSA measurement combined with the Gleason score (histological classification) of the tumor improves staging accuracy.[32] The reference standard for lymph node staging remains operative lymphadenectomy. Bone is the commonest site of metastatic spread from a prostatic carcinoma primary; radionuclide scintigraphy is the investigation of choice for detecting such lesions; a PSA of > 100 ng/mL is nearly 100% predictive for metastasis.[29]

Patients with good performance state, organ-confined disease, and a life expectancy of > 10 years are candidates for aggressive therapy by means of a radical (total) prostatectomy or radical radiotherapy.[29] Watchful monitoring is another option in a selected subgroup. Those patients with advanced disease or limited life expectancy are treated with antiandrogen therapy, palliative radiotherapy, hormonal manipulation, or watchful monitoring.

> **Summary points:**
> - Clinical presentation of prostate carcinoma overlaps with BPH
> - The life-time risk of developing prostate cancer is 30% for microscopic disease and 10% for clinically significant disease
> - Diagnosis for prostate carcinoma includes digital rectal examination, prostate specific antigen measurement, and trans-rectal ultrasound-guided prostate biopsy
> - Following diagnosis of prostate carcinoma, the stage of the disease has a major impact on the selection of appropriate treatment and prognosis

Focal Renal Lesions

Advances in imaging have had a major impact in the diagnosis and evaluation of focal renal lesions; a number of lesions are detected incidentally following imaging of the abdominal structures for other unrelated reasons. A simplified classification of renal tumors is given in Table 7.7.

Simple renal cysts are the commonest benign lesion, and renal cell carcinoma accounts for the majority of malignant renal tumors. Renal cysts are a common incidental finding and are considered to be a part of normal aging. Occasionally a simple renal cyst may cause pain, renal obstruction, or become infected. Ultrasound will evaluate renal cysts to identify those that are simple in nature or identify suspicious features such as septations, internal echoes, or calcification to recommend further imaging with CT. The Bosniak classification of renal cysts is a useful guide to determine malignant potential.[36,37]

Many clinically detected renal cell carcinomas (RCCs) are metastatic at diagnosis. One of the most valuable clinical benefits of ultrasound in urological practice is the role in early detection of renal cell cancer. This is particularly important, as surgery in the early stage of the disease is the best curative option for an RCC. RCC, once called the "internist's tumor" due to its protean manifestations, now rightly deserves to be called the "radiologist's tumor," as up to 80% of asymptomatic RCCs are now diagnosed incidentally with ultrasound. Ultrasound screening for RCCs is limited to high-risk groups, as the cost–benefit of ultrasound in this scenario is unproved.[38]

The classic clinical triad of loin pain, mass, and hematuria is seen in only a small number of patients with an RCC, though single symptoms are common. Weight loss, fatigue, malaise, and nausea are some of the other nonspecific symptoms, but are features of advanced disease. Paraneoplastic syndromes may be seen in up to 40% of patients. Stauffer syndrome is a unique paraneoplastic syndrome characterized by liver dysfunction, fever, weight loss, and fatigue, which is reversible in 60–70% of patients following nephrectomy, thought to be due to cytokine production by bulky necrotic tumors.[39,40] Differential diagnosis of RCC includes angiomyolipoma, oncocytoma, renal infarction, column of Berthin hypertrophy, xanthogranulomatous pyelonephritis, renal abscess, and an arteriovenous fistula (AVF); following renal biopsy.

Ultrasound will demonstrate a renal mass as small as 1.5 cm with 80% accuracy.[41] The main strength of ultrasound is the ability to differentiate solid and cystic components of a lesion with ease. Furthermore, ultrasound readily demonstrates tumor extension into the renal vein or inferior vena cava (IVC) but is less accurate in demonstrating thrombus below the IVC tumor. Large lymph nodes (> 1 cm) can also be detected with ultrasound. Ultrasound guidance may help in tumor biopsy in inconclusive cases as well as for cryosurgical or radiofrequency (RF) ablation of an RCC.[42,43] With nephron-sparing surgery, intraoperative ultrasound is useful to detect small tumor masses.

Overall, ultrasound is inadequate for the complete evaluation and staging of renal tumors; CT imaging is currently the standard for evaluating renal masses, being 72–90% accurate in staging renal carcinoma.[41] Other benign renal lesions such as angiomyolipoma and oncocytoma may also be differentiated due to their characteristic features, such as fat aggregation and central stellate scarring, respectively.[41] A central tumor location suggests a TCC and the diagnostic accuracy in such instances is increased with urine cytology, retrograde pyelography, and ureterorenoscopy.

Table 7.7 Pathological classification of renal tumors

Malignant
- Renal cell carcinoma (RCC)*
- Upper tract transitional cell carcinoma (TCC)*
- Lymphoma*
- Leiomyosarcoma
- Hemangiopericytoma
- Liposarcoma
- Rhabdomyosarcoma
- Schwannoma
- Osteosarcoma
- Fibrous histiosarcoma
- Neurofibrosarcoma
- Metastatic disease
- Invasion by adjacent neoplasm
- Carcinoid
- Adult Wilms tumor
- Mesoblastic nephroma
- Leukemia

Benign
- Simple cyst*
- Angiomyolipoma*
- Oncocytoma*
- Pseudotumour
- Renninoma
- Pheochromocytoma
- Leiomyoma
- Hemangioma
- Cystic nephroma
- Fibroma
- Arteriovenous malformation
- Renal artery aneurysm

Inflammatory
- Abscess*
- Pyelonephritis*
- Xanthogranulomatous pyelonephritis
- Infected renal cyst
- Tuberculosis
- Rheumatic granuloma

*Most common causes

MR imaging is presently considered a supplementary imaging modality for characterizing renal masses that are not fully assessed with CT imaging. MR imaging is also useful when CT is contraindicated due to iodinated contrast allergy or renal insufficiency. The overall accuracy of differentiating tumors confined to the kidney (Stage < T2) versus those with extracapsular spread (Stage T3) is higher with MR imaging than with CT imaging.[41,44] Apart from demonstrating angiomyolipoma (fat content well seen), the most significant role of MR imaging is the accuracy in differentiating IVC tumor from thrombus.[45] Following radical nephrectomy, patients are monitored for local tumor recurrence, metachronous tumor in the contralateral kidney, and for metastasis. Ultrasound combined with a chest radiograph or CT imaging of the abdomen may be used for this purpose. Five-year disease-free survival for localized (Stage T1–2) and advanced (Stage T3–4 or M+) disease is approximately 50–90% and 0–13%, respectively.[46]

Summary points:
- Lesions are detected incidentally following imaging for unrelated reasons
- Cysts are the most common benign lesion and renal cell carcinoma the most common malignant tumor
- Clinically detected renal cell carcinomas are metastatic at diagnosis
- Clinical triad of loin pain, mass, and hematuria is seen rarely in patients with a renal cell carcinoma
- 80% of asymptomatic renal cell carcinomas are diagnosed incidentally with ultrasound

Urogenital Trauma

All trauma patients are initially assessed according to the Advanced Trauma and Life Support (ATLS) protocol. In addition to baseline trauma investigations, urine analysis, hematocrit, and serum creatinine are particularly valuable in the assessment urinary tract injuries.

Renal Injury

Approximately 8–10% of abdominal injuries involve the kidneys.[47] Most patients with renal trauma do not require imaging or active intervention; the likelihood of a significant renal injury in an adult with microscopic hematuria due to trauma is minimal in the absence of hypovolemic shock.[48] Any pre-existing renal anomalies will make significant renal injury more likely. Guidelines for assessing both the adult and pediatric renal trauma patient have been issued by the European Association of Urology (Table 7.8).[48]

Table 7.8 **Indications for renal imaging following trauma**

Adults
- Blunt trauma with microscopic hematuria and hypotension
- Rapid deceleration injury or significant associated injury
- Macroscopic hematuria
- Penetrating injury

Children
- Blunt and penetrating trauma with any level of hematuria
- Associated significant abdominal injury regardless of urine analysis findings
- Rapid deceleration injuries, fall from a height, or direct flank trauma

The ideal imaging modality in trauma patients should provide accurate assessment of the specific injury, as well as associated injuries; CT is regarded as the reference standard. Ultrasound has limited value due to the inability for detailed assessment and the difficulty in obtaining a good acoustic window in a trauma patient. If patients are not hemodynamically stable enough for a CT examination, a focussed assessment with sonography in trauma (FAST) examination is of value particularly when combined with an intraoperative single abdominal radiograph following a bolus of intravenous iodinated contrast media. Again the use of microbubble ultrasound contrast media may play a role in the assessment of blunt trauma to solid abdominal organs.[49]

Although sensitivity for IVU in renal trauma is reported at 95%, there is lack of specificity and the ability to detect associated injuries.[48] Identification of renal tract injury with CT imaging is estimated at 95.6%, whereas with ultrasound specificity is reported at 78.8%.[48] With the availability of CT imaging, the use of angiography in renal trauma is largely limited to selective renal arterial embolization to halt continuing hemorrhage. Selective renal arterial embolization is a safe alternative to renal exploration, as the risk of nephrectomy is high with surgical exploration.[50] Most renal injuries may be managed nonoperatively.

Ureteral Injury

Traumatic ureteric injuries are rare, accounting for 1% of urinary tract injuries, whereas iatrogenic ureteric injury is more frequently encountered.[51] The diagnosis of ureteric injury requires a high degree of clinical suspicion, as there are no specific signs and symptoms. Urinary extravasation (including fistula) and features of upper renal tract obstruction are suggestive. Most ureteric injuries are diagnosed following imaging, most often on a CT examination. When CT imaging findings are inconclusive, a plain abdominal radiography at 30 minutes after iodinated contrast (administered for the CT examination) may provide a more detailed view of any extravasation of contrast media.[48] Retrograde pyelography is the reference standard in evaluating ureteric injury.

Prompt attention to ureteric injury is vital for renal preservation and prevention of complications related to continuing urine extravasation. Principles of management include early diagnosis, surgical reconstruction or repair, drainage, antibiotic therapy, and possible stenting of the repaired ureteric segment.

Bladder Injury

The urinary bladder occupies both the abdomen and pelvis and may be involved in injuries related to either; 70–90% of bladder injuries are associated with pelvic fractures.[52] Hematuria in the presence of a pelvic fracture, abdominal tenderness, and distension with inability to void are highly suggestive of a bladder injury. Cystography (on a CT examination or via conventional retrograde bladder filling) is the imaging method of choice. A minimum of a plain radiograph, a view with a bladder filled with contrast, and a view following bladder voiding should be performed. Ultrasound and IVU are thought to be suboptimal for the assessment of bladder injury. Extraperitoneal rupture of the bladder due to blunt trauma may be managed with bladder catheter drainage alone, whereas intraperitoneal rupture and penetrating injuries often need surgical closure.

Genital Injury

A high proportion (30–60%) of all urinary tract injury is associated with genital injury.[48] Blunt trauma to the erect penis may result in corporal fracture, which often occurs during sexual activity.[53] Patients usually complain of a "cracking" noise associated with sudden detumescence and penile swelling (the "aubergine sign"). There may be an associated urethral injury. The diagnosis of a penile fracture is often clinical.

MR imaging and ultrasound are both useful in ascertaining integrity of the tunica albuginea, especially when clinical assessment is difficult in the presence of a large hematoma.[54] A penile fracture must be differentiated from rupture of the dorsal vein of penis, as management is different. An ascending urethrogram should be performed if urethral injury is suspected. Early surgical repair is the preferred management of a penile fracture, as if surgical repair is performed early, the majority of patients will avoid significant erectile dysfunction that is known to be associated with this injury.[55]

Following blunt injury, the testis may be contused, ruptured, or dislocated. Patients present with a painful and swollen scrotum. Rarely testicular tumors present as swellings only brought to the patient's attention following trauma.[56] The accuracy of ultrasound in the assessment of testicular injury is debatable, though probably the commonest imaging modality used. Most penetrating injuries to the genitalia are associated with other organ injury, the choice of imaging guided by the clinical picture but not delaying urgent surgical exploration.

> **Summary points:**
> - 8–10% of abdominal injuries involve the kidneys
> - Pre-existing renal anomalies will make significant renal injury more likely
> - Traumatic ureteric injuries are rare
> - 70–90% of bladder injuries are associated with pelvic fractures
> - Early surgical repair of a penile fracture is indicated

Penile and Scrotal Abnormalities

Testis

There are a number of causes of testicular pain (Table 7.9). The presentation of a patient with acute scrotal pain is a potential emergency as it is imperative to manage testicular torsion correctly to avoid irreversible ischemic injury to the testis. Testicular infarction may occur within a few hours following initial symptoms.

The classic clinical presentation of testicular torsion is acute scrotal pain, nausea, and vomiting.[57] However, not all patients will have testicular symptoms; pain may be referred to the lower quadrant of the abdomen. The affected testis is often "high-riding" and lies in the transverse plane and the spermatic cord feels tender and indurated at the site of torsion. With late presentation the overlying scrotal skin may be discolored. With torsion of the appendix of testis or epididymis, tenderness may be more localized than with testicular torsion. Acute lower ureteric obstruction can be referred to the ipsilateral testis, but in such an instance the testis is not normally tender to palpation. Epididymo-orchitis is an important differential diagnosis, but the history of pain

Table 7.9 Differential diagnosis of acute scrotal pain

Testicular torsion
• Torsion of the appendix of testis
• Torsion of the appendix of epididymis
• Epididymo-orchitis
• Infected hydrocele
• Obstructed hernia
• Vasculitis
• Dermatological problems of the scrotum

in patients with epididymo-orchitis tends to be less acute and progressing over time.[58]

When there is significant clinical doubt, a testicular color Doppler ultrasound may be useful, as it demonstrates blood flow to the testis and may identify epididymo-orchitis.[59] Nuclear medicine imaging may also assess testicular blood flow, though is impractical due to its relative unavailability in an emergency setting. It must be emphasized that no imaging examination is reliable enough to rule out testicular torsion and the diagnosis is mainly based on clinical suspicion.[60] Prompt surgical exploration should be carried out in such instances and if testicular torsion is confirmed, both testes should be fixed to prevent subsequent torsion.

The presence of scrotal discomfort, pain, or a mass is a frequent urological referral. Hydrocele, varicocele, and cysts of the epididymis are common benign conditions occurring at all ages, but a testicular tumor, the main concern of this group of patients, has a peak incidence in the third and fourth decades. Testicular tumors account for about 10% of cancer deaths in males of this age group.[61] Testicular tumors usually present as a painless testicular swelling; other symptoms are less common and include localized pain (27%), gynecomastia (7%), and may mimic epididymo-orchitis in 10% of patients.[56] Clinical examination of the scrotum often reveals the diagnosis. Ultrasound is the imaging modality of choice for the initial assessment of scrotal pathology; accuracy is further enhanced by the use of color Doppler ultrasound. Ultrasound is particularly useful in evaluating the testis when a tense hydrocele prevents adequate palpation. Color Doppler ultrasound is useful in the differentiation of inflammatory change from tumor masses. Subclinical varicoceles may be demonstrated on ultrasound; the significance of treating varicoceles remains uncertain.[62,63] Epididymal cysts do not require treatment unless large or symptomatic.

Ultrasound is sensitive in demonstrating testicular tumors, although MR imaging is arguably superior due to greater accuracy with local tumor staging and the ability to differentiate seminomatous from nonseminomatous tumors.[64] MR imaging is not routinely performed in the staging of testicular tumors, as tumor markers (alpha-fetoprotein [AFP], human beta-chorionic gonadotropin [beta-HCG], lactate dehydrogenase [LDH]) along with clinical and ultrasound local assessment is adequate in the majority of patients. CT imaging is the recommended modality for staging the retroperitoneum and chest.

Treatment options for testicular tumors vary according to the stage of disease. Platinum-based chemotherapy and radiotherapy has improved the overall survival of patients with testicular malignancy to over 90%.[65,66] The risk of contralateral testicular tumor varies from 2.5–5%, more likely with a morphologically abnormal testis or in the presence infertility.[56] Testicular microlithiasis is recognized as a risk factor for the development of a testicular tumor, and these patients should be offered ultrasound and clinical surveillance.[67]

A number of patients present with chronic testicular pain (chronic orchalgia) in whom no abnormality can be demonstrated, a difficult clinical problem in which to offer any treatment.[68]

Penile carcinoma is rare in the developed countries. Penile carcinoma is related to penile hygiene and is almost never seen in males who have been circumcised at a young age. The tumor may begin as a small painless papule or ulcer. Delayed presentation is common, with approximately 50% of patients demonstrating palpable lymph nodes, which may be inflammatory or malignant, at the time of presentation. MRI is gerally accepted as the staging modality of choice.

Erectile Dysfunction

Although penile erection is a predominantly neurovascular event, there are many causes of erectile dysfunction, which may be classified as psychogenic, neurogenic, hormonal, or vascular. Primary assessment of a patient with erectile dysfunction includes a detailed interview focussed on the medical and psychosexual history, physical examination, and appropriate baseline investigations. If a vascular abnormality is suspected, a color and spectral Doppler ultrasound is useful in assessing cavernosal arterial blood flow. Cavernosography may be used when venous leak is suspected from the initial ultrasound, to visualize the abnormal draining veins. Revascularization surgery of the penis and procedures for venous leak are undertaken with varying success.[69,70]

Infertility

Infertility is defined as the inability to achieve conception after one year of unprotected intercourse.[63] Often patients are investigated sooner than the one-year period as female fertility declines after age 35. There are a number of factors contributing to male and female infertility. The main purpose of evaluating patients with infertility is to detect treatable causes, advise on suitable alternate conception methods for those with uncorrectable problems, diagnose potentially life-threatening conditions that may underlie infertility, and to identify genetic abnormalities that may affect the offspring.

The initial assessment includes a complete reproductive history and a focused physical examination, particular emphasis being given to secondary sexual characteristics, testicular size, and the presence of a scrotal varicocele. On rectal examination, a palpable nodule or cyst may suggest a müllerian duct cyst. Two semen analyses are performed as a basic investigation, and other investigations will include a reproductive hormone profile and postejaculatory semen analysis. Any immunological or genetic investigations are performed as the clinical history and examination dictates. TRUS is useful to demonstrate ejaculatory duct cysts or ejaculatory duct obstruction. Scrotal ultrasound is used to evaluate the testes when physical examination is inconclusive, documenting testicular volume as this is important in infertility.[71] Subclinical varicoceles may be demonstrated. Testicular tumors and microlithiasis are found in 0.5% and 5% of subfertile males, respectively.[67]

Summary points:
- Acute scrotal pain is an emergency as testicular torsion must be managed correctly
- Hydroceles, varicoceles, and cysts of the epididymis are common benign conditions
- Testicular tumors present as a painless testicular swelling; other symptoms are less common
- Chronic orchalgia is a difficult clinical problem in which to offer any treatment
- Penile carcinoma is related to penile hygiene and is not seen in circumcised males

References

1. Naber KG, Bergman B, Bishop MC, et al. EAU guidelines for the management of urinary and male genital tract infections. Urinary Tract Infection (UTI) Working Group of the Health Care Office (HCO) of the European Association of Urology (EAU). Eur Urol 2001; 40:576–588.
2. Busch R, Huland H. Correlation of symptoms and results of direct bacterial localization in patients with urinary tract infections. J Urol 1984;132:282–285.
3. Kangarloo H, Gold RH, Fine RN, Diament MJ, Boechat MI. Urinary tract infection in infants and children evaluated by ultrasound. Radiology 1985;154:367–373.
4. Huang JJ, Tseng CC. Emphysematous pyelonephritis: clinicoradiological classification, management, prognosis, and pathogenesis. Arch Intern Med 2000;160:797–805.
5. Kass EJ, Kernen KM, Carey JM. Paediatric urinary tract infection and the necessity of complete urological imaging. BJU Int 2000;86:94–96.
6. Hardeman SW, Husmann DA, Chinn HK, Peters PC. Blunt urinary tract trauma: identifying those patients who require radiological diagnostic studies. J Urol 1987;138:99–101.
7. Mentzel HJ, Vogt S, Patzer L, et al. Contrast-enhanced sonography of vesicoureterorenal reflux in children: preliminary results. AJR Am J Roentgenol 1999;173:737–740.
8. Anderson RA. A complementary approach to urolithiasis prevention. World J Urol 2002;20:294–301.
9. Tiselius H-G, Ackermann D, Alken P, Buck C, Conort P, Gallucci M. EAU Guidelines on Urolithiasis. EAU Update Series. 2001. http://www.uroweb.org/files/uploaded_files/urolithiasis.pdf
10. Morse RM, Resnick MI. Ureteral calculi: natural history and treatment in an era of advanced technology. J Urol 1991;145:263–265.
11. Riedmiller H, Androulakakis P, Beurton D, Kocvara R, Gerharz E. EAU guidelines on paediatric urology. Eur Urol 2001;40:589–599.
12. Dhillon HK. Prenatally diagnosed hydronephrosis: the Great Ormond Street experience. Br J Urol 1998;81(Suppl 2):39–44.
13. Gray Sears CL, Ward JF, Sears ST, Puckett MF, Kane CJ, Amling CL. Prospective comparison of computerized tomography and excretory urography in the initial evaluation of asymptomatic microhematuria. J Urol 2002;168:2457–2460.
14. Khadra MH, Pickard RS, Charlton M, Powell PH, Neal DE. A prospective analysis of 1,930 patients with hematuria to evaluate current diagnostic practice. J Urol 2000;163:524–527.
15. Sultana SR, Goodman CM, Byrne DJ, Baxby K. Microscopic haematuria: urological investigation using a standard protocol. Br J Urol 1996;78:691–696.
16. Goessl C, Knispel HH, Miller K, Klan R. Is routine excretory urography necessary at first diagnosis of bladder cancer? J Urol 1997;157:480–481.
17. Oosterlinck W, Lobel B, Jakse G, Malmstrom P-U, Stockle M, Sternberg C. EAU Guidelines on Bladder Cancer. EAU Update Series. 2001. http://www.uroweb.org/files/uploaded_files/bladdercancer.pdf
18. Ragde H, Kenny GM, Murphy GP, Landin K. Transrectal ultrasound microbubble contrast angiography of the prostate. Prostate 1997;32:279–283.
19. Oosterlinck W. Guidelines on diagnosis and treatment of superficial bladder cancer. Minerva Urol Nefrol 2004;56:65–72.
20. Koch WF, Ezz eD, de Wildt MJ, Debruyne FM, de la Rosette JJ. The outcome of renal ultrasound in the assessment of 556 consecutive patients with benign prostatic hyperplasia. J Urol 1996;155:186–189.
21. Speakman MJ, Kirby RS, Joyce A, Abrams P, Pocock R. Guideline for the primary care management of male lower urinary tract symptoms. BJU Int 2004;93:985–990.
22. Blake C, Abrams P. Noninvasive techniques for the measurement of isovolumetric bladder pressure. J Urol 2004;171:12–19.
23. Manieri C, Carter SS, Romano G, Trucchi A, Valenti M, Tubaro A. The diagnosis of bladder outlet obstruction in men by ultrasound measurement of bladder wall thickness. J Urol 1998;159:761–765.
24. Kaefer M, Barnewolt C, Retik AB, Peters CA. The sonographic diagnosis of infravesical obstruction in children: evaluation of bladder wall thickness indexed to bladder filling. J Urol 1997;157:989–991.
25. Lepor H, Williford WO, Barry MJ, et al. The efficacy of terazosin, finasteride, or both in benign prostatic hyperplasia. Veterans Affairs Cooperative Studies Benign Prostatic Hyperplasia Study Group. N Engl J Med 1996;335:533–539.
26. Buck AC. Phytotherapy for the prostate. Br J Urol 1996;78:325–336.
27. Neal DE. The national prostatectomy audit. Br J Urol 1997;79(Suppl 2):69–75.
28. Malek RS, Kuntzman RS, Barrett DM. High-power potassium-titanyl-phosphate laser vaporization prostatectomy. J Urol 2000;163:1730–1733.

29. Aus G, Abbou CC, Pacik D, et al. EAU Guidelines on Prostate Cancer. EAU Update Series. 2003. http://www.uroweb.org/files/uploaded_files/prostatecancer.pdf
30. Oyen RH. Imaging modalities in diagnosing and staging carcinoma of the prostate. In: Petrovich Z, Baert L, Brady LW, eds. Carcinoma of the prostate. Innovation and management. Berlin: Springer Verlag: 1996:65–96.
31. Keetch DW, Catalona WJ, Smith DS. Serial prostatic biopsies in men with persistently elevated serum prostate specific antigen values. J Urol 1994;151:1571–1574.
32. Partin AW, Yoo J, Carter HB, et al. The use of prostate-specific antigen, clinical stage and Gleason score to predict pathological stage in men with localized prostate cancer. J Urol 1993;150:110–114.
33. May F, Treumann T, Dettmar P, Hartung R, Breul J. Limited value of endorectal magnetic resonance imaging and transrectal ultrasonography in the staging of clinically localized prostate cancer. BJU International 2001;87:66–69.
34. Mufti G, Naseem MS, Masood S, Patel H, Reddy K. Preoperative imaging of pelvic urological malignancies: is it accurate? BJU International 2002;90(Suppl 2):199.
35. Frauscher F, Klauser A, Halpern EJ. Advances in ultrasound for the detection of prostate cancer. Ultrasound Q 2002;18:135–142.
36. Bosniak MA. The use of the Bosniak classification system for renal cysts and cystic tumors. J Urol 1997;157:1852–1853.
37. Leder RA. Radiological approach to renal cysts and the Bosniak classification system. Curr Opin Urol 1999;9: 129–133.
38. Zhan X, Sidhu PS, Muir GH. Screening for renal cell carcinoma using ultrasonography; a feasibility study. BJU Int 2003;92:1047–1048.
39. Gold PJ, Fefer A, Thompson JA. Paraneoplastic manifestations of renal cell carcinoma. Semin Urol Oncol 1996;14:216–222.
40. Strohmaier WL, Bichler KH. Paraneoplastic syndrome in kidney cancer. Med Klin (Munich) 1989;84:86–89.
41. Roy C, Buy X, el Ghali S. Imaging in renal cell cancer. EAU Update Series 2003;1:209–214.
42. Abe M, Saitoh M. Selective renal tumour biopsy under ultrasonic guidance. Br J Urol 1992;70:7–11.
43. Brausi M, Castagnetti G, Gavioli M, Peracchia G, de Luca G, Olmi R. Radiofrequency (RF) ablation of renal tumours does not produce complete tumour destruction: results of a phase II study. Euro Urol Suppl 2004;3: 4–17.
44. Semelka RC, Shoenut JP, Magro CM, Kroeker MA, MacMahon R, Greenberg HM. Renal cancer staging: comparison of contrast-enhanced CT and gadolinium-enhanced fat-suppressed spin-echo and gradient-echo MR imaging. J Magn Reson Imaging 1993;3:597–602.
45. Aslam SA, Teh J, Nargund VH, Lumley JS, Hendry WF, Reznek RH. Assessment of tumor invasion of the vena caval wall in renal cell carcinoma cases by magnetic resonance imaging. J Urol 2002;167:1271–1275.
46. Mickisch G, Carballido J, Hellsten S, Schulze H, Mensink H. Guidelines on renal cell cancer. Eur Urol 2001;40:252–255.
47. Sahin H, Akay AF, Yilmaz G, Tacyildiz IH, Bircan MK. Retrospective analysis of 135 renal trauma cases. Int J Urol 2004; 1:332–336.
48. Lynch D, Martinez-Pineiro L, Plas E, Serafetinidis E, Turkeri L, Hohenfellner M. EAU Guidelines on Urological Trauma. EAU Update Series. 2003. http://www.uroweb.org/files/uploaded_files/guidelines/urotrauma.pdf.
49. Kraemer N, Cosgrove DO, Blomley MJ. Microbubble ultrasound demonstrates liver trauma. J Trauma 2004;56:913–914.
50. Hagiwara A, Sakaki S, Goto H, et al. The role of interventional radiology in the management of blunt renal injury: a practical protocol. J Trauma 2001;51:526–531.
51. Dobrowolski Z, Kusionowicz J, Drewniak T, et al. Renal and ureteric trauma: diagnosis and management in Poland. BJU Int 2002;89: 748–751.
52. Flancbaum L, Morgan AS, Fleisher M, Cox EF. Blunt bladder trauma: manifestation of severe injury. Urology 1988;31: 220–222.
53. Mansi MK, Emran M, el Mahrouky A, el Mateet MS. Experience with penile fractures in Egypt: long-term results of immediate surgical repair. J Trauma 1993;35:67–70.
54. Uder M, Gohl D, Takahashi M, et al. MRI of penile fracture: diagnosis and therapeutic follow-up. Eur Radiol 2002;12:113–120.
55. Gontero P, Sidhu PS, Muir GH. Penile fracture repair: assessment of early results and complications using color Doppler ultrasound. Int J Impot Res 2000;12:125–128.
56. Laguna MP, Pizzocaro G, Klepp O, Algaba F, Kisbenedek L, Leiva O. EAU guidelines on testicular cancer. Eur Urol 2001; 40:102–110.
57. Cole FL, Vogler R. The acute, nontraumatic scrotum: assessment, diagnosis, and management. J Am Acad Nurse Pract 2004;16:50–56.
58. Knight PJ, Vassy LE. The diagnosis and treatment of the acute scrotum in children and adolescents. Ann Surg 1984;200:664–673.
59. Chou CC, Chen CS, Chu SH, Lai MK. Color Doppler sonography in differentiation between testicular torsion and epididymoorchitis: report of three cases. Changgeng Yi Xue Za Zhi 1996;19:90–94.
60. Sidhu PS. Clinical and imaging features of testicular torsion: role of ultrasound. Clin Radiol 1999;54:343–352.
61. Buse S, Lurati G, Schmid HP. Testicular tumors—a current review. Schweiz Rundsch Med Prax 2003;92:1989–1997.
62. Kass EJ, Chandra RS, Belman AB. Testicular histology in the adolescent with a varicocele. Pediatrics 1987;79:996–998.
63. Weidner W, Colpi GM, Hargreave TB, Papp GK, Pomerol JM, Ghosh C. EAU guidelines on male infertility. Eur Urol 2002; 42:313–322.
64. Thurnher S, Hricak H, Carroll PR, Pobiel RS, Filly RA. Imaging the testis: comparison between MR imaging and US. Radiology 1988;167:631–636.
65. Miron L. The current therapeutic strategy in testicular cancer. Rev Med Chir Soc Med Nat Iasi 1995;99:29–39.
66. Loehrer PJ, Sr., Williams SD, Einhorn LH. Status of chemotherapy for testis cancer. Urol Clin North Am 1987;14: 713–720.
67. Miller FN, Sidhu PS. Does testicular microlithiasis matter? A review. Clin Radiol 2002;57:883–890.
68. Hayden LJ. Chronic testicular pain. Aust Fam Physician 1993;22:1357–9.
69. Michal V, Kramar R, Pospichal J, et al. Vascular surgery in the treatment of impotence; its present possibilities and prospects. Czech Med 1980;3:213–217.
70. Sarramon JP, Malavaud B, Bertrand N, Rischmann P. Vascular microsurgery in the treatment of vasculogenic erectile dysfunction: clinical experience apropos of 115 operations performed according to 2 different surgical techniques. Prog Urol 1999;9:707–714.
71. Schutte B. New diagnostic procedures in assessing male fertility. Z Hautkr 1989;64:292;295–298.

8 Focal Lesions of the Kidney
M. J. Weston

Introduction

Many focal renal lesions are detected incidentally during investigation for other symptoms. Ultrasound is commonly used in the investigation of diverse abdominal and pelvic symptoms; the kidneys are seen as part of the ultrasound examination. The most likely finding is of a simple renal cyst, and ultrasound has a high degree of accuracy in cyst characterization.[1] The mode of presentation of renal tumors gives prognostic information; those that are found incidentally do better than those who present with symptoms.[2] It is important for the ultrasonologist to recognize which lesions can be ignored and which need further action.

Renal Cysts

Simple Cysts

Simple renal cysts are common in older patients; they are a normal part of the process of aging and are the commonest renal mass in adults. A recent prevalence study using ultrasound showed that 5.1% of people in the fourth decade of life have at least one cyst; this increases sevenfold to 36.1% in the eighth decade of life.[3] The same study also showed that cysts were twice as common in men as in women. Furthermore, there is an average yearly increase in size of 6.3%. Uncomplicated cysts are usually asymptomatic and do not require any treatment. Large cysts are likely to be symptomatic with pressure effects on adjacent structures, leading to discomfort, hematuria, hypertension, and urinary obstruction. Symptomatic renal cysts can be treated using ultrasound-guided aspiration and instillation of either absolute alcohol alone or alcohol and tetracycline.[4,5] Success in relieving symptoms is said to be between 75 and 95%.

The ultrasound features are of a hypoechoic fluid collection arising from the kidney with the following characteristics (Fig. 8.**1**):
- No internal echoes
- A rounded or ovoid shape
- An imperceptible, smooth wall, with a sharply-defined distal margin
- Increased through transmission of sound

There are technical factors that influence these appearances. Reverberation echoes from the skin surface or strong superficial reflectors may appear within the cyst. These echoes fade out the deeper into the cyst they go. Harmonic imaging will reduce this effect. Cysts < 2 cm in size may show apparent internal echoes from partial volume effects from adjacent solid tissue. Remember that the ultrasound beam has width.

Multiple Simple Cysts

The presence of more than one simple cyst in a kidney becomes commoner with increasing age. These cysts retain the characteristics of a simple cyst (Fig. 8.**2**). Some medical syndromes produce multiple cysts, but once established these syndromes have innumerable cysts affecting both kidneys equally. In contrast, multiple simple cysts affect the two kidneys in an asymmetric way and always remain countable in number.

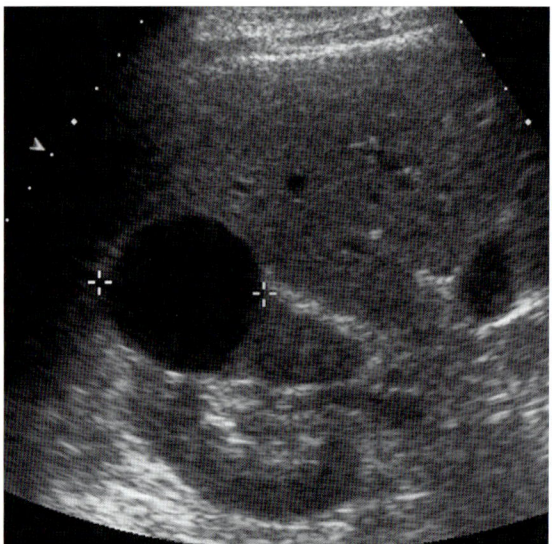

Fig. 8.**1 Simple cortical cyst** (between cursors), demonstrating the characteristic features of a cyst: No internal echoes, an ovoid shape, an imperceptible, smooth wall, and increased through transmission of sound

Complicated Cysts

Septations

Fine septations of < 1 mm thickness do not stop a simple cyst from being regarded as simple. Thicker septations, particularly those with nodular thickening, are suspicious for malignancy and require further investigation (Fig. 8.3). Rarely, a cyst may change over time to become more septated and show malignant features.[6] Computed tomography (CT) imaging is advocated for any cyst that deviates from being simple.[7] Some authors advocate the use of Doppler studies or microbubble contrast-enhanced Doppler studies of septated lesions. It has been shown that flow in the septa, particularly high-velocity, pulsatile flow is a marker for malignancy.[8,9]

Hemorrhage

Internal echoes within a cyst are usually the result of either infection or hemorrhage (Fig. 8.4). The rate of hemorrhage into simple cysts is usually quoted as 6%, though the relevant studies were performed 30 years ago, predating sophisticated ultrasound. Cysts of polycystic kidney disease suffer a greater rate of hemorrhagic complication, in part due to the large size of the kidneys and their vulnerability to trauma. The appearance of a hemorrhage will vary with time. A fresh hemorrhage is anechoic, gaining echoes over time. Eventually, clot retraction, nodule and septum formation, calcification, and thickening of the cyst wall will occur. Hemorrhagic cysts are associated with malignancy;[10] they may themselves mimic features of malignancy that lead to unnecessary surgery.[11] Aspiration cytology is unhelpful because of the frequency of false negative results. If CT or magnetic resonance (MR) imaging do not show any overt features of malignancy, then follow-up of hemorrhagic cysts with serial ultrasound imaging is prudent.

Infection

Infection of a cyst can occur via hematogenous spread or via iatrogenic cyst puncture. An infected cyst may be indistinguishable from a simple cyst but is likely to show a complex echo pattern. The contents may be highly reflective (Fig. 8.4), there may be fluid–fluid levels with dependant debris and there may be contained gas. The wall of the cyst becomes thicker and may appear nodular due to adherent inflammatory tissue and an infected cyst will have clinical features of an abscess. Both are characterized by fever and flank pain resistant to antibiotic therapy. Aspiration and drainage are required for diagnosis and treatment.[12]

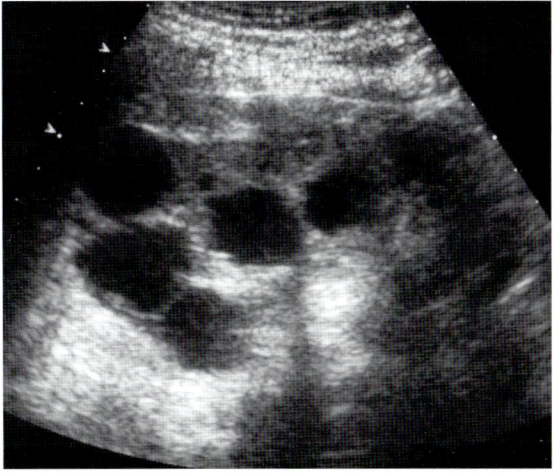

Fig. 8.2 **Five simple cysts of similar size in the kidney of a 60-year-old.** All demonstrate the typical features of a simple cyst

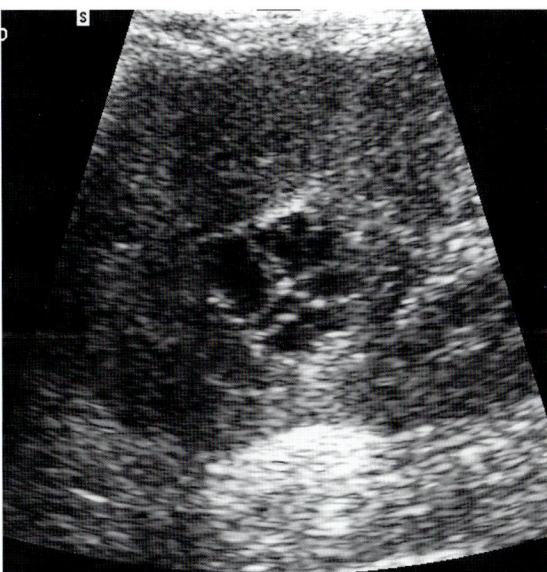

Fig. 8.3 **Septated cyst.** The septations in this cyst are thicker than 1 mm, and therefore the lesion requires further investigation

Hydatid (echinococcosis) cysts of the kidney represent a rare form of renal infection. Renal involvement occurs in only 4% of confirmed hydatid disease.[13] The ultrasound appearances are nonspecific, but daughter cysts within the main cyst and fine wall calcification may aid in the diagnosis.

Calcification

There is eggshell-like mural calcification in about 3% of simple cysts (Fig. 8.5). The majority represent calcification that has occurred as a result of bleeding or inflammation and is seen as a thin, bright margin to the cyst.[14]

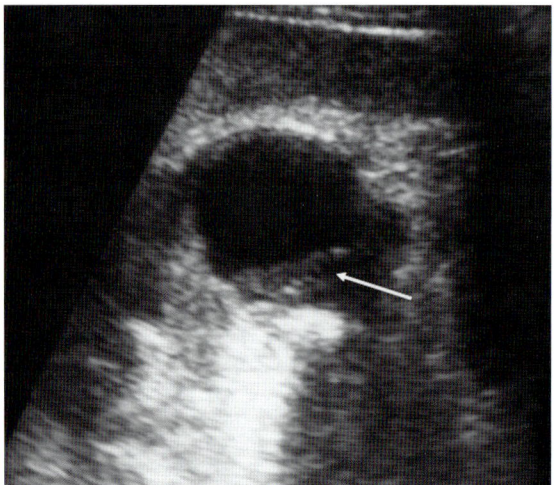
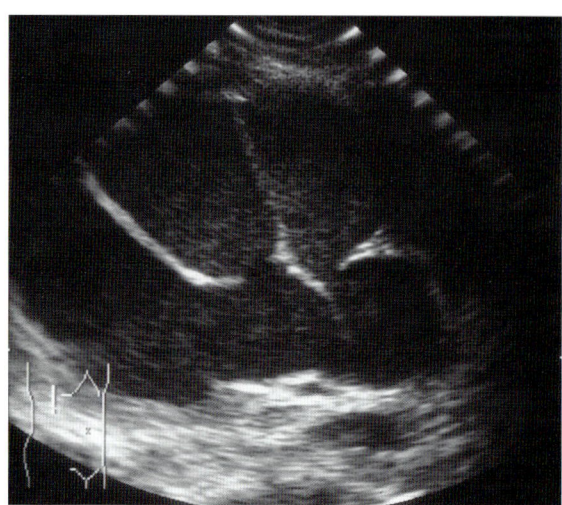

Fig. 8.4 **a** A fluid–debris level (arrow) within a cyst following recent intracystic hemorrhage. **b** Pyonephrosis in a longstanding hydronephrosis. Note that there is little or no remaining renal cortex. The fine echoes within the fluid indicate the presence of pus, blood, or other debris. The clinical picture is needed to aid in the differentiation of these entities

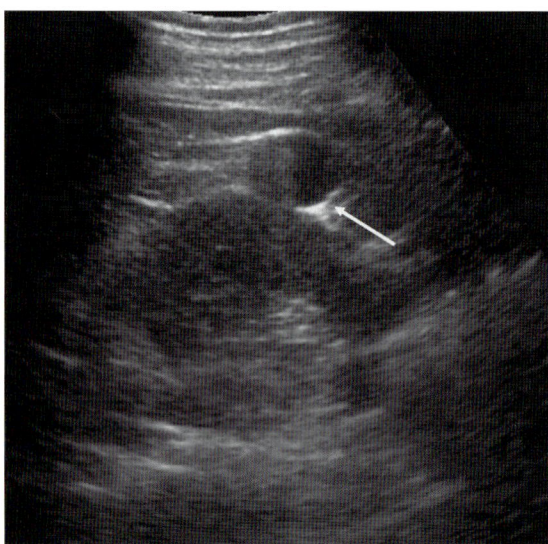

Fig. 8.5 **Calcified wall of a hemorrhagic cyst** (arrow) **at the upper aspect of the left kidney.** (Courtesy of Dr. G.M. Baxter)

Bright foci in the cyst walls or septa that show ringdown artifact are often seen but do not correlate with calcification on CT images.[15] There is an association of renal cyst calcification with malignancy, but this is much less important in the diagnosis than the presence of soft-tissue nodules.[16] Milk of calcium cysts contain a colloidal suspension of calcium crystals; these often show a dependant layer of high-reflective material on ultrasound, enough to cause shadowing.[17] Milk of calcium cysts may masquerade as renal calculi but represent a calyceal diverticulum that has lost its communication with the collecting system.[18] A milk of calcium cyst is usually asymptomatic.

Differential Diagnosis of Renal Simple Cysts

Calyceal and Renal Pelvic Diverticula

Fluid-containing lesions that communicate with the renal collecting system can be indistinguishable from simple cysts on ultrasound alone. Contrast-enhanced CT or urography is required to show the communication.

Hydronephrosis Duplex System

Diagnostic confusion can arise in both directions; peripelvic cysts may mimic hydronephrosis and obstructed calyces may mimic a cyst.[19,20] Likewise, the obstructed upper moiety of a duplex kidney may simulate an upper-pole renal cyst, especially if the surrounding cortex has become atrophic and nonfunctioning (Fig. 8.6). Conventionally, intravenous urography (IVU) is needed to establish the diagnosis. Nicolau et al. have claimed that measuring the size of the cystic structure on ultrasound before and after a 1.5 L fluid load will reliably distinguish between a cyst and renal obstruction; an increase in size of the lesion indicates renal obstruction.[21] Most authors prefer the greater certainty afforded by urography or contrast-enhanced CT imaging.

Lymphatic Cysts

Cysts in the renal sinus are produced in two forms: Parapelvic and peripelvic.[22] Parapelvic cysts are parenchymal in origin and are usually solitary and are seen in about 1.5% of autopsies. Peripelvic cysts are thought to arise by lymphatic ectasia and are usually multiple and

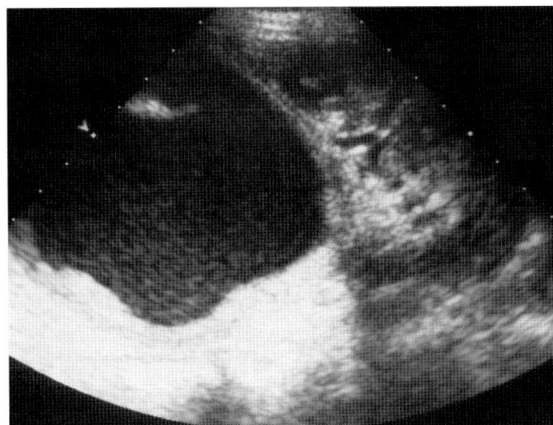

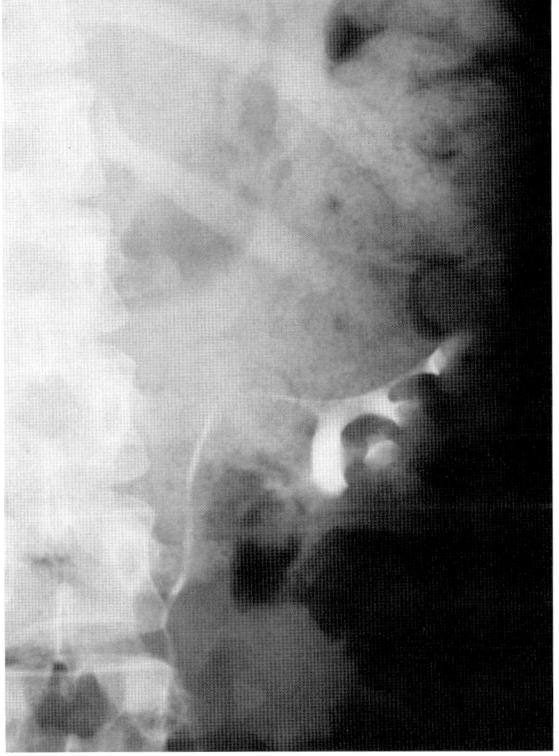

Fig. 8.6 **a** Obstructed upper moiety of a duplex kidney. Atrophy of the renal cortex around the upper moiety has occurred. The fluid within the dilated collecting system contains echoes indicating pus, blood, or other debris. In this case, the upper moiety was infected. **b** IVU in the same patient, demonstrating the typical "drooping flower head" sign of a normal lower moiety being displaced by the nonfunctioning upper moiety

septated. Peripelvic lymphangiectasia is rare and is associated with perirenal lymphatic cysts, as well as perivascular cysts (probably dilated lymph vessels).[23,24] The perirenal cysts appear to arise in a capsular location rather than a cortical location.

Hematoma

A recent hematoma may be indistinguishable from a cyst. The diagnosis should be suspected in the light of a history of trauma and serial ultrasound will show the development of echoes within the lesion as the hematoma matures.

Arteriovenous Malformations and Aneurysms

Arteriovenous malformations and aneurysms may appear identical to a simple cyst on gray-scale ultrasound but will present no diagnostic difficulty if Doppler ultrasound imaging is used.[25] Occasionally CT will misinterpret a venous varix as an enhancing mass.[26]

Multilocular Cystic Nephroma

This is a rare lesion that appears as a discrete, space-occupying mass with a thick capsule and consisting of several noncommunicating cysts of varying size separated by fibrous septa (Fig. 8.7).[27,28] If the cysts are

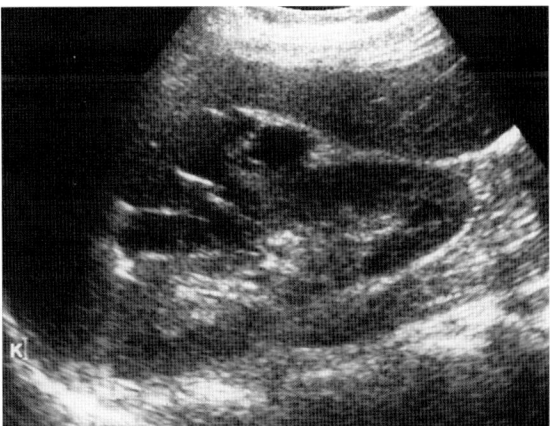

Fig. 8.7 **Example of a multilocular cystic nephroma.** The cysts are contained within the one lesion

small, the lesion may appear as a more solid mass. Multilocular cystic nephromas are predominantly found in young males or older females. There is pathological disagreement on their origin and this has led to a confusing array of synonyms: Benign cystic nephroma, cystic hamartoma, multilocular cystadenoma, cystic Wilms tumor, benign cystic differentiated nephroblastoma, and segmental polycystic kidney, to name a few. Whatever the name given, it is not possible for ultrasound or CT to distinguish the lesion from a cystic renal cell carcinoma (RCC).

Cystic Malignancy (Table 8.1)

The seminal paper by Bosniak on the classification of renal cysts and the likelihood of malignancy was based on CT imaging, but the findings can be extrapolated to ultrasound.[29] The initial premise was to identify reliably lesions that did not require surgery. Cysts are graded from I to IV depending on their internal complexity, with Grade I being a simple cyst and Grade IV being complex with solid areas. Approximately 60% of Grade III lesions and almost 100% of Grade IV lesions are malignant. Grades I and II can be left alone, whereas Grades III and IV require surgery. This approach has been shown to succeed,[30] though some modifications to the classification have evolved. Biopsy of Grade III lesions is advocated to prevent unnecessary surgery[31] and follow-up of moderately complex lesions (Grade IIF) is advised, as the absence of change supports benign disease.[32]

Table 8.1 Bosniak classification of renal cystic masses: CT criteria

Category 1	Cystic masses with well-defined margins, homogeneous, of water density, with no contrast enhancement
Category 2	Cystic masses showing a few thin septa (< 1 mm) or thin fine calcifications, or appearing as hyperdense cysts
Category 3	Cystic masses showing more extensive thickened and irregular calcifications, uniform wall thickening, and thickened and irregular or multiple septa (> 1 mm)
Category 4	Cystic masses having irregular thickened walls or solid elements and possibly having enhancement of cyst walls, septa, or solid areas

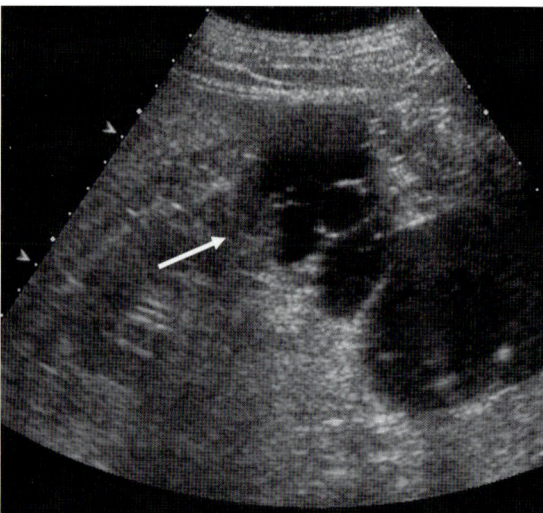

Fig. 8.8 Thickening of the upper cyst wall (arrow) in a large cystic renal carcinoma of the midaspect of the right kidney

Most cystic renal carcinomas (50%) are unilocular and represent necrosis within the renal tumor.[33] Ultrasound shows a thick, uneven wall with the cystic component containing echoes. Next most common (30%), the mass has several cystic spaces with thick nodular intervening masses containing adenocarcinoma. In 20%, there is a solid mass within the wall of a cyst (Fig. 8.8); this feature is usually caused by asymmetric necrosis. Rarely, the lesion is a unilocular cystadenocarcinoma with a thin layer of clear cells in the walls. Multilocular cystadenocarcinoma represents only 3% of renal cell tumors but follows a relatively benign clinical course.[34]

Congenital Cystic Renal Disease

Polycystic Kidney Disease

Autosomal recessive polycystic kidney disease (ARPKD) may present in utero or in childhood. The kidneys are symmetrically enlarged, smooth, and are of increased reflectivity due to the multiple tiny cysts being too small to individually resolve, but providing numerous reflective interfaces. However, a few small discrete cysts may be seen and a low-reflective rim may develop around the kidneys. Generally, ARKPD patients diagnosed in utero have a poor prognosis and may succumb from underdeveloped lungs caused by lack of amniotic fluid (Fig. 8.9). ARKPD patients diagnosed at an older age generally have better renal function but suffer from portal hypertension as a consequence of hepatic cysts and periportal fibrosis. Those ARKPD patients that survive the perinatal period have a better prognosis than is generally perceived.[35]

Autosomal dominant polycystic kidney disease (ADPKD) usually presents in the fourth or fifth decade of life with renal impairment, hypertension, hematuria, and abdominal pain. ADPKD may also be detected serendipitously during ultrasound imaging for other reasons. Screening of offspring of affected ADKPD adults is normally performed with ultrasound. Renal cysts are rare below age 30; finding two or more renal cysts in this age group with a family history of ADPKD indicates that the patient is also affected.[36] Once the condition is established, innumerable cysts of varying sizes disrupt the normal architecture of the kidneys and both kidneys become considerably enlarged (Fig. 8.10). The size of the kidneys is related to renal function and hypertension; an increase in cyst volume correlates with decline in renal function.[37] Liver cysts occur in up to 67% and increase in size and number with age. Women suffer more severe polycystic liver disease than men.[38] Seminal vesicle cysts occur in 40% of men, and rarely cysts may occur in the pancreas, spleen, and ovary.[39]

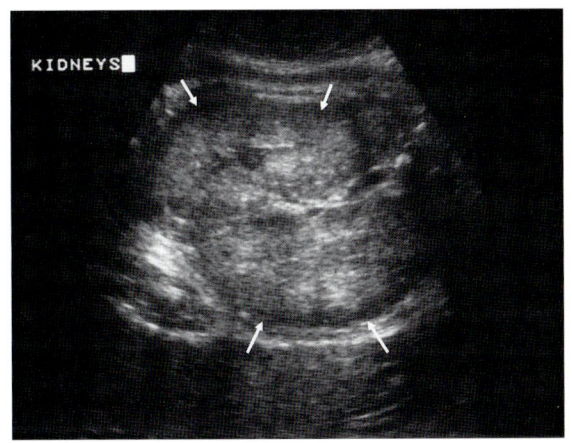
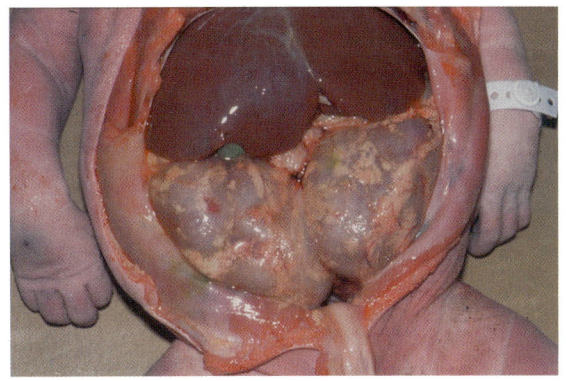

Fig. 8.9 **a** Autosomal recessive polycystic kidneys diagnosed in utero. Both kidneys are symmetrically enlarged with smooth surfaces and a bright texture. A hypoechoic rim (arrows) has developed around each kidney. The lack of amniotic fluid shows the kidneys are not functioning. **b** Autopsy of the newborn child. The baby died at birth due to lack of lung development as a consequence of the lack of amniotic fluid. The kidneys are shown to fill the abdomen and to have a smooth outline with no macroscopic cysts

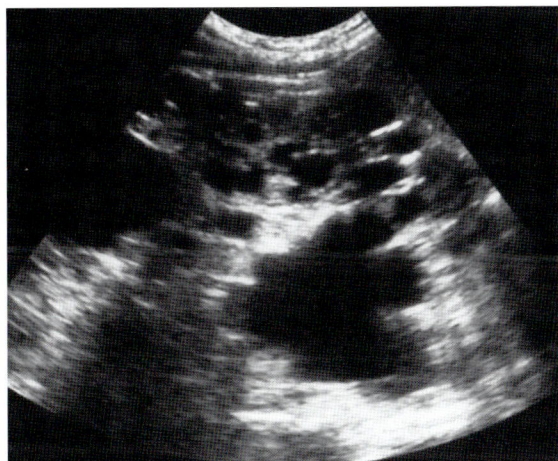
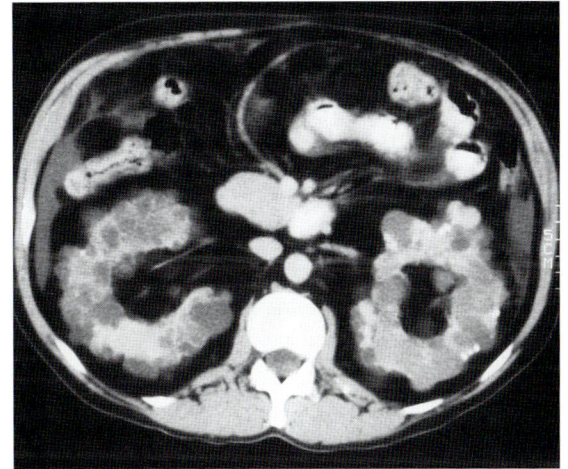
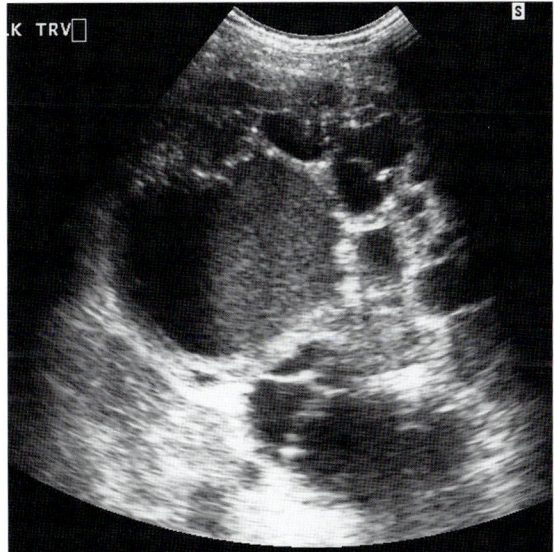

Fig. 8.10 **a** Longitudinal image through the right kidney in a patient with ADPKD. **b** CT image of ADPKD, demonstrating numerous cysts throughout both kidneys with disruption of the normal renal architecture. **c** One of the cysts in this autosomal dominant polycystic kidney shows a fluid–debris level. The clinical history and outcome were of hemorrhage into the cyst rather than infection

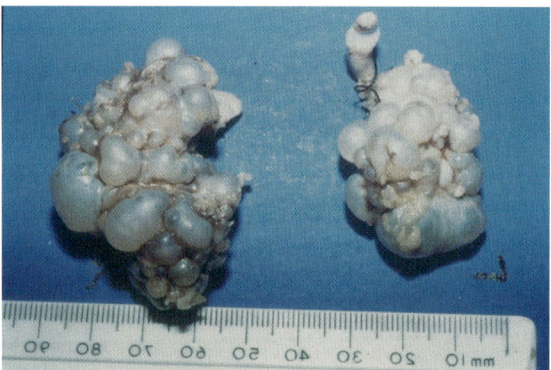

Fig. 8.**11 Autopsy specimen from a fetus affected with bilateral multicystic dysplastic kidneys.** There are cysts of different sizes distorting the renal outline. Note how this differs from the image of autosomal recessive polycystic kidneys shown in Fig. 8.**9b**

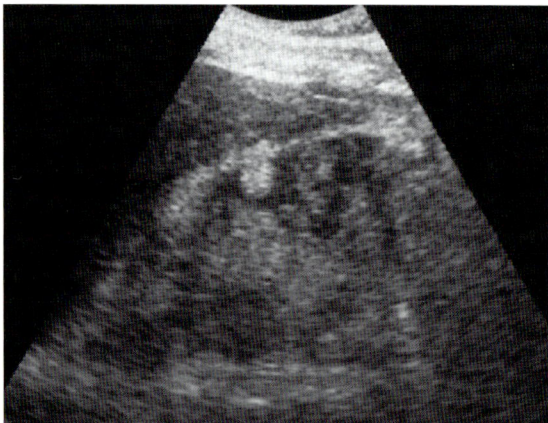

Fig. 8.**12 Patient with tuberous sclerosis where the kidneys are affected by innumerable angiomyolipomata**

Hemorrhage or infection of the cysts of polycystic kidney disease may occur and demonstrate similar signs to the same process that may occur in other simple cysts (Fig. 8.**10**). It can be difficult to assess which of the many cysts present in polycystic disease is giving rise to the symptoms. Calculi are seen in up to 20% of patients.[40]

Multicystic Dysplastic Kidney

Multicystic dysplastic kidney is thought to occur as a result of ureteric atresia during early fetal life. The kidney or part of the kidney affected is nonfunctioning; consequently, bilateral multicystic dysplastic kidneys are not compatible with life (Fig. 8.**11**). An affected kidney is replaced by a mass of cysts of varying sizes; it usually undergoes atrophy during childhood. The clinical relevance is the association with disorders of the contralateral kidney. This can occur in up to 40% and usually takes the form of pelviureteric obstruction or vesicoureteric reflux (VUR). Such reflux causes the contralateral kidney to have reduced growth.[41] Multicystic dysplastic kidney may affect one part of a duplex kidney. Most cases are sporadic, but there are occasional instances of familial recurrence.[42]

Von Hippel–Lindau Disease

Von Hippel–Lindau disease is inherited in an autosomal dominant fashion with variable expression and penetrance. It usually manifests after the second decade of life and features one or more of the following: Renal cysts (75%), cerebellar hemangioblastoma (35–60%), retinal angiomatosis (50%), renal adenocarcinoma (25–45%), and pheochromocytoma (10%). The renal cysts may be the first manifestation of the disease; ultrasound of the abdomen is advocated as a screening tool in those at risk. Cysts are usually cortical and between 0.5 and 3.0 cm in size. Cysts may also develop in the pancreas, liver, and adrenals. The renal adenocarcinoma that occurs is bilateral in 75% and multifocal within one kidney in about 87% of cases. These patients are usually offered nephron-sparing surgery. MR imaging is the best tool for screening known affected kidneys for the development of carcinoma.[43]

Tuberous Sclerosis

Tuberous sclerosis is characterized by mental retardation, seizures, and cutaneous adenoma sebaceum. It is an autosomal dominant hereditary neurocutaneous disorder. Renal cysts and angiomyolipomas may be the earliest or only manifestation of the disease in childhood. Angiomyolipomas occur in 80% of patients and may be too numerous to count; cysts occur in 47% of cases (Fig. 8.**12**). Both cysts and angiomyolipomas increase in size and number with increasing age.[44] There is a small incidence of renal adenocarcinoma developing.[45]

Medullary Cystic Disease Complex

This is a group of rare disorders comprising juvenile nephronophthisis, medullary cystic renal degeneration, and renal retinal dysplasia. Presentation is in childhood or young adulthood with renal failure. The kidneys are small and smooth with cortical atrophy, although the cortex is usually bright on ultrasound. There may be multiple cysts of 1–2 cm diameter lying in the medulla or at the corticomedullary junction (thought to be dilated distal convoluted tubules).[14]

> **Summary points:**
> - Simple cysts are well-defined and anechoic. Thin septa 1 mm thick or less are allowed
> - Simple cysts gradually increase in size and number with age
> - Complex cysts with thick septa, internal echoes, and areas of calcification need further investigation

Benign Solid Lesions

Adenoma

The diagnosis of a renal adenoma is no longer a consideration on imaging. Previously solid lesions < 3 cm in size were thought to be benign and larger lesions malignant. It is now clear that an adenoma cannot be distinguished from an adenocarcinoma even on histology and therefore the distinction based entirely on size criteria is untenable. However, it is documented that small solid renal tumors grow slowly, usually < 0.5 cm per year, and that these tumors virtually never metastasize when < 3 cm.[46] Consequently, "watchful waiting" is appropriate, especially in elderly patients or those that might not survive surgery. Small cortical tumors in the donor kidney are sometimes found incidentally during surgery for transplantation, not having shown up on imaging studies; the risk of malignant transformation with immunosuppression is not quantifiable so the kidney is not transplanted.[47]

Oncocytoma

Oncocytomas are commoner in men, usually asymptomatic, and most often found serendipitously in the sixth and seventh decade. These tumors contain oncocytes, large cells that have a granular eosinophilic cytoplasm. Oncocytomas represent up to 6% of all renal tumors and generally follow a benign course without metastasis.[48] On ultrasound appearances are varied; oncocytomas may be isoreflective, have reduced or increased reflectivity. A characteristic feature is a central stellate scar, and microbubble contrast enhancement may show a "spoke-wheel" pattern, more typically found on angiography (Fig. 8.13). There are no reliable imaging features that allow an oncocytoma to be distinguished from renal adenocarcinoma.[49] Hemorrhage is rare. Biopsy is unhelpful, as oncocytoma rests are occasionally found in renal adenocarcinomas. There are reports of oncocytomas of unusual appearance mimicking other lesions and the final diagnosis can only be made after the entire tumor is examined by histology.[50]

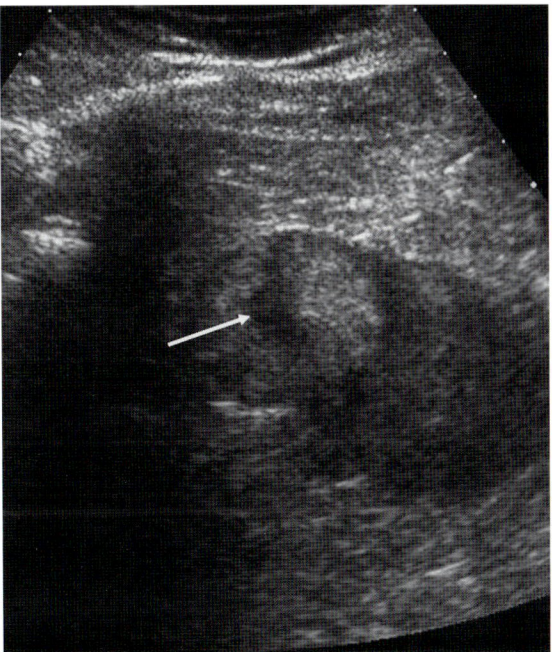
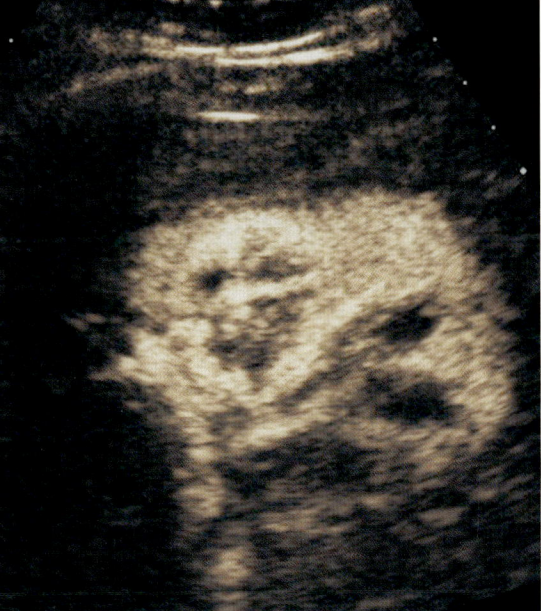

Fig. 8.13 **a** A well-circumscribed high-reflective lesion arising from the upper aspect of the left kidney, demonstrating a central low-reflective "scar" (arrow). **b** Following the administration of SonoVue (Bracco, Milan, Italy), and using low mechanical index (MI) imaging (CPS, Acuson, Siemens, Mountain View, CA), a typical "spoke-and-wheel" effect is demonstrated in keeping with an oncocytoma. (Courtesy of Dr. P.S. Sidhu)

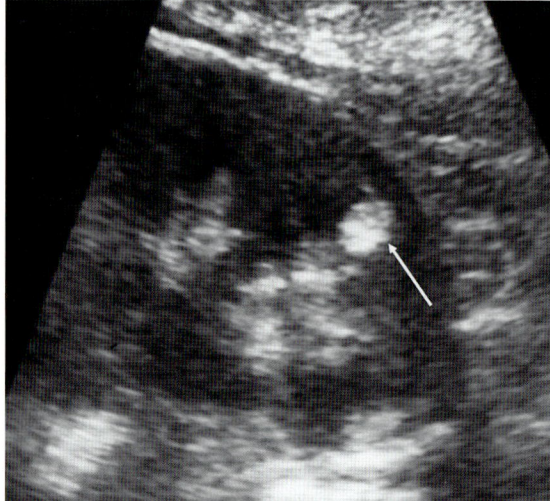

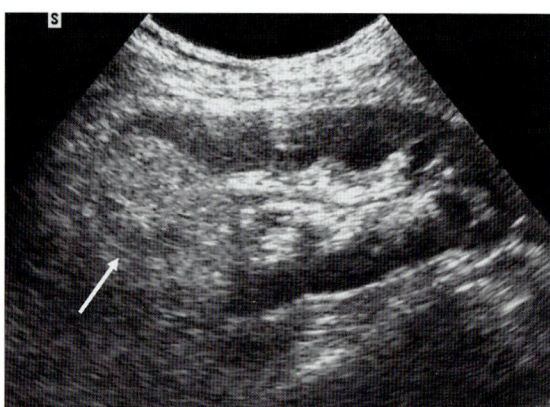

Fig. 8.14 **a** A small cortical angiomyolipoma (arrow) within the kidney. **b** A larger, exophytic angiomyolipoma (arrow). The fat content of this lesion needs to be confirmed with CT imaging, as some RCCs may be as reflective as this

Angiomyolipoma

Angiomyolipomas are benign hamartomatous lesions of the kidney; the tumors contain varying proportions of blood vessels, smooth muscle, and fat. They may occur as single or multiple lesions in one or both kidneys; 50% of patients with renal angiomyolipomas will have tuberous sclerosis. Those tumors that are not associated with tuberous sclerosis are most commonly found in middle-aged women and are usually unilateral. The angiomyolipomas seen in tuberous sclerosis had been thought to be small and asymptomatic, but at least one series has shown large symptomatic tumors presenting with pain, hematuria, and fever.[51] Angiography often reveals aneurysmal dilation of the tumoral arteries; this explains the association of angiomyolipomas with spontaneous renal bleeding confined to the subcapsular and perirenal space (Wunderlich syndrome).[52] The likelihood of spontaneous bleeding increases once the tumor is > 4 cm and there is an aneurysm > 5 mm in size.[53]

The ultrasound features are characteristically of a highly reflective cortical mass, some of which may be exophytic (Fig. 8.**14**). The brightness of the lesion is similar to renal sinus fat. The fat content of the tumor contributes to the high reflectivity of the lesion; a third may show acoustic shadowing. Bleeding into the tumor alters the appearance and may make diagnosis difficult. Some renal adenocarcinomas are as reflective as angiomyolipomas.[54] The diagnosis of angiomyolipoma may be confirmed by CT or MR imaging, demonstrating the fat content of the tumor. Biopsy is rarely useful.[55] Small tumors do not need to be treated, whereas large tumors need to be surgically removed using nephron-sparing techniques to prevent complications. Actively bleeding angiomyolipomas may be treated with coil embolization during catheter angiography.

Summary points:
- Benign
- Carry a risk of bleeding
- May be the earliest manifestation of tuberous sclerosis
- Large lesions can mimic carcinoma and vice-versa

Focal Infection/Inflammatory Pseudotumour

There are several synonyms: Lobar nephronia, acute focal pyelonephritis, focal bacterial nephritis, and pseudoabscess. Essentially the condition is a focal area of pyelonephritis in a lobar distribution; it forms part of the diagnostic continuum of acute pyelonephritis and represents an inflammatory mass that does not contain pus amenable to percutaneous or surgical drainage.[56] Ultrasound features are of a loss of corticomedullary differentiation in the affected segment and a mass or wedge-shaped area that can be of high, low or mixed reflectivity (Fig. 8.**15**).[57] Since the clinical presentation is one of infection, the diagnosis is not usually in doubt. Tissue-harmonic imaging gives increased contrast resolution and is said to allow up to 97% of kidneys with acute pyelonephritis to show focal changes. Serial ultrasound during appropriate antibiotic treatment will show focal changes resolve, although progression to an abscess will occur if treatment is not adequate.

Fig. 8.15 **Focal infection. a** The patient presented with clinical features typical of infection, and the ultrasound image demonstrates a mass extending from the medulla into the cortex (arrow). This represents an area of acute focal pyelonephritis. **b** The same patient, one week later, demonstrates persistence of the abnormality. Resolution of the appearances of the mass may be slow despite appropriate antibiotics. Progression to an abscess has not occurred. **c** High-reflective fungus balls within the pelvicalyceal system of an immunocompromized child (between cursors)

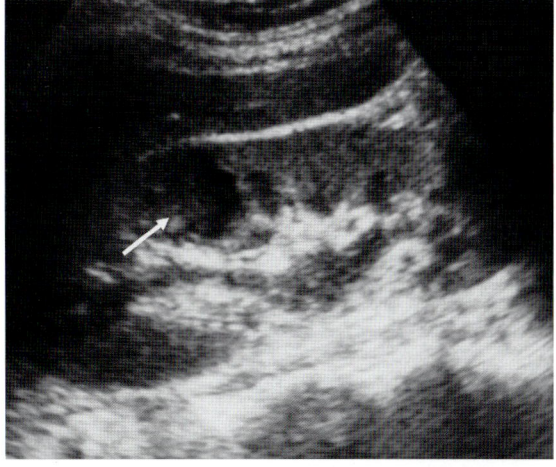

Malignant Tumors

Renal Adenocarcinoma

Ninety percent of adult primary renal tumors are renal adenocarcinomas. There is a male to female preponderance of two to one; multiple tumors are found in one kidney in 5% of cases, and 1–2% have bilateral tumors.[58] There is an association with von Hippel–Lindau disease and tuberous sclerosis. Common symptoms at presentation are painless hematuria, flank pain, and a palpable mass together with anorexia and weight loss. The proportion of tumors < 3 cm in size is rising entirely as a result of detection as an incidental finding during imaging for other indications.[59] Ultrasound screening programs have been advocated; one trial involving 9959 volunteers yielded only nine renal adenocarcinomas. The sensitivity at one-year follow-up was 82% and the positive predictive value of positive findings was 50%.[60]

Ultrasound features are of a solid tumor mass which may be of increased, decreased, or similar reflectivity as the normal renal cortex. Larger tumors are more likely to be isoreflective, whereas tumors < 3 cm in size are more likely to be of increased reflectivity relative to the renal parenchyma (Fig. 8.16). Larger tumors are more

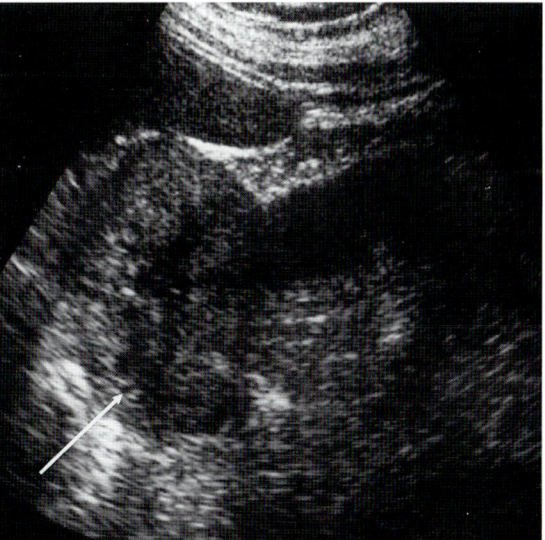

Fig. 8.16 **A large, high-reflective, exophytic RCC (arrow). Larger tumors are more usually echo-poor (see Fig. 8.17);** the reflectivity of the lesion does not correlate with the type of RCC

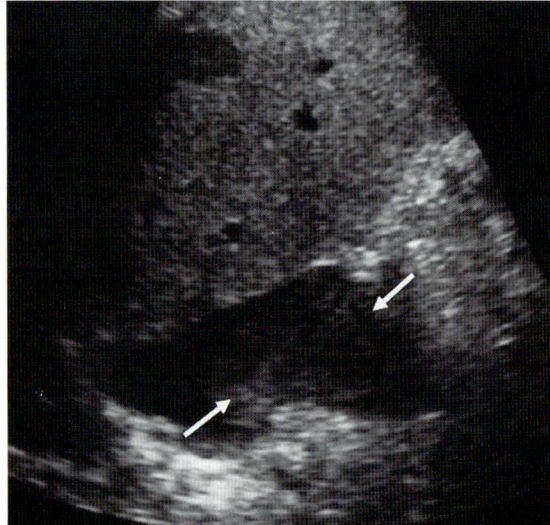

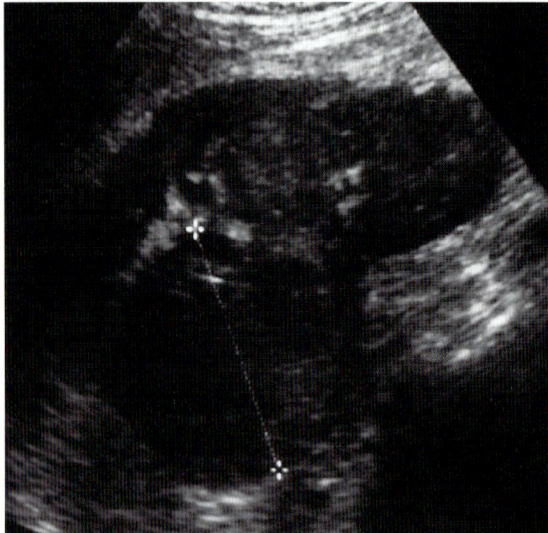

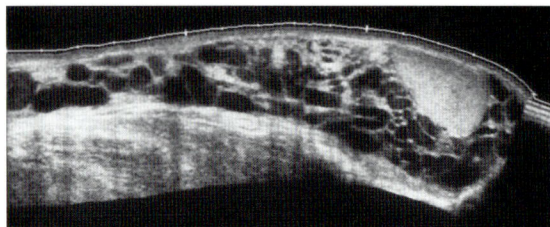

Fig. 8.17 **a** An area of high reflectivity (arrows) within a dilated IVC, representing tumor thrombus which has extended from the kidney. **b** The primary tumor in the kidney shows the typical hypoechoic pattern seen in larger RCCs (between cursors). **c** A large varicocele of the scrotum. Varicoceles may occur following obstruction of the left renal vein by tumor-thrombus spreading from an RCC

likely to show hemorrhage or central necrosis. Rimlike calcification occurs in a small proportion; however, central calcification is more strongly predictive of adenocarcinoma. The pattern on ultrasound does not bear any useful relationship to the type of renal adenocarcinoma. Color and spectral Doppler ultrasound features of high-velocity and turbulence are nonspecific for malignancy,[61] though some authors believe Doppler ultrasound is useful in cystic lesions.[8]

The differential diagnosis of a solid or partly solid mass on ultrasound includes various tumors, hematomas, infections, and pseudotumors such as a prominent column of Bertin. It has been hoped that ultrasound microbubble contrast agents would, together with harmonic imaging, improve diagnostic certainty with ultrasound, but initial reports show that differential diagnosis remains difficult.[62] This lack of specificity on ultrasound means that all masses should be evaluated further with CT or MR imaging. Both CT and MR perform equally well in characterizing and local staging of a tumor; multichannel helical CT takes less time to examine the whole abdomen.[63]

Local spread of renal adenocarcinoma is into the renal vein with progressive extension into the inferior vena cava (IVC; Fig. 8.17) or even the right atrium. Indeed, late recurrence of tumor can occur within the IVC.[64] Local spread also occurs to the retroperitoneal lymph nodes and into adjacent organs. Fixity of the kidney relative to the liver during respiration or ultrasound palpation is a sign of local invasion. Renal adenocarcinoma may metastasize to any distant organ but there is a predilection for lung metastases.

Percutaneous renal biopsy is not generally indicated, as the ultrasound and CT features are sufficient to confirm the need for surgical resection. Those patients who are not destined for surgery but still require a histological diagnosis before immunotherapy or chemotherapy can undergo a biopsy, usually with accuracy.[65]

Renal Pelvic Tumors

Tumors of the renal pelvis represent 10% of solid renal tumors, with the majority of these being transitional cell carcinomas (TCCs); the remainder are mostly squamous cell carcinoma. TCC is much less common in the upper renal tracts than in the bladder, as the urothelium of the upper tracts represents a much smaller surface area with urine in contact with it for a shorter period than in the bladder. Any patient with TCC of the bladder has a 4% risk of developing an upper renal tract tumor.[66] If the upper tract tumor is the presenting lesion, there is a 30% risk of developing a bladder tumor and a 6% risk of developing a tumor in the contralateral kidney.[67]

Men are affected more often than women, and peak incidence is between age 40 and 70. The most common presenting symptom is hematuria. There is still debate as to whether patients with hematuria should be investigated with ultrasound or IVU. However, since upper tract TCCs are so much less common than bladder tumors or renal adenocarcinomas, most authorities agree that ultrasound should be the primary imaging tool.[68]

The ultrasound features of renal pelvic TCC are quite variable depending on whether the tumor is sessile or papillary and whether it is causing hydronephrosis. Large tumors are seen as discrete, low-reflective, solid masses within the renal pelvis and may cause dilation of the calyces (Fig. 8.**18**). Blood clots, sloughed papillae, and fungus balls may show similar features. Fat within the normal renal sinus may appear relatively low-reflective and can mimic tumor. However, posterior acoustic shadowing, an indistinct posterior wall, and traversing hilar vessels all point to it being a normal renal sinus (Fig. 8.**18**).[69] Color Doppler ultrasound does not help in the evaluation of TCC, as tumor grade, stage, and size are not related to vascularity.[70] Metastases are primarily to lymph nodes, bone, and lung.

Lymphoma

The kidneys do not contain lymphatic tissue. Primary renal lymphoma is a contested diagnosis and certainly very rare.[71] Secondary involvement of the kidney by lymphoma, particularly non-Hodgkin lymphoma, is seen in up to a third of cases. Ultrasound usually shows either multiple, small, low-reflective masses or diffuse enlargement of the kidney due to infiltration.[72] It is less common to find a focal solitary mass.[73] Rarely, lymphoma may manifest as a rind of low-reflective tissue surrounding the kidney. Most diagnoses are made as part of CT staging of known disease.

Metastases

Autopsy studies show that the kidney is the fifth most common site for metastases. However, metastases are diagnosed much less commonly during life. The common primary sites are lung, breast, and the contralateral kidney. Ultrasound typically shows multiple masses, which are usually low-reflective. Less commonly, a metastasis may present as a solitary renal mass (Fig. 8.**19**). If a patient is known to have another primary tumor, even one in remission, then a renal biopsy is needed to distinguish a metastasis from a renal adenocarcinoma.

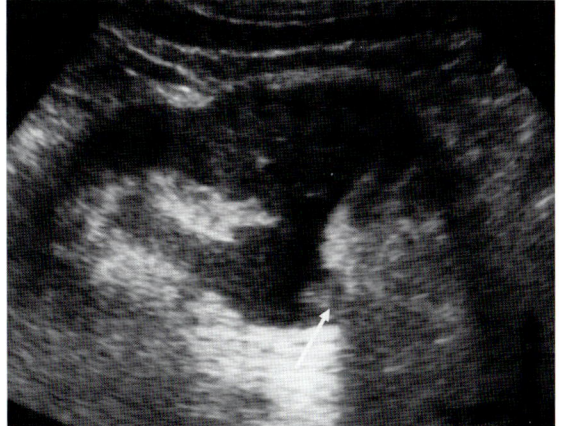

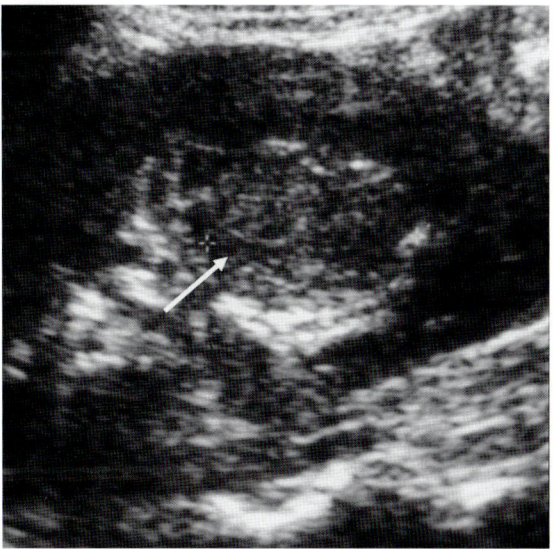

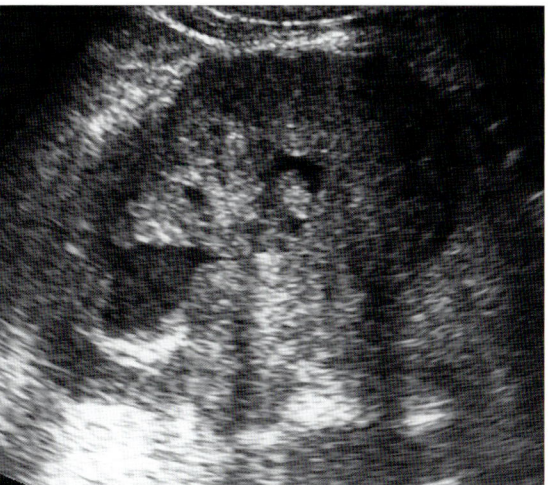

Fig. 8.**18** **a** A small TCC (arrow) causing obstruction at the pelviureteric junction. **b** A TCC filling and distending the lower pole calyx of the kidney (arrow). **c** Large TCC filling the renal pelvis. Note that the posterior margin of the lesion is well-defined, with no posterior acoustic shadowing, and there is a visible distended calyx. These features distinguish the tumor from normal renal sinus fat

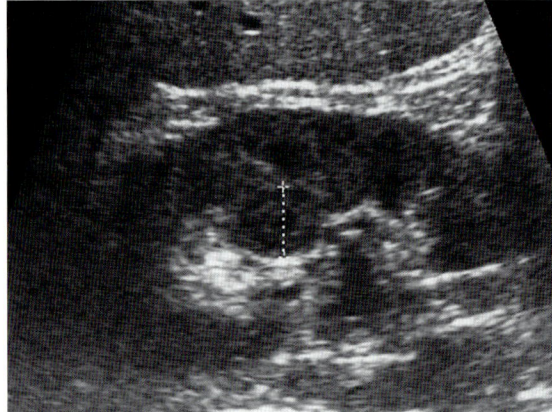

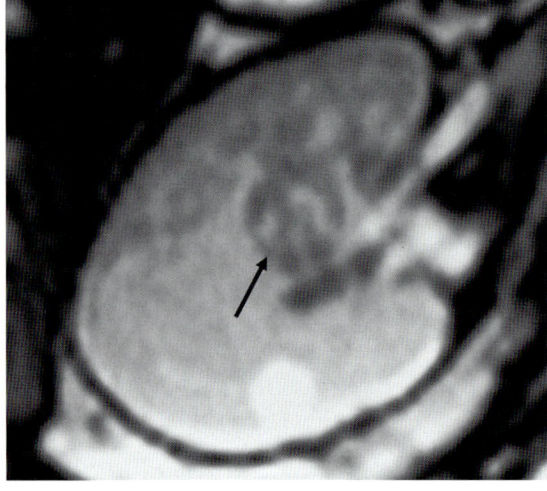

Fig. 8.19 **a** A focal mass of mixed reflectivity (between cursors) in the right kidney representing a metastasis from a carcinoma of the cervix. **b** MR imaging in the transverse plane, demonstrating the metastatic lesion seen on ultrasound (arrow). There is a simple cyst, indicated by the well-circumscribed area of high signal

Sarcoma

Sarcomas represent only 1% of renal malignancies. The ultrasound appearances of a sarcoma are common to other tumors and diagnosis is usually only made following resection. The commonest form of sarcoma in the kidney is a leiomyosarcoma which may be solid or occasionally cystic.[74] Prognosis is poor, with five-year survival rates of about a third.

Other Rare Renal Tumors

There are many different tumors that can affect the kidney, of which the following are the most common: Sarcoid, splenosis, fibroma, leiomyoma, lipoma, hemangiopericytoma, hemangioma, lymphangioma, pheochromocytoma, reninoma, plasmacytoma, carcinoid, and adult Wilms tumor.

> **Summary points:**
> Clinical history and features are needed for diagnosis
> - RCC (represents the vast majority)
> - TCC
> - Lymphoma
> - Metastases
> - Inflammatory pseudotumours
> - Sarcomas and other rare tumors

Renal Trauma

The classification of injuries to the kidney is detailed in Table 8.**2**.[75] The majority of traumas to the kidney are blunt, such as occur in road-traffic accidents, sports, falls, and fights. Kidneys with an underlying pathology are more likely to be injured, usually because the kidney is enlarged and consequently less protected by surrounding structures. Patients with hematuria after minimal-force, blunt abdominal trauma are particularly worthy of suspicion for an underlying pathology.[76] Penetrating injuries are less common and, in the United Kingdom, more likely to be iatrogenic after renal biopsy or nephrostomy than following a gunshot or stab wound (Fig. 8.**20**).

CT imaging is the examination method of choice in suspected renal trauma because of excellent sensitivity and the ability to image trauma to other organs.[77] There has been a resurgence of interest in the use of ultrasound with the advent of focused assessment sonography in trauma (FAST). Ultrasound has the potential advantage of being readily available at the patient's bedside. However, there are limitations. Ultrasound visualization of the kidneys may be poor in an immobile patient with extensive bruising. Major renal parenchyma injuries may not be visible.[78] Hemoperitoneum cannot be relied on to indicate renal injuries as it occurs in less than 50% of renal injuries.[79] Ultrasound may have a role in the early triage of patients, as, although it is often normal in renal trauma, it is more likely to be abnormal in category 2 or greater injuries.[80] Since a negative ultrasound does not exclude renal injury, if the clinical and laboratory parameters remain of concern, a CT examination should be done.

Intrarenal or extrarenal fluid following trauma may represent either blood or urine. Hemorrhage, while still fluid, will appear low-reflective. Echoes develop as the blood forms a hematoma. Finally, as resolution progresses over several weeks, the hematoma again becomes low-reflective and appears as a simple fluid col-

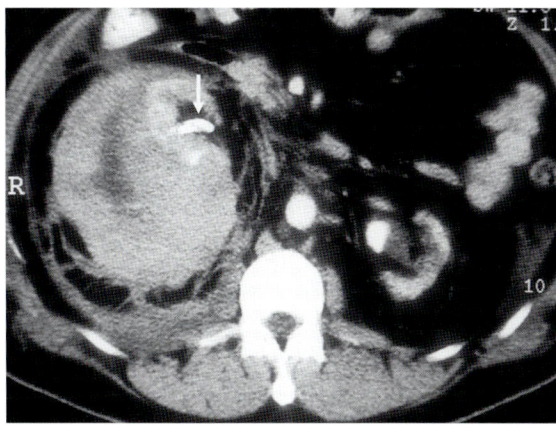
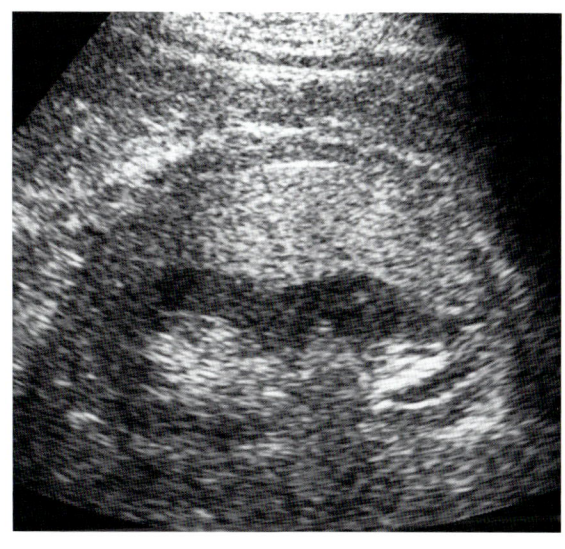

Fig. 8.20 **a** CT image of a large perinephric hematoma following placement of a nephrostomy tube (arrow). **b** Ultrasound image of a subcapsular hematoma. The kidney is flattened by an echogenic collection of blood

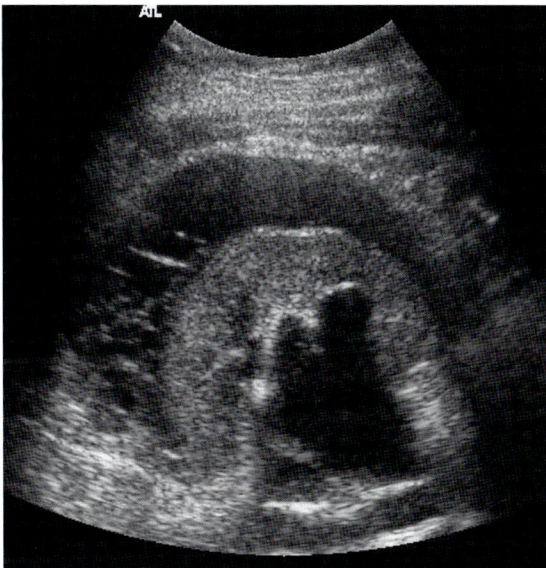

Fig. 8.21 **Perinephric urinoma in a hydronephrotic kidney.** The clinical history should distinguish this lesion from a post-traumatic hematoma

Table 8.2 **Classification of renal injury**[75]

Category 1	Minor injuries (75–85%): Contusions, superficial lacerations, and small perinephric bleeds. Conservative management
Category 2	Major injuries (10%): Deep lacerations communicating with the pelvicalyceal system. Conservative management in most cases
Category 3	Catastrophic injuries (5%): Shattered kidney and renal pedicle injury. Surgical management
Category 4	Avulsion of the pelviureteric junction or renal pelvic laceration (rare). Surgical management

lection. Lacerations are seen as linear areas of discontinuous parenchyma. A subcapsular collection will cause the kidney to become flattened. A "shattered" kidney will appear as several fragments of disorganized tissue in the renal bed surrounded by fluid and hematoma.

Color Doppler may show if the kidney is still perfused but is not reliable at confirming the converse; technical factors may limit the machine's ability to detect blood flow. Penetrating injuries, particularly renal biopsy, can produce arteriovenous fistulae (AVF). Color Doppler will show perivascular tissue vibration artifact and spectral Doppler will show high velocities in the feeding artery and transmission of pulsation into the draining venous spectral Doppler waveform. Muscular crush injuries cause rhabdomyolysis and secondary renal failure. The renal resistive index provides prognostic information in this circumstance.[81]

It has been advocated that ultrasound is a good tool to follow up the resolution of perinephric collections (Fig. 8.21) and perfusion anomalies. However, if the clinical course is uncomplicated following blunt abdominal trauma, follow-up imaging does not aid management.[82] Drainage of symptomatic perinephric collections can be guided percutaneously by ultrasound.

Summary points:
- Underlying pathology makes renal damage more likely
- FAST has a role in immediate triage
- Ultrasound is poor at detecting renal injuries
- Hemoperitoneum occurs in less than 50% of renal injuries
- Color Doppler can confirm perfusion of the kidney

References

1. Rodriguez R, Fishman EK, Marshall FF. Differential diagnosis and evaluation of the incidentally discovered renal mass. Semin Urol Oncol 1995;13:246–253.
2. Lee CT, Katz J, Fearn PA, Russo P. Mode of presentation of renal cell carcinoma provides prognostic information. Urol Oncol 2002;7:135–140.
3. Terada N, Ichioka K, Matsuda Y, Okubo K, Yoshimura K, Arai Y. The natural history of simple renal cysts. J Urol 2002;167:21–23.
4. Paananen I, Hellstrom P, Leinonen S, et al. Treatment of renal cysts with single-session percutaneous drainage and ethanol sclerotherapy: long-term outcome. Urology 2001; 57:30–33.
5. Liatsikos EN, Siablis D, Karnabatidis D, et al. Percutaneous treatment of large symptomatic renal cysts. J Endourol 2000;14:257–261.
6. Sakai N, Kanda F, Kondo K, Fukuoka H, Tanaka T. Sonographically detected malignant transformation of a simple renal cyst. Int J Urol 2001;8:23–25.
7. Ooi GC, Sagar G, Lynch D, Arkell DG, Ryan PG. Cystic renal cell carcinoma: radiological features and clinico-pathological correlation. Clin Radiol 1996;51:791–796.
8. Hirai T, Ohishi H, Yamada R et al. Usefulness of color Doppler flow imaging in differential diagnosis of multilocular cystic lesions of the kidney. J Ultrasound Med 1995;14:771–776.
9. Kim AY, Kim SH, Kim YJ, Lee IH. Contrast-enhanced power Doppler sonography for the differentiation of cystic renal lesions: preliminary study. J Ultrasound Med 1999;18: 581–588.
10. Gooding GA. Sonography of hemorrhagic cysts with computed tomographic correlation. J Ultrasound Med 1986;5: 699–702.
11. Fujii Y, Higashi Y, Owada F, Arisawa C, Horiuchi S. Benign hemorrhagic renal cysts mimicking cystic renal cell carcinoma. Hinyokika Kiyo 1993;39:1113–1117.
12. Frishman E, Orron DE, Heiman Z, Kessler A, Kaver I, Graif M. Infected renal cysts: sonographic diagnosis and management. J Ultrasound Med 1994;13:7–10.
13. Zmerli S, Ayed M, Horchani A, Chami I, El Ouakdi M, Ben Slama MR. Hydatid cyst of the kidney: diagnosis and treatment. World J Surg 2001;25:68–74.
14. Schild HH, Mildenberger P, Schweden FJ. Cystic renal diseases. In: Computed tomography in Urology. Schild HH, Schweden FJ, Lang EK, eds. Stuttgart: Georg Thieme Verlag: 1992:81–102
15. Thurston W, Wilson SR. The urinary tract. In: Diagnostic ultrasound. 2nd ed. Rumack CM, Wilson SR, Charboneau JW, eds. St. Louis: Mosby: 1998:373.
16. Israel GM, Bosniak MA. Calcification in cystic renal masses: is it important in diagnosis? Radiology 2003;226:47–52.
17. Yeh HC, Mitty HA, Halton K, Shapiro R, Rabinowitz JG. Milk of calcium in renal cysts: new sonographic features. J Ultrasound Med 1992;11:195–203.
18. Melekos MD, Kosti PN, Zarakovitis IE, Dimopoulos PA. Milk of calcium cysts masquerading as renal calculi. Eur J Radiol 1998;28:62–66.
19. Patel U, Huntley L, Kellett MJ. Sonographic features of renal obstruction mimicked by peripelvic cysts. Clin Radiol 1994;49:481–484.
20. Zinn HL, Becker JA. Peripelvic cysts simulating hydronephrosis. Abdom Imaging 1997;22:346–347.
21. Nicolau C, Vilana R, Del Amo M, et al. Accuracy of sonography with a hydration test in differentiating between excretory renal obstruction and renal sinus cysts. J Clin Ultrasound 2002;30:532–536.
22. Amis ES, Cronan JJ. The renal sinus: an imaging review and proposed nomenclature for sinus cysts. J Urol 1988;139: 1151–1159.
23. Murray KK, McLellan GL. Renal peripelvic lymphangiectasia: appearance at CT. Radiology 1991;180:455.
24. Honma I, Takagi Y, Shigyo M, et al. Lymphangioma of the kidney. Int J Urol 2002;9:178–182.
25. Mishal J, Lebovici O, Bregman L, London D, Yoffe B, Sherer Y. Huge renal arteriovenous malformation mimicking simple parapelvic cyst. Clin Imaging 2000;24:166–168.
26. Deibler AR, Nadig SN, Curry N, Bissada NK, Hull GW. Intrarenal varix presenting as an enhancing renal mass with calcifications. J Urol 2001;166:997–998.
27. Dalla-Palma L, Pozzi-Mucelli F, di Donna A, Pozzi-Mucelli RS. Cystic renal tumours: US and CT findings. Urol Radiol 1990;12:67–73.
28. Canakli F, Tekdogan UY, Ergul G, Aslan Y, Atan A. Cystic nephroma: a rare clinical entity. Int Urol Nephrol 2002;34: 19–21.
29. Bosniak MA. The current approach to renal cysts. Radiology 1986;158:1–10.
30. Aronson S, Frazier HA, Baluch JD, Hartman DS, Christenson PJ. Cystic renal masses: usefulness of the Bosniak classification. Urol Radiol 1991;13:83–90.
31. Harisinghani MG, Maher MM, Gervais DA, et al. Incidence of malignancy in complex renal masses (Bosniak category III): should imaging-guided biopsy precede surgery? AJR Am J Roentgenol 2003;180:755–758.
32. Israel GM, Bosniak MA. Follow-up CT of moderately complex cystic lesions of the kidney (Bosniak category IIF). AJR Am J Roentgenol 2003;181:627–633.
33. Hartman DS, Davis CJ, Johns T, Goldman SM. Cystic renal carcinoma. Urology 1986;28:145–153.
34. Nassir A, Jollimore J, Gupta R, Bell D, Norman R. Multilocular cystic renal cell carcinoma: a series of 12 cases and review of the literature. Urology 2002;60:421–427.
35. Guay-Woodford LM, Desmond RA. Autosomal recessive polycystic kidney disease: the clinical experience in North America. Pediatrics 2003;111:1072–1080.
36. Ravine D, Gibson RN, Walker RG, Sheffield LJ, Kincaid-Smith P, Danks DM. Evaluation of ultrasonographic diagnostic criteria for autosomal dominant polycystic kidney disease. Lancet 1994;343:824–827.
37. King BF, Reed JE, Bergstralh EJ, Sheedy PF II., Torres VE. Quantification and longitudinal trends of kidney, renal cyst, and renal parenchyma volumes in autosomal dominant polycystic kidney disease. J Am Soc Nephrol 2000; 11:1505–1511.
38. Nicolau C, Torra R, Bianchi L, et al. Abdominal sonographic study of autosomal dominant polycystic kidney disease. J Clin Ultrasound 2000;28:277–282.
39. Belet U, Danaci M, Sarikaya S, et al. Prevalence of epididymal, seminal vesicle, prostate, and testicular cysts in autosomal dominant polycystic kidney disease. Urology 2002; 60:138–141.

40. Segal AJ, Spataro RF, Barbaric ZL. Adult polycystic kidney disease: a review of 100 cases. J Urol 1977;118:711.
41. Fanos V, Sinaguglia G, Vino L, Pizzini C, Portuese A. Multicystic dysplastic kidney and contralateral vesicoureteral reflux. Renal growth. Minerva Pediatr 2001;53:95–98.
42. Belk RA, Thomas DF, Mueller RF, Godpole P, Markham AF, Weston MJ. A family study and the natural history of prenatally detected unilateral multicystic dysplastic kidney. J Urol 2002;167:666–669.
43. Choyke PL, Glenn GM, Walther MM, Patronas NJ, Linehan WM, Zbar B. von Hippel-Lindau disease: genetic, clinical, and imaging features. Radiology 1995;194:629–642.
44. Caspar KA, Donnelly LF, Chen B, Bissler JJ. Tuberous sclerosis complex: renal imaging findings. Radiology 2002;225:451–456.
45. Saito M, Kakinuma H, Linuma M, et al. A case of renal cell carcinoma in tuberous sclerosis. Nippon Hinyokika Gakkai Zasshi 2003;94:634–638.
46. Bosniak MA, Birnbaum BA, Krinsky GA, Waisman J. Small renal parenchymal neoplasms: further observations on growth. Radiology 1995;197:589–597.
47. Jones JR, Woodside KJ, Early MG, Gugliuzza KK, Daller JA. Renal cortical adenoma incidentally found during living donor nephrectomy. Prog Transplant 2003;13:94–96.
48. Romis L, Cindolo L, Patard JJ, et al. Frequency, clinical presentation and evolution of renal oncocytomas: multicentric experience from a European database. Eur Urol 2004;45:53–57.
49. Goiney RC, Goldenberg L, Cooperberg PL, et al. Renal oncocytoma: sonographic analysis of 14 cases. AJR Am J Roentgenol 1984;143:1001–1004.
50. Sekido N, Kawai K, Takeshima H, Akaza H, Koiso K. Renal oncocytoma mimicking hemorrhagic renal cyst. Int J Urol 1995;2:336–338.
51. Tong YC, Chieng PU, Tsai TC, Lin SN. Renal angiomyolipoma: report of 24 cases. Br J Urol 1990;66:585–589.
52. Albi G, del Campo L, Tagarro D. Wünderlich's syndrome: causes, diagnosis and radiological management. Clin Radiol 2002;57:840–845.
53. Yamakado K, Tanaka N, Nakagawa T, Kobayashi S, Yanagawa M, Takeda K. Renal angiomyolipoma: relationships between tumor size, aneurysm formation, and rupture. Radiology 2002;225:78–82.
54. Forman HP, Middleton WM, Melson GL, McClennan BL. Hyperechoic renal cell carcinoma: increase in detection at US. Radiology 1993;188:431–434.
55. Nelson CP, Sanda MG. Contemporary diagnosis and management of renal angiomyolipoma. J Urol 2002;168:1315–1325.
56. Montejo M, Santiago MJ, Aguirrebengoa K, Garcia B, Goicoetxea J, Martin A. Acute focal bacterial nephritis: report of four cases. Nephron 2002;92:213–215.
57. Dubbins P. Ultrasound in acute urinary tract infection. BMUS Bulletin 2003;11:25–29.
58. Thoenes W, Storkel S, Rumpelt HJ. Histopathology and classification of renal cell tumours. Pathol Res Pract 1986;181:125.
59. Curry N. Small renal masses (lesions less than 3 cm): imaging evaluation and management. AJR Am J Roentgenol 1995;164:355–362.
60. Filipas D, Spix C, Schulz-Lampel D, et al. Screening for renal cell carcinoma using ultrasonography: a feasibility study. BJU Int 2003;91:595–599.
61. Kier R, Taylor KJW, Feyock AL, Ramos IM. Renal masses: characterization with Doppler US. Radiology 1990;176:703–707.
62. Quaia E, Siracusano S, Bertolotto M, Monduzzi M, Mucelli RP. Characterization of renal tumours with pulse inversion harmonic imaging by intermittent high mechanical index technique: initial results. Eur Radiol 2003;181:143–145.
63. Walter C, Kruessell M, Gindele A, Brochhagen HG, Gossmann A, Landwehr P. Imaging of renal lesions: evaluation of fast MRI and helical CT. Br J Radiol 2003;76:696–703.
64. Ioannis V, Panagiotis S, Anastasios A, et al. Tumor extending through inferior vena cava into the right atrium. A late recurrence of renal cell carcinoma. Int J Cardiovasc Imaging 2003;19:179–182.
65. Rybiki FJ, Shu KM, Cibas ES, Fielding JR, van Sonnenberg E, Silverman SG. Percutaneous biopsy of renal masses: sensitivity and negative predictive value stratified by clinical setting and size of masses. AJR Am J Roentgenol 2003;180:1281–1287.
66. Yousem DM, Gatewood OM, Goldman SM, et al. Synchronous and metachronous transitional cell carcinoma of the urinary tract: prevalence, incidence and radiographic detection. Radiology 1988;167:613–618.
67. Kang CH, Yu TJ, Hsieh HH, et al. The development of bladder tumors and contralateral upper tract tumors after primary transitional cell carcinoma of the upper urinary tract. Cancer 2003;98:1620–1626.
68. Datta SN, Allen GM, Evans R, Vaughton KC, Lucas MG. Urinary tract ultrasonography in the evaluation of haematuria - a report of over 1,000 cases. Ann R Coll Surg Engl 2002; 84:203–205.
69. Seong CK, Kim SH, Lee JS, Kim KH, Sim JS, Chang KH. Hypoechoic normal renal sinus and renal pelvis tumors: sonographic differentiation. J Ultrasound Med 2002;21:993–999.
70. Horstman WG, McFarland RM, Gorman JD. Color Doppler sonographic findings in patients with transitional cell carcinoma of the bladder and renal pelvis. J Ultrasound Med 1995;14:129–133.
71. Stallone G, Infante B, Manno C, Campobasso N, Pannarale G, Schena FP. Primary renal lymphoma does exist: case report and review of the literature. J Nephrol 2000;13:367–372.
72. Obrador GT, Price B, O'Meara Y, Salant DJ. Acute renal failure due to lymphomatous infiltration of the kidneys. J Am Soc Nephrol 1997;8:1348–1354.
73. Chepuri NB, Strouse PJ, Yanik GA. CT of renal lymphoma in children. AJR Am J Roentgenol 2003;180:429–431.
74. Dominici A, Mondaini N, Nesi G, Travaglini F, Di Cello V, Rizzo M. Cystic leiomyosarcoma of the kidney: an unusual clinical presentation. Urol Int 2000;65:229–231.
75. Federle MP. Evaluation of renal trauma. In: Pollack HM, ed. Clinical urography. Philadelphia: WB Saunders: 1990:1472–1494.
76. Chopra P, St-Vil D, Yazbeck S. Blunt renal trauma—blessing in disguise? J Pediatr Surg 2002;37:779–782.
77. Vasile M, Bellin MF, Helenon O, Mourey I, Cluzel P. Imaging evaluation of renal trauma. Abdom Imaging 2000;25:424–430.
78. Perry MJ, Porte ME, Urwin GH. Limitations of ultrasound evaluation in acute closed renal trauma. J R Coll Surg Edinb 1997;42:420–422.

79. Shanmuganathan K, Mirvis SE, Sherbourne CD, Chiu WC, Rodriguez A. Hemoperitoneum as the sole indicator of abdominal visceral injuries: a potential limitation of screening abdominal US for trauma. Radiology 1999;212:423–430.
80. McGahan JP, Richards JR, Jones CD, Gerscovich EO. Use of ultrasonography in the patient with acute renal trauma. J Ultrasound Med 1999;18:207–213.
81. Keven K, Ates K, Yagmurlu B, et al. Renal Doppler ultrasonographic findings in earthquake victims with crush injury. J Ultrasound Med 2001;20:675–679.
82. Mizzi A, Shabani A, Watt A. The role of follow-up imaging in paediatric blunt abdominal trauma. Clin Radiol 2002;57:908–912.

9 Diseases of the Collecting System and Ureters

P. L. Allan

Introduction

The pelvicalyceal system and ureter transport urine from the collecting tubules in the renal medullary pyramids to the bladder. The renal pelvis and calyces lie in the center of the kidney, surrounded by the fat of the renal sinus, which also contains the segmental arteries and veins.

Obstruction

One of the most common reasons for requesting a renal tract ultrasound is to confirm or exclude obstruction, either as a cause of renal failure or as a source of possible renal colic. Obstruction can be acute, as in the case of an impacted ureteric calculus, or develop more slowly, as in cases of ureteric transitional cell carcinoma (TCC). It is important to distinguish between dilatation of the collecting system due to obstruction and nonobstructive dilatation, which can result from several causes, including diuresis or a distended bladder; these situations are discussed in more detail below. Conversely, significant obstruction may be present with only minimal dilatation of the collecting system; this situation occurs most commonly with recent acute obstruction but can also be seen in cases of retroperitoneal fibrosis. Therefore, although ultrasound is sensitive for the detection of renal dilatation, it is essential that the ultrasound appearances are interpreted in the light of the clinical picture, rather than in isolation.[1]

Acute Obstruction

In the early stages of acute, severe obstruction, there may be a reflex decrease in the production of urine,[2] which can last for two to three hours. This means that significant dilatation of the pelvicalyceal system may not be apparent in these early stages[3] and a repeat ultrasound examination five to eight hours after the onset of symptoms should be considered in appropriate cases.

The earliest sign of obstruction on ultrasound is "splitting" of the collecting system within the sinus fat.[4] This becomes more marked if significant obstruction persists, with increasing prominence of the collecting system (Fig. 9.**1**). In addition, the high intrarenal pressure can produce some thinning of the parenchyma and an increase in overall renal size; both of these will return to normal after early relief of the obstruction. Extravasation of urine into the perirenal tissues may occur if obstruction persists, in one study with computed tomography (CT), 22% of patients had moderate or severe perinephric fluid collections after four hours of obstruction.[5] This perinephric fluid can also be identified on ultrasound (Fig. 9.**2**) and in a few cases a significant urinoma may develop.

Once pelvicalyceal dilatation has been identified, it is important to try and ascertain the level of obstruction and, if possible, the cause. In the first instance it is worth looking in the pelvis, as a dilated lower ureter with a calculus (Fig. 9.**3**) or a pelvic mass may be identified behind the bladder; alternatively a bladder tumor may be seen. Careful scanning of the para-aortic and paracaval areas may show a dilated ureter, or identify a mass causing the obstruction; although overlying bowel gas makes visualization of these areas more difficult.

In patients with a duplex system (see below), only one of the moieties may be affected by obstruction and distinction from changes resulting from reflux will depend on the clinical situation.

The use of ultrasound together with a plain film of the abdomen and pelvis (kidneys, ureter, bladder [KUB]) has been shown to be accurate in the diagnosis of renal colic and is a viable alternative to the intravenous urogram for the diagnosis of ureteric colic arising from calculi.[6]

An obstructed system is often infected to a greater or lesser degree. If the obstruction is not relieved, this can result in pyonephrosis, which, in turn, can produce septicemia. Pyonephrosis is recognized on ultrasound by identification of echogenic material within the dilated collecting system (Fig. 9.**4**); some layering out of the debris may also be observed.[7] In patients with infection by gas-forming bacteria, emphysematous pyelitis, the gas can obscure the view of the dilated collecting system unless an appropriate scan plane is used to scan from the side rather than from a superior approach. Debris may not be apparent in some patients, leading to a false negative examination; conversely

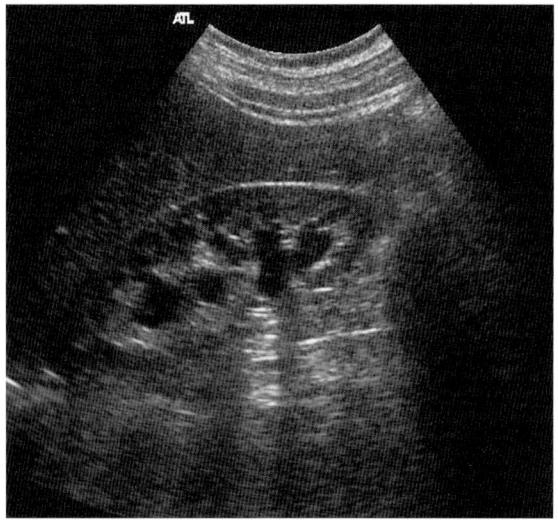
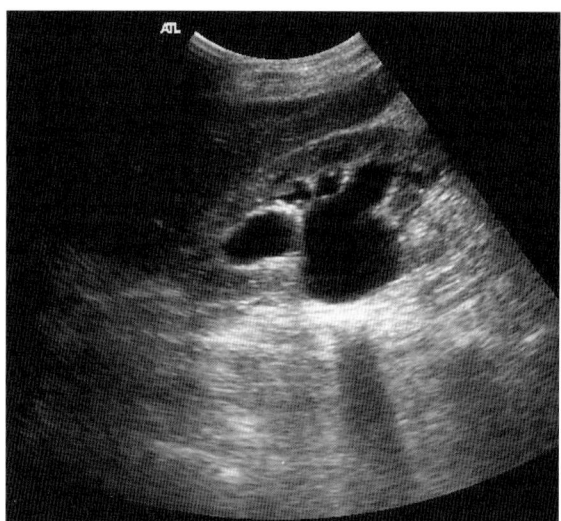
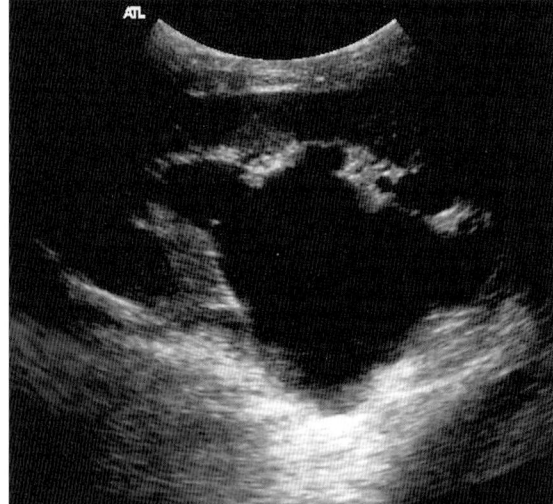

Fig. 9.1 Varying degrees of obstructive dilatation of the collecting system. a Mild. b Moderate. c More marked

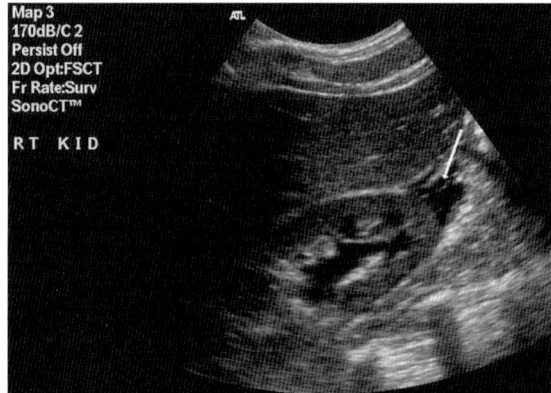

Fig. 9.2 Mild to moderate splitting of the pelvicalyceal system in a patient with acute ureteric obstruction with a small collection of urine at the lower pole (arrow)

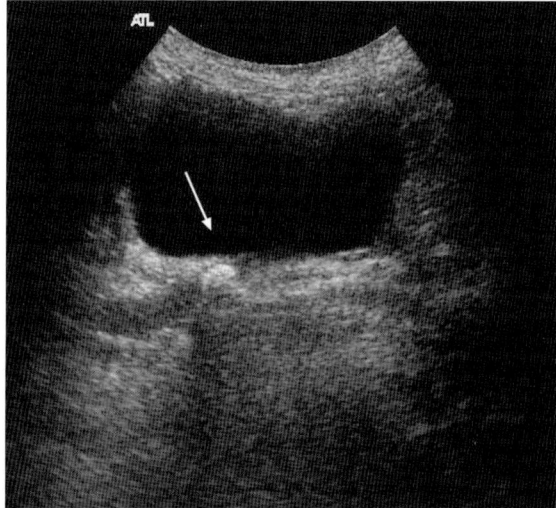

Fig. 9.3 A calculus (arrow) in a dilated ureter impacted at the vesicoureteric junction (VUJ)

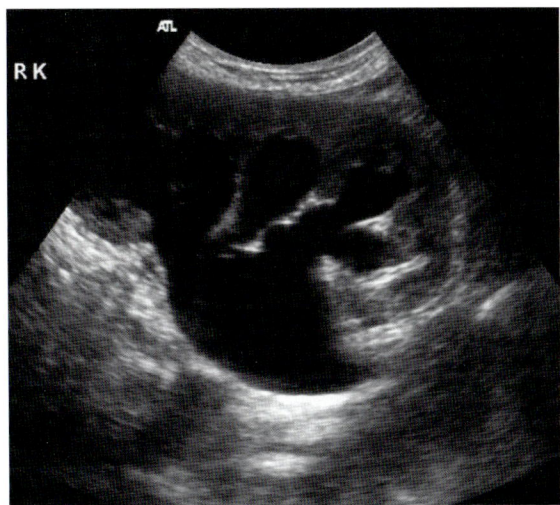

Fig. 9.4 **Pyonephrosis. a** Original scan showing hydronephrosis with some associated loss of cortex. This was treated with nephrostomy and ureteric stenting. **b** One year later the patient presented with septicemia and features suggestive of a pyonephrosis on ultrasound. This was secondary to a blocked stent. A nephrostomy was inserted, the pus drained, and the patient improved. Thick turbid echoes (arrows) can be seen in both the renal pelvis and calyces consistent with pus. Cf. the "clean" hydronephrosis in a

echoes may be seen in a dilated, but uninfected, renal pelvis as a result of hemorrhage. It is therefore important to carry out diagnostic aspiration if infection is suspected on clinical grounds.

Other Ultrasound Techniques in the Diagnosis of Obstruction

Other ultrasound techniques which may be used in the assessment of possible acute ureteric obstruction include assessment of the intrarenal resistive index (RI), identification of ureteric jets in the bladder, and diuretic-enhanced sonography.

Doppler findings: The pathophysiological effects arising from acute obstruction are complex.[8] There is a transient increase in renal blood flow two to four hours after the onset of obstruction; following this, three to five hours after obstruction, various circulating and local factors produce vasoconstriction. If obstruction persists, then profound renal vasoconstriction develops after 18–24 hours which persists until the obstruction is relieved. Even then, residual long-term damage may result from this relative ischemia. In addition, dilatation of the collecting system resulting from acute obstruction produces an increase in intrarenal pressure. These changes result in a decrease in diastolic arterial blood flow, which occurs approximately six hours after the onset of obstruction and can be detected by an increase in the RI in the intrarenal arteries;[9] the measurement should be made in the segmental, interlobar, or arcuate arteries, as the RI tends to be higher in the larger vessels at the renal hilum. In nonobstructed kidneys without any other pathology, the RI is < 0.7 and the difference between the RI for the two kidneys is < 0.1. An RI > 0.7 and/or a difference of > 0.1 in the RI between the two kidneys (Fig. 9.**5**) is therefore indicative of obstruction.[4,10,11]

It should be remembered that the RI tends to increase with age, and values of 0.7, or higher, are not excessive in a 70-year-old patient;[12] in this situation, the difference in RI between the two sides is therefore the more important criterion for diagnosis. Similarly, the RI in young children (< 4–5 years) is relatively high.[4,13] In very early cases of obstruction, the RI may not yet have increased for the reasons described above.[8] The presence of parenchymal disease may also lead to an increase in the RI, although the changes are bilateral in these cases and there is no significant difference between the two sides. The use of nonsteroidal anti-inflammatory drugs (NSAIDs) to treat the pain of renal colic has been shown to decrease the RI in obstructed kidneys, and although a difference between the obstructed and nonobstructed sides persists, this is less marked than in untreated patients.[14,15]

Ureteric jets: Examining the lower bladder with color Doppler will show jets of urine coming from the ureters. The frequency of these depends on the degree of hydration/diuresis of the patient, but in normal circumstances they should be symmetrical in shape and of similar frequency bilaterally (Fig. 9.**6**).[16] The presence of an obstructing calculus will reduce the frequency, or stop these jets; edema of the vesicoureteric junction (VUJ) can result in alteration to the shape and direction of the jets (Fig. 9.**7**).[17] It has been noted that pressure from the uterus can affect the ureteric jets on one side

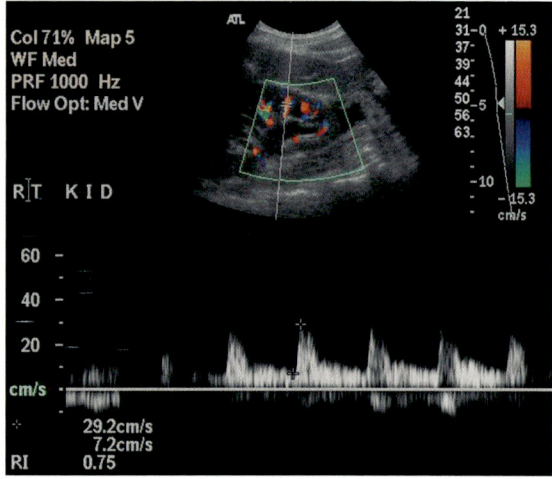
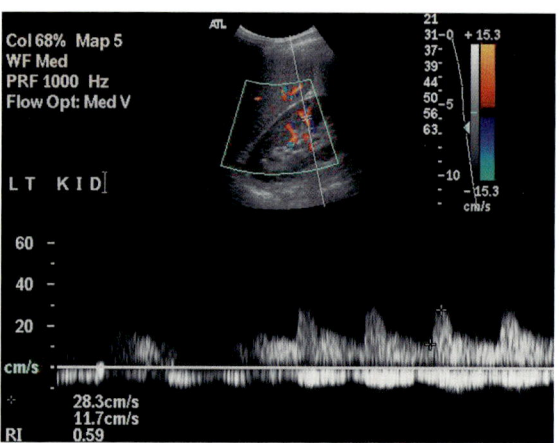

Fig. 9.5 **a** An obstructed kidney in which the RI is 0.75. **b** The contralateral kidney with an RI of 0.59

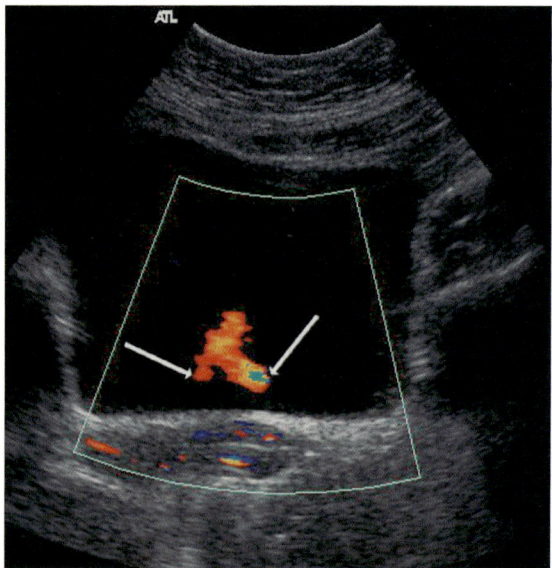

Fig. 9.6 **Normal, symmetrical ureteric jets in the bladder** (arrows)

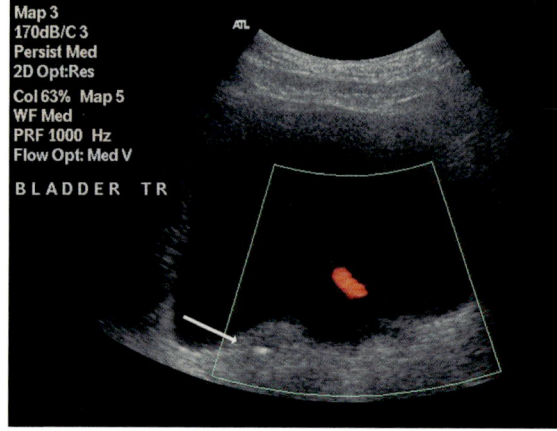

Fig. 9.7 **A transverse scan of the bladder showing a calculus impacted at the right VUJ** (arrow). Despite scanning for several minutes a right ureteric jet was not identified

or the other,[18] and third trimester patients with possible renal colic should be examined in the decubitus position to relieve this pressure.[19] Congenital abnormalities of the VUJ may also result in abnormally shaped, or misdirected jets.

Diuretics: Diuresis-enhanced ultrasound of a kidney with possible obstruction may occasionally be of value. If there is minimal dilatation of the collecting system but a strongly suggestive history for obstruction, or if there is difficulty in distinguishing between a possible parapelvic cyst and an obstructed system, then scanning after a fluid load and an injection of a diuretic (40 mg frusemide) may show a distinct increase in the degree of dilatation in the presence of obstruction.[20]

Measurement of the RI in the affected kidney may also show an increase in the presence of obstruction to > 0.75, whereas the RI in an unobstructed kidney will remain below this level.[21]

Chronic Obstruction

In long-standing, severe obstruction there is loss of parenchyma due to atrophy, which can be variable in extent. Dilatation of the collecting system is variable but can be very marked.[4] In some severe cases, no recognizable cortex remains and a cystic mass represents the massively dilated collecting system (Fig. 9.**8**).

Pelvicalyceal Dilatation Without Obstruction

It is important to distinguish between obstructive and nonobstructive dilatation of the collecting system: The former needs continuing monitoring and possible intervention, whereas, with the latter, time can be taken to discover the cause and subsequent management decisions can be made at a more leisurely pace.

Asymptomatic dilatation of the renal collecting system is not uncommon in pregnancy; it can be detected as early as 12–14 weeks gestation. By 36 weeks gestation, dilatation can be seen in two thirds of subjects more commonly on the right side.[22,23] This is due to a variety of factors, including a 20–25% increase in the circulating blood volume, increased cardiac output, generalized vasodilatation, and parenchymal hypertrophy. In addition, the presence of a large pelvic mass in the later stages of pregnancy and hormonal factors all contribute to dilatation of the renal collecting systems. Following delivery, the renal parenchymal volume returns to normal within a few days, although the collecting system changes can take a few weeks and some residual prominence may persist for longer. A diagnostic dilemma can occur if a pregnant woman develops symptoms that may be due to renal colic. Intrarenal resistance indices are not normally altered by pregnancy,[24,25] so assessing the inter-renal RI difference (see above) may be of value in this type of case as they should be equal and similar to those of a nonpregnant woman; a difference of > 0.1 between the two kidneys would be indicative for obstruction. Examination of intravesical ureteric jets may also contribute to the diagnosis but, as noted above, care is required in making the assessment.[18,19]

In patients with a fluid load, diuresis, and a full bladder, there is physiological dilatation of the pelvicalyceal system (Fig. 9.9). In these circumstances, the bladder should be emptied and the kidneys re-examined: Normal kidneys should show a marked improvement in the degree of dilatation.

In children particularly, prominent vessels in the renal sinus may cause problems but these can be identified easily on spectral or color Doppler (Fig. 9.10);[26] very occasionally an intrarenal artery aneurysm may cause a problem. A prominent extrarenal pelvis, or parapelvic cysts may also produce an appearance suggestive of dilatation, but careful scanning should resolve these problems: In cases of obstruction the cystic areas in the kidney are seen to be in continuity with each other, whereas with parapelvic cysts these will appear separate. If concern persists, then scanning following a fluid load and administration of a diuretic may clarify the situation.[20] Other abnormalities in the region of the collecting system can simulate obstruction. These include papillary necrosis, reflux nephropathy, and calyceal diverticula.

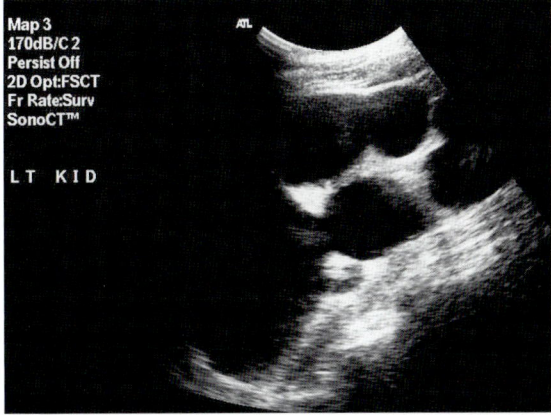

Fig. 9.**8 Chronic obstruction resulting in marked dilatation of the collecting system and atrophy of the renal parenchyma**

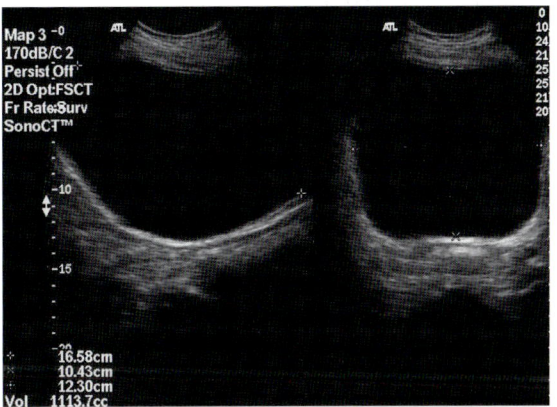

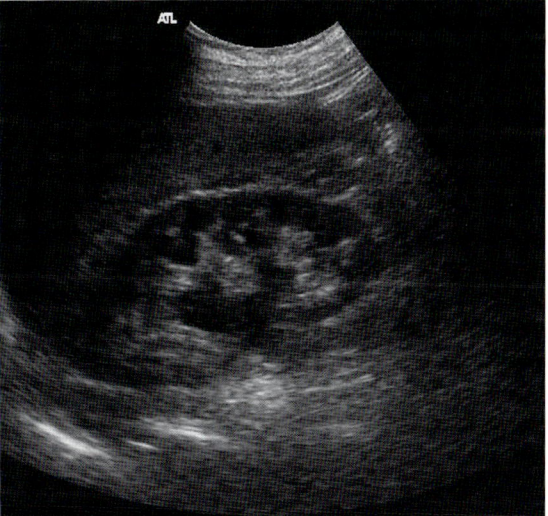

Fig. 9.**9 Renal collecting system dilatation in a patient with retention. a** Dilated bladder of more than 1100 mL. **b** Mild dilatation of the collecting system which resolved following catheterization

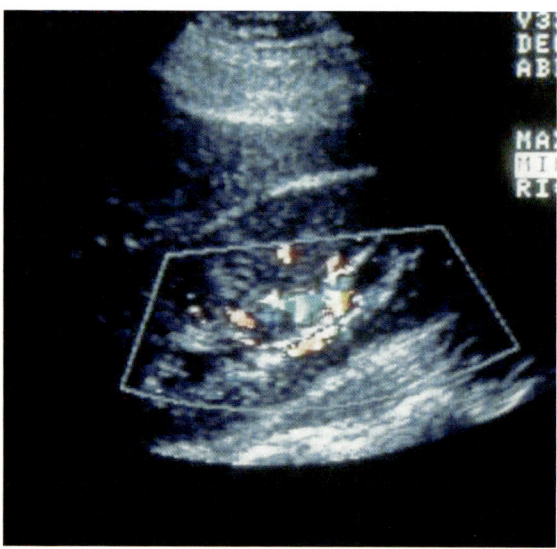

Fig. 9.10 **a** There is some apparent splitting of the renal sinus echoes. **b** Color Doppler shows that this appearance is due to prominent blood vessels, rather than to a dilated collecting system

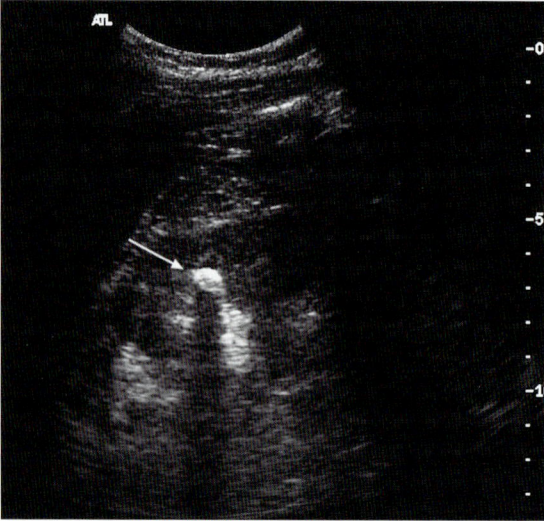

Fig. 9.11 **An intrarenal calculus** (arrow) **showing dense, "clean" acoustic shadowing**

Calculi

Renal calculi form in the pelvicalyceal system, where they can cause problems with infection and hemorrhage. If they pass down into the ureter, they produce obstruction which may be partial or complete. Hematuria can also result from damage to the ureteric mucosa. Stasis, infection, and imbalance of urinary minerals can all predispose to calculi. They are more common in males (2–4:1), Caucasians, and in warm countries, where a degree of dehydration is more likely. They are usually formed from minerals containing calcium, phosphate, urate, or cysteine.

On ultrasound, tiny calyceal calculi of < 2–3 mm may be difficult to distinguish from the surrounding renal fat as they are smaller than the ultrasound beam width and will not cast an acoustic shadow;[27] ultrasound will therefore miss a significant proportion of these small calculi.[28] Larger intrarenal calculi will be seen as echogenic foci with well-defined, "clean," acoustic shadows (Fig. 9.11) and ultrasound will detect some 90% of calculi > 5 mm.[29] Conversely, large staghorn calculi in the renal pelvis may be overlooked for two reasons: Firstly, they are so large and echogenic that the unwary mistake them for renal sinus fat; secondly, some are made up of softer aggregates of mineral and debris and may be surprisingly trans-sonic in nature (Fig. 9.12).[30] Whilst calculi can be identified in the calyces and renal pelvis, they are more difficult to identify within the ureters, as these are often obscured by bowel gas. In the pelvis, they

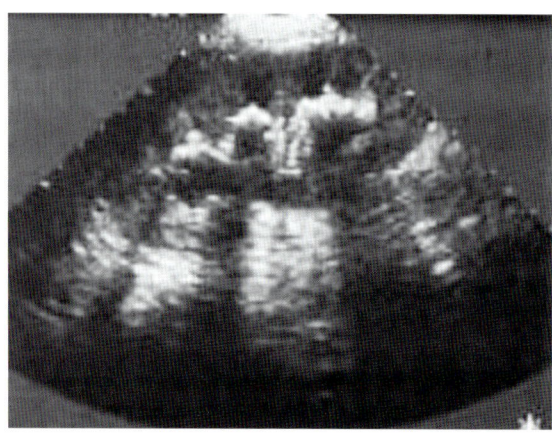

Fig. 9.12 **A staghorn calculus showing acoustic shadowing from much of the area of the renal sinus.** (Image courtesy of Dr. S.A. Moussa)

may be identified in the region of the VUJ, if impacted in a patient with renal colic (Figs. 9.**3** and 9.**7**).

Many renal calculi and some ureteric calculi are treated with extracorporeal shock-wave lithotripsy (ESWL) and ultrasound is valuable for localizing the calculi during therapy sessions, as well as identifying problems following treatment. Foremost amongst these is the development of ureteric obstruction following fragmentation of an intrarenal calculus.[31]

> **Summary points:**
> - Hydronephrosis can be easily diagnosed with ultrasound. However, it cannot distinguish obstructed from nonobstructed systems—clinical correlation is required
> - In suspected pyonephrosis diagnostic aspiration ± drainage is required
> - RI maybe helpful in differentiating obstructive from nonobstructive hydronephrosis
> - Ultrasound should be able to differentiate a prominent extrarenal pelvis or parapelvic cyst from pelvicalyceal dilatation in the majority
> - Ultrasound can miss small calculi (< 2–3 mm) and huge staghorn calculi in the kidney

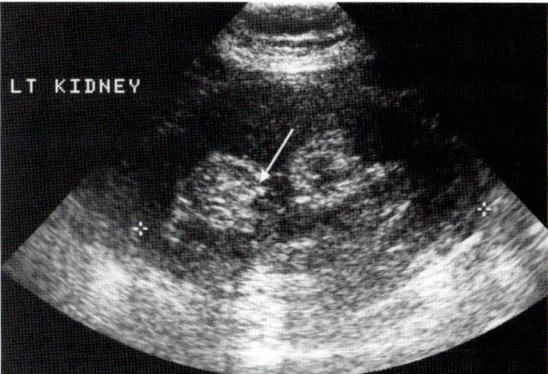

Fig. 9.**13 Duplex collecting system with clear interruption of the sinus echo complex** (arrow)

Congenital Abnormalities

Duplex Systems

Partial duplex collecting systems are not usually recognized on ultrasound, but full duplex systems may be identified by division of the renal sinus into two components with parenchymal tissue lying between them (Fig. 9.**13**); a double renal pelvis may also be identified if the collecting systems are prominent due to diuresis or a degree of obstruction. Often, however, an uncomplicated duplex system will not be recognized on ultrasound. Significant duplex systems occur in about one in 150 births, they are more common in females and are usually unilateral (6:1 unilateral:bilateral).[32] The ureters may join somewhere along the length of their course, or be inserted separately into the bladder; in this case the upper moiety ureter is inserted into the bladder more inferiorly. In males it is always inserted above the external sphincter, but in females it may insert into the urethra or the vagina, producing incontinence. The upper moiety (lower ureteric insertion) is more often associated with obstruction and ureteroceles, whereas the lower moiety (upper insertion) is more prone to reflux as it tends to have a shorter intramural course in the bladder. Duplex systems can show differential changes in cases of obstruction and reflux with the two components being affected differently, so that only one moiety shows dilatation or scarring. With severe changes, it may be difficult to distinguish the affected moiety so that the presence of a complicated duplex kidney is not recognized.

Ectopic Ureters and Ureteroceles

Ectopic insertions of the ureters into the bladder may be associated with single ureters as well as duplex systems; 10% are bilateral and they are more common in females (7:1).[32] In many cases, ectopic ureters do not cause problems and may only be recognized incidentally if ureteric jets are being checked in cases of possible obstruction, in which case an abnormal location may be recognized; abnormalities of direction and shape of the jet may also be apparent. The point of insertion into the bladder is usually inferior to the normal site and may even be into the urethra or vagina, which results in incontinence in females as noted above.

Simple ureteroceles occur at normally sited ureteric insertions and ectopic ureteroceles at abnormally sited insertions. Ureteroceles are more common in females (4:1) and 10% are bilateral.[32] The abnormal insertion of the ureter into the bladder results in an intravesical segment of dilated terminal ureter, which can be seen on or behind the posteroinferior wall of the bladder. It may be seen to change in size with ureteric peristalsis.

Vesicoureteric Reflux

Vesicoureteric Reflux (VUR) is due to a congenital abnormality at the VUJ, with the ureter taking a less oblique intramural course which allows reflux of urine into the ureter as bladder pressure rises. The prevalence of VUR in normal children has been estimated to be

0.4–1.8%, but a review of the literature suggests that the true prevalence may be significantly higher than traditional estimates.[33] It is more common in boys than girls but in many cases the reflux is mild and resolves by age two years.[34] However, it is important to distinguish between simple reflux and reflux nephropathy, in which scarring of the renal parenchyma results from intrarenal reflux associated with infection. Renal scarring is most likely to occur in children with VUR if they get a urinary tract infection (UTI) during the first six months of life; it is rare for it to occur in children over age five, but they remain vulnerable.[35]

Detection of VUR has primarily been by micturating cystography with five grades of reflux recognized.[36] More recently it has been proposed that instilling an ultrasonic contrast agent instead into the bladder and scanning the retrovesical and renal areas during micturition allows detection of reflux by the presence of contrast echoes in the retrovesical lower ureters or in the collecting system. This is particularly useful as a screening tool to identify children with reflux as it does not involve radiation. Those who have a positive or borderline result can then go on to other imaging as necessary.[37] It has been shown that the use of harmonic imaging to detect contrast agent further improves detection.[38] As an alternative, color Doppler can also be used with or without echo-enhancing agents to detect VUR into the kidneys.[39,40]

Pelviureteric Junction Obstruction

Pelviureteric junction (PUJ) obstruction is usually congenital in origin, and abnormalities of the ureteric musculature can be seen histologically at the point of narrowing with a preponderance of longitudinal fibers and a reduction or absence of circular muscle fibers.[41] It can also result from adhesions, aberrant vessels,[42] and kinking of the upper ureter. It must be distinguished from a prominent, ectatic extrarenal pelvis, or a parapelvic cyst. In cases of true PUJ obstruction, there is associated dilatation of the intrarenal component of the collecting system, including the calyces, whereas in a case of an ectatic extrarenal pelvis these are normal. Assessment of the RI before and after a fluid load and injection of a diuretic may also be of value in distinguishing an obstructed system.[21,43]

Congenital Megaureter

Congenital megaureter is a dilated but unobstructed ureter with no apparent cause, often without reflux and with normal renal function. In some cases it can be attributed to an adynamic segment of the lower ureter. It should be distinguished from ureteric dilatation secondary to bladder outlet obstruction, reflux, or a ureterocele. It is important that reflux or obstruction are excluded as patients with asymptomatic, nonobstructive dilatation can then be managed conservatively.[44]

Summary points:
- A duplex collecting system may result in incontinence in the female depending upon site of ureteric insertion
- Ureteroceles are commoner in females
- Renal scarring secondary to infection and VUR is uncommon after age five years
- Ultrasonic contrast agents maybe helpful in the diagnosis of VUR

Tumors of the Collecting System and Ureters

Transitional Cell Carcinoma

Transitional cell carcinomas (TCCs) account for some 90% of uroepithelial tumors. They can affect any part of the urinary tract from the calyces down to the bladder. They may present with hematuria or obstruction, depending on their location and size. Small pelvicalyceal tumors are not usually apparent on ultrasound unless there is dilatation of the collecting system. One study reported that ultrasound picked up only 36% of cases, whereas retrograde pyelography identified 89%;[45] larger lesions may be seen as a hypoechoic mass within the renal sinus area (Fig. 9.**14**), but distinction from a RCC may be impossible based on the ultrasound appearances. In addition, differentiation of associated blood clot may be difficult. As with bladder TCCs, encrustation of the tumor surface with mineral deposits may occur, leading to confusion with an intrarenal calculus.[46] Small lesions may produce localized dilatation of calyces or of a portion of the pelvicalyceal system. Infiltrative forms of the tumor replace sinus fat, have ill-defined margins, and tend to preserve the reniform shape of the kidney;[47] however, it is difficult to distinguish them from other infiltrative processes such as lymphoma.

Ureteric TCCs are more difficult to identify as much of the ureter may be obscured by bowel gas. They usually present with hematuria or flank pain, and ultrasound will show a varying degree of dilatation of the collecting system and the ureter above the lesion. If the lesion is identified, it appears as an intraluminal, hypoechoic, soft-tissue mass,[48] but careful, persistent scanning may be required to show these lesions.

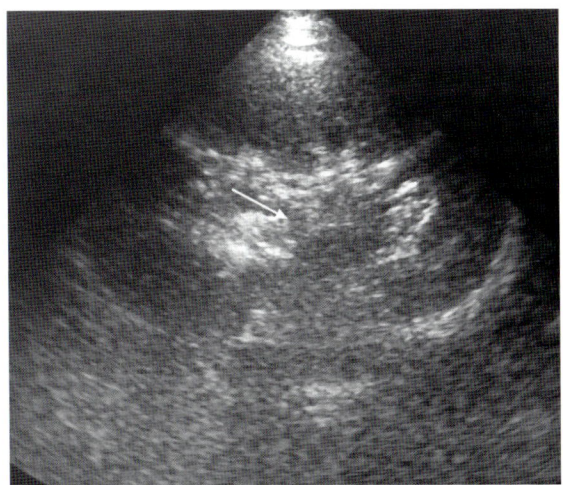
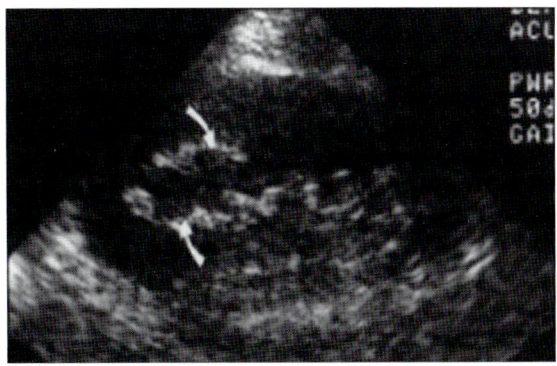

Fig. 9.**14 Two examples of TCC in the renal pelvis. a** An ill-defined mass amongst the sinus echoes (arrow). **b** A similar area of low echogenicity in the upper renal sinus echoes in a different kidney (arrows) (Courtesy of Dr. S.A. Moussa)

Other Malignant Lesions

Approximately 10% of primary uroepithelial malignancies are squamous cell tumors; adenocarcinomas account for less than 1% of lesions. Lymphoma can affect the kidney diffusely or as a focal lesion, and distinction from other pathologies is usually not possible on the ultrasonic appearances of the kidney alone.[49]

Secondary tumors arising within the ureters or renal pelvis are rare, but obstruction of the ureters by extrinsic malignant disease in the para-aortic or pelvic regions is a common cause of obstruction in oncological practice.

Miscellaneous Disorders

Retroperitoneal Fibrosis

Retroperitoneal fibrosis results from a chronic inflammatory and fibrotic process which extends through the retroperitoneal tissues, usually in a perivascular distribution;[50] as regards its cause, there is evidence of an underlying immune reaction. This can be primary, when it may be stimulated as a reaction to atheroma and its constituents, or secondary to a wide variety of inflammatory and infective conditions. The chronic inflammatory process can also be triggered by malignancy and some drug therapies, such as methysergide.

The ureters are involved in the inflammatory and fibrotic process, usually in the middle third but it can be anywhere along their course. CT is the modality of choice for assessment, but ultrasound can show an extensive, well-defined, smooth-margined, retroperitoneal mass centered over the sacral promontory and enveloping the aorta and inferior vena cava (IVC), obliterating adjacent tissue planes.[51] Associated dilatation of the renal pelvicalyceal system will also be seen in the majority of patients, but retroperitoneal fibrosis can produce significant functional obstruction with only minimal hydronephrosis,[52] and is a recognized cause of a false negative diagnosis of obstruction with ultrasound. This finding is thought to be because the obstruction is functional in nature with loss of peristaltic activity in the ureter as a result of inflammation, rather than a structural stenosis secondary to fibrosis within the ureter.[50]

Inflammatory Disorders of the Ureters

A wide variety of disparate disorders, predominantly inflammatory, may affect the ureters.[53] These conditions usually produce changes in the bladder and renal pelvicalyceal system, although local inflammatory processes in the retroperitoneum may affect the ureter directly. Acute edematous inflammation may go on to fibrotic change, with resultant stricture formation and obstruction. In acute inflammation, ureteric peristalsis may be impaired significantly as a result of mural inflammation or bacterial endotoxins; this results in dilatation of a functional nature.

These inflammatory disorders include infections such as acute pyelonephritis, tuberculosis, schistosomiasis, and cytomegalovirus in immunocompromised patients; radiation ureteritis may result from para-aortic or pelvic treatments. However, specific details of changes within the ureter are not visible on ultrasound and the resulting dilatation of the pelvicalyceal system is the main feature on examination.[53] Other inflammatory conditions which may affect the ureter include malacoplakia, keratinizing desquamative squamous metaplasia (KDSM), eosinophilic segmental ureteritis, and ureteritis cystica

> **Summary points:**
> - Ultrasound is poor in the detection of TCC of the renal tract
> - Secondary tumors of the ureter and renal pelvis are rare; extrinsic ureteric compression is common in oncological practice
> - Retroperitoneal fibrosis may be primary or secondary
> - Hydronephrosis maybe absent on ultrasound despite significant functional obstruction in retroperitoneal fibrosis

References

1. Amis ES Jr, Cronan JJ, Pfister RC, Yoder IC. Ultrasonic inaccuracies in diagnosing renal obstruction. Urology 1982; 19:101–5.
2. Catalano C, Comuzzi E, Davi L, Fabbian F. Reflex anuria from unilateral ureteral obstruction. Nephron 2002;90:349–51.
3. Curry NS, Gobien RP, Schabel SI. Minimal-dilatation obstructive nephropathy. Radiology 1982;143:531–4.
4. Platt JF. Urinary obstruction. Radiol Clin Nth Am 1996;34: 1113–29.
5. Varanelli MJ, Coll DM, Levine JA, Rosenfield AT, Smith RC. Relationship between duration of pain and secondary signs of obstruction on unenhanced helical CT. Am J Roentgenol 2001;177:325–30.
6. Dalla Palma L, Stacul F, Bazzocchi M, Pagnan L, Festini G, Marega D. Ultrasonography and plain film versus intravenous urography in ureteric colic. Clin Radiol 1993;47: 333–6.
7. Yoder IC, Lindfors KK, Pfister RC. Diagnosis and treatment of pyonephrosis. Radiol Clin North Am 1984;22:407–14.
8. Mostbeck GH, Zontsich T, Turetschek. Ultrasound of the kidney: obstruction and medical diseases. Eur Radiol 2001; 11:1878–89.
9. Opdenakker L, Oyen R, Vervloessem I, Goethuys H, Baert AL, Baert LV, Marchal G. Acute obstruction of the renal collecting system: the intrarenal resistive index is a useful yet time-dependent parameter for diagnosis. Eur Radiol 1998;8:1429–32.
10. Platt JF, Rubin JM, Ellis JH. Acute renal obstruction: evaluation with intrarenal duplex Doppler and conventional ultrasound. Radiology 1993;186:685–8.
11. Rodgers PM, Bates JA, Irving HC. Intrarenal Doppler ultrasound studies in normal and acutely obstructed kidneys. Br J Radiol 1992;65:207–12.
12. Zubarev AV. Ultrasound of the renal vessels. Eur Radiol 2001;11:1902–15.
13. Gill B, Palmer LS, Koenigsberg M, Laor E. Distribution and variability of resistive index values in undilated kidneys in children. Urology 1994;44:897–901.
14. Shokeir AA, Abdulmaaboud M, Farage Y, Mutabagani H. Resistive index in renal colic: the effect of nonsteroidal anti-inflammatory drugs. BJU Int 1999;84:249–51.s
15. Kmetec A, Peskar-Babnik D, Butorovic-Ponikvar J. Time-dependent changes of resistive index in acute renal obstruction during nonsteroidal drug administration. BJU Int 2002;89:847–50.
16. Cox IH, Erickson SJ, Foley WD, Dewire DM. Ureteric jets: evaluation of normal flow dynamics with color Doppler sonography. Am J Roentgenol 1992;158:1051–5.
17. Burge HJ, Middleton WD, McClennan BL, Hildebolt CF. Ureteral jets in healthy subjects and in patients with unilateral ureteral calculi: comparison with color Doppler US. Radiolgy 1991;180:437–42.
18. Burke BJ, Washowich TL. Ureteral jets in normal second- and third-trimester pregnancy. J Clin Ultrasound 1998;26: 423–6.
19. Wachsberg RH. Unilateral absence of ureteric jets in the third trimester of pregnancy: pitfall in color Doppler US diagnosis of urinary obstruction. Radiology 1998;209: 279–81.
20. Nicolau C, Vilana R, Del Amo M, Anguera A, Sala X, Pages M, Arguis P, Bru C. Accuracy of sonography with a hydration test in differentiating between excretory renal obstruction and renal sinus cysts. J Clin Ultrasound 2002;30:532–6.
21. Mallek R, Bankier AA, Etele-Hainz A, Kletter A, Mostbeck GH. Distinction between obstructive and nonobstructive hydronephrosis: value of diuresis duplex Doppler sonography. AJR Am J Roentgenol 1996;166:113–117.
22. Cietak KA, Newton JR. Serial qualitative maternal nephrosonography in pregnancy. Br J Radiol 1985;58:399–404.
23. Faundes A, Bricola-Filho M, Pinto e Silva JL. Dilatation of the urinary tract during pregnancy: proposal of a curve of maximal calyceal diameter by gestational age. Am J Obstet Gynaecol 1998;178:1082–6.
24. Nazarian GK, Platt JF, Rubin JM, Ellis JH. Renal duplex Doppler sonography in asymptomatic women during pregnancy. J Ultrasound Med 1993;12:441–4.
25. Hertzberg BS, Carroll BA, Bowie JD, Paine SS, Kliewer MA, Paulson EK, Weber TM, Gimenez EI. Doppler ultrasound assessment of maternal kidneys: analysis of intrarenal resistivity indexes in normal pregnancy and physiologic pelvicaliectasis. Radiology 1993;186:689–92.
26. Scola FH, Cronan JJ, Schepps B. Grade 1 hydronephrosis: pulsed Doppler US evaluation. Radiology 1989;171: 519–20.
27. Rubin JM, Adler RS, Bude RO, Fowlkes JB, Carson PL. Clean and dirty shadowing at US: a reappraisal. Radiology 1991; 181:231–6.
28. Fowler KA, Locken JA, Duchesne JH, Williamson MR. US for detecting renal calculi with nonenhanced CT as a reference standard. Radiology 2002;222:109–13.
29. Middleton WD, Dodds WJ, Lawson TL, Foley WD. Renal calculi: sensitivity for detection with US. Radiology 1988; 167:239–44.
30. Zwirewich CV, Buckley AR, Kidney MR, Sullivan LD, Rowley VA. Renal matrix calculus. Sonographic appearance. J Ultrasound Med 1990;9:61–4.
31. Vorwerk D, Auffermann W, Fischer N. Diagnosis of obstruction and stone passage following ESWL therapy. ROFO (German) 1987;147:294–7.
32. Neild GH. Congenital abnormalities of the renal tract. In: Comprehensive clinical nephrology, 2nd ed. Johnson RJ, Feehally J, eds. Mosby: 2003:677–94.

33. Sargent MA. What is the normal prevalence of vesicoureteral reflux? Pediatr. Radiol 2000;30:587–93.
34. Lynn K. Vesicoureteral reflux and reflux nephropathy. In: Comprehensive clinical nephrology, 2nd ed. Johnson RJ, Feehally J, eds. Mosby: 2003:779–91.
35. Smellie JM, Ransley PG, Normand IC, Prescod N, Edwards D. Development of new renal scars: a collaborative study. Br Med J 1985;290:1957–60.
36. International Reflux Study Committee. Medical versus surgical treatment of primary vesicoureteral reflux: a prospective international reflux study in children. J Urol 1981; 125:277–83.
37. Darge K Troeger J, Duetting T, Zieger B, Rohrschneider W, Moehring K, Weber C, Toenshoff B. Reflux in young patients: comparison of voiding US of the bladder and retrovesical space with echo enhancement versus voiding cystourethrography for diagnosis. Radiology 1999;210:201–7.
38. Darge K, Zieger B, Rohrschneider W, Ghods S, Wunsch R, Troeger J. Contrast-enhanced harmonic imaging for the diagnosis of vesicoureteral reflux in pediatric patients. Am J Roentgenol 2001;177:1411–5.
39. Kosar A, Yesildag A, Oyar O, Perk H, Gulsoy U. Detection of vesico-ureteric reflux in children by colour-flow Doppler ultrasonography. BJU Int 2003;91:856–9.
40. Galia M, Midiri M, Pennisi F, Farina R, Bartolotta TV, De Maria M, Lagalla R. Vesicoureteral reflux in young patients: Comparison of voiding color Doppler US with echo enhancement versus voiding cystourethrography for diagnosis or exclusion. Abdom Imaging 2004;29:303–308.
41. Harris PG. Urinary tract obstruction. In: Comprehensive clinical nephrology, 2nd ed. Johnson RJ, Feehally J, eds. Mosby: 2003:745–58.
42. Veyrac C, Baud C, Lopez C, Couture A, Saguintaah M, Averous M. The value of colour Doppler sonography for identification of crossing vessels in children with pelvi-ureteric junction obstruction. Pediatr Radiol 2003;33:745–51.
43. Renowden SA, Cochlin DL. The potential use of diuresis Doppler sonography in PUJ obstruction. Clin Radiol 1992; 46:94–6.
44. Simoni F, Vino L, Pizzini C, Benini D, Fanos V. Megaureter: classification, pathophysiology, and management. Pediatr Med Chir 2000;22:15–24.
45. Paivansalo M Merikanto J, Myllyla V, Hellstrom P, Kallionen M, Jalovaara P. Radiological and cytological detection of renal pelvic transitional-cell carcinoma. ROFO 1990;153: 266–70.
46. Janetschek G, Putz A, Feichtinger H. Renal transitional cell carcinoma mimicking stone echoes. J Ultrasound Med 1988;7:83–6.
47. Hartman DS, Davidson AJ, Davis CJ Jr, Goldman SM. Infiltrative renal lesions: CT-sonographic-pathologic correlation. Am J Roentgenol 1988;150:1061–4.
48. Hadas-Halpern I, Farkas A, Patlas M, Zaghal I, Sabak-Gottschalk S, Fisher D. Sonographic diagnosis of ureteral tumours. J Ultrasound Med 1999;18:639–45.
49. Tornroth T, Heiro M, Marcussen N, Franssila K. Lymphomas diagnosed by percutaneous kidney biopsy. Am J Kid Dis 2003;42:960–71.
50. Kottra JJ, Dunnick NR. Retroperitoneal fibrosis. Radiol Clin Nth Am 1996;34:1259–75.
51. Rubenstein WA, Gray G, Auh YH, Honig CL, Thorbjarnarson B, Williams JJ, Haimes AB, Zirinsky K, Kazam E. CT of fibrous tissues and tumors with sonographic correlation. Am J Roentgenol 1986;147:1067–74.
52. Lalli AF. Retroperitoneal fibrosis and inapparent obstructive uropathy. Radiology 1977;122:339–42.
53. Wasserman NF. Inflammatory disease of the ureter. Radiol Clin Nth Am 1996;34:1131–56.

10 Diseases of the Bladder and Prostate

U. Patel

Introduction

Of all the radiological modalities, ultrasound is ideally suited for evaluation of the lower urinary tract, as it does not involve ionizing radiation, is reproducible and, apart from transrectal ultrasound (TRUS), is a noninvasive investigation. As a screening or first-line examination, ultrasound is unrivaled. The present chapter will detail the diagnostic value of lower urinary tract ultrasound.

Anatomy of the Bladder and Prostate

The Urinary Bladder

The bladder develops from the urogenital sinus, but the base (or bladder trigone) is of mesonephric duct origin. The median umbilical ligament is a fibrous cord anterior to the bladder and develops from the urachus.

The bladder lies centrally in the pelvis[1] and, although extraperitoneal, the peritoneum reflects over its superior surface (Fig. 10.1). The bladder base or trigone lies inferiorly and is indistinguishable from the rest of the bladder, except it may be slightly raised, particularly in the male because of the prostate gland. The ureters enter the trigone approximately 2 cm either side of the midline and are identifiable as a slight "corrugation" as they traverse diagonally through the bladder wall. With full distension, the normal bladder neck may be seen as a slightly open funnel at the base of the bladder. These structures, the trigone, ureters, and bladder neck, are the only fixed landmarks seen on bladder ultrasound. The bladder wall is muscular and has three parts: The outer longitudinal muscle layer, the middle circular muscle, and an inner longitudinal layer.

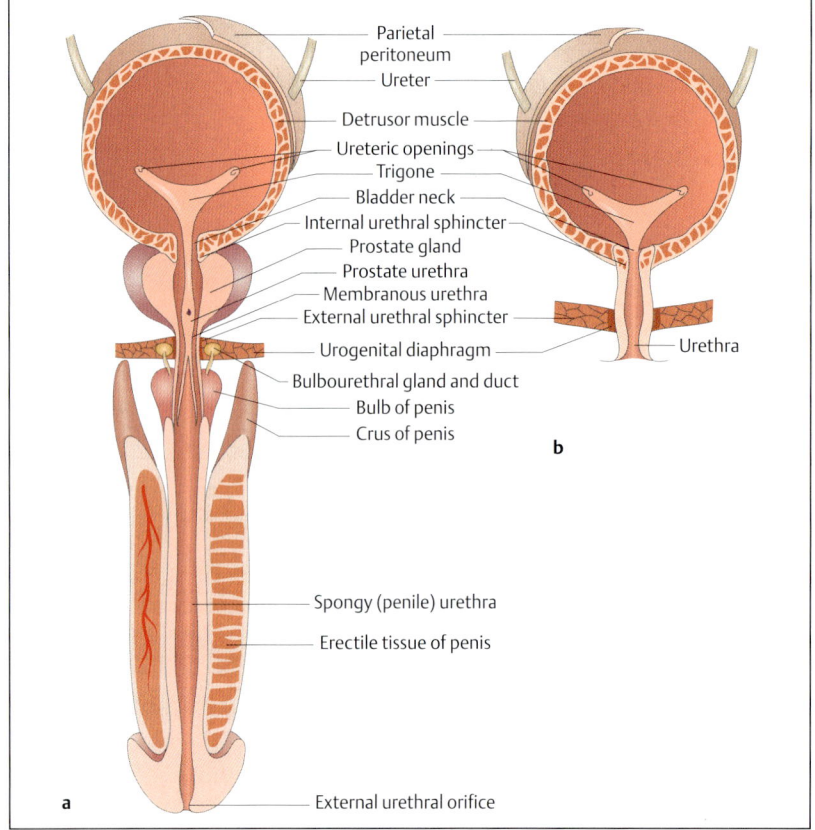

Fig. 10.1 Depiction of the gross anatomy of the male (a) and female (b) bladder

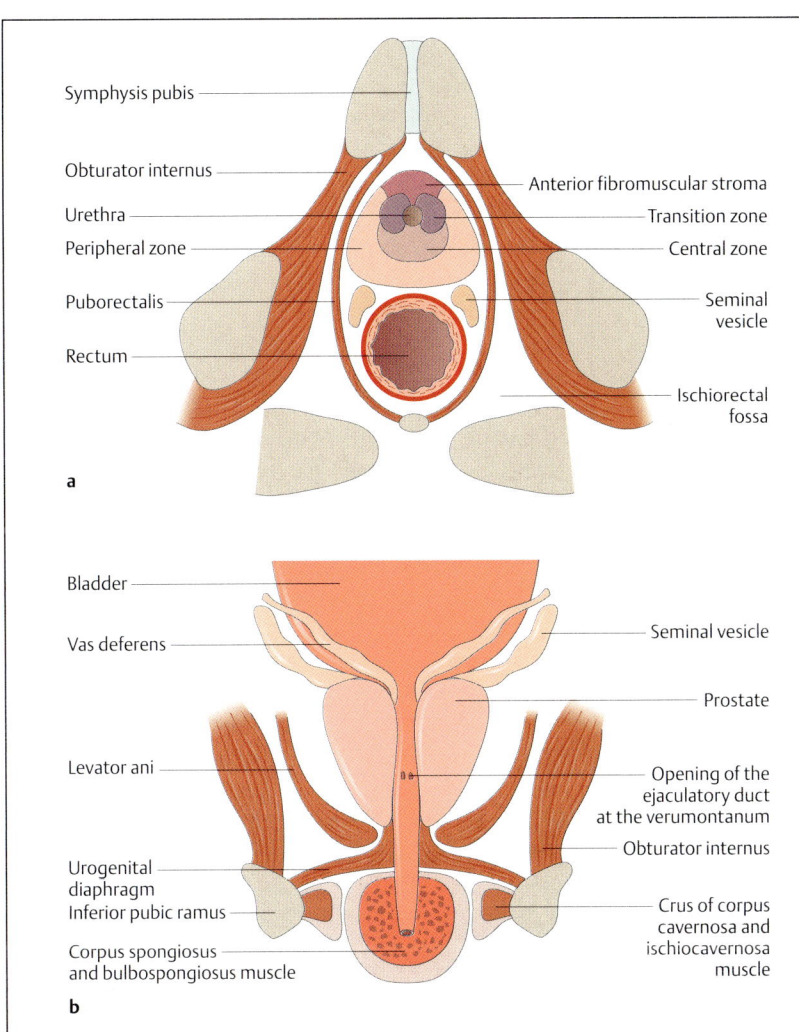

Fig. 10.2 **Anatomical depiction of the prostate gland. a** Axial plane. **b** Coronal plane

The urothelium (transitional cell epithelium) lines the inner muscle layer and is continuous with the urothelium of the ureters and urethra. The muscles around the bladder neck fuse to form the internal urethral sphincter, which encircles the upper prostatic urethra. In the female the external urethral sphincter lies just below the bladder neck and the uterus posteriorly; in the male the prostate gland lies between the bladder neck and the external urethral sphincter, with the seminal vesicles and rectum as the posterior structures (the rectovesical pouch lies in between).

The Prostate

Embryologically, the prostate gland develops from outgrowths of the urogenital sinus and the embryological prostatic urethra.

Gross Anatomy of the Prostate

Postpuberty the gland has a volume of up to 25 mL. The prostate gland measures approximately 3.5 cm in length or height, 4.0 cm in width, and 2.5 cm anteriorly to posteriorly in depth, or the size and shape of a walnut. For unknown reasons, though presumably hormones play a role, the prostate gland increases in size and changes shape with age unless the man has been castrated before puberty, in which case the gland does not mature.

The prostate gland is a retroperitoneal structure, lying anterior to the rectum and inferior to the bladder (Fig. 10.2). Between the gland and the rectum lies Denonvillier fascia; this is an obliterated peritoneal plane. The shape of the prostate gland conforms to the anatomical limitations of the deep pelvic boundaries and has the appearance of an inverted cone or pyramid. On the sides of the prostate gland lie the levator ani and obturator internus muscles. The superior margin, or the

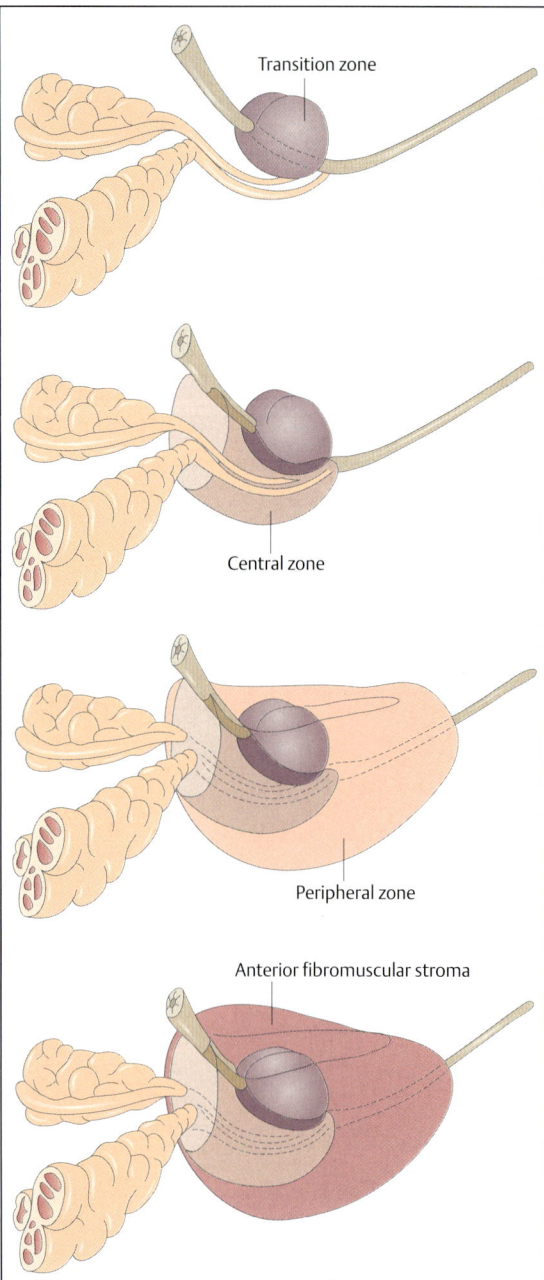

Fig. 10.3 Anatomical depiction of the zonal anatomy of the prostate gland

ment. Beyond a certain size, the prostate gland will preferentially enlarge superiorly, protruding into the bladder base, the so-called median lobe enlargement. In the past, the prostate gland was considered a lobar structure, with right and left lobes, and a midline median lobe. Lobar anatomy is no longer thought to be an accurate representation in the adult, and the gland is now split into glandular zones. The neurovascular bundles contain the branch arteries, veins, and nerves, and lie posterolaterally.

Zonal Anatomy of the Prostate

Anatomically the gland may be divided into zones,[2,3] which is more important than the gross anatomy, as zonal anatomy may be visualized on ultrasound and has a bearing on disease distribution and biopsy technique. Three glandular zones may be defined: The central, the peripheral, and the periurethral transition zones. There is a further anterior nonglandular area called the fibromuscular stroma (Fig. 10.3). The line between the peripheral and central/transition zones, referred to as the "surgical" capsule, separates the inner from the outer gland of the prostate and represents the line of dissection during certain surgical operations.

The peripheral zones account for 75% of the prostate mass in young men, but with increasing age the transitional zone increases in size due to benign prostatic hyperplasia (BPH) whilst the central zone atrophies and the peripheral zone remains static. Therefore, for clinical purposes the important regions are the peripheral and transition zones. A separate terminology divides the gland into the peripheral and central glands (or the outer and inner glands), indicating that it is impossible to identify the central zone as a separate structure. The peripheral and central zones are terminologically incorporated into a single unit, namely the peripheral or outer gland.

base of the prostate gland, lies immediately below the bladder. The most inferior part of the prostate gland, paradoxically the apex of the gland, lies just above the urogenital diaphragm, a fibrous supporting ring which also contains the urethra and the external urethral sphincter. The "prostate capsule" is not a true fibroelastic capsule but a loose compression of the periprostatic fat and stroma, through which pass the neurovascular bundles and the ejaculatory ducts.

The deep pelvis is a restricted space and insufficient to accommodate significant prostate gland enlarge-

> **Summary points:**
> - The prostate gland is split into three glandular zones: Central, peripheral, and transition zones
> - The prostate gland has the appearance of an inverted pyramid
> - The prostate gland has a normal volume of 25 mL
> - The prostate gland capsule is not a true fibroelastic capsule but is made up of periprostatic fat and stroma
> - The line between the peripheral and central/transitional zones (surgical capsule) separates inner from outer gland

Anatomy of the Prostatic Urethra

The prostatic urethra runs in the midline through the gland from the base of the bladder to the urogenital diaphragm (Figs. 10.**2**, 10.**3**). The prostatic urethra has no lumen at rest, but during micturition the cross-sectional area varies from round to triangular in the midportion. The triangulated portion is the verumontanum, and the ejaculatory ducts drain at this site. There is a variable amount of smooth muscle around the urethra and together with the urothelial margin, despite being collapsed; the urethra is visible on ultrasound. The external sphincter, and to a lesser extent the bladder neck, maintain continence.

Anatomy of the Seminal Vesicles and Ejaculatory Ducts

The seminal vesicles are paired sacs of variable shape and size that lie behind the bladder and above the prostate gland (Figs. 10.**2**, 10.**3**). A degree of asymmetry is common. Embryologically, the seminal vesicles represent outsourcings of the vasa deferens and when fully formed merge with the vas deferens to form the ejaculatory ducts, which enter the base of the prostate gland. The ejaculatory ducts run through the prostate in the central zone, in a close midline position. The normal nondilated ejaculatory ducts are difficult to separate from each other and commonly the two are referred to as the ejaculatory duct complex. The course of the ejaculatory ducts is anterior and they communicate with the posterior urethra at the verumontanum.

Ultrasound of the Bladder and Prostate Gland

Functionally the bladder and prostate gland are intimately linked, but ultrasound examination of the two requires separate approaches; transabdominal ultrasound imaging for the bladder and TRUS imaging for the prostate gland. Although in certain situations the alternative ultrasound imaging approach may be informative for either structure.

Ultrasound of the Bladder

Technique (Table 10.1)

A full bladder is essential and a 3.5–5 MHz curved array probe is used. Only in a well-distended bladder can wall abnormalities be recognized, otherwise apparent focal wall masses or diverticula may be simulated by invagi-

Table 10.**1** Ultrasound of the bladder

Preparation:	Full bladder; at least 200 mL, preferably > 400 mL
Position:	Supine (or oblique/decubitus)
Transducer:	3.5–5 MHz curved array transducer. 7.5–10 MHz may be useful for the anterior wall (± harmonic/pulse-inversion imaging)
Method:	Image systematically in both axial and longitudinal planes
Images:	Axial and longitudinal positions
Assess:	

1. Bladder wall
    a) Thickness: Normally < 3 mm (range: 3–5 mm) when well-distended
    b) Trabeculation
    c) Focal masses: Location, solid or cystic, continuation above bladder wall, acoustic shadowing, mobile (use decubitus imaging)
2. Diverticula
    Location, size of diverticulum and neck, calculus, or mass within
3. Bladder base
    a) Ureteric orifices and intramural ureter, calculi, ureterocele, jets
    b) Bladder neck
    c) Base elevation; prostate enlargement
4. Scrutinize the blind areas (± harmonic/pulse-inversion imaging)
    a) Assess anterior wall using a 5–7.5 MHz transducer
    b) Lateral walls; angulate the transducer
    c) Bladder base: Transrectal transducer if suspicion persists
5. Bladder volume = height × width × depth × 0.52
6. Urinary flowmetry and postvoid residue (if appropriate)

nations of the bladder wall. Supine position is adequate, but lateral scanning can help identify mobile calculi. A systematic method should be used: First the bladder is imaged in an axial plane and note made of any asymmetry of the wall. The normal bladder wall is smooth and thin. The normal wall thickness is quoted as 3–5 mm and measures < 3 mm when well-distended.[4] Next, the bladder is imaged in the longitudinal plane. Asymmetry of the bladder wall is again assessed. In the midline, the bladder neck is seen as a short funnel. The lower ureters should be particularly scrutinized and both axial and longitudinal views are useful. Again, asymmetry is important and calculi lodged in the ureters may be suspected by a prominence of the intramural portion of the ureters. Transrectal imaging may also be used to visualize the intramural ureter and ureteric orifice.

Often bladder ultrasound is combined with measurement of urinary flow rates and bladder emptying as the ultrasound cystodynamogram. Such "functional" ultrasound is useful in the assessment of bladder outflow obstruction.

Ultrasound Appearances of the Normal Bladder

The normal bladder wall is smooth and any focal variation in wall thickness should be scrutinized for mucosal-based masses or diverticula (Fig. 10.**4**). Occasionally the

10 Diseases of the Bladder and Prostate

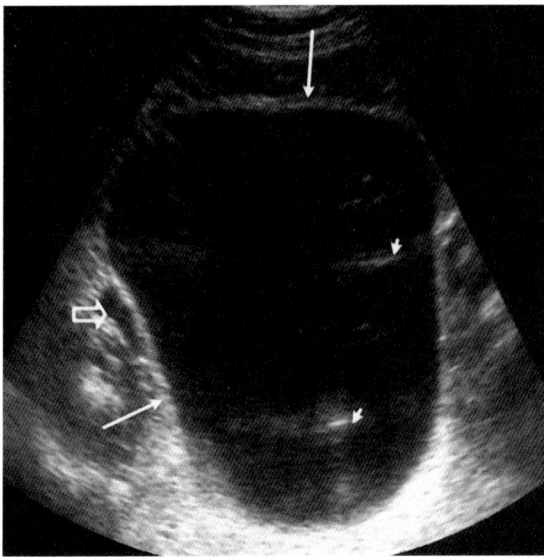

Fig. 10.**4 Ultrasound image in the axial plane of a normal, well-distended bladder**, demonstrating the thin bladder wall (long arrows) and the iliac vessels (open arrow). Reverberation artifact is present within the lumen of the bladder (short arrows)

Table 10.**2 Transrectal ultrasound examination of the prostate**

Preparation:	None specific
Position:	Left lateral position
Transducer:	5–10 MHz axial/longitudinal or end-firing transducer
Method:	Image gland in both planes, base to apex and side to side
Images:	Recorded in a) Transverse/axial planes; base, mid, and apex b) Longitudinal/sagittal planes; midline, left, and right parasagittal
Assess:	1. Measure prostate volume (height × width × length × 0.52) 2. Note reflectivity, nodules, and gland symmetry 3. Evaluate the prostate capsule 4. Scrutinize blind areas in both planes: Posterolateral margins (also sometimes called anterior horns), base, apex, and far anterior gland (decrease frequency to 5–7.5 MHz) 5. Neurovascular bundle symmetry 6. Seminal vesicle and ejaculatory duct assessment 7. Color Doppler imaging (transducer movement, calcification, and biopsy will result in artifact signals)

N.B.: Prostate gland volume is more accurately measured by planimetry. The formula above becomes increasingly inaccurate with glands > 80 mL.

different layers of the bladder wall can be differentiated but not sufficiently well for accurate analysis (e.g., for staging of bladder cancer). Well-distended, the ovoid shape of the bladder in the longitudinal plane and quadrangle in the axial plane is apparent. The bladder base is smooth in outline and the intramural ureters seen as linear "corrugations" along the bladder base. In the absence of an enlarged prostate gland the bladder base should not be elevated. Urine appears completely echo-free, but occasionally the more concentrated urine may layer posteriorly or be seen as a high-reflective "jet" as it ejects from the ureter.[5]

The echo-free urine makes bladder-wall analysis straightforward; but marked reverberation artifact may be seen and the anterior wall, lateral wall, and base of the bladder may be difficult to visualize. Suspected abnormalities of the anterior wall should be evaluated with a higher frequency probe (7.5–10 MHz); the base may be better evaluated by transrectal imaging. Tissue-harmonic imaging helps to better define the bladder wall and reduce reverberation artifacts.

On color Doppler ultrasound the normal bladder wall does not demonstrate color signal, but urine may be seen ejecting from the ureteric orifices as "color jets."[6] Differences in the specific gravity between the ejecting urine and the bladder urine may account for the visualization of these jets on B-mode imaging alone.[7] Visualization of jets is improved by hydration (500 mL of water before imaging or use of intravenous hydration or diuretic agents). Normal jets are well-defined, generally symmetrical cones of color turbulence, directed anteromedially.

■ Transrectal Ultrasound of the Prostate Gland

Technique (Table 10.2)

Although the prostate gland may be visualized on transabdominal imaging, the views are often inadequate for diagnosis; dimensions may be measured, albeit inaccurately. In contrast, the prostate may be visualized in great detail using a transrectal probe. A variety of transducer designs are now available, each requiring a different method for imaging and transducer movement. Most radiology departments prefer the more versatile end-firing transducer which requires a fanning or rocking motion, unlike the simple advancement or rotation movements necessary for true axial/longitudinal transducers. These modern transducers image at a frequency of 5–10 MHz, but are often also capable of multifrequency imaging and prostate biopsy. A 7.5–10 MHz transducer is adequate for most prostate glands, but large prostate glands require 5 MHz to inspect the anterior structures or the bladder neck.

The left lateral patient position is best for imaging the prostate via the transrectal route. A lubricated, condom-covered transducer is inserted into the anus and directed slightly posterior to follow the natural contour of the lower rectum. Deep inspiration through an open mouth helps to relax the anal sphincter. The transducer should be advanced about 10 cm beyond the anal margin and the prostate gland examined in a systematic manner (Table 10.2). Magnification should be adjusted until the entire prostate gland is visualized on the ultrasound monitor. The prostate gland should be examined in the axial plane from the base to the apex. The reflectivity of the glandular zones should be compared between the two sides and note made of any asymmetry. The prostate gland should then be examined in the longitudinal plane and asymmetry again noted. Unlike the bladder, color flow imaging may be of diagnostic value and in the axial plane any focal color Doppler signal asymmetry noted. Following full examination, prostate gland biopsies may be obtained.

Ultrasound Appearances of the Normal Prostate Gland

In the young man, the prostate gland may be homogenous and the zones difficult to differentiate (Fig. 10.5), but normally the peripheral zone is hyperreflective relative to the central and transition zones. This echo-differentiation enhances further with glandular enlargement as the peripheral zone is compressed. Usually the central and transition zones cannot be separated from each other and the anterior fibromuscular stroma is not readily defined. Although there is no histological prostate capsule, the distinction between the gland and surrounding fat is so distinct that a "sonographic" capsule may be seen. The levator ani muscles

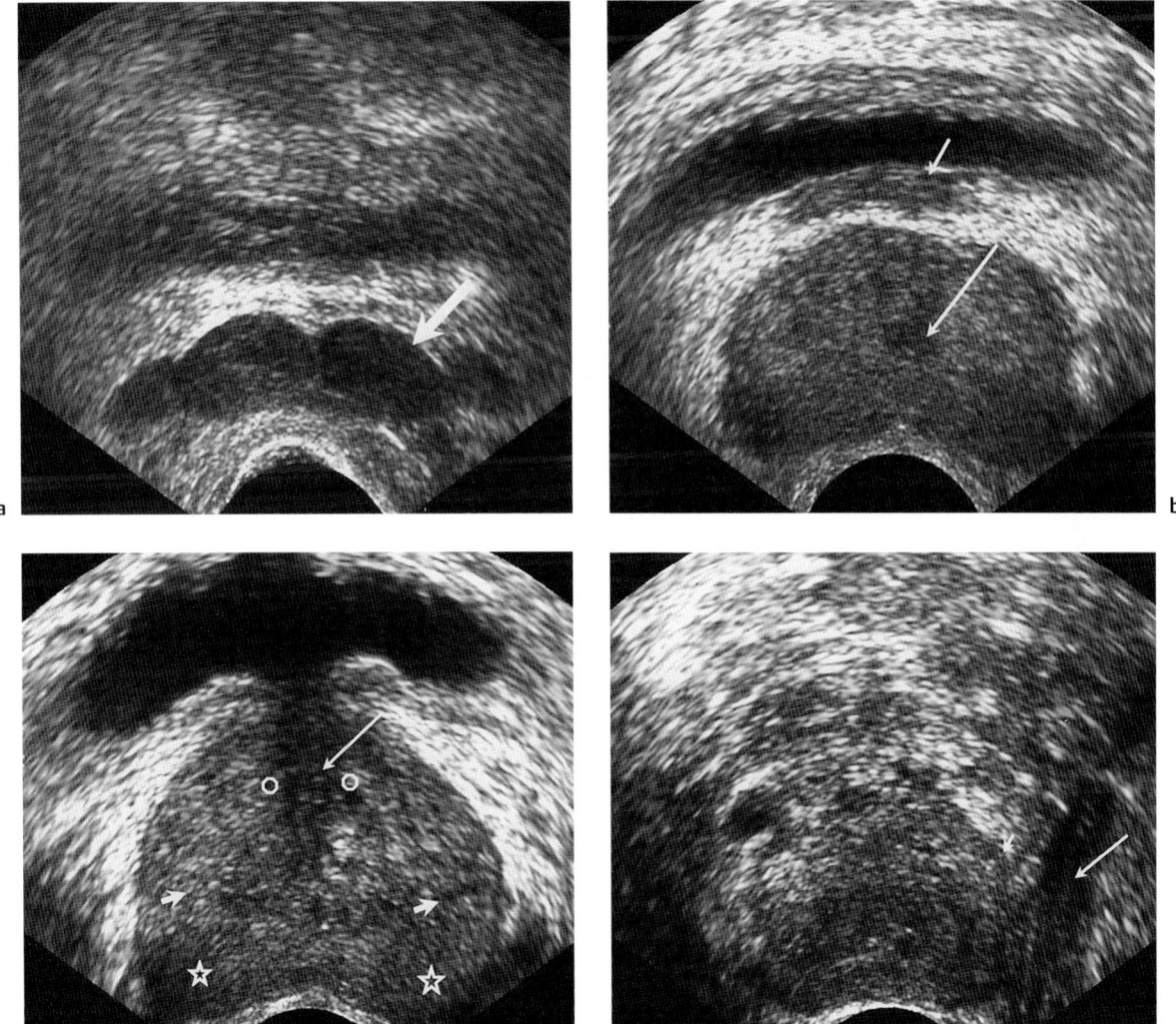

Fig. 10.5 **Ultrasound appearances, in the transverse plane at several levels, of the normal prostate gland and seminal vesicles. a** The seminal vesicles (arrow) lie posterior to the bladder base. **b** The base of the prostate gland, demonstrating the ejaculatory ducts (long arrow) and the seminal vesicles (small arrow). **c** The midportion of the prostate gland, demonstrating the urethra with surrounding low-reflectivity representing hypertrophy of the urethral muscles (long arrow). The peripheral zone (star), central zone (short arrow), and the transitional zone (open circle) are all demonstrated. **d** The apex of the prostate gland, demonstrating the apical portion (short arrow) and the levator ani muscle (long arrow).

Fig. 10.**5e, f** see next page

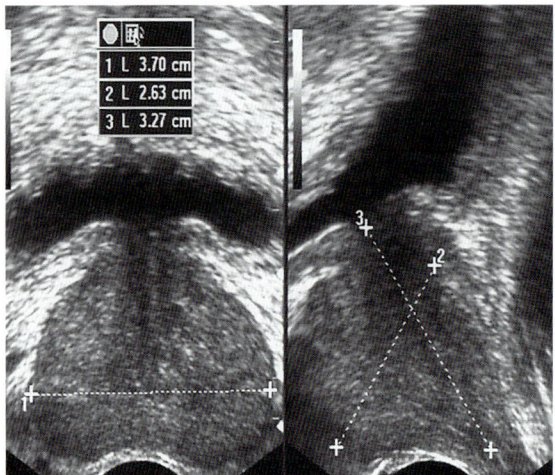
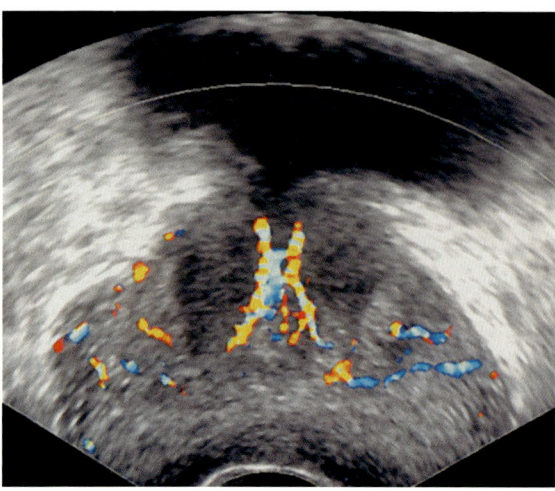

Fig. 10.**5e, f**
e The dimensions of the prostate gland are measured in three directions to give an estimation of the gland volume (see Table 10.**2**). **f** Normal prostate gland vascularity with symmetrical flow around the urethra, periphery, and the intersection of peripheral and central zones is demonstrated on a color Doppler image

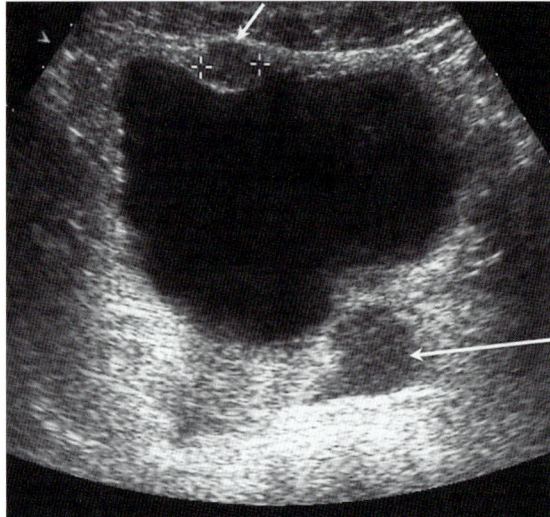

Fig. 10.**6 A longitudinal view of the bladder with a solid urachal remnant** (short arrow) **at the upper aspect and the normal prostate gland at the lower aspect of the bladder** (long arrow)

are seen as linear echogenic boundaries of the prostatic bed. The urethra is seen as a line of mixed echogenicity, even though it has no lumen at "rest." With muscular hypertrophy the urethra and bladder neck become increasingly of low reflectivity, with acoustic shadowing, a common finding with prostate gland enlargement. Just beyond the apex, the periurethral tissues are hypoechoic due to the external urethral sphincter. Highreflective, nonshadowing foci may be seen within the ducts of the inner gland, so-called corpora amylacea, representing mucoproteins of no clinical significance. Scattered areas of calcification are also sufficiently common to be considered a "normal" finding. More focal calcification may represent prostatitis or calculi within the ejaculatory ducts or urethra; only very rarely is prostate carcinoma calcified.

On color Doppler ultrasound the normal gland has marked vascular signals from the neurovascular bundles, the anterior venous plexus, the periurethral tissues, and vessels traversing the inner gland. Importantly, like the overall gland reflectivity, parenchymal vascularity should be symmetrical.[8]

> **Summary points:**
> - The peripheral zone accounts for 75% of the volume of the prostate gland in young men
> - The transition zone increases in benign prostatic hypertrophy, the central zone atrophies, and the peripheral zone remains stable
> - The clinically important zones are the transition and peripheral zones
> - The peripheral zone of the prostate gland is high-reflective compared to the central/transition zone
> - There is marked but symmetrical vascularity of the prostate as seen on color Doppler ultrasound

Ultrasound of the Abnormal Bladder (Table 10.3)

Congenital Anomalies

Bladder agenesis is rare but duplication is slightly more common. Bladder duplication often presents with an incomplete septum; a complete septum dividing the bladder is very unusual.[9] Congenital bladder anomalies, for example bladder extrophy, are usually identified in early childhood. However, urachal abnormalities may go undetected in childhood and present in the adult. A urachus may fail to involute and be seen as a patent tube (50%), a cyst in the midline (30%), a midline urachal sinus (15%), an anterior bladder diverticulum, or an area of thickening.[10,11] There is an increased incidence of adenocarcinoma or calculus formation within a urachal remnant, and when a urachus is encountered, a soft-tissue mass or calculus should be carefully sought (using a 7.5–10 MHz linear array transducer; Fig. 10.**6**). Congenital diverticula are rare, but the Hutch diverticulum is characteristically wide-mouthed, small, and near the ureteric orifices.

> **Summary points:**
> - There is a higher incidence of adenocarcinoma or calculus formation in an urachal remnant
> - A persistent urachus may take the form of a tube, a cyst, a sinus, or anterior bladder-wall thickening/ diverticulum

Acquired Diverticula

These are pulsion diverticula, secondary to the high voiding pressures of bladder outflow obstruction (Fig. 10.**7**). Acquired diverticula are usually associated with generalized bladder-wall thickening and trabeculation, have a narrow neck, and may be quite large. Any diverticula should be carefully examined for calculi and primary bladder tumors. When present, bladder diverticula, especially if there is a narrow neck, should be reported to the cystoscopy operator to allow for careful examination of mucosal-based lesions within the diverticula. A large diverticulum may act as a reservoir, resulting in incomplete emptying or "*pis en deux*," recognized by comparing the prevoid and postvoid dimensions of the diverticulum.[12] Such dynamic information is helpful when a patient is being considered for resection of a diverticulum, for example in those with recurrent infections or calculi.

Table 10.**3** Abnormalities of the bladder

1. **Diffuse bladder-wall thickening**
   a) Bladder outflow obstruction: Trabeculated, small or large volume, diverticula, ureteric dilatation, enlarged prostate, bladder neck may be open or closed
   b) Neurogenic bladder: Trabeculated wall, small volume, ureteric dilatation (sometimes bladder is thin-walled and large)[15]
   c) Tuberculosis: Small volume, ureteric strictures, rarely intravesical tuberculoma[18,19]
   d) Schistosomiasis: Chronic, due to ova in the submucosa, focal masses may be seen, calcification[20,21]
   e) Acute cystitis: Due to E. coli, fungal infection, emphysematous (air in bladder wall);[17] there may be lobulated masses
   f) Hemorrhagic cystitis: May be drug-induced with lobulated masses
   g) Chronic cystitis: Interstitial cystitis, small, thick-walled[22]
2. **Focal bladder-wall thickening**
   a) TCC: Usually polypoid or "frondlike," rarely plaque ± calcification
   b) Squamous cell carcinoma: Associated with Schistosomiasis,[21] leukoplakia, chronic calculus disease, long-term catherization, or squamous metaplasia
   c) Adenocarcinoma: Arises from urachal remnant, anterior wall
   d) Leiomyoma, pheochromocytoma, lymphoma: No typical features
   e) Infections: Tuberculosis, acute schistosomiasis, malacoplakia,[22] cystitis, cystica glandularis[23]
   f) Amyloidosis
   g) Endometriosis[24]
   h) Hemangioma: Serpiginous, cystic areas[27]
3. **Intraluminal abnormalities**
   a) Calculus: Shadow-casting, "twinkle" artifact
   b) Thrombus: High-reflective rim or layers of different reflectivity
   c) Fungus balls
   d) Indwelling catheter or foreign body
4. **Abnormalities of bladder outline**
   a) Diverticula: May contain calculus, tumor
   b) Dilated ureters
   c) Ureterocele (may contain calculus)
   d) Urachal remnant cyst: Anterior wall
   e) Reimplanted ureters: Focal thickening or reflective nodule

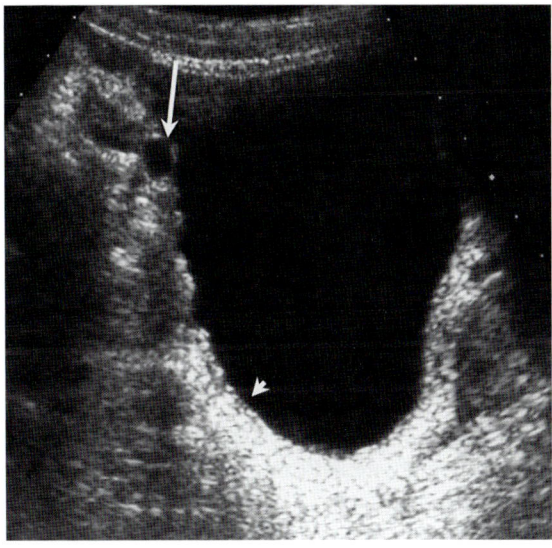

Fig. 10.**7** **Thickened irregular bladder wall** (short wall) **with a small diverticulum** (long arrow) **in a patient with prostate gland enlargement, outflow obstruction, and high-pressure voiding**

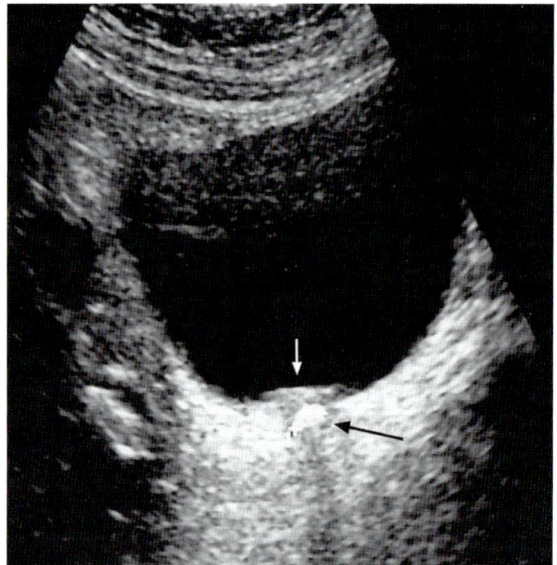 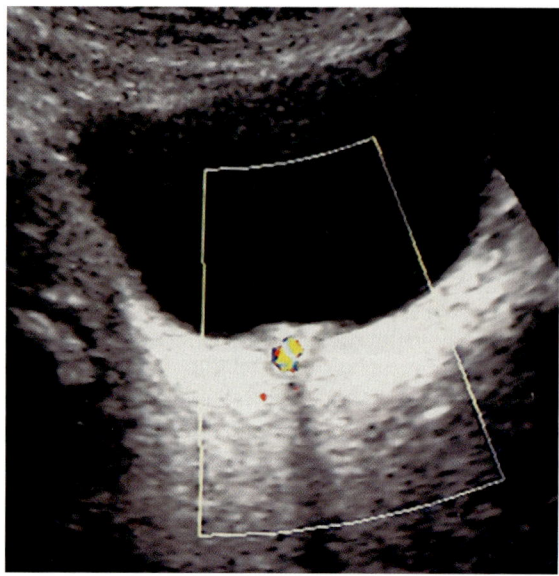

Fig. 10.8 a Image of the bladder demonstrating a calculus (long arrow and calipers) lodged in the ureteric orifice causing hematuria. The blood can be seen layering over the posterior surface of the bladder (short arrow). b The "twinkle" artifact due to the calculus is demonstrated on the color Doppler ultrasound image

wall (Fig. 10.9). A smooth, high-reflective rim may be seen and layers of high and low reflectivity have been described with bladder hematomas.[15] Occasionally when a hematoma is adherent to the bladder wall, it may be indistinguishable from a bladder tumor. Color Doppler ultrasound is not always useful in differentiating a hematoma from a mass, as color Doppler signals from true bladder tumors are often not present (Fig. 10.10). Extravagant enlargement of the prostate gland may protrude asymmetrically into the bladder and again be indistinguishable from a bladder tumor.

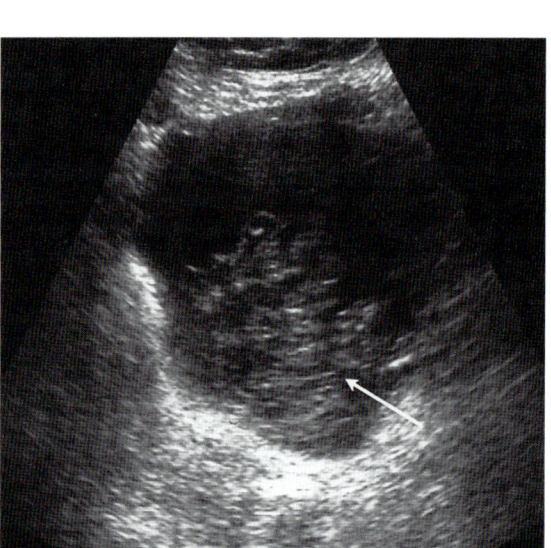

Fig. 10.9 A large hematoma is present in the bladder, which demonstrates features of some age, with organization occurring (arrow). A blood clot is usually mobile, but may be adherent and indistinguishable from bladder carcinoma

Filling Defects or Intravesical Masses

An intravesical mass is an uncommon finding (Table 10.3). Calculi are more common, recognized as mobile, high-reflective areas causing posterior acoustic shadowing often demonstrating the "twinkle" artifact (Fig. 10.8) which may be related to calculi hardness, more common with oxalate stones.[13,14] A hematoma may be mobile or form a layer in the dependent area of the bladder and subsequently adhere to the bladder

Diffuse Bladder-Wall Abnormalities (Table 10.3)

The bladder wall decreases in thickness (range: 3–5 mm) as the bladder fills to 50% of the total volume, and then remains constant. With a full bladder the bladder wall should be smooth and measure < 3 mm in thickness. Diffuse thickening is usually due to muscular hypertrophy, a compensatory phenomenon secondary to significant outflow obstruction which is often due to prostate gland enlargement or urethral stricture but is also seen with a neurogenic bladder.[16] Trabeculation, diverticula, or calculi may be seen as associated findings (Fig. 10.7). Correlation with flowmetry and bladder volume is important (Table 10.4). Infective cystitis does not usually cause any abnormalities on ultrasound, but occasionally masses or pseudotumours are seen.[17] Severe infection may result in emphysematous cystitis (usually in diabetics with E. coli infections), recognized as bladder-wall thickening with areas of high reflectivity not casting prominent shadows, representing pockets of air.[18] Hemorrhagic cystitis may occur

Table 10.4 **Patterns seen during ultrasound cystodynamograms of patients with benign prostatic hyperplasia (BPH) and prostate gland enlargement**

1. **Normal flow rate—normal ultrasound anatomy—complete emptying**
Seen in men voiding with high bladder pressures against outflow obstruction as well as unobstructed normal men.
2. **Low flow rate—thickened bladder wall—elevated bladder base—complete bladder emptying**
Characteristic of bladder outflow obstruction due to BPH. Prostate cancer alone is an uncommon cause of outflow obstruction.
3. **Low flow rate—thickened bladder wall—elevated bladder base—incomplete bladder emptying**
Suggests severe outflow obstruction with detrusor decompensation resulting in residual urine. Such men complain of *pis en deux*, i.e. having to urinate within a few minutes.
4. **Low flow rate—normal bladder wall—elevated bladder base—incomplete emptying**
Suggests a failing bladder due to obstruction
5. **Low flow rate—thickened bladder wall—large postvoid residue and dilated distal ureters**
This is an important combination to recognize, indicating high-pressure chronic retention. This condition can be lethal because of progressive renal failure

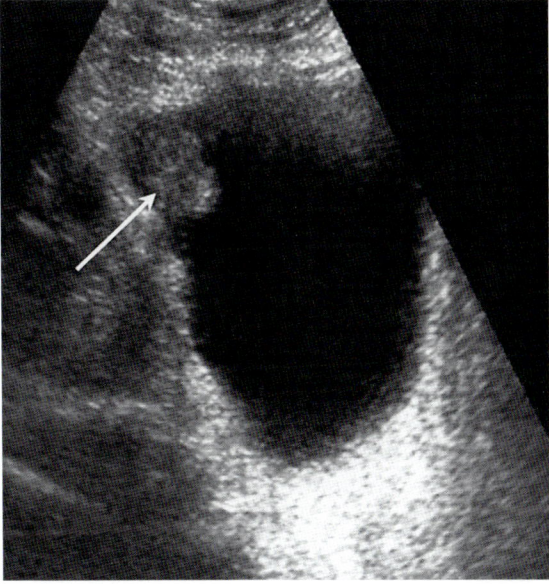

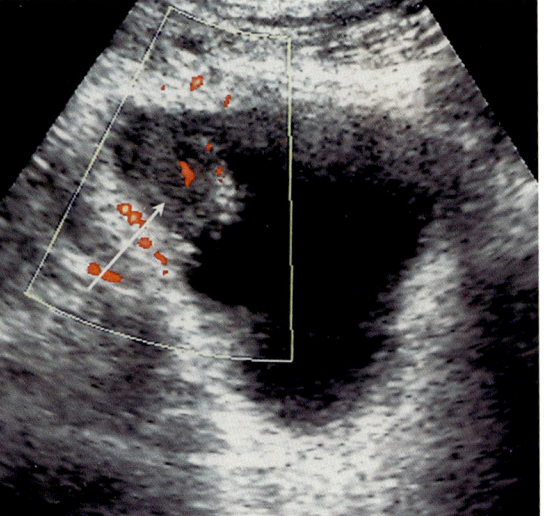

Fig. 10.10 **a** A focal mass arising from the anterior bladder wall (arrow). **b** The mass demonstrates a mildly increased vascularity on color Doppler ultrasound although most bladder masses are poorly vascular

after bone-marrow transplantation, cyclophosphamide therapy, or de novo, where diffuse thickening may be associated with intraluminal lobulated masses.[19] Cyclophosphamide cystitis may be calcified. Further causes of bladder-wall calcification are transitional cell carcinoma (TCC) in < 1%, tuberculosis, and schistosomiasis. Other causes of diffuse bladder-wall thickening are rare (Table 10.3).[20–26]

Focal Bladder-Wall Abnormalities

Over 95% of focal bladder-wall lesions are due to TCC, which accounts for 2–4% of all cancers. The vast majority of TCCs present symptomatically with macroscopic hematuria. TCCs are commonly seen on ultrasound as "frondlike" projections but may also present as a plaque or polyp (Fig. 10.10). Rarely a TCC may calcify. If there is dilatation of the distal ureter the implication is of involvement of the ureteric orifices by tumor. Note should be made of the number and location of lesions and conveyed to the cystoscopy operator. Focal lesions may not be identified if present within diverticula, in an urachal remnant, on the anterior bladder wall, or arising from the bladder base adjacent to an enlarged prostate gland. These areas should be carefully inspected in a patient with macroscopic hematuria. The sensitivity of ultrasound for the diagnosis of bladder TCC is reported to be as high as 90%, identifying more bladder lesions than intravenous urography (IVU).[27–29] However, a single study had an 11% false positive rate due to bladder-wall trabeculation, hematoma, and calculi or focal cystitis.[30] Small lesions are more difficult and the true positive rate for lesions of < 5 mm was only 38%.[30] A recent study of 1000 patients reported a sensitivity of only 63% and specificity of 99% for all bladder tumors.[31] Consequently, bladder ultrasound is not recommended for exclusion of a bladder tumor in patients with macroscopic hematuria; cystoscopy is necessary in all.[32] Recurrent TCC is frequent and subsequent surveillance is better performed by cystoscopy. However, in those not suitable for cystoscopy, ultrasound surveillance with urinary cytology has a sensitivity of 74% for identifying recurrent disease.[33] Ultrasound is unreliable at staging bladder tumors and is not used routinely; accuracy being only about 55%.[34] Endoscopic ultrasound is thought to be more accurate but is invasive and in practice computed tomography (CT)/magnetic resonance (MR) imaging is necessary.[35]

Schistosomiasis may be suspected if multiple, or more rarely solitary, focal lesions are seen in a patient from an endemic area, with evidence of ureteric obstruction or renal pelvicalyceal dilatation. The commonest ultrasound feature is bladder-wall thickening, which may be diffuse and rarely calcified. All these ultrasound features improve with chemotherapy, even the calcification. However, cystoscopy should be performed as schistosomiasis has a known association with squamous cell carcinoma, which has a similar appearance on ultrasound.[23,36] Rarely, a squamous carcinoma may develop in patients with a chronic indwelling bladder catheter. These patients are also prone to chronic cystitis, which may present on ultrasound as a focal bladder-wall thickening rather than generalized thickening. Hemangiomata have been described as serpiginous, cystic areas.[37] Malacoplakia causes multiple focal lesions with increased color Doppler signal, but diffuse or irregular wall thickening may also be seen.[38] Further causes of focal thickening are listed in Table 10.**3**.

Postoperative Bladder Appearances

Reimplanted ureters may be seen as focal, high-reflective or fusiform thickening of the intramural tunnel of the ureter or the trigone.[39] Immediately following transurethral resection of the prostate (TURP) a hematoma may be seen. Later, the TURP defect is seen as a widened bladder neck. Prostate regrowth may obliterate this defect, but this is not sufficiently reliable to diagnose recurrent outflow obstruction and correlation with flowmetry is necessary (Table 10.**4**). In comparison, bladder neck incision may be barely visible even if there has been good functional outcome. The augmented bladder may be structurally bizarre,[40] depending on the amount and type of bowel used; peristalsis may be seen. Bladder lesions may be simulated by the folds of the bowel mucosal or by mucus strands. There is also an increased incidence of carcinoma after colonic augmentation, TCC may occur in the remnant bladder, and calculi may also be seen. Ultrasound is a useful investigation for the augmented bladder, but volume estimation is less accurate, as the reconstructed bladder is of a more complex shape.

Interventional Ultrasound of the Bladder

Occasionally ultrasound guidance may be necessary for suprapubic catheterization if the bladder is of small volume. An area close to the midline and just above the symphysis pubis is chosen, as this route will be extraperitoneal. Transabdominal needle biopsy of a bladder mass is rarely necessary and, furthermore, there is a risk of tumor seeding. The transabdominal route or the transrectal route may be used to puncture a nondeflating balloon of a urinary catheter. A fine needle (22-gauge) is directed into the balloon and the balloon contents aspirated. Occasionally the transabdominal route may be used to create a large (30-Fr) track for endoscopic lithotripsy. Transabdominal high-intensity frequency ultrasound (HIFU) ablation of prostate and bladder tumors is currently under investigation.

Summary points:
- The bladder wall should be < 3 mm thick with a full bladder
- Hemorrhagic cystitis occurs with cyclophosphamide therapy, seen as diffuse bladder-wall thickening
- 95% of focal bladder-wall thickening is due to a TCC
- The majority of TCCs present with hematuria
- Ultrasound is 90% sensitive for the detection of a TCC
- Cystoscopy is always necessary in the presence of macroscopic hematuria

The Abnormal Prostate and Ejaculatory Mechanism

Developmental Anomalies

The seminal vesicles, vasa, and/or ejaculatory duct may be absent as a combined maldevelopment of the woolfian duct. This may additionally affect the bladder trigone, which may be deficient with a wide bladder neck. These wolffian duct anomalies are rare, but abnormalities of the müllerian duct development are commonly seen as midline cystic structures on TRUS (Fig. 10.**11**). These cystic structures are round in the axial plane and teardrop-shaped on longitudinal imaging, often extending above the prostate gland. The majority are incidental findings, may be slightly thick-walled, but are always low-reflective unless bleeding has occurred or the cyst is infected (Fig. 10.**11**). Occasionally calcification may be present. Clinical symptoms include hematospermia or obstructive infertility; giant cysts may obstruct urinary flow which is usually seen in teenagers. Bilateral müllerian cysts may be associated with unilateral renal agenesis. Tumors of müllerian remnants are extremely rare.

Müllerian cysts do not communicate with the urethra, unlike a persistent prostatic utricle (or "utricle cyst"). Utricles do not extend beyond the gland and in practice it is difficult to differentiate a persistent utricle from a small müllerian remnant cyst on TRUS. Persistent utricles are often associated with hypospadias or genital anomalies. Very rarely, the prostate may be hypoplastic, for example in the prune belly syndrome.

Benign Acquired Abnormalities

Benign Prostate Hyperplasia/Benign Prostate Hypertrophy

Beyond age 40 the prostate will enlarge and above age 50 over 50% of men will have some degree of benign prostatic hypertrophy. Both the glandular and stromal elements enlarge, particularly within the transition zone and the periurethral glands, but it may also affect the peripheral zone. The exact cause of this hypertrophy is unknown, but hormones play a role. Hypertrophy may be diffuse or develop as distinct adenomas (Fig. 10.12). In addition, there is hypertrophy of the periurethral muscle spiral as a result of the associated outflow obstruction and the higher voiding pressures needed to maintain flow rates. There is no clear relation between the degree of prostate and periurethral muscle spiral hypertrophy and reduced urinary flow. A variety of ultrasound abnormalities are seen (Table 10.5). Some men present with irritative symptoms (frequency, nocturia) rather than significantly reduced flow rates, whereas others may present with urgency and stress incontinence due to secondary detrusor instability (or overactive bladder). Therefore, the entire symptom complex secondary to prostate gland enlargement is now referred to as lower urinary tract symptoms (LUTS). As well as LUTS, the other pressing difficulty is differentiation of benign hyperplastic nodules from the 10–20% of prostate carcinomas that arise from the transitional or central zones (Fig. 10.12).

For the evaluation of the patient with BPH, the most useful radiological investigation is the ultrasound cystodynamogram (USCD). TRUS does not provide any extra information in the evaluation of the patient presenting with reduced flow rates or LUTS, but the size of the prostate gland may be accurately measured (Fig. 10.5). The correlation between the ultrasound-measured volume and true prostate weight is estimated at between

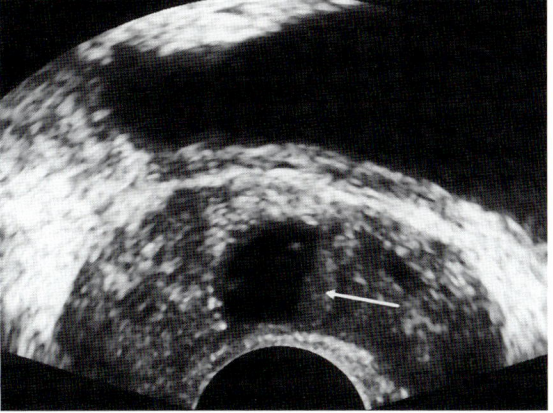

Fig. 10.11 **Axial view of the base of the prostate gland.** A large müllerian remnant cyst (arrow) with evidence of internal hemorrhage. The patient was examined in the left lateral position accounting for the position of the fluid–blood layer

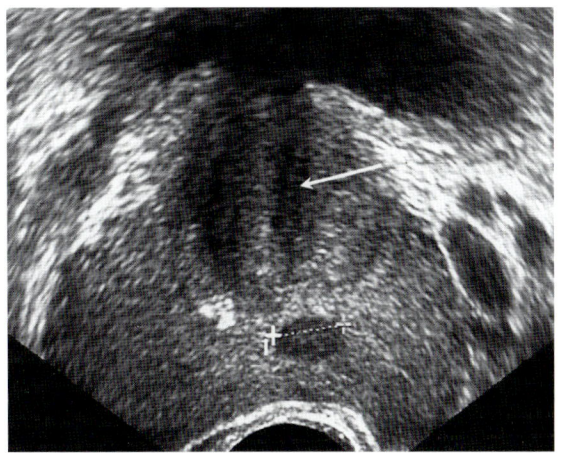

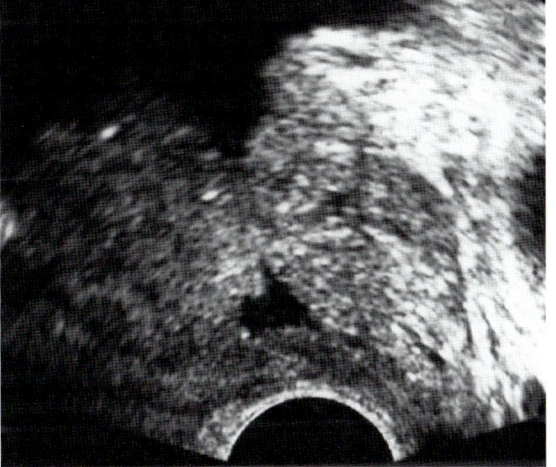

Fig. 10.12 **Two patients demonstrating benign prostatic hypertrophy. a** Inner gland enlargement with hypertrophy of the transition zone (arrow) and a nodule in the peripheral zone (calipers). Hyperplastic nodules (or adenomas) are usually of mixed reflectivity or isoreflective and located in a central position. Occasionally nodules are of low reflectivity, located in the periphery, and are indistinguishable from prostate carcinoma. Biopsy is then necessary. **b** A longitudinal view in another patient, demonstrating regrowth of benign prostate hyperplasia (BPH) after a previous transurethral resection of the prostate (TURP)

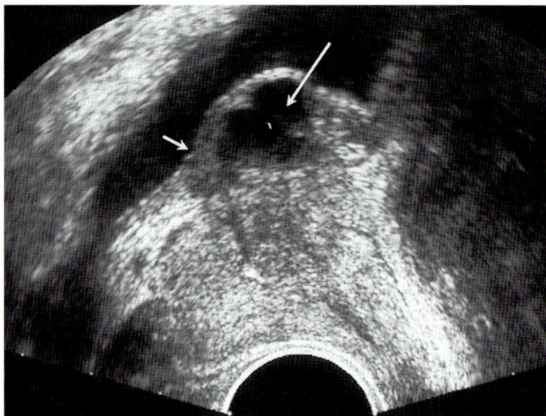

Fig. 10.13 Longitudinal view demonstrating a cyst (long arrow) arising centrally from the prostate gland and close to the bladder neck (short arrow). Occasionally such cysts can obstruct urine flow by a "ball–valve" action

0.82 and 0.99. The correlation is poorer for large prostate glands (>100 mL), as large glands deviate from the semi-ellipsoid shape assumed by the formula used for volume calculation. Volume estimation is important as a prostate gland in excess of 100 mL is better managed by retropubic prostatectomy, rather than a transurethral resection (TUR). There are rare occasions when TRUS provides useful information, as when an obstructing cyst at the bladder neck is a cause for LUTS (Fig. 10.13). Such cysts may be aspirated under TRUS-guidance to relieve obstructive symptoms, but the benefit is temporary. The value of TRUS for evaluation of recurrent outflow obstruction after TURP has also not been proved (Fig. 10.12b). On imaging, regrowth with restriction of the bladder neck may be seen, but does not directly influence management as much as uroflowmetry and postvoid residue estimations. Furthermore, TRUS is not of proved value in the follow-up of the patient on conservative or pharmacological management of known BPH and LUTS. 5α-reductase agents such as finasteride can decrease the prostate gland size by about 25%, but this information does not directly influence management.

> **Summary points:**
> - Over age 50, 50% of men will have benign prostatic hypertrophy
> - LUTS describes frequency, nocturia, urgency, and stress incontinence secondary to benign prostatic hypertrophy
> - The prostate gland may be unremarkable on ultrasound in the presence of prostatitis
> - The majority of prostate cysts are benign; position determines the cause
> - The commonest prostate cyst is a müllerian duct remnant

Prostatitis

The clinical, pathological, and ultrasound features of prostatitis vary widely. Acute prostatitis is uncommon but can occur in the young man, and is due to infection by the usual urinary tract organisms (*E. coli*, *Enterococci*, and anaerobic bacteria). Systemic clinical signs of infection are present, and the prostate gland is exquisitely tender on digital rectal and TRUS examination. On TRUS with color Doppler imaging the prostate gland demonstrates increased generalized or focal vascularity (Table 10.5, Fig. 10.14). The prostate gland is of focal or gener-

Table 10.5 Common benign prostate pathology and TRUS features

Pathology	Site	TRUS features
BPH Correlation between TRUS findings of BPH, prostate volume, and outflow obstruction is poor. Uroflowmetry correlation is necessary (see Table 10.4)	Transition zone or periurethral glands	• Gland enlargement (>25mL) • Heterogeneous changes in 2/3, homogenous in rest • Thinning of the peripheral zone • Nodules in the transitional zone: Low, high, or mixed reflectivity with defined boundary (unlike malignancy) • Capsule may bulge but is always intact • Cystic degeneration of nodules Bladder base is elevated ("median lobe" enlargement)
Acute or chronic prostatitis Data on many of these features are not established. Clinical correlation is necessary	Peripheral zone or transition/central zone	**Acute** • Diffuse or focal low reflectivity • Focal or generalized Increased vascularity • Abscess (focal, thick-walled, low-reflective area) **Chronic** • High-reflective foci • Prominence of the periprostatic venous plexus • Thickening of the "capsule" of the gland • Prominent calcification of inner gland • Mild/moderate increase color Doppler flow (focal or global).

alized, decreased reflectivity and the capsule is thick or ill-defined. An abscess may be identified as a focal cystic degenerative area with a thick capsule, and containing air. A prostate gland abscess may be drained by TRUS-guided aspiration (Fig. 10.**15**).[41] Paradoxically the prostate may be entirely unremarkable on ultrasound in the presence of prostatitis.

Chronic prostatitis is more common and is usually nonbacterial; chemical prostatitis due to reflux of urine or agents such as *Chlamydeous* or *Ureaplasma* may play a role. Clinical symptoms are generally vague and persistent perineal pain is commonest. On TRUS, the appearances are as nonspecific as the symptoms; distension of the periprostatic veins, dystrophic inner gland, and periurethral calcification or high-reflective capsule thickening have been described.[42,43] In practice, TRUS findings need to be correlated with the clinical findings and biochemistry of prostate secretions after transrectal digital massage. On USCD, reduced urine flow rates and incomplete bladder emptying may be seen. Although midline cysts are often seen, presumed to be either müllerian cysts or more likely persistent utricles, the relationship with prostatitis is not established.

Less common causes of prostatitis are eosinophilic prostatitis or granulomatous infections. Most granulomatous infections are idiopathic but tuberculosis, either infective or the result of bacille Calmette–Guérin (BCG) instillation to treat bladder TCC, may be a cause. On TRUS, the gland may be of diffusely decreased reflectivity or characteristically a mixed-reflective nodule may be seen in the peripheral zone and may be mistaken for prostate carcinoma (Fig. 10.**16**). Biopsy is nec-

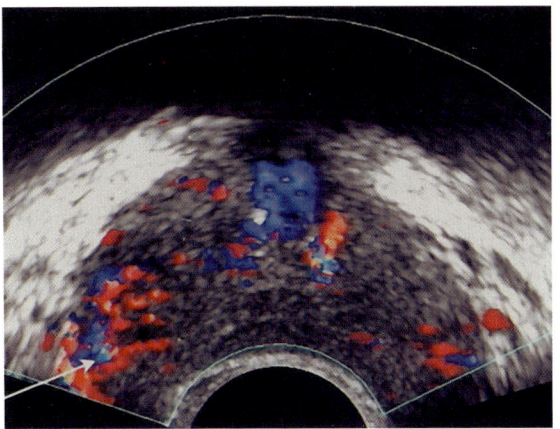

Fig. 10.**14 Axial color Doppler ultrasound image of the prostate gland in acute prostatitis.** There is a focus of increased vascularity in the right peripheral zone (arrow). This finding is, however, uncommon and most patients with prostatitis (acute or chronic) will demonstrate either normal or a minimal increase in vascularity

essary to establish the diagnosis. Caseating tuberculous nodules are rarely seen.

Cysts of the Prostate Gland and Associated Structures

The vast majority of prostate cysts are benign and location determines the cause (Table 10.**6**, Fig. 10.**17**). The commonest prostate cyst in a young man is a cyst of the müllerian remnants followed by cysts of the utricles. In the older man, cystic change usually represents areas of degeneration as a part of BPH. Multiple cysts of the seminal vesicles are seen with adult polycystic kidney

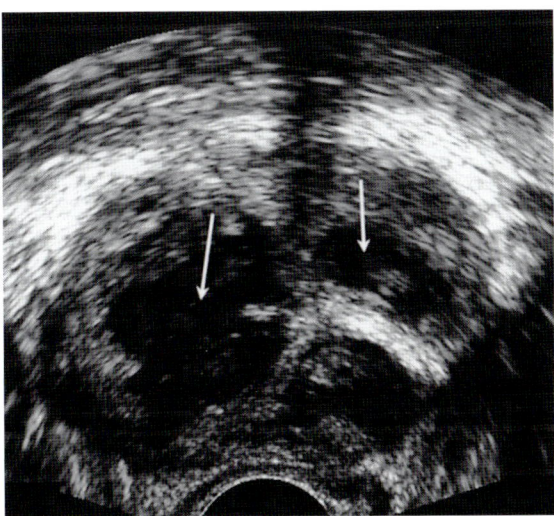

Fig. 10.**15 Transverse image through the prostate gland demonstrating multiple prostate abscesses** (arrows)

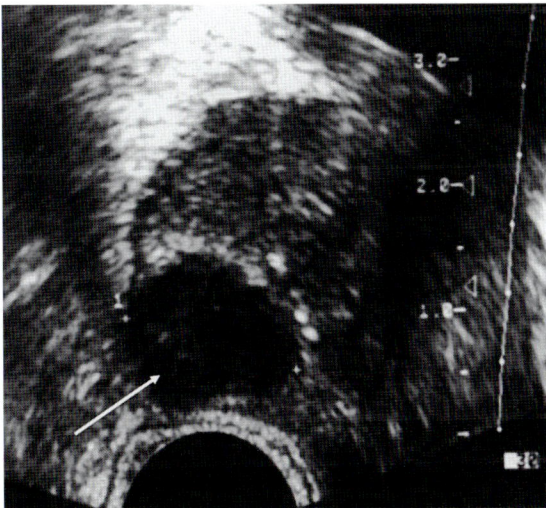

Fig. 10.**16 A large low-reflective nodule in the right peripheral zone** (arrow) **representing an area of granulomatous prostatitis on histology.** However, it is indistinguishable from prostate carcinoma on ultrasound

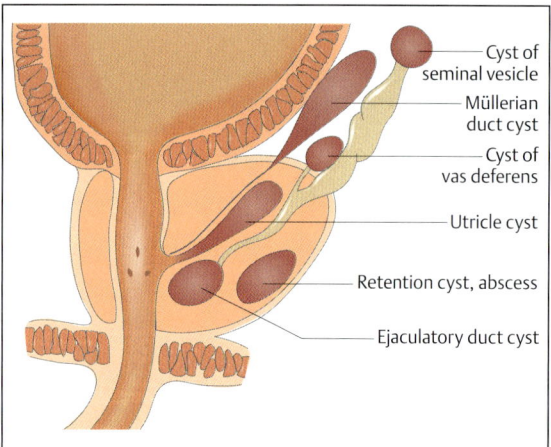

Fig. 10.**17** The typical locations of the various types of cysts in the prostate gland and its appendages as seen on TRUS examination

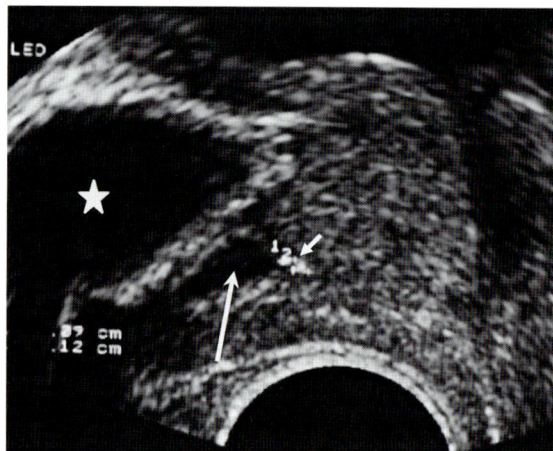

Fig. 10.**18** A longitudinal image demonstrating a dilated ejaculatory duct (long arrow) and seminal vesicle (star) secondary to two ejaculatory duct calculi (short arrow)

Table 10.**6** Cysts of the prostate gland and associated structures

Developmental

1. Müllerian duct cysts
Midline, usually extend above the gland and may be large, contain no sperm, and no communication with urethra

2. Utricle "cysts"
Not a true cyst. Lie in the midline, at the level of the verumontanum, intraglandular, rarely contain sperm, communicate with the urethra, and are usually < 1 cm in diameter. Known association with hypospadias or ambiguous genitalia

Acquired

1. Duct ectasia
Mild distension of normal ducts and is common

2. Ejaculatory duct cysts
Usually just lateral to midline, occur postinflammation or TURP. Contain sperm or calculi with seminal vesicle dilatation

3. Cystic degeneration of BPH nodules
Commonest cysts and found in the transitional zone

4. Retention cysts
Due to dilatation of gland acini and may cause obstruction if located close to the bladder neck ("ball–valve" obstruction)

5. Cavitary prostatitis
Multiple cysts due to prolonged inflammation (rare)

6. Abscess
Thick-walled, septated cysts occurring following prostatitis. Commoner in diabetics and after bladder catheterization

7. Cystic prostate cancer (very rare)

disease and renal maldevelopment, but are otherwise asymptomatic.

Transrectal Ultrasound and Evaluation of Male Infertility

Transrectal ultrasound (TRUS) may provide useful information in men with low or absent sperm by excluding obstruction of the ejaculatory ducts.[44] Obstruction of the ejaculatory ducts is suggested by dilatation of the ducts and/or seminal vesicles (Fig. 10.**18**). Mild vesicular distension may be seen with normal physiological storage of seminal fluid, and isolated vesicular distension needs to be differentiated from normal physiological distension by postejaculatory imaging. True obstruction may be as a consequence of calculi in the ducts with associated duct stricturing. Occasionally a large müllerian remnant cyst may obstruct the ducts or the seminal vesicles. Vasa and ejaculatory ducts may all be absent as part of a generalized maldevelopment of the embryological wolffian duct. Chronic hematospermia may be investigated with transrectal ultrasound.[45]

Malignant Acquired Abnormalities

Carcinoma of Prostate

Prostate carcinoma is the second most common male cancer, with over 80% originating in the peripheral zone; the remainder arise in the central/transition zone or are peripheral zone tumors preferentially infiltrating in an anterior direction.[46] On ultrasound the peripheral zone is the most homogenous of the zones, and even in the presence of marked hyperplasia most carcinomas should be readily identified. However, in practice the ultrasound appearances of prostate carcinomas are highly variable, ranging from low-reflective to high-reflective, or as is most often the case, isoreflective and barely visible (Fig. 10.**19**). Ultrasound evaluation is therefore difficult and a meta-analysis indicated the positive predictive value of TRUS for detection of prostate carcinoma was only 6%.[47] Table 10.**7** shows the various ultrasound appearances that may be en-

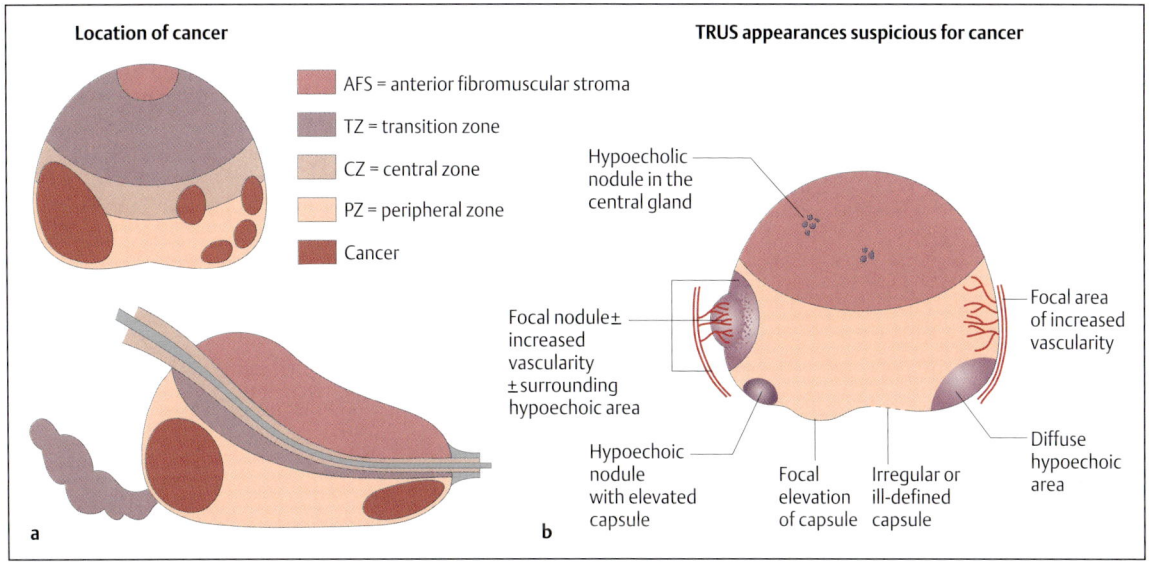

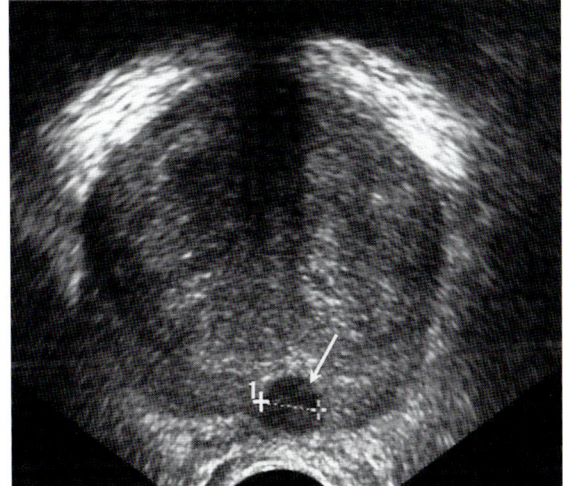

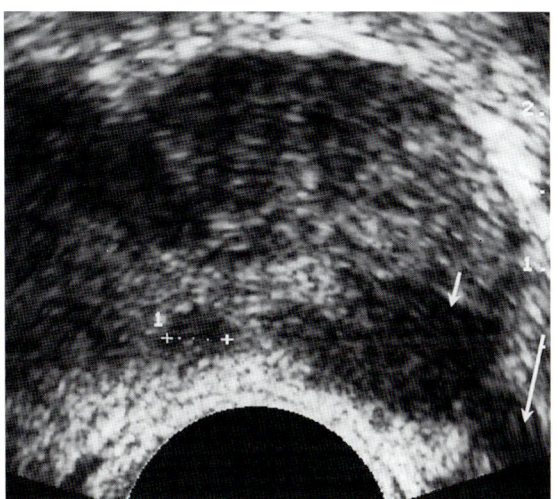

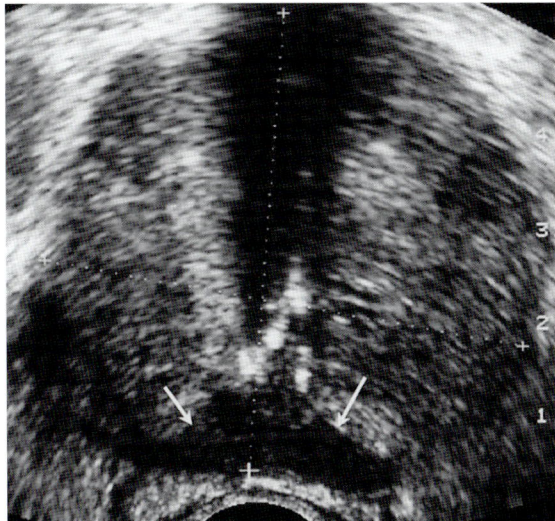

Fig. 10.**19 Distribution and typical appearances of prostate carcinoma on TRUS. a** The distribution of prostate carcinoma in relation to the zones of the prostate gland. **b** The various appearances of prostate carcinoma. Most tumors diagnosed in the modern era (particularly if PSA < 5 ng/mL) are either iso-reflective or demonstrate only subtle changes on ultrasound. **c** There is a nodule close to the midline in the peripheral zone (arrow and cursors) representing a T1/2 tumor. **d** A T3 tumor with irregular, diffuse reflectivity changes of the left peripheral zone (short arrow) and involvement of the adjacent neuro-vascular bundle (long arrow). A further separate nodule is present in the right peripheral zone (calipers). **e** An extensive tumor involving both lobes, with low-reflective texture of both peripheral zones (arrows)

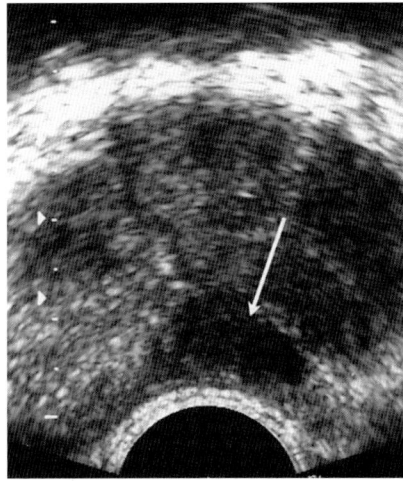 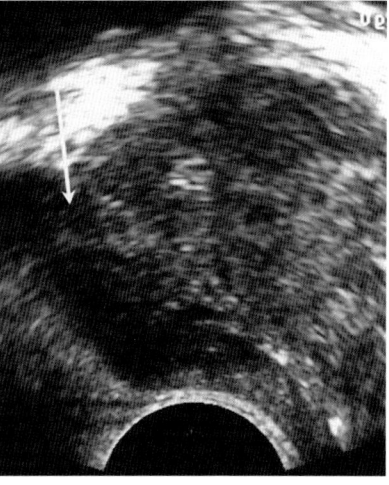

Fig. 10.**20 The importance of imaging in both planes when prostate carcinoma is suspected is demonstrated** (Table 10.**3**). The left-hand axial image demonstrates a nodule in the peripheral zone (arrow: a T1/2 lesion). However, on the right-hand image, on the longitudinal view, the nodule is demonstrated to extend into the seminal vesicle (arrow): a T3 lesion

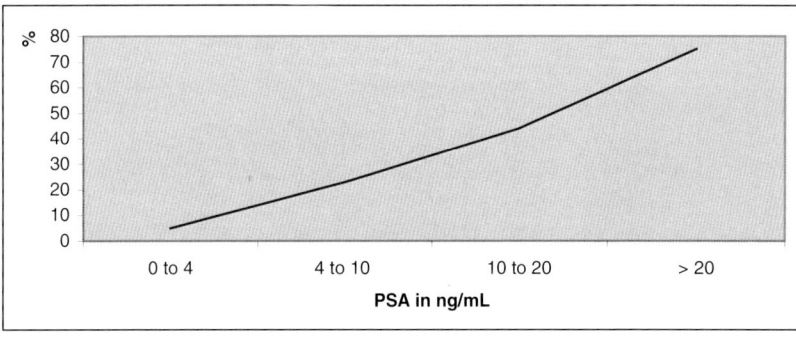

Fig. 10.**21 The visibility of prostate carcinoma on TRUS according to the PSA level** (based on the author's unpublished data)

countered and the diagnostic accuracy. Often the abnormality is subtle, and careful examination is important. The posterolateral aspects, apices and the base of the prostate gland close to the seminal vesicles are areas of higher carcinoma incidence. These are relatively "blind" areas and should be examined in multiple orientations, comparing the two sides of the gland (Fig. 10.**20**). However, even those abnormalities described on ultrasound are not specific, as inflammation, hyperplasia, and necrosis may all appear similar and mimic carcinoma. Visibility on ultrasound is partly related to the tumor stage and prostate-specific antigen (PSA) level. With the down-migration of clinical stage at presentation, reflecting the increase in PSA testing and case-finding, the number of isoreflective carcinomas diagnosed is increasing (Fig. 10.**21**).

Examination of prostate gland vascularity using color Doppler ultrasound[48–50] improves the specificity of carcinoma detection by about 5–10% but not sufficiently to obviate biopsy. This performance is only slightly improved by the use of power Doppler or by the use of ultrasound microbubble contrast media (Fig. 10.**22**).[51] Three general color Doppler flow patterns have been described: 1) increased focal flow, 2) increased flow around a nodule, and 3) asymmetric flow with increased number and size of vessels on the side harboring tumor. When seen in association with a low-reflective nodule any of these flow patterns are highly suggestive of carcinoma. With the more difficult isoreflective nodule, color Doppler flow is often disappointing. Simple three-dimensional (3-D) TRUS systems are now becoming available but their value remains uncertain (Fig. 10.**23**). Hence, in current practice, TRUS is inaccurate for confident diagnosis or exclusion of prostate carcinoma.[47] A prostate biopsy is necessary to confirm suspected malignancy and exclude low-volume or isoreflective carcinoma in all patients with a clinical suspicion of tumor, either because the PSA is elevated or the gland is nodular or hard on digital rectal examination.

Summary points:
- Prostate carcinoma is the second most common male malignancy
- 80% of prostate carcinoma originates in the peripheral zone
- Most prostate carcinomas in the peripheral zone are isoreflective to normal prostate tissue
- Color Doppler US improves the specificity of carcinoma detection
- Prostate biopsy is always necessary to diagnose prostate carcinoma

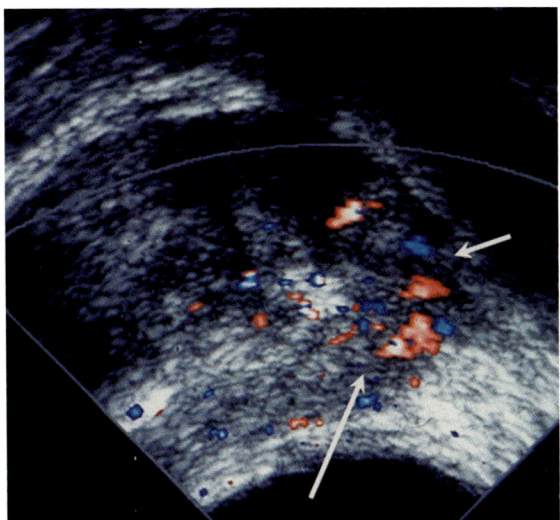

Fig. 10.22 **Imaging of prostate carcinoma** (arrows) **on color Doppler ultrasound** (either conventional, power, or microbubble contrast-enhanced ultrasound) may improve TRUS specificity by 5–10% but does not obviate the need to perform a biopsy

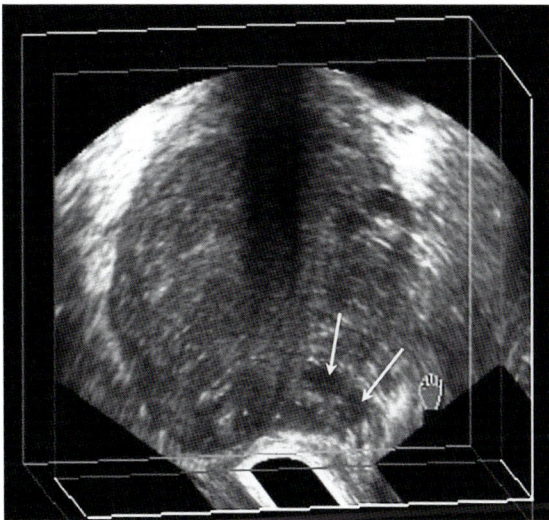

Fig. 10.23 **3-D reformatted ultrasound images of the prostate gland with a low-reflective area of prostate carcinoma present** (arrows). 3-D ultrasound has yet to find a role in routine practice

Table 10.7 **TRUS features of prostate carcinoma**

Prostate carcinoma	TRUS features
Diagnosis There is a correlation between PSA level (and tumor stage) and ultrasound appearances (Fig. 10.21). Below 10 ng/mL, less than 30% are visible but the figure rises to > 75% if PSA level is > 20 ng/mL. In practice most tumors are not visualized as the median PSA is < 15 ng/mL and falling with increased "case-finding" or "de facto" screening	**Strongly suggestive** • Low-reflective nodules with indistinct edge in PZ • Diffuse low reflectivity in PZ • Nodule with surrounding altered reflectivity • Low-reflective area in PZ with increased vascularity **Moderately suggestive** • Low-reflective or isoreflective focal bulge of the PZ • Irregular or ill-defined capsule **Weakly suggestive** • Low-reflective nodule in the inner gland • Focal increase in vascularity of an isoreflective area in the PZ • Focal increase in vascularity in the inner gland
Staging Accuracy: 50–92% for extracapsular extension; 78% for seminal vesicle extension. MRI is more accurate	**Extracapsular extension** • Irregular, low-reflective bulge of capsule • Infiltration into periprostatic fat **Neurovascular bundle** • Asymmetry • Enlargement **Seminal vesicle involvement** • Loss of angle between seminal vesicle and base of gland • Enlargement of seminal vesicle **High Gleason grade** • High color Doppler flow may signify higher Gleason grades

PZ = peripheral zone; TZ = transitional zone; CZ = central zone; PSA = prostate-specific antigen

Staging of Prostate Carcinoma

Known prostate carcinoma may be locally staged with TRUS but only with limited accuracy, namely 50–92% for extracapsular extension and 78% for seminal vesicle extension (Table 10.7).[52–54] In clinical practice, staging is better carried out with MR or CT imaging, combined with an isotope bone scan. Clinical outcome of prostate carcinoma is also dependent on the histological or Gleason score determined from the prostate biopsies.[55] Further but less specific measures of clinical outcome are the number of prostate biopsies that reveal carcinoma, the percentage of the core length involved by carcinoma, and whether biopsies from both lobes were positive.

Follow-up of Prostate Carcinoma

TRUS is of limited value and cannot replace PSA-level monitoring. Following radiotherapy, the prostate gland may vary from diffusely low-reflective or resemble a mixed-reflective pattern, with or without a prominent "capsule." The value of color Doppler ultrasound has not been established. After prostatectomy, nodular areas in the prostate bed may denote residual tumor and may be subject to a biopsy.

> **Summary points:**
> - TRUS has limited accuracy for local staging of prostate carcinoma
> - Staging of prostate carcinoma is better with CT or MRI
> - Staging is also dependent on the histology (Gleason score)

Unusual Transrectal Ultrasound Abnormalities

Other rare prostate abnormalities may be demonstrated and their ultrasound appearances are described in Table 10.**8**.

Transrectal Ultrasound-Guided Intervention

Prostate Biopsy

A prostate biopsy can be performed by the transrectal or transperineal route. Modern transducers allow biopsy by the transrectal route, and the transperineal route is normally reserved for brachytherapy implantation. The advantage of the transrectal route is ease and relative comfort for the patient but at the risk of infection and rectal bleeding. All patients should have antibiotic prophylaxis; the agent of choice varies but the use of a 5-quinolone is a common choice. The evidence for the use of an antianerobic agent as well is less strong. Local anaesthetic is also increasingly used.[56,57] Table 10.**9** lists the preprocedural and equipment details.

The number of biopsies necessary to confidently exclude clinically significant prostate carcinoma is a matter of continuing debate. Subjecting only visible abnormalities to biopsy is highly inaccurate, and a systematic sampling technique is necessary to identify the sonographically invisible cancers. Six cores, targeted onto the peripheral zone, was the practice standard but studies suggest that this may miss 19–31% of tumors, and increasingly eight, 10, 12, or more biopsies are being advocated.[58–65] More cores may identify extra tumors, but there is a concern that these may be insignificant carcinomas and diagnosed at the expense of extra complications.[58] A summary of the principles of prostate biopsy (or more accurately sampling) and the different biopsy policies are detailed in Figure 10.**24**. Currently it is advocated that at least octant biopsies be performed as standard practice, but with large prostate glands (> 80 mL) or in those undergoing repeat biopsies 12 or more cores should be considered to include the inner gland.

Biopsy of the Postprostatectomy Bed

After total prostatectomy the PSA level should be undetectable. If not, or if the PSA starts rising after a nadir,

Table 10.8 Unusual abnormalities of the prostate gland

Abnormality	TRUS findings
Tuberculosis (may be secondary to intravesical BCG for treatment of bladder carcinoma)	Similar to prostatitis
Sarcoidosis	Nonspecific
Infarction (particularly following bladder catheterization)	Low-reflective nodules
Lymphoma (usually non-Hodgkin lymphoma)	Large, low-reflective masses throughout the gland with periprostatic infiltration
Leukemia	Nonspecific
Metastasis (lung or melanoma)	Nonspecific
Comedocarcinoma	Low-reflective nodules with multiple, small, low-reflective foci
Other rare cancers	Nonspecific

Table 10.**9** Preparation and equipment necessary for TRUS-guided prostate biopsy[4]

- Stop anticoagulation (warfarin) until international normalized ratio (INR) < 1.3. Stop clopidogrel for seven days. Evidence suggests that aspirin may be continued safely.[76] Commence antibiotics at least one hour before biopsy
- Biopsy attachment: Either a disposable unit or a reusable metal guide
- 15–20–cm, 22-gauge spinal needle, 10-mL syringe, and 1% plain lignocaine (or lidocaine) for local anesthesia
- Sterile 18-gauge biopsy needle, with biopsy "gun" or device. Needle length longer than the length of the biopsy guide (16 cm long). Seminal vesicle biopsies are easier with a 20-cm needle length. Core length of the needle "notch" should be 1.5–2.0 cm, but seminal vesicle biopsy requires a shorter length of 1 cm
- Separate pots with formalin–saline solution for each core so the anatomical position of the tumor is known
- A small pot of sterile saline to "swizzle" and clean the needle tip in order to remove the formalin between biopsies

Principles:
- Coverage should be maximized for the peripheral zone and areas of high tumor incidence; the apex, postero-lateral margins, and the medial base.
- Systematic strategies perform better than guided biopsies as most carcinomas are iso-reflective and prostate carcinoma is often multifocal.
- The classical sextant biopsy pattern may miss 20–30% of carcinomas; at the moment 8 biopsies are a common choice (with additional cores through focal abnormalities).
- Transitional zone biopsies have a low pick rate (2–8%) and should be reserved for repeat biopsies.
- For large glands or repeat biopsies (rising PSA or previous PIN) more than 8 should be taken (12 biopsies) and the transitional zone included.
- For staging biopsies the base of the seminal vesicles and the prostate capsule should be sampled.

Complications:
- Hematuria in 12.5–80%; hematospermia in 5.1–89% and between 1.3 and 37% notice rectal bleeding (pooled data from existing literature).
- Serious hemorrhage is usually due to heavy rectal bleeding and occurs in 0.2–1%.
- Septicemia in 1–2%.
- Urinary retention appears to be higher with >12 biopsies and if urethra is transgressed with deep inner gland biopsies.

Sextant biopsy pattern: This is the modified version of the classical pattern described; the middle biopsies were moved laterally and the trajectories directed obliquely to increase sampling of the peripheral zone (70). However, even this pattern misses many carcinomas.

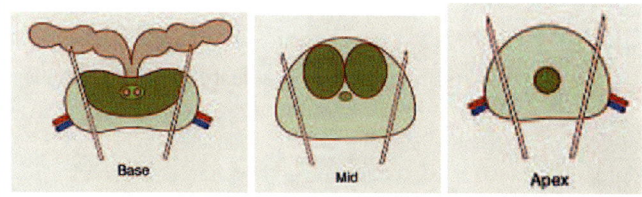

Alternative biopsy patterns described to improve sampling

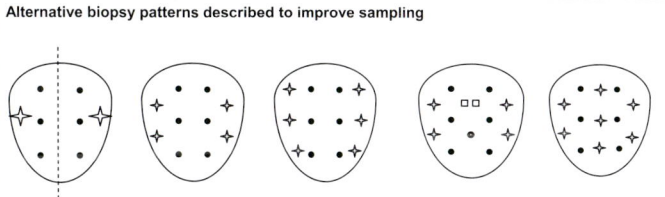

Notes: **8 PZ biopsies:** improved detection rate from 85% to 97% (71). **10 PZ biopsies:** 20% improved accuracy (60, 72). Ravery et al (72) however reported only a 3% improvement. **12 biopsies;** 12 biopsies targeted onto the PZ and TZ, 20% improved accuracy (65) but increased hematospermia and rectal bleeding (73) (recommended for large glands and repeat biopsies). **11 core multi-site:** sampling of anterior TZ, midline of the gland as well 4 lateral PZ biopsies (74). 33% improved diagnosis, the extra PZ biopsies contributing most to improved diagnosis. TZ biopsies have a low positive rate (between 2 and 10%) and advocated only for repeat biopsies. **"5 Region Biopsy":** 13 biopsies of the peripheral zone (75), improved diagnostic rate by 35%, but high hematuria rate (80%) because of midline biopsies. **Other patterns:** saturation biopsies where 24 to 30 cores taken under sedation/anesthesia with high urinary retention rate. Staging biopsies target the capsule and seminal vesicles. Transurethral biopsies for sampling gland immediately anterior to the urethra.

Fig. 10.**24 The principles of prostate biopsy**

concern is raised about residual prostate carcinoma. This may be due to bony or lymph node metastasis, but if appropriate investigations (isotope bone scan and CT or MR imaging) are negative there may be residual/recurrent disease at the anastomosis (Fig. 10.**25**). The anastomosis and surrounding tissues may be of mixed reflectivity and asymmetric due to either normal postoperative fibrosis or recurrent tumor; and biopsy is necessary for differentiation.[66,67] At least two cores should be taken, one from either side and just above the anastomosis.

Summary points:
- Prostate biopsy is nearly always performed by TRUS
- Prophylactic antibiotics and local anaesthetic are administered
- The peripheral zone of the prostate is targeted for systematic biopsy
- The number of samples obtained varies from six to 12;
- Subjecting visible abnormalities to biopsy is inaccurate
- More biopsy cores diagnose more tumors

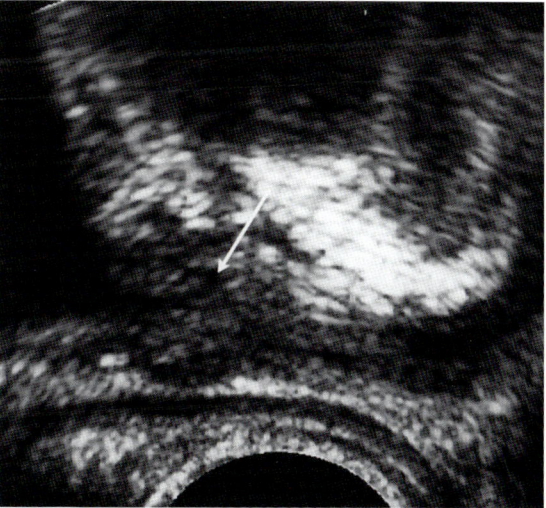

Fig. 10.**25 Normal TRUS views of the postradical prostatectomy bed.** The arrow points to the perianastomotic tissues. The appearances can be variable and biopsy is necessary to exclude recurrent disease

Drainage of Prostate Abscess, Cyst, or Seminal Vesicles

Drainage procedures may be carried out under transrectal guidance in the left lateral position after antibiotic coverage, although a more purist approach would be via the transperineal route in order to decrease the risk of introduced infection or contamination. A long-shaft (20 cm), 20–22-gauge needle can be accurately guided into the suspected fluid collection and aspirated. If necessary iodinated contrast medium may be injected via the indwelling needle to assess for communication with the ejaculatory ducts or urethra, or in suspected cases of obstructive infertility.[68] This requires fluoroscopic facilities.

Prostate Brachytherapy

Implantation of radioactive seeds (normally ^{132}I) for the treatment of gland-confined prostate carcinoma has become an accepted procedure. Recent data show that more than 85% of T1 and T2 tumors are disease-free at 10-year follow-up.[69] Dedicated equipment is necessary, namely a transperineal transducer, a brachytherapy gantry and grid, and the appropriate radiotherapy planning software. The technique is merely an extension of transperineal biopsy but requires spinal or general anaesthetic as 20–30 needle insertions (to deliver 100–120 seeds) are required.

Prostate Ablation

Many minimally invasive techniques have been tried for ablation of prostate tissue for the treatment of BPH or prostate cancer, for example microwave heating, cryotherapy, HIFU, transurethral needle ablation (TUNA), and laser ablation. All are successful to a variable degree but none has been overwhelmingly so. TRUS can contribute in the planning or execution of many of these techniques.

References

1. Hayes WS. The urinary bladder. In: Davidson AS, Hartman DS, eds. Radiology of the kidney and urinary tract. Philadelphia: WB Saunders: 1994:607–610.
2. McNeal JE. The zonal anatomy of the prostate. Prostate 1981;2:35–49.
3. McNeal JE. Regional morphology and pathology of the prostate. Am J Clin Pathol 1968;49:347–357.
4. Manieri C, Carter SSC, Romano G, Trucchi A, Valenti M, Tubaro D. The diagnosis of bladder outlet obstruction in men by ultrasound measurement of bladder wall thickness. J Urol 1998;159:761–765.
5. Price CI, Adler RS, Rubin JM. Ultrasound detection of differences in density: explanation of ureteric jet phenomenon and implications for new ultrasound applications. Invest Radiol 1989;24:876–883.
6. Patel U, Kellett MJ. Ureteric drainage and peristalsis post-stenting. Br J Urol 1996;77:530–535.
7. Baker SM, Middleton WD. Color Doppler sonography of ureteral jets in normal volunteers: importance of relative specific gravity in the urine and bladder. AJR Am J Roentgenol 1992;159:773–775.
8. Patel U, Rickards D. The diagnostic value of colour Doppler flow in the peripheral zone of the prostate with histological correlation. Br J Urol 1994;74:590–595.
9. Friedland GW, Devries PA, Nino-Murcia M, et al. Congenital anomalies of the urinary tract. In: Pollack HM, ed. Clinical urography: An atlas and textbook of urologic imaging. Philadelphia: WB Saunders: 1990:559–787.
10. Spataro RF, Davis RS, McLachlan MS, Linke CA, Barbaric ZL. Urachal abnormalities in the adult. Radiology 1983;149:659–663.
11. Bouvier JF, Pascaud E, Mailhes F, Pascaud JL, Hummel P, Rousseau J. Urachal cysts in the adult: ultrasonic diagnosis. J Clin Ultrasound 1984;12:48–50.
12. Rifkin MD, Needleman L, Kurtz AB, et al. Sonography of non-gynaecologic cystic masses of the pelvis. AJR Am J Roentgenol 1984;142:1169–1174.
13. Rosenfield AT, Taylor KJW, Weiss RM. Ultrasound evaluation of bladder calculi. J Urol 1979;121:119–120.
14. Chelfouh N, Grenier N, Higueret D, et al. Characterization of urinary calculi: in vitro study of "twinkling artifact" revealed by color-flow sonography. AJR Am J Roentgenol 1998;171:1055–60.
15. Lam AH, Tang S. Sonographic findings in bladder haematoma. Australas Radiol 1994;38:48–50.
16. Amis ES, Blaivas JG. Neurogenic bladder simplified. Radiol Clin North Am 1991;29:571–580.
17. Stark GL, Feddersen R, Lowe BA, Benson CT, Black W, Borden TA. Inflammatory pseudotumor (pseudosarcoma) of the bladder. J Urol 1989;141:610–612.
18. Kauzlaric D, Barmeir E. Sonography of emphysematous cystitis. J Ultrasound Med 1985;4:319–320.
19. Cartoni C, Arcese W, Avvisati G, Corinto L, Capua A, Meloni G. Role of ultrasonography and follow-up of haemorrhagic cystitis after bone marrow transplantation. Bone Marrow Transplant 1993;12:463–467.
20. Das KM, Indudhara R, Vaidyanathan S. Sonographic features of genitourinary tuberculosis. AJR Am J Roentgenol 1992;158:327–329.
21. Premkumar A, Lattimer J, Newhouse JH. CT and sonography of advanced urinary tract tuberculosis. AJR Am J Roentgenol 1987;148:65–69.
22. Buchanan WM, Gelfand M. Calcification of the bladder in urinary Schistosomiasis. Trans R Soc Trop Med Hyg 1970;64:593–596.
23. Al-Ghorab MM. Radiological manifestations of genito-urinary bilharziasis. Clin Radiol 1968;19:100–111.
24. Curran FT. Malakoplakia of the bladder. Br J Urol 1987;59:559–563.
25. Raja G, Anson KA, Patel U. Cystitis Cystica and Cystitis Glandularis—Presentation with acute ureteric obstruction. Clin Radiol Extra 2003;58:43–44.

26. Kumar R, Haque AK, Cohen MS. Endometriosis of the urinary bladder demonstrated by sonography. J Clin Ultrasound 1984;12:363–365.
27. Abu Yousef MM, Narayana AS, Brown RC, et al. Urinary bladder tumours studied by cystosonography Part I. Detection. Radiology 1984;153:223–226.
28. Itzchak Y, Singer D, Fischelovitch Y. Ultrasonographic detection of bladder tumours 1. Tumour detection. J Urol 1981;26:31–33.
29. Brun B, Gammelgaard J, Christoffersen J. Transabdominal dynamic ultrasonography in the detection of bladder tumours. J Urol 1984;132:19–20.
30. Malone PR, Weston-Underwood J, Aron PM, Wilkinson KW, Joseph AE, Riddle PR. The use of abdominal ultrasound in the detection of early bladder tumours. Br J Urol 1986; 58:520–522.
31. Datta SN, Allen GM, Evans R, Vaughton KC, Lucas MG. Urinary tract ultrasonography in the evaluation of haematuria—a report of over 1000 cases. Ann R Coll Surg of Engl 2002;84:203–205.
32. RCR working party. Making the best use of a department of clinical radiology. 5th ed. London: The Royal College of Radiologists: 2003.
33. Vallencien G, Veillon B, Charton M, Brisset JM. Can transabdominal ultrasonography of the bladder replace cystoscopy in the follow-up of superficial bladder tumors. J Urol 1986;136:32–34.
34. Singer D, Itzchak Y, Fischelovitch Y. Ultrasonographic assessment of bladder tumours. II Clinical staging. J Urol 1981;26:34–36.
35. Devonec M, Chapelon JY, Codas H, Dubernard JM, Revillard JP, Cathignol D. Evaluation of bladder cancer with a miniature high frequency transurethral ultrasonographic probe. Br J Urol 1987;59:550–553.
36. Doehring E, Ehrich JH, Bremer HJ. Reversibility of urinary tract abnormalities due to schistosoma haematobium infection. Kidney Int 1986;30:582–585.
37. Pakter R, Nussbaum A, Fishman EK. Hemangioma of the bladder: sonographic and computerized tomography findings. J Urol 1988;140:601–602.
38. Steele B, Vade A, Lim-Dunham J. Sonographic appearance of bladder malacoplakia. Pediatr Radiol 2003;33:253–255.
39. Zerin JM, Smith JD, Sanvordenker JK, Bloom DA. Sonography of the bladder after ureteral reimplantation. J Ultrasound Med 1992;11:87–91.
40. Hertzberg BS, Bowie JD, King LR, Webster GD. Augmentation and replacement cystoplasty: sonographic findings. Radiology 1987;165:853–856.
41. Papanicolaou N, Pfister RC, Stafford SA, Parkhurst EC. Prostatic abscess: imaging with transrectal sonography and MR. AJR Am J Roentgenol 1987;149:981–982.
42. Griffiths GJ, Crooks AJ, Roberts EE, et al. Ultrasonic appearances associated with prostatic inflammation: a preliminary study. Clin Radiol 1984;35:343–345.
43. Doble A, Carter SS. Ultrasonographic findings in prostatitis. Urol Clin North Am 1989;16:763–772.
44. Kuligowska E, Baker CE, Oates RD. Male infertility: role of transrectal ultrasound in diagnosis and management. Radiology 1992;185:353–360.
45. Worischeck JH, Parra RO. Chronic haematospermia: assessment by transrectal sonography. Urology 1994;43:515–520.
46. McNeal JE, Redwine EA, Freiha FS, Stamey TA. Zonal distribution of prostatic adenocarcinoma. Correlation with histological pattern and direction of spread. Am J Surg Pathol 1988;12:897–906 .
47. Coley CM, Barry MJ, Fleming C, Mulley AG. Early detection of prostate cancer. Part 1: prior probability and effectiveness of tests. Ann Intern Med 1997;126:394–406.
48. Kelly IM, Lees WR, Rickards D. Prostate cancer and the role of color Doppler US. Radiology 1993;189:153–6.
49. Alexander AA. To color Doppler image the prostate or not: that is the question. Radiology 1995;195:11–13.
50. Newman JS, Brea RL, Rubin JM. Prostate cancer: diagnosis with color Doppler sonography with histological correlation of each biopsy site. Radiology 1995;195:86–90.
51. Halpern EJ, Rosenberg M, Gomella LG. Prostate cancer: contrast-enhanced US for detection. Radiology 2001;219: 219–25.
52. Rifkin MD, Zerhouni EA, Gatsonis CA, et al. Comparison of magnetic resonance imaging and ultrasonography in staging early prostate cancer. Results of a multi-institutional co-operative trial. N Engl J Med 1990;323:621–626.
53. Hamper UM, Sheth S, Walsh PC, Holtz PM, Epstein JI. Carcinoma of the prostate: value of transrectal sonography in detecting extension into the neurovascular bundle. AJR Am J Roentgenol 1990;155:1015–1019.
54. Terris MK, McNeal JE, Stamey TA. Invasion of the seminal vesicles by prostate cancer: detection with transrectal sonography. AJR Am J Roentgenol 1990;155:811–815.
55. Partin AW, Yoo J, Carter HB et al. The use of prostate specific antigen, clinical stage and Gleason score to predict pathological stage in men with localized prostate cancer. J Urol 1993;150:110–114.
56. Seymour H, Perry MJA, Lee-Elliot C, Dundas D, Patel U. Pain after transrectal ultrasonography-guided prostate biopsy: the advantages of periprostatic local anaesthesia. BJU Int 2001;88:540–544.
57. Lee-Elliot C, Dundas D, Patel U. Randomized trial of lidocaine vs. lidocaine/bupivacaine periprostaticInjection on longitudinal pain scores after prostate biopsy. J Urol 2004;171:247–250.
58. Klein EA, Zippe CD. Transrectal ultrasound guided prostate biopsy—defining a new standard. J Urol 2000;163: 179–180.
59. Stamey TA. Making the most of six systematic sextant biopsies. Urology 1995;45:2–12.
60. Presti JC, Chang JJ, Bhargava V Shinohara K. The optimal systematic prostate biopsy should include 8 rather than 6 biopsies: results of a prospective clinical trial. J Urol 2000; 163:163–166.
61. Djavan B, Ravery V, Zlotta A, et al. Prospective evaluation of prostate cancer detected on biopsies 1, 2, 3 and 4: when should we stop? J Urol 2001;166:1679–1683.
62. Borboroglu PG, Comer SW, Riffenburgh RH, Amling CL. Extensive repeat transrectal ultrasound-guided prostate biopsy in patients with previous benign sextant biopsies. J Urol 2000;163:158–62.
63. Stewart CS, Leibovich BC, Weaver AL, Lieber MM. Prostate cancer diagnosis using a saturation needle biopsy technique after negative sextant biopsies. J Urol 2001;166: 86–91.
64. Terris MK, Pham QT, Issa MM, Kabalin JN. Routine transition zone and seminal vesicle biopsies in all patients undergoing TRUS-guided prostate biopsies are not indicated. J Urol 1997;157:204–206.
65. Durkan GC, Sheikh N, Johnson P, Hildreth AJ, Greene DR. Improving prostate cancer detection with an extended-core transrectal ultrasonography-guided prostate biopsy protocol. BJU Int 2002;89:33–39.

66. Wasserman NF, Kapoor DA, Hildebrandt WC, et al. Transrectal ultrasound in evaluation of patients after radical prostatectomy. Part 1: Normal post-operative anatomy. Radiology 1992;185:361–366.
67. Wasserman NF, Kapoor DA, Hildebrandt WC, et al. Part 2: TRUS and biopsy findings in the presence of residual and early recurrent prostatic cancer. Radiology 1992;185:367–377.
68. Meacham RB, Townsend RR, Drose JA. Ejaculatory duct obstruction: diagnosis and treatment with transrectal sonography. AJR Am J Roentgenol 1995;165:1463–1466.
69. Ragde H, Korb L. Brachytherapy for clinically localized prostate cancer. Semin Surg Oncol 2000;18:45–51.
70. Norberg M, Egevad L, Holmberg L, Sparen P, Norlen BJ, Busch C. The sextant protocol for ultrasound-guided core biopsies of the prostate underestimates the presence of cancer. Urology 1997;50:562–566.
71. Chang JJ, Shinohara K, Bhargava V, Presti JC. Prospective evaluation of lateral biopsies of the peripheral zone for prostate cancer detection. J Urol 1998;160:2111–2114.
72. Ravery V, Billebaud T, Toublanc M, et al. Diagnostic value of ten systematic transrectal ultrasound guided prostate biopsies. Eur Urol 1999;35:298–303.
73. Naughton CK, Ornstein DK, Smith DS, Catalona WJ. Pain and morbidity of transrectal ultrasound-guided prostate biopsy: a prospective randomized trial of 6 versus 12 cores. J Urol 2000;163:168–171.
74. Babaian RJ, Toi A, Kamoi K, et al. A comparative analysis of sextant and an extended 11 core multisite directed biopsy strategy. J Urol 2000;163:152–157.
75. Eskew LA, Bare RL, McCullough DL. Systematic 5-region prostate biopsy is superior to sextant method for diagnosing carcinoma of the prostate. J Urol 1997;157:199–202.
76. Maan Z, Cutting CW, Patel W. Morbidity of transrectal ultrasound (TRUS) guided prostate biopsies in patients following continued use of low-dose aspirin. BJU Int 2003;91:798–800.

11 Diseases of the Testis and Epididymis

P. S. Sidhu

Introduction

The superficial nature of the scrotal sac and contents lends itself to detailed and precise imaging with ultrasound. As a consequence, ultrasound is firmly established as the first-line and often only imaging modality employed in the assessment of scrotal abnormalities. Recent technical advances in transducer design and image processing have further improved ultrasound diagnosis of diseases of the scrotal contents. This chapter will deal with aspects related to the testis and epididymis, detailing both normal ultrasound features and those features related to disease processes.

Normal Anatomy

During the seventh month of fetal development, as a result of the rapid growth of the fetal body and failure of growth of the gubernaculum testis, the testes descend into the scrotal sac. A dense layer of fibrous connective tissue called the tunica albuginea forms a capsule that covers the testis. The testis is then further covered by a reflected fold of the processes vaginalis that becomes the visceral layer of the tunica vaginalis, with the remainder of the peritoneal sac forming the parietal layer of the tunica vaginalis. The visceral layer of the tunica vaginalis covers the testes and the epididymis, whereas the parietal reflection covers the anterior and lateral parts of the testes and the epididymis, leaving a "bare area" to which the mesentery of the testis is attached. A reflection of the tunica albuginea forms the mediastinum testis, within which the rete testis forms (Fig. 11.1).[1]

The arterial supply to the scrotal sac and contents arise from three sources: The *testicular artery* (arising from the aorta and supplying the testis), the *cremasteric artery* (a branch of the inferior epigastric artery, supplying the scrotal sac and the coverings of the spermatic cord), and the *artery to the ductus deferens* (arising from

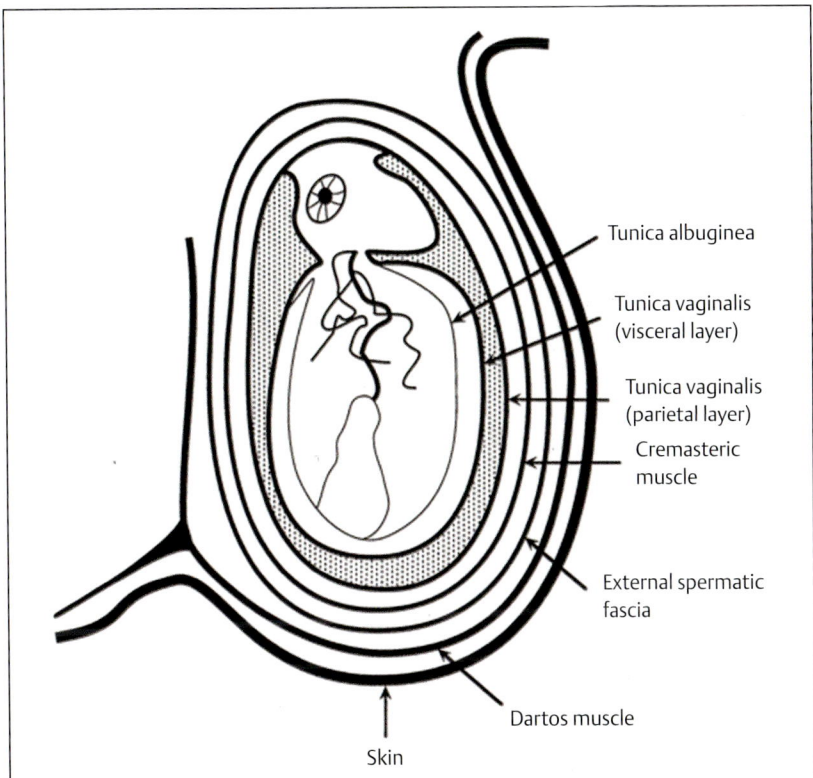

Fig. 11.1 **Anatomical layers surrounding the normal testis.** The shaded area between the two layers of the tunica vaginalis is the area of fluid accumulation giving rise to a hydrocele (shaded area, potential space for fluid accumulation). (Source: Sidhu PS. Clinical and imaging features of testicular torsion: role of ultrasound. Clin Radiol 1999;54: 134–143)

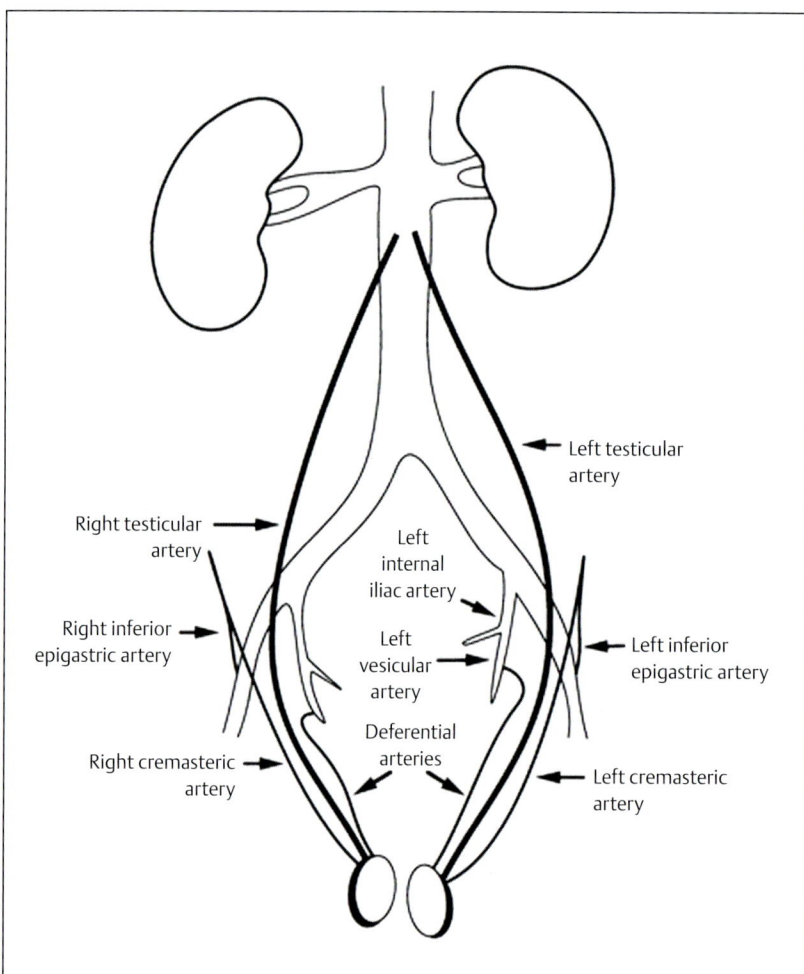

Fig. 11.2 Normal arterial anatomy of the testis. (Source: Sidhu PS. Clinical and imaging features of testicular torsion: role of ultrasound. Clin Radiol 1999;54: 134–143)

the superior vesicle artery) (Fig. 11.2). Veins exit the testes at the mediastinum; join the veins draining the epididymis to form the pampiniform plexus at the superior aspect of the testes. The cremasteric plexus (mainly draining extratesticular blood) lies posterior to the pampiniform plexus. The right testicular vein drains directly into the inferior vena cava (IVC) below the level of the right renal vein, whereas the left testicular vein drains into the left renal vein (Fig. 11.3). These three arteries and the veins are loosely held together by connective tissue along with nerves, lymph vessels, and the ductus deferens in the spermatic cord.[2] Although there are anastomoses between these arteries, these are not sufficient to prevent testicular ischemia when the testicular artery is compromised.

Summary points:
- The tunica albuginea covers the testis; a reflection forms the mediastinum testis
- Two layers of tunica vaginalis (visceral and parietal) leave a small bare area
- Three arteries supply the scrotum: The testicular artery, the cremasteric artery, and the artery to the ductus deferens
- Pampiniform plexus drains into the testicular vein

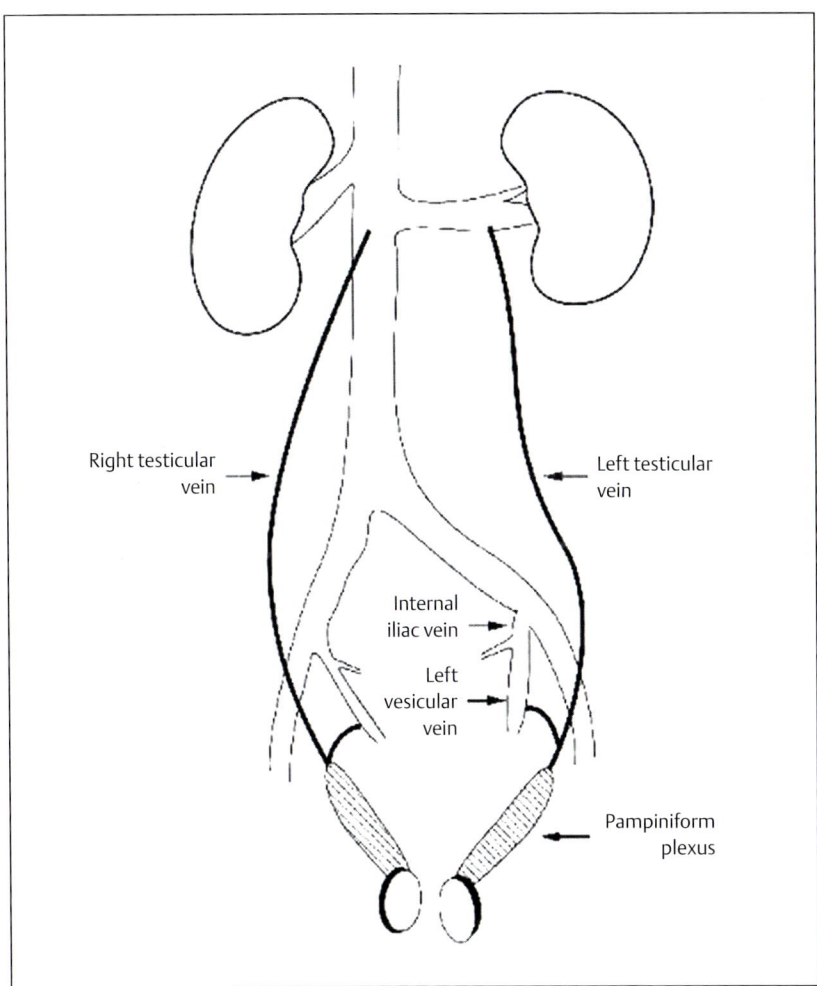

Fig. 11.3 Normal venous drainage of the testis. (Source: Sidhu PS. Clinical and imaging features of testicular torsion: role of ultrasound. Clin Radiol 1999;54: 134–143)

Ultrasound Examination Technique

Examination should always take place in a private setting, with the person undertaking the examination using a gloved hand for the examination. A chaperone should be present. The ultrasound gel should be warm, and copious amounts applied. The scrotal sac may be held in a stable position by placing paper towels beneath the sac, and the penis should be held against the anterior abdominal wall, by the patient, and preferably covered with paper towels. By crossing the legs the patient is able to provide for more a stable position for the examination. A high-frequency linear array probe (7–12 MHz) should be used, with sensitive color and spectral Doppler capabilities. Typically the probe length should be such as to allow longitudinal length measurements of the testis. Initially both testes are examined in the transverse plane, in order to produce the "spectacle" view to allow comparison of testicular parenchyma features, which is important if a unilateral global testicular problem is suspected (Fig. 11.4). The examination of the entire scrotal sac should include both the transverse and longitudinal planes, documenting any abnormalities present. Testicular volume may be calculated and color Doppler ultrasound will confirm vascular supply.

Summary points:
- In US examination of the testes, a high-frequency linear array transducer is used
- Sensitive color Doppler facility
- "Spectacle" transverse view through both testes is essential

Normal Ultrasound Appearances of the Testis and Epididymis

The testes are homogenous and of medium-level reflectivity (Fig. 11.5). At birth the testis measures approximately 1.5 cm in length and 1.0 cm in width, and before

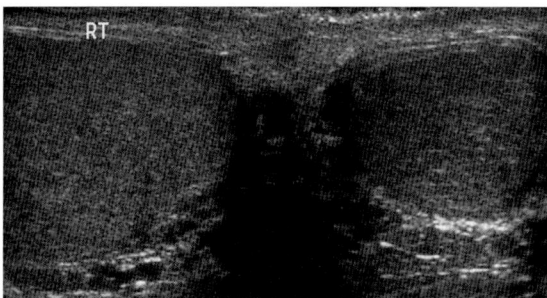

Fig. 11.4 Transverse view through both the testes. The "spectacle view" allows comparison of the reflectivity of the two testes, of particular importance in infiltrative lymphoma and leukemia. In this example there is atrophy and altered reflectivity of the left testis following surgery for cryptorchidism

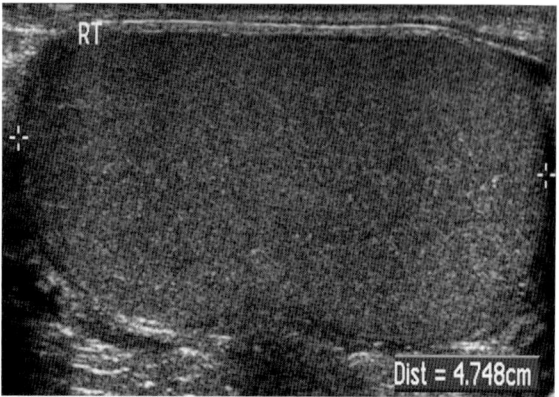

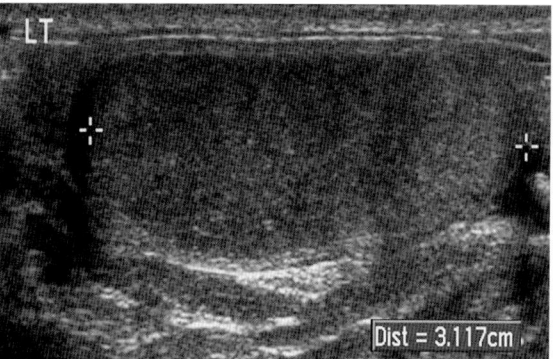

Fig. 11.5 a The right testis from the same patient as in Fig. 11.4. It measures 4.7 cm in length and demonstrates normal, smooth reflectivity.
b The left testis in the same patient is smaller, measuring 3.1 cm, and demonstrates a less uniform reflectivity

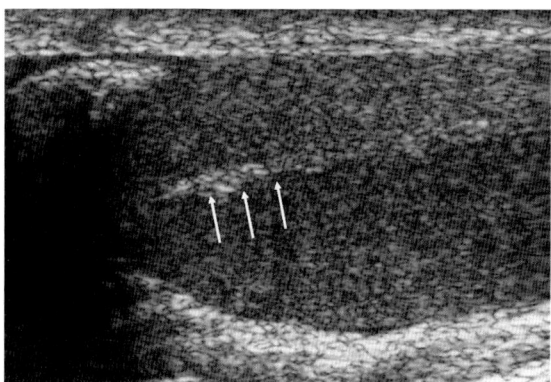

Fig. 11.6 The mediastinum testis is seen as a highly reflective linear structure at the posterior–superior aspect of the testicle (arrows) draining the seminiferous tubules of the testes into the rete testis

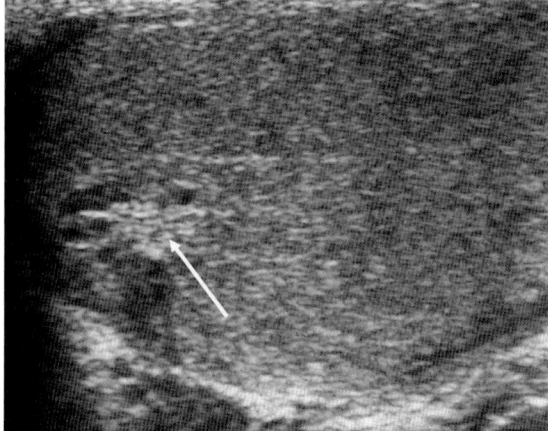

Fig. 11.7 The rete testis is a low-reflective area at the hilum of the testis with fingerlike projections into the parenchyma (arrow)

age 12 the testicular volume is 1–2 mL. In the adult, testicular length may be up to 5 cm. Volume measurement is calculated using the formula length × width × height × 0.51. A total volume (both testis) of > 30 mL is indicative of normal function.[3] A testicular volume > 2 mL allows reliable appreciation of intratesticular color Doppler flow.[4] The mediastinum testis is seen as a highly reflective linear structure at the posterior–superior aspect of the testicle, draining the seminiferous tubules of the testes into the rete testis (Fig. 11.6). The rete testis is a low-reflective area at the hilum of the testis with fingerlike projections into the parenchyma (Fig. 11.7).[5] Apart from these projections, the parenchyma of the testis should remain of homogenous reflectivity. The appendix testis (a vestigial remnant of the müllerian duct) is present in the majority of patients, most commonly at the superior testicular pole or in the groove between the testis and the head of the epididymis medially.[6] There is marked variation in the size and appearance of an appendix testis; it is usually oval, although a stalklike cystic structure is occasionally seen (Fig. 11.8).

The epididymis is 6–7 cm in length. The head (globus major) is a pyramid-shaped structure lying superior to the upper pole of the testis. The body courses along the posterolateral aspect of the testicle. The tail (globus minor) is slightly thicker than the body and can be seen as a curved structure at the inferior aspect of the testicle where it becomes the proximal portion of the ductus deferens. The body and tail are of similar or slightly lower reflectivity when compared with the testis, whilst the head is of slightly higher reflectivity (Fig. 11.**9**). Color Doppler signal may be identified in the normal epididymis.[7] The appendix epididymis is not as frequently seen as the appendix testis.[8] It is part of the mesonephric (wolffian duct), and projects from the epididymis from different sites, most commonly the head. It usually has a stalklike appearance. The globus major measures 10–12 mm in diameter, the body less than 4 mm (average: 1–2 mm) in diameter.[9]

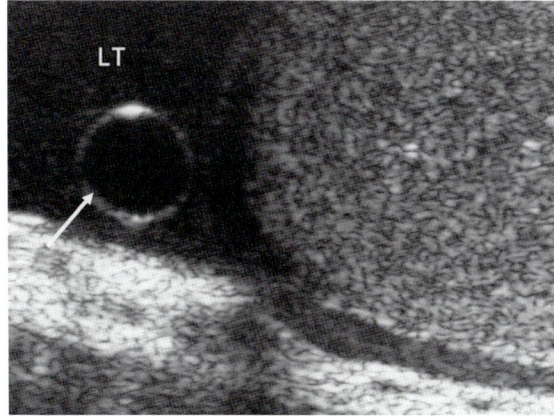

Fig. 11.**8** There is marked variation in the size and appearance of an appendix testis. It is usually oval, although a stalklike cystic structure is occasionally seen (arrow)

Summary points:
- The normal testis is of medium-level, smooth reflectivity
- The mediastinum testis is a linear, high-reflective structure
- The epididymal head is a pyramidal structure; the epididymal body is of lower reflectivity
- The testicular and epididymal appendix are present at the superior aspect

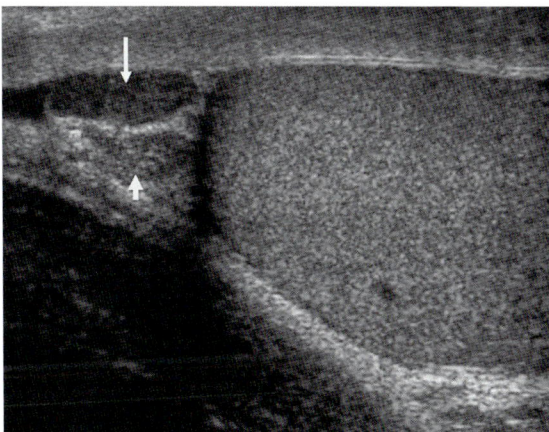

Fig. 11.**9** Changes in reflectivity of the epididymis. The low reflectivity of the body (long arrow) alters in the head of the epididymis (short arrow) to a higher reflectivity

Intratesticular Abnormalities

Normal Variants

Transmediastinal Artery

An intratesticular artery traverses the testis in a centrifugal direction in a reported 52% of patients, unilaterally in half.[10] The artery is readily identified with color Doppler ultrasound, and returns a low-resistance spectral Doppler waveform (Fig. 11.**10**).

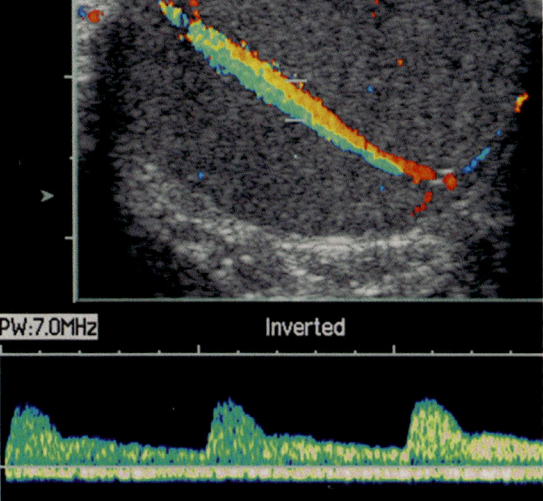

Fig. 11.**10** Color and spectral Doppler ultrasound of transmediastinal vessels demonstrate the normal low-resistance pattern of the testicular artery and a normal venous waveform pattern

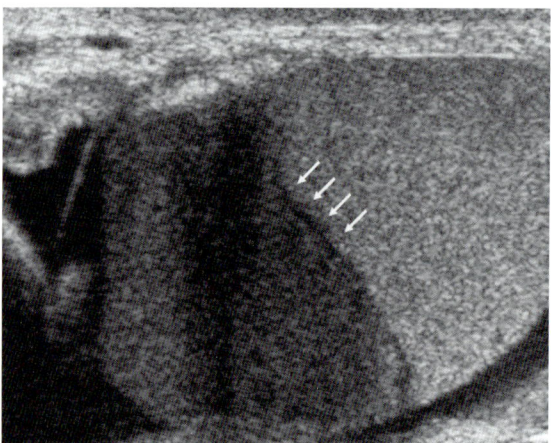 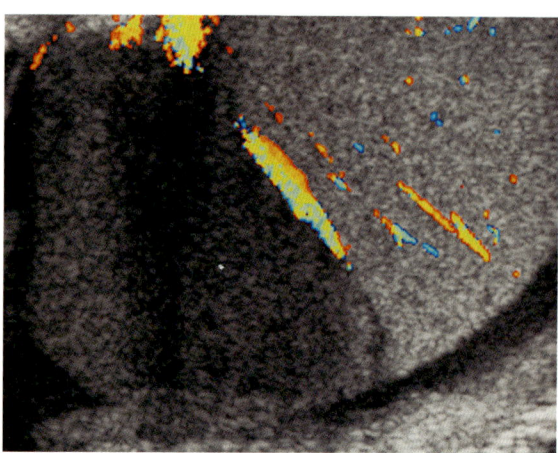

Fig. 11.**11 a** There is a well-demarcated, low-reflective appearance generated through the testis (arrows) which does not appear to be related to a pathological cause. **b** Following the use of color Doppler ultrasound, the cause of this appearance is a prominent transmediastinal artery and vein

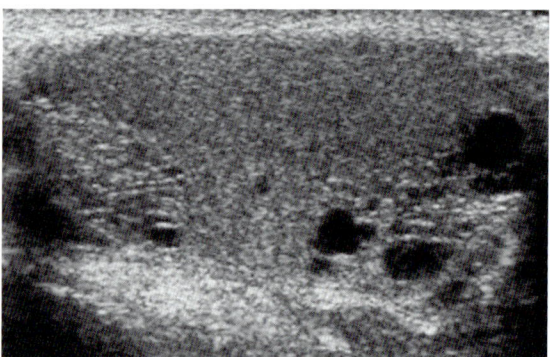

Fig. 11.**12** A florid example of a rete testis, with a number of cysts of varying size present adjacent to the mediastinum of the testis

Two-Tone Testis

The term "two-tone" describes the appearance of an artifact within the testis where an intratesticular artery produces acoustic shadowing, resulting in a discreet uniform area of decreased reflectivity posterior to the artery (Fig. 11.11). This artifact is caused by refractive shadowing at both edges of the intratesticular artery.[11] The reflectivity of the remainder of the testis is normal. The use of color Doppler ultrasound readily confirms the presence of the intratesticular artery as being the source of the artifact.

Rete Testis

The rete testis is located in the mediastinum testis (Fig. 11.12). Microscopically the rete testis is composed of three parts: The septal (interlobular) portion containing the tubuli recti, the tunical (mediastinal) portion consisting of a network of channels, and the extratesticular rete, comprising the irregular-shaped lacunar spaces which connect to the efferent ducts.[12] Seminiferous tubules contained within 250 lobules join the tubuli recti, and the efferent ducts drain out into the epididymis. On ultrasound, the rete testis has a spectrum of appearances ranging from a faintly visible ill-defined area of decreased reflectivity (18% of patients) at the testicular hilum to a coarse tubular appearance with fingerlike projections into the parenchyma.[5]

Appendix Testis

A remnant of the paramesonephric and mesonephric ducts may remain to form the appendix testis (hydatid of Morgagni) and appendix epididymis, respectively. Three further appendages, not seen on ultrasound, have been identified microscopically: The paradidymis (appendix of the cord or organ of Giraldés) arising from the spermatic cord and the superior and inferior vas aberrans of Haler.[13] The appendix testis is found at the upper pole of the testis in the groove between the testis and the laterally situated head of the epididymis. The appendix testis can measure between 1 and 7 mm in length, and may be present in up to 92% of patients, bilaterally in 69%.[14] The appendix testis is usually of similar reflectivity to the head of the epididymis, best seen in the presence of a hydrocele, with a variable morphology, most commonly being oval-shaped and sessile, but it may appear "stalklike" and pedunculated, cystic, or even calcified.[6] The "stalklike" and cystic appendices are associated with an increased likelihood of appendiceal torsion, recognized as a cause of acute scrotal pain.[15] The epididymal appendix is less frequently seen on ultrasound (6%), has a length of between 3 and 8 mm, is more frequently stalked, and, like the testicular appendix, may undergo torsion, although less commonly so.[14] On occasion both an epididymal

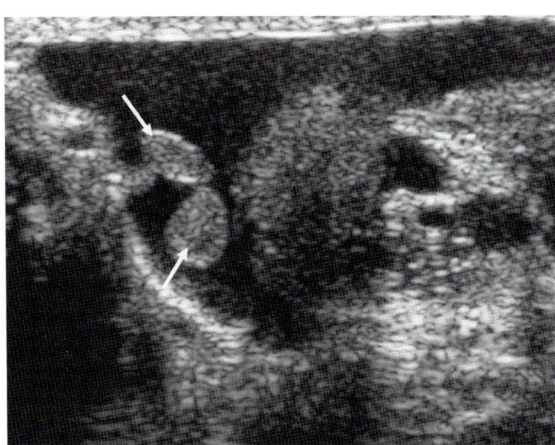

Fig. 11.13 Two areas (arrows) arising from the upper aspect of the testis. Both are isoreflective to the epididymal head, surrounded by a small hydrocele. The image demonstrates both the appendix testis and the appendix epididymis; differentiation is not possible on this image

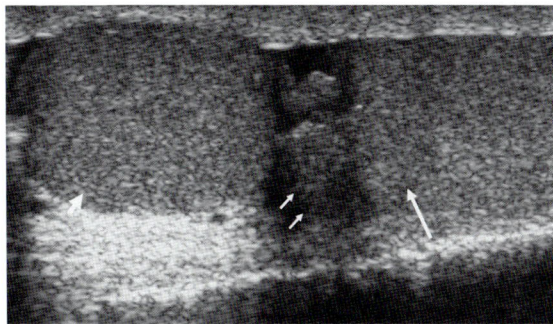

Fig. 11.14 A normal testis (long arrow) with a normal epididymal head (short arrows) and a further mass. It is isoreflective to the normal testis (arrowhead) lying in a superior position, representing an extra testicle: Polyorchidism

and testicular appendage may be seen in the same patient (Fig. 11.13).

Polyorchidism

Polyorchidism (more than two testes) is a rare condition and most commonly involves a bifid or duplicated testis with a single epididymis, with a uniform surrounding tunica albuginea (Fig. 11.14).[16,17] Less common is a complete duplication of the testis and epididymis. On ultrasound, the extra testis demonstrates reflectivity identical to the normal testis.[18]

Intratesticular Focal Lesions

Testicular Tumors

Testicular carcinoma represents 1% of all neoplasm in men and is the most common malignancy in the 15–34-year-old age group.[19] A second peak prevalence occurs in the 71–90-year-old age group, with metastasis and lymphoma most common. There has been an unexplained increase in the prevalence of testicular carcinoma over the last 70 years, and testicular carcinoma is predominantly a cancer of white males. The most common presenting symptom is a painless scrotal mass; only 10% of patients present with pain. A smaller number of patients present with metastases or rarely with endocrine abnormalities such as gynecomastia. Survival rates for testicular carcinoma approach 95%.[19]

There are well-documented risk factors for the development of testicular carcinoma, namely previous testicular tumor, family history, cryptorchidism, infertility, and intersex syndromes. Testicular tumors may

Table 11.1 Classification of testicular tumors[24]

Germ cell tumors
Precursor lesions
Intratubular germ cell neoplasia
Tumors of one histological type
Seminoma
Embryonal carcinoma
Yolk sac tumor
Choriocarcinoma
Teratoma
Mature
Immature
With malignant transformation
Tumors of more than one histological type
Sex cord and stromal tumors
Leydig cell tumor
Sertoli cell tumor
Granulosa cell tumor
Fibroma-thecoma
Tumors with both sex cord and stromal cells and germ cells
Gonadoblastoma
Lymphoid and hematopoietic tumors
Lymphoma
Leukemia
Metastasis

be divided into germ cell and nongerm cell tumors; 95% of testicular tumors are germ cell tumors which arise from spermatogenic cells. Nongerm cell tumors derive from sex cords (Sertoli cells) and stroma (Leydig cells); these tumors are malignant in 10% of cases. Lymphoma, leukemia, and metastases may manifest as testicular tumors (Table 11.1).

Most testicular tumors are of homogenous, low reflectivity in comparison to the surrounding testicular parenchyma, although a wide range of appearances oc-

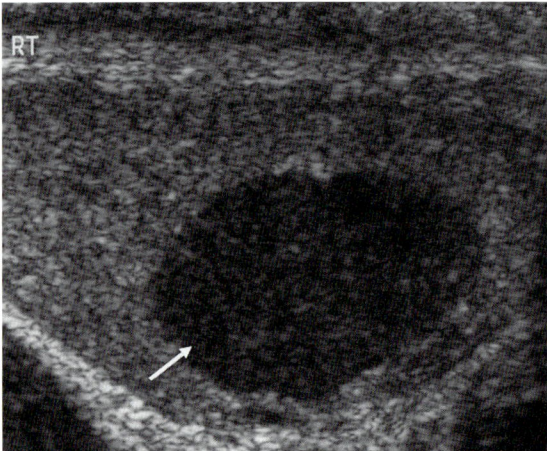

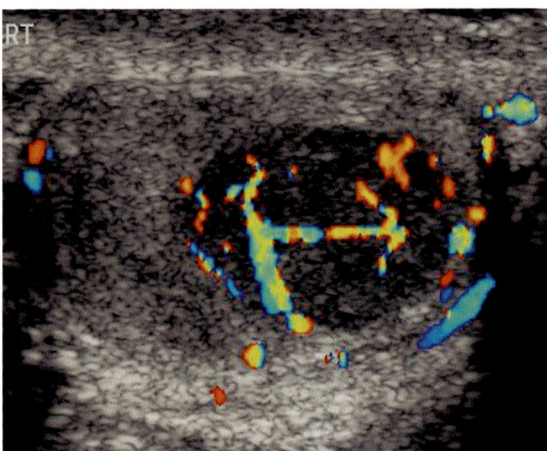

Fig. 11.15 **a** A low-reflective mass lying within testicular parenchyma, with a well-delineated border (arrow) demonstrating features of a seminoma. **b** Following the addition of color Doppler ultrasound, there is intralesional vascularity demonstrated in the seminoma

cur, including high-reflective, heterogeneous lesions with areas of calcification and cystic change.[20] Larger tumors demonstrate increased vascularity,[21] although with the newer high-frequency transducers, malignant vascularity may be identified in small-volume tumors.[22,23]

Summary points:
- Testicular tumors = 1% of all male neoplasm
- Higher incidence in the 15–34-year-old age group
- Increasing in prevalence for unknown reasons
- Cancer of white males
- Commonly presents as a painless scrotal mass

Germ Cell Tumors

The precursor of germ cell tumors is thought to be intratubular germ cell neoplasia; if development is along a "unipotential" gonadal line, a seminoma will form, but if development occurs along a "totipotential" gonadal line, a nonseminomatous tumor will develop.[24] The "totipotential" cells may remain undifferentiated (embryonal carcinoma), develop toward embryonic differentiation (teratoma) or extraembryonic differentiation (yolk sac tumors, choriocarcinoma). Multiple histological types occur together (mixed germ cell tumor), as these "totipotential" cells develop along multiple pathways.[25]

Most germ cell tumors spread via the lymphatic system rather than hematogenous, except for choriocarcinoma. Normally testicular lymphatic drainage follows the testicular vein, occurring in a predictable pattern. Orchidectomy for all testicular tumors is performed through an inguinal approach to avoid skin involvement and spread to the external iliac nodes. Staging of testicular carcinoma follows the tumor, node, metastasis (TNM) classification.[24] Tumor markers play an important role in diagnosis, staging, prognosis, and follow-up of germ cell tumors.[26] The most important tumor markers are alpha-fetoprotein (AFP), human chorionic gonadotrophin (HCG), and lactate dehydrogenase (LDH).

Seminomatous Germ Cell Tumors

Seminoma is the most common pure germ cell tumor, accounting for up to 50% of cases, occurring in a slightly older patient group of age 40. The ultrasound appearances reflect the uniform cellular nature of the tumor; they are uniformly of low reflectivity, although larger tumors may be heterogeneous, lobulated, or present as multinodular areas in continuity (Fig. 11.15). These tumors are extremely radiosensitive.

Nonseminomatous Germ Cell Tumors

Mixed Germ Cell Tumors
Mixed germ cell tumor contains more than one germ cell component; any combination of cell type can occur. The average age of presentation is 30 years. These tumors constitute up to 60% of all germ cell tumors and are more common than the pure histological forms of testicular tumors (Fig. 11.16).

Embryonal Carcinoma
This is the second most common pure germ cell tumor after seminoma; embryonal carcinoma is present in 87% of mixed germ cell tumors, but in the pure form accounts for 2% of all testicular tumors. Embryonal carcinoma affects younger men (age 25–35) and tends to be more aggressive. These tumors are often hetero-

geneous, ill-defined, blending imperceptibly into adjacent testicular parenchyma.

Choriocarcinoma
Choriocarcinoma is a rare tumor, occurring in a pure form in < 1% of patients, but in a mixed germ cell tumor in 8% of patients, where it is highly malignant. Choriocarcinoma carries the worst prognosis of any germ cell tumor; a high level of HCG confers a poor prognosis.

Yolk Sac Tumor
Yolk sac tumors account for 80% of childhood (< age two) tumors but is rare in adults. Elevation of AFP levels is present. The imaging features are nonspecific, often just testicular enlargement in children.

Teratoma
Teratoma is the second most common testicular tumor in children (< age four), and teratoma cells occur in over 50% of adult cases of mixed germ cell tumors. A teratoma tends to be a complex tumor, and the ultrasound features are those of a well-defined complex mass with cystic change (Fig. 11.**17**). Calcification may be present. In the prepubertal testes a pure teratoma runs a benign course and testis-sparing surgery may be undertaken. This is not true for the postpubertal teratoma, which will metastasize irrespective of the histological features.

Epidermoid Cyst
The pathogenesis of an epidermoid cyst is uncertain; it either arises from monodermal development of a teratoma or as a result of squamous metaplasia of surface mesothelium. These are benign lesions with no malignant potential.[27] Epidermoid cysts comprise 1% of all testicular tumors and are true cysts, containing a cheesy laminated material. On ultrasound, epidermoid cysts are well-circumscribed with a high-reflective border and internal laminations giving an "onion-ring" appearance (Fig. 11.**18**).[28]

"Regressed" or "Burnt-out" Germ Cell Tumors
Patients may present with widespread metastases but no primary tumor except for an area of calcification within the testis.[29] The pathogenesis of this phenomenon may be the result of a high metabolic rate of the tumor, which outgrows its blood supply and involutes (Fig. 11.**19**).

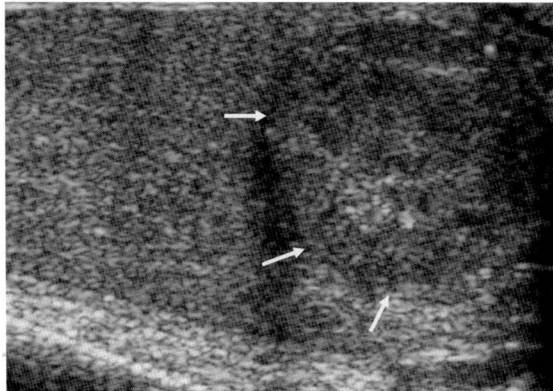

Fig. 11.**16 A focal mass** (arrows), **a mixed germ cell tumor, is present at the lower aspect of the testis**, heterogeneous but mainly high reflectivity and is not as clearly defined as the example of the seminoma in Fig. 11.**15**

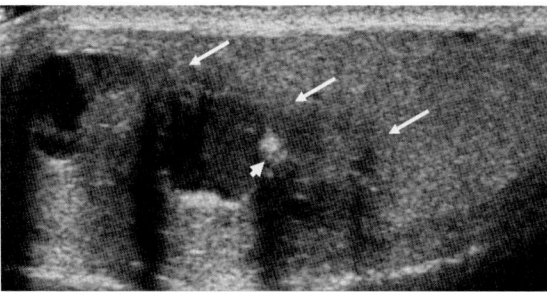

Fig. 11.**17 A lobulated mass at the upper aspect of the testis** (arrows) **demonstrating cystic change and focal calcification** (arrowhead). A teratoma

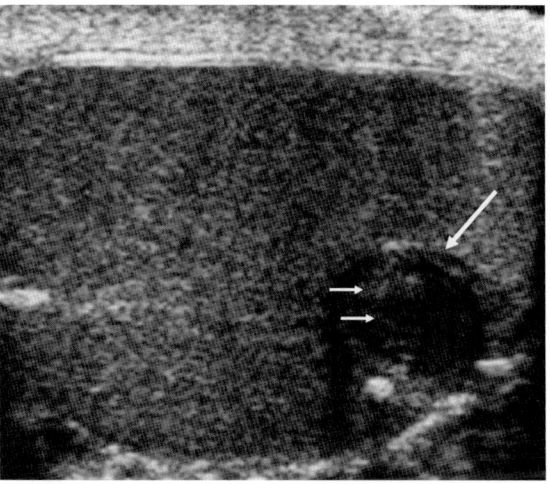

Fig. 11.**18 An epidermoid cyst** (long arrow). It demonstrates a well-circumscribed, low-reflective appearance with a high-reflective border and internal laminations (small arrows) giving an "onion-ring" appearance

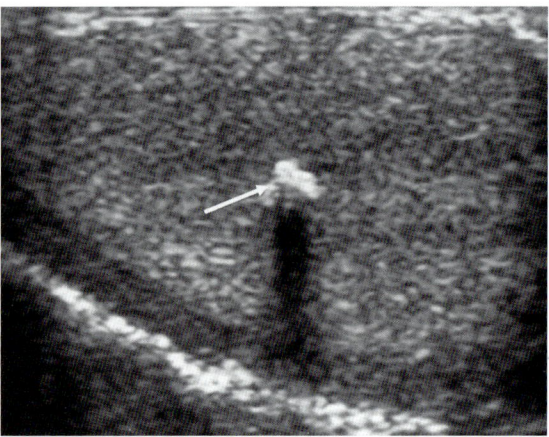

Fig. 11.19 A focal clump of calcification (arrow) is present in the central aspect of the testis on ultrasound in a patient with a retroperitoneal germ cell tumor. A "burnt-out" testicular tumor

> **Summary points:**
> - Unipotential gonadal cell line develops into a seminoma
> - Totipotential gonadal cell line develops into nonseminoma
> - Multiple histological cell types occur together: Mixed germ cell tumor
> - Tumor spread is via the lymphatic system

Nongerm Cell Tumors

The prevalence of nongerm cell tumors is higher in the pediatric age group, constituting 30% of all testicular tumors. Nearly all nongerm cell tumors are benign, but there is no clear ultrasound criterion that allows differentiation from malignant testicular tumors. Leydig cell tumors occur across all age groups and account for 3% of all testicular tumors. Patients demonstrate symptoms related to androgen or estrogen secretion by the tumor, which includes precocious virilization, gynecomastia, or decreased libido. On ultrasound Leydig cell tumors are small, commonly of low reflectivity with cystic change.[30] Use of color Doppler ultrasound may demonstrate poor internal color Doppler flow with increased peripheral vascularity in Leydig tumors when small, but vascularity increases with tumor size (Fig. 11.20).[31] Sertoli cell tumors constitute 1% of all testicular tumors, and are less likely than Leydig cell tumors to secrete hormones. On ultrasound the Sertoli cell tumors are well-circumscribed, round, and lobulated.

Lymphoma
Testicular lymphoma may be the primary site of involvement, the initial manifestation of widespread disease, or the site of recurrence. Testicular lymphoma, which accounts for 5% of testicular tumors, is the most common testicular tumor in the over 60-year-old age group. The ultrasound appearances of testicular lymphoma are similar to germ cell tumors: Discrete, low-reflective lesions with increased color Doppler flow but complete testicular involvement may be seen, emphasizing the need to compare the reflectivity of both testes (Fig. 11.21).[32]

Leukemia
Primary leukemia of the testis is rare, although a common site of recurrence in children. The ultrasound appearances are very variable, being unilateral or bilateral, diffuse or focal, low- or high-reflective.[33]

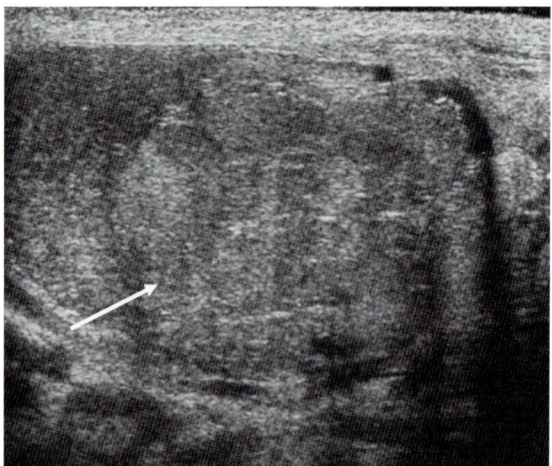

a

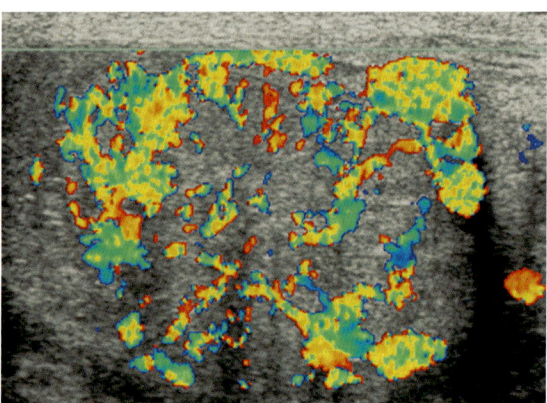

b

Fig. 11.20 **a** A large, mixed-reflective, heterogeneous tumor at the lower aspect of the testis which on histological examination was found to be a Leydig cell tumor. **b** The same Leydig cell tumor demonstrating increased color Doppler flow in both a peripheral and central distribution

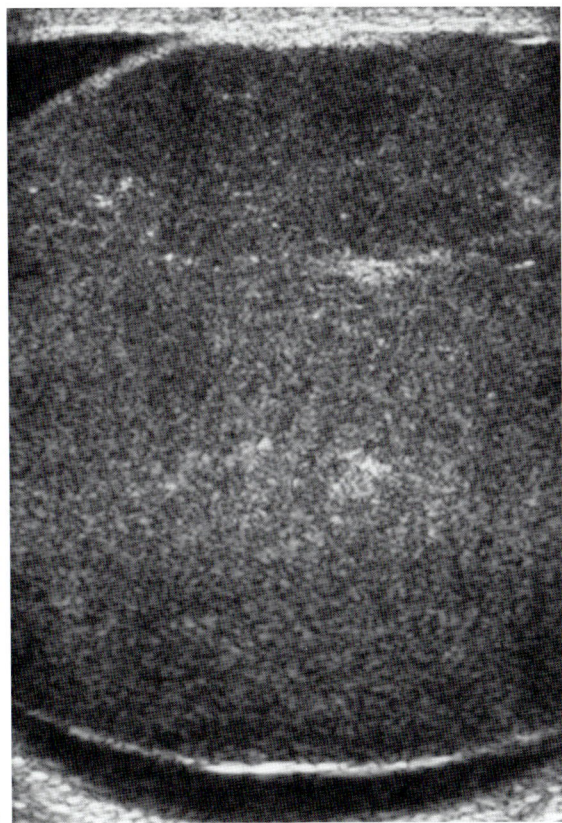
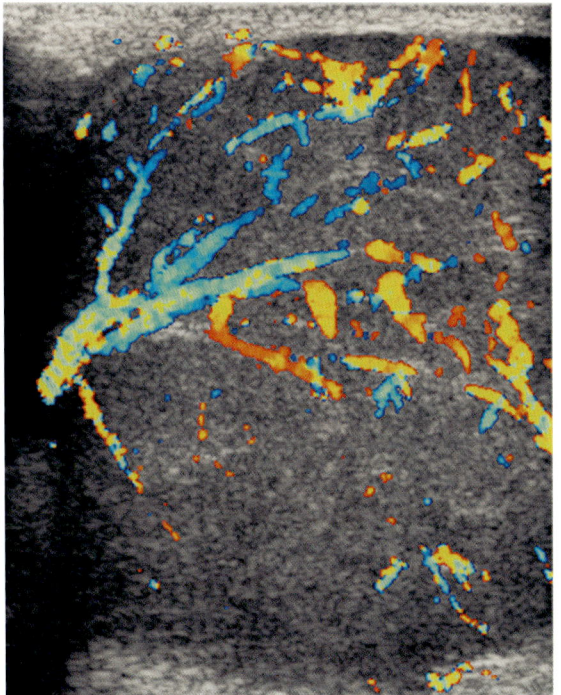

Fig. 11.**21 a** There is enlargement of the testis, with a uniform low-reflective appearance with a surrounding hydrocele in a patient with testicular lymphoma. **b** Color Doppler ultrasound demonstrates a markedly abnormal vascular pattern to the lymphoma infiltrated testis

Metastasis
Metastasis to the testis is unusual, with the most frequent primary sites being the prostate, lung, melanoma, colon, and kidney.[34] Metastasis usually occurs in advanced disease and is indistinguishable on ultrasound from primary tumors of the testis (Fig. 11.**22**).

Splenogonadal Fusion
Splenogonadal fusion is a rare condition where an accessory spleen exists within the scrotum or pelvis fused to the gonadal organs; the majority of cases occur on the left side. Splenogonadal fusion is far more common in males, where presentation is usually with a scrotal mass.[35] Two types of splenogonadal fusion are described: Continuous and discontinuous.[36] In the more common continuous type, a cord connects the normal and ectopic spleen; this cord may be beaded with small splenunculi. In the discontinuous type no cord is present. There are several recognized associations with splenogonadal fusion: Inguinal hernia and cryptorchidism are the most common, with micrognathia, peromelia, cleft palate, cardiac defects, and several other rarer congenital anomalies also reported. The appearance of splenogonadal fusion on ultrasound resembles a mass within the scrotal sac of low reflectivity in comparison to the normal testicular parenchyma.[37,38]

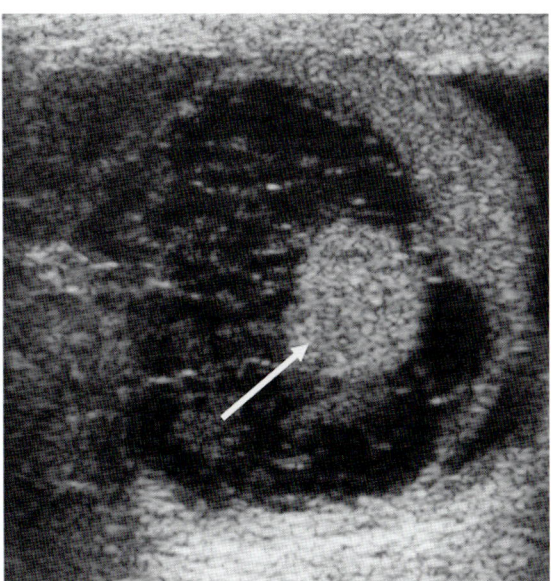

Fig. 11.**22 A secondary lesion** (arrow) **from a prostate primary in the testis with surrounding cystic degeneration**

The mass may not be seen separate to the testis and as such will be readily confused with a primary testicular tumor (Fig. 11.**23**). Color Doppler ultrasound flow in the abnormal tissue assumes a pattern similar to that seen

164 11 Diseases of the Testis and Epididymis

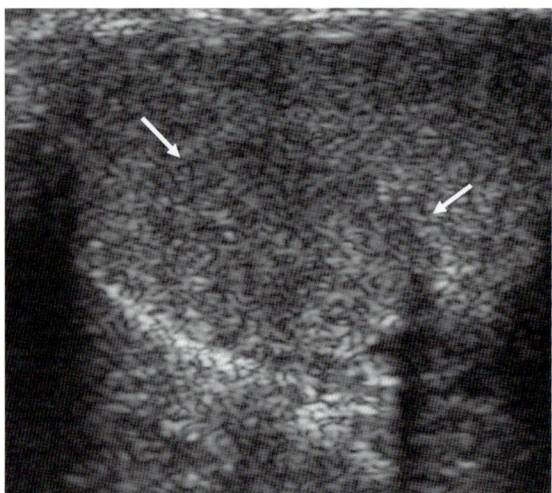
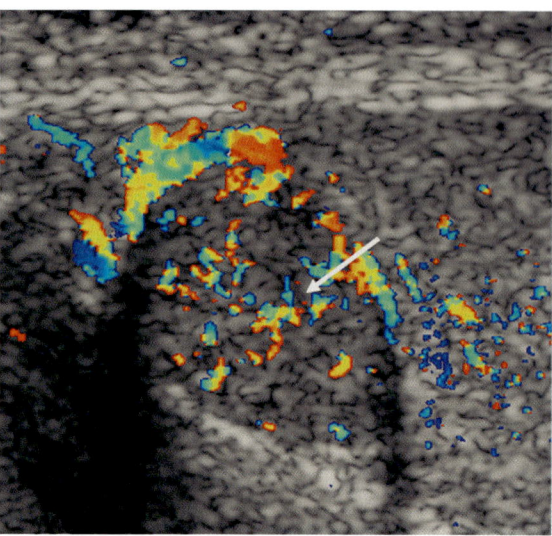

Fig. 11.23 **a** A subtle, defined lesion at the upper aspect of the testis (arrows) which has the appearance of a primary testicular tumor. **b** Color Doppler ultrasound of the abnormality demonstrates abnormal vascularity within the tumor. Orchidectomy was performed, and histology demonstrated a splenogonadal fusion as the cause for these appearances. (Reproduced with permission from the Editor of the Journal of Ultrasound in Medicine)[39]

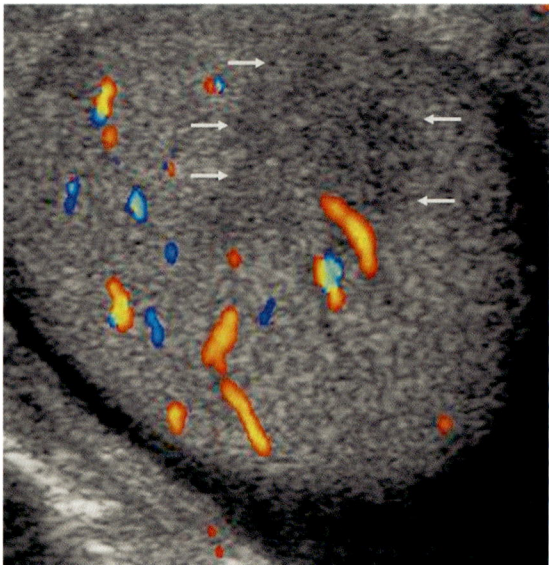

Fig. 11.24 **A focal area of low reflectivity** (arrows), **assuming a "wedge-shape," in a testis of a patient complaining of acute testicular pain.** The color Doppler appearances demonstrate absence of flow to the area, suggesting a segmental infarction as the cause of the appearances

in the central aspect of the normal testis or that seen in splenic tissue.[39]

Adrenal Rest Cells
Adrenal rest cells arise within the testis as a tumourlike abnormality in response to elevated circulating adenocorticotrophic hormone (ACTH). The adrenal rest cells migrate with the gonadal tissue during fetal life. These tumors usually appear as focal, low-reflective abnormalities with abnormal color flow and are often bilateral.[40,41]

Segmental Infarction
Global testicular infarction is well-recognized, usually as a result of torsion of the spermatic cord, severe epididymo-orchitis, or trauma.[42] Segmental testicular infarction is, however, rare and is usually diagnosed following orchidectomy.[43] The predisposing factors to segmental infarction include polycythemia, intimal fibroplasia of the spermatic artery, sickle cell disease, hypersensitivity angiitis, and trauma, although the majority is idiopathic in origin.[44] Segmental testicular infarction is characterized by poor or absent flow on color Doppler ultrasound in a focal, low-reflective area with no posterior acoustic enhancement,[45,46] although a high-reflective abnormality has been documented.[47] Focal expansion of a pole of the testis may mimic a primary testicular tumor and color Doppler ultrasound provides a useful discriminatory tool (Fig. 11.24).[44,48]

Summary points:
- Ultrasound is unable to differentiate germ cell from nongerm cell tumors
- Higher prevalence of non-germ cell tumors in the pediatric age group
- Nearly all non-germ cell tumors are benign
- Lymphoma occurs in the > 60yr old age group

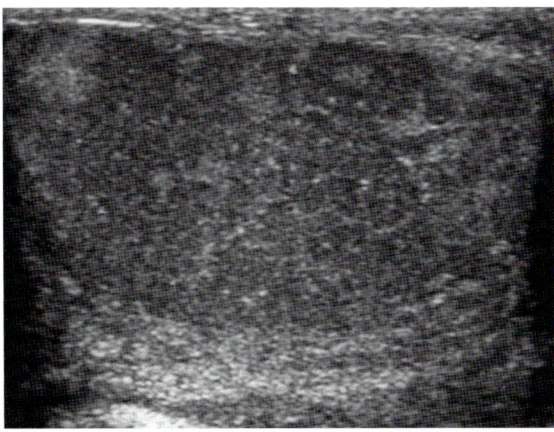

Fig. 11.25 Testicular atrophy in an 80-year-old man, demonstrating a heterogeneous appearance

Other Tumourlike Testicular Lesions

A number of other focal testicular lesions may cause clinical and ultrasound confusion: Granulomatous epididymo-orchitis,[49] sarcoidosis,[50] tubular ectasia,[5] and cysts either intraparenchymal or adjacent to the tunica albuginea.[51]

Diffuse Testicular Change

Atrophy

Testicular atrophy may occur following cryptorchidism, inflammation, torsion, trauma, hypothyroidism, estrogen treatment, liver cirrhosis, hypopituitary disease, and aging. The testis is globally reduced in size, usually unilateral, with changes in testicular reflectivity related to the underlying cause, but usually of lower reflectivity. While volume and vascularity of the testis are reduced, the epididymis remains normal. Atrophy is a natural phenomenon of aging, where changes in the normal testis reflectivity, usually of a heterogeneous nature, may occur (Fig. 11.25).[52]

Orchitis and Abscess Formation

Pure orchitis is uncommon; the testis is frequently involved when epididymitis occurs resulting in epididymo-orchitis. Pure orchitis most often arises as a result of the paramyxovirus causing mumps.[53] On ultrasound, the testis is enlarged with either diffuse low reflectivity with pure orchitis or more commonly focal areas of low reflectivity when associated with epididymitis. Abscess formation may occur, where the abscess demonstrates peripheral but no internal color Doppler signals (Fig. 11.26).[54]

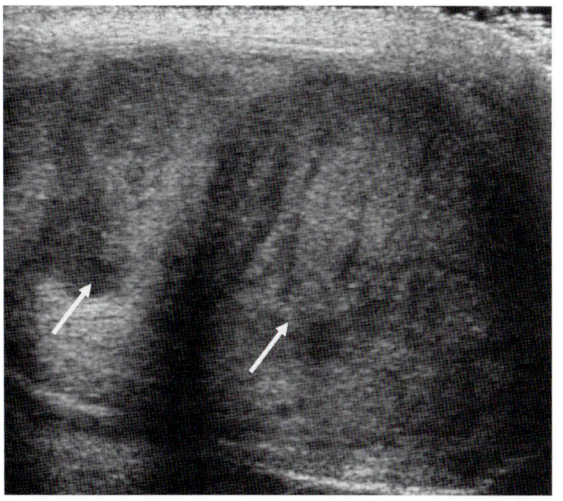

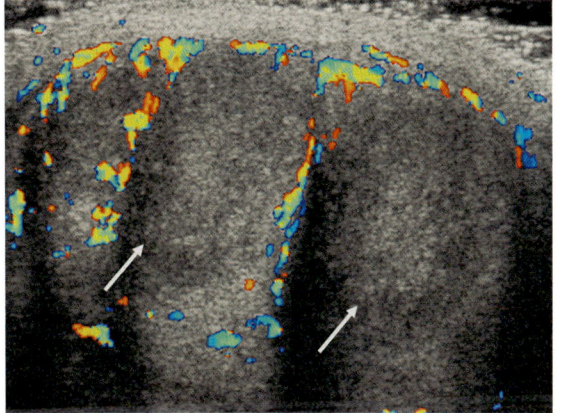

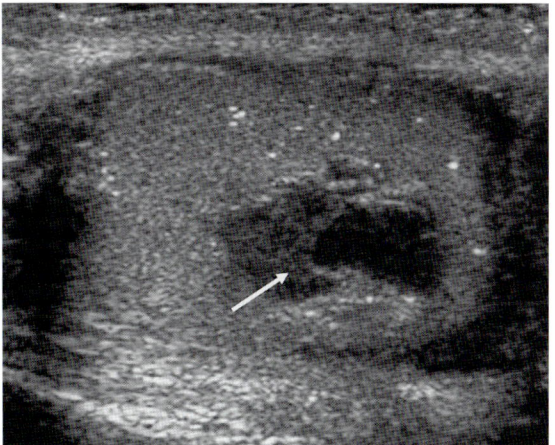

Fig. 11.26 a Two poorly defined heterogeneous areas in the testis, mainly of high reflectivity (arrows) in a patient with pyuria and a painful scrotum. b Color Doppler ultrasound demonstrates absence of color signal within these mass lesions, with increased flow around the periphery. The patient responded to antibiotic therapy: Intratesticular abscesses. c In a separate patient, an irregular, mixed reflective lesion is present representing a chronic testicular abscess (arrow). Incidental testicular microlithiasis is present

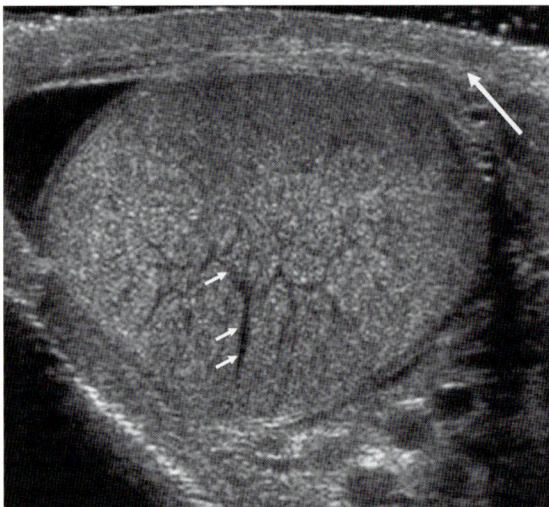

Fig. 11.27 **Following surgery to the prostate, a patient developed scrotal swelling.** On ultrasound there is thickening of the scrotal skin (long arrow), a small hydrocele, and there is intratesticular serpiginous low reflectivity (short arrows) following anatomical boundaries: Intratesticular edema

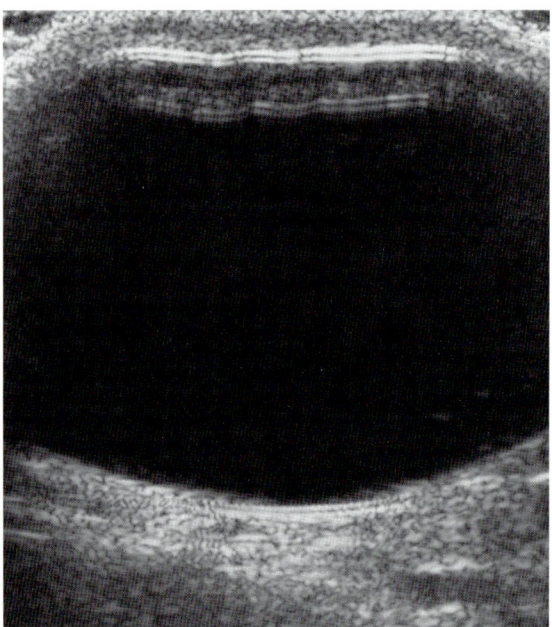

Fig. 11.28 **A silicone testicular prosthesis demonstrating some reverberation artifact, and uniform low reflectivity**

Postoperative Testis

Following surgery to the pelvis, prostate, and scrotum, edema of the scrotal wall is a frequent finding causing thickening visible on ultrasound. Often there is edema of the testicular parenchyma causing a characteristic "crazy-paving" appearance as the edema follows anatomical boundaries (Fig. 11.27).

Testicular Prosthesis

Following orchidectomy, patients may elect to have a testicular prosthesis inserted, normally made of silicon. A testicular prosthesis has a characteristic appearance on ultrasound (Fig. 11.28).

Microlithiasis and Macrocalcification

Testicular microlithiasis describes the appearance of multiple tiny bright foci, measuring 1–2 mm in diameter, which may be unilateral or bilateral (Fig. 11.29). The number of calcified foci and the pattern of distribution can vary, being either very diffuse or more peripherally clustered.[55] Testicular microlithiasis is characterized by the formation of microliths from degenerating cells in the seminiferous tubules. Acoustic shadowing is not seen, probably due to the small size of the calcifications. Although usually an incidental finding during the investigation of testicular symptoms, testicular microlithiasis has been associated with various medical conditions, including infertility, cryptorchidism, Klinefelter syndrome, Down syndrome, and pulmonary alveolar microlithiasis.[56]

Testicular microlithiasis has also been found in association with benign and malignant tumors in the testis, with reports indicating seminoma as the commonest tumor to occur in association with testicular microlithiasis (Fig. 11.30).[57] Furthermore, a high number of patients with intratubular germ cell neoplasia have testicular microlithiasis; approximately 50% of patients with intratubular germ cell neoplasia develop testicular cancer within five years.[58] As a consequence, the significance of finding isolated testicular microlithiasis is as yet uncertain; surveillance with ultrasound on an annual basis is advocated.[59]

The association of testicular macrocalcification with benign testicular lesions is well-documented and can be found in association with intratesticular cysts and epidermoid tumors. Benign intratesticular tumors, commonly derived from the Sertoli and Leydig cells of the seminiferous tubules, are difficult to distinguish from malignant tumors, and these too demonstrate calcification. Large, smooth, curvilinear calcification at the periphery of a tissue mass has been shown in Sertoli cell tumors. Granulomatous disease within the testes can also present with a low-reflective mass and areas of calcification within.[60] The presence of macrocalcification in association with malignant tumors has also been raised, particular with the entity of "burnt-out" tumors (Fig. 11.31).[61]

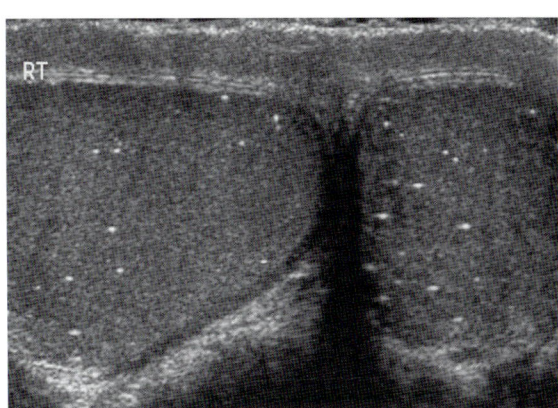

Fig. 11.**29** **Bilateral testicular microlithiasis.** Small, high-reflective areas measuring 1–2 mm without evidence of posterior acoustic shadowing

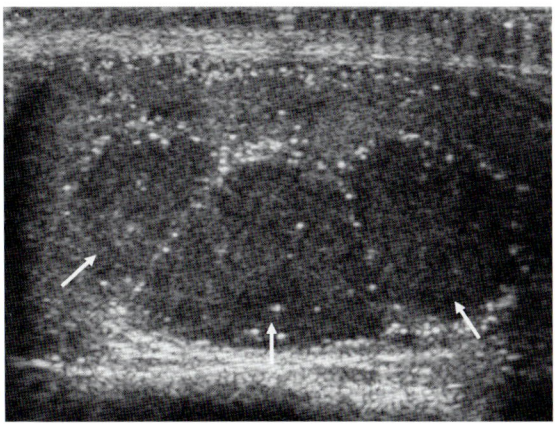

Fig. 11.**30** **Florid testicular microlithiasis with three seminomas** (arrows) **seen on ultrasound.** There is an increased prevalence of primary testicular tumors in the presence of testicular microlithiasis

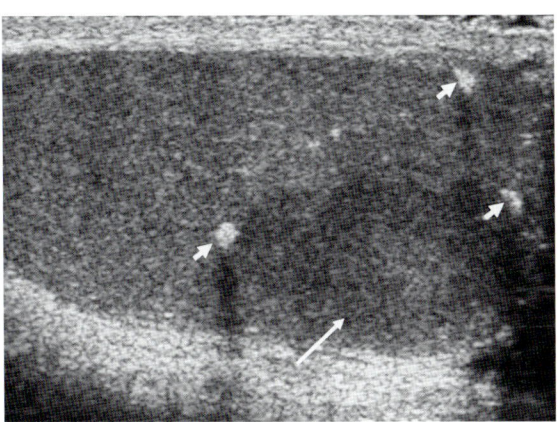

Fig. 11.**31** **A seminoma is present in the lower aspect of the testis** (long arrow), with focal areas of macrocalcification lying outside the tumor margins (arrowheads)

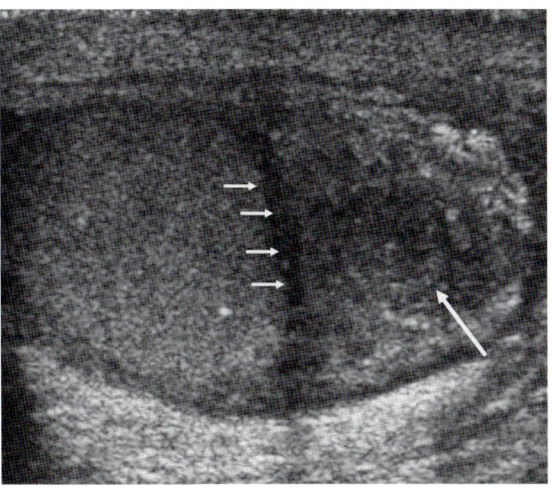

Fig. 11.**32** **Ultrasound of the testis following trauma**, demonstrating a fracture line (short arrows) through the midaspect of the testis and disruption of the lower testicular pole with a heterogeneous appearance of hemorrhage

Summary points:
- In testicular microlithiasis, small (1–2 mm), high-reflective areas with no posterior acoustic shadowing are seen
- Bilateral or unilateral
- Associated with an increased prevalence of testicular malignancy
- High numbers of patients with testicular microlithiasis have intratubular germ cell neoplasia
- Annual ultrasound surveillance is suggested

Trauma

Trauma from a variety of causes but mainly from a sporting injury may be responsible for testicular contusion, hematoma, fracture, or rupture (Fig. 11.**32**). Testicular rupture is a surgical emergency. On ultrasound, in testicular rupture, there is discontinuity of the tunica albuginea, irregular heterogeneous testicular margins, a hematocele, and diminished color Doppler flow to the affected area.[62,63] Direct visualization of a fracture site is unusual; more often parenchyma heterogeneous areas are seen. A hematoma will initially be seen as a high-reflective area, but with evolution of the hematoma over time will subsequently manifest as a low-reflective, complex cystic structure.

Extratesticular Abnormalities

Inguinal Hernia

Physical examination is normally sufficient to arrive at the diagnosis of an intrascrotal inguinal hernia; ultrasound may be useful in the difficult cases. On ultrasound the hernia contains bowel or omentum, giving rise to peristalsis of fluid-filled loops of bowel, air within bowel, or high-reflective omental fat.

Hydrocele

Between the two layers of the tunica vaginalis, there is normally a little serous fluid, and this may be visualized in up to 85% of asymptomatic men.[9] When the collection of fluid becomes large, a hydrocele develops, the commonest cause of a painless scrotal swelling. A hydrocele is normally of low reflectivity, with posterior acoustic enhancement, but may contain multiple echoes in the presence of cholesterol crystals (Fig. 11.**33**).[64] Hydroceles may be idiopathic or develop secondary to trauma (hematocele), infection (pyocele), torsion, tumor, or be congenital (secondary to a patent processes vaginalis). The testis is normally displaced to the posterior aspect of the scrotal sac in the presence of a hydrocele, in contrast to the inferior position when a large epididymal cyst causes displacement of the testis.

Spermatic Cord

The spermatic cord runs from the deep inguinal ring into the scrotum. The principal artery of the spermatic cord is the testicular artery, but also present are the artery to the vas deferens and the cremasteric artery. Although it is not possible to identify a named artery within the spermatic cord, color Doppler is able to demonstrate the three individual arteries within the spermatic cord (Fig. 11.**34**).[65] Despite anastomoses existing between the testicular, deferential, and cremasteric arteries, one of the arteries will consistently show a significantly lower resistive index (RI) than the other two arteries.

Spermatic Cord Torsion

Testicular torsion occurs when the spermatic cord is twisted; the correct term is spermatic cord torsion.[66] A narrow mesenteric attachment from the spermatic cord to the testes and epididymis is regarded as the dominant cause, a slender attachment occurring as a result of a small testicular bare area. This allows the testes to fall forward within the cavity of the tunica vaginalis and then to rotate like a "bell-clapper," the "intravaginal" type of torsion, as the gubernaculum is fixed to the scrotal wall, preventing the rotation of the tunica vaginalis.[67] In neonates, the gubernaculum is not attached to the scrotal wall and the entire testes, epididymis, and the tunica vaginalis twist in a vertical axis on the spermatic cord, which is termed "extravaginal" torsion.[68] Neonatal torsion is rare, occurring in the prenatal period and being associated with an inguinal hernia.[69] Factors other than an anatomical anomaly may predispose to spermatic cord torsion since the incidence of torsion (0.025%) is far less than the incidence of "bell-clapper" deformities.[70]

Two factors are of importance in spermatic cord torsion: The extent of the spermatic cord twist (90° to three complete twists) and the duration of the torsion. The initial disruption will be to the venous and lymphatic drainage, rather than to the arterial input of the testes, and venous infarction occurs earlier.[71] Scrotal edema is an early feature as the lower pressure cremasteric venous plexus is the first vascular channel to be affected. Areas of testicular infarction begin to appear within two hours of complete occlusion of the testicular artery, irreversible ischemia occurs after six hours, and complete infarction is established by 24 hours.[72] Intra-

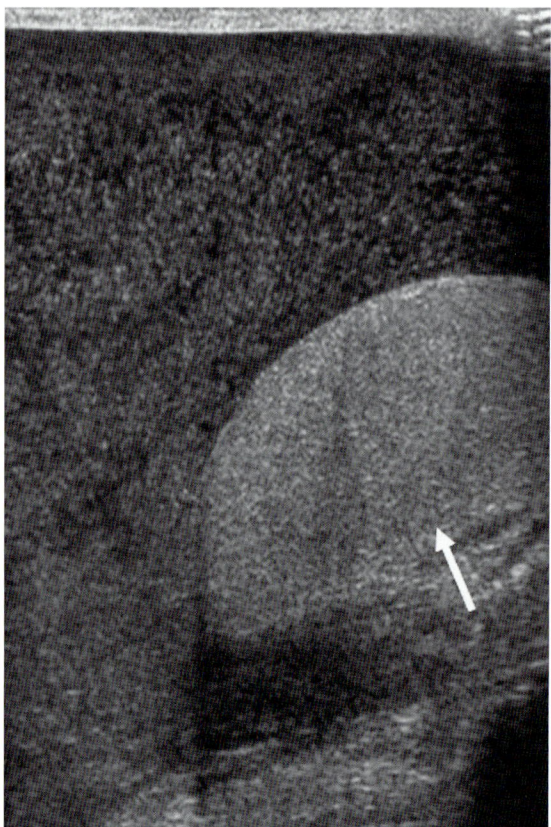

Fig. 11.**33** The testis (arrow) is displaced inferiorly by a large hydrocele with extensive, highly reflective material within the hydrocele representing cholesterol crystals

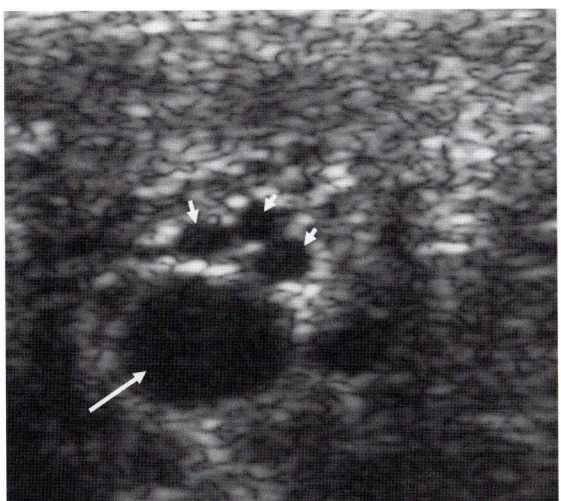
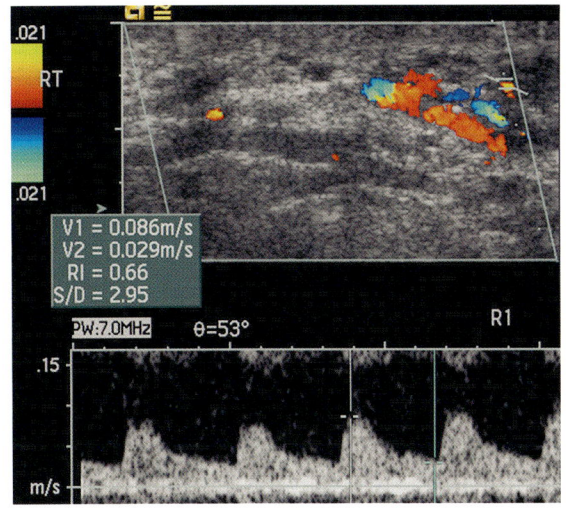
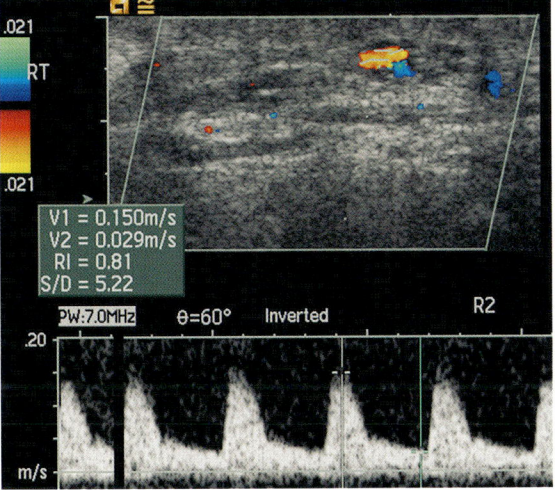

Fig. 11.**34 a** A transverse image through the spermatic cord, demonstrating the testicular vein (long arrow) and the three arteries (short arrows) that are present in the spermatic cord: The *testicular artery*, the *cremasteric artery*, and the *artery to the ductus deferens*. **b** Spectral Doppler analysis of one of the arteries in the spermatic cord demonstrates a low resistance pattern (RI = 0.66), implying that this is the testicular artery. **c** Spectral Doppler analysis of one of the arteries in the spermatic cord demonstrates a high resistance pattern (RI = 0.81), implying that this is either the cremasteric artery or the artery to the ductus deferens

vaginal torsion most commonly occurs between age 12 and 18, with a reported incidence of one in 4000 males younger than age 25.[73] Torsion commonly arises as puberty approaches, when testicular volume may increase by a factor of five, thereby increasing the propensity of the testis to fall forward and rotate.

Clinically, intravaginal torsion presents with pain of sudden or insidious onset and is followed by swelling of the ipsilateral scrotum. The main clinical dilemma remains the distinction between spermatic cord torsion and acute epididymo-orchitis. Establishing the diagnosis is important since in acute epididymo-orchitis, resolution with minimal intervention is the rule unless complications, such as an abscess, supervene. By contrast, surgery is mandatory for torsion. The diagnostic dilemma is compounded by the occasional similarity in clinical presentation: Fever and pyuria may occur in both conditions.[74]

In spermatic cord torsion, ultrasound appearances are variable depending on the time elapsed from the onset of symptoms. With the development of congestion and infarction, the testes appear abnormally enlarged with decreased reflectivity (Fig. 11.**35**).[75] The tunica albuginea and the mediastinum testis appear of relative high reflectivity, and a small amount of fluid may pool in the lower pole of the sac of the tunica vaginalis. Later, as infarction is established, hemorrhage may cause increased reflectivity and heterogeneity; this is particularly true in missed torsion and "chronic" torsions (symptoms present for > 10 days). Enlarged, thrombosed pampiniform plexus veins, within the spermatic cord, may be visible and there may be an abrupt change in caliber of the spermatic cord below the point of torsion. This results in an enlarged, twisted spermatic cord superior and posterior to the epididymal head, containing round anechoic structures representing veins.[76] This may resemble the whirlpool pattern encountered with magnetic resonance (MR) imaging (Fig. 11.**36**). Skin thickening of the scrotum may be present as a manifestation of venous congestion.

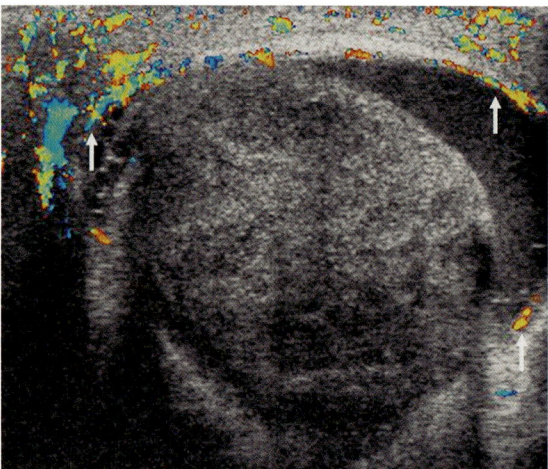

Fig. 11.35 In acute testicular torsion, the testis is enlarged and heterogeneous with a surrounding hydrocele. No color Doppler flow is identified within the testis, but there is color Doppler signal within the paratesticular tissues (arrows)

infarction.[79] In these cases, a reversal of diastolic flow in the testicular artery is thought to be characteristic of venous thrombosis and, when combined with the gray-scale and color Doppler ultrasound appearances of the inflamed epididymis, should allow a correct diagnosis to be reached.[80,81] Currently, there is no single clinical feature or imaging examination that can reliably distinguish torsion from other causes of testicular pain.[42]

- Spermatic cord torsion occurs commonly between age 12 and 18 years
- A "bell-clapper" deformity predisposes to torsion
- Testicular ischemia depends on the extent and duration of the torsion
- Diagnosing torsion is a clinical skill
- Ultrasound is able to differentiate acute epididymitis as a cause of pain

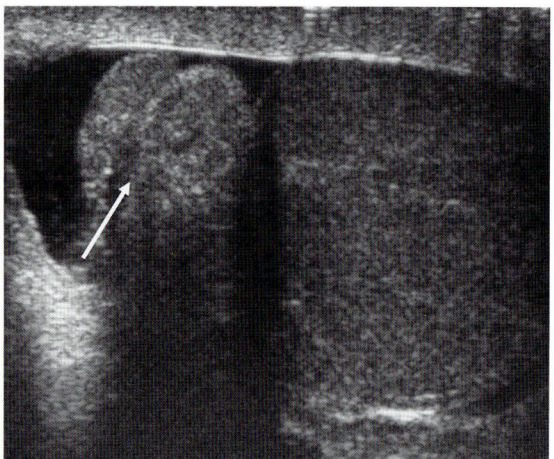

Fig. 11.36 The appearance of a "whirlpool" above the testis (arrow), and separate from the epididymis, which represents the torsed spermatic cord

The basis for the ultrasound diagnosis of spermatic cord torsion is the absence or decreased flow in the symptomatic testis compared to the asymptomatic testis. Color Doppler ultrasound allows visualization of intratesticular blood flow; in torsion blood flow is either reduced or absent, whereas it may be increased in epididymo-orchitis.[77,78] Therefore, color Doppler ultrasound is most useful in rapidly differentiating acute spermatic cord torsion from epididymo-orchitis. Although color Doppler ultrasound is of value in the adult testes, it is less sensitive for the detection of blood flow in children, since symmetry of blood flow is less well-established and is dependent on testicular size.[4] A further limitation with color Doppler ultrasound is the entity of epididymo-orchitis complicated by testicular

Spontaneous Detorsion

A pitfall of the use of color Doppler ultrasound in the assessment of the acute scrotum and in the desire to exclude the presence of spermatic cord torsion, is the entity of a spontaneous detorsion. The susceptible testis undergoes torsion and then spontaneously untwists, resulting in hyperemia of the previously ischemic testis. On ultrasound, the B-mode appearances may be unremarkable, but an increase in color Doppler flow may resemble acute epididymo-orchitis, resulting in a misinterpretation and possible severe consequences for the patient.

Torsion of an Appendage

Torsion of the testicular (or epididymal) appendage is considered to be more common than spermatic cord torsion and an important differential diagnosis among boys under age 13 who present acutely with a painful scrotum. Although most frequently presenting in patients of between age seven and 13, torsion of a testicular appendage can occur at any age. The onset may be associated with trauma or exercise, with pain, erythema, tenderness, and scrotal swelling common presenting symptoms.[42] In light-skinned individuals the palpable, infracted, tender appendage may be visible at the upper pole of the testis; this "blue-dot" sign is reported to occur in up to 21% of patients presenting with torsion of an appendage.[82]

With torsion of a testicular appendage, the testis itself usually appears normal on ultrasound with a normal, low-resistance arterial supply. There is often an associated localized upper-pole hydrocele and an inflammatory reaction in the epididymis, which is often enlarged. The torsed appendage may have a variable appearance, most commonly of increased homogenous reflectivity, although up to 30% are reported as being of low reflectivity surrounded by an area of increased perfusion (Fig. 11.**37**).[77] Color Doppler studies may demonstrate an avascular mass separate from the testis and epididymis and an inflammatory reaction, with increased blood flow in adjacent structures. With time the appendix becomes increasingly of higher reflectivity, indicating the onset of calcification, eventually completely detaching itself. The loose calcified body may be termed a "scrotal pearl," although the origins of these scrotal pearls are uncertain as they may also arise from detached calcified areas of tunica albuginea. These are usually solitary, round, and measure up to 1 cm in diameter, producing acoustic shadowing. Scrotal calculi may occasionally be palpable but are often found in association with a secondary hydrocele (Fig. 11.**38**).[83]

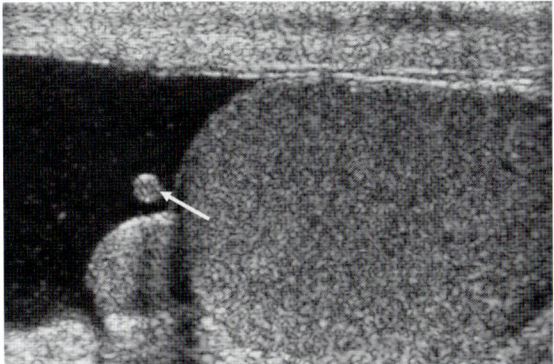

Fig. 11.**37** A hydrocele surrounds the upper aspect of the testis, with a prominent appendix testis (arrow). Appearances are those of torsion of an appendix in a patient with the appropriate symptoms of sudden onset of testicular pain

Summary points:
- Torsion of an appendage is more common in the 7–13-year-old age group
- Testis is normal on ultrasound
- Highly reflective appendage with a surrounding hydrocele
- Surgical exploration is not indicated

Epididymis

Varicocele

A varicocele is present in up to 15% of adult male patients.[84] This abnormal dilatation of veins arises more often on the left as a consequence of the angle at which the left testicular vein enters the left renal vein. The normal veins of the pampiniform plexus measure 0.5–1.5 mm and a vein diameter of > 2 mm should be considered abnormal.[85] On ultrasound, a varicocele consists of multiple, low-reflective serpiginous tubular structures of varying size, best seen superior and lateral to the testis. If large the varicocele may extend to the inferior aspect of the testis (Fig. 11.**39**). Tumbling low-level echoes may be identified on real-time imaging, secondary to low flow. Ultrasound in the supine and erect positions as well as following the Valsalva maneuver will help identify the varicocele and document retrograde filling. Examination of the left kidney is advocated in the presence of a varicocele that has recently arisen in patients over age 40 to exclude a renal tumor, without much supporting evidence as to the prevalence of this association. Occasionally an intratesticular varicocele may occur (Fig. 11.**40**).[86] Iden-

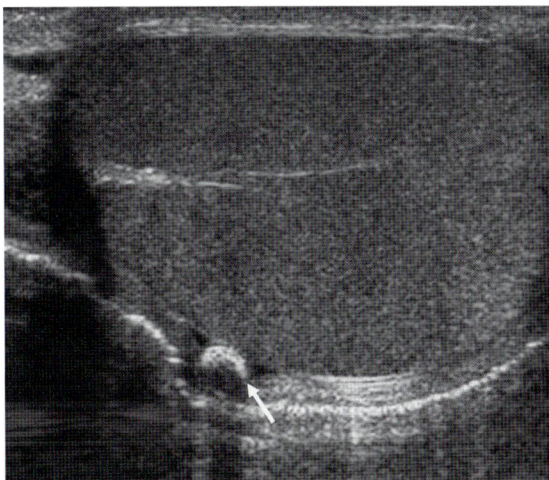

Fig. 11.**38** The highly reflective area (arrow) lying free within the scrotal sac represents a "scrotal pearl"

tification of a varicocele in patients being investigated for infertility may be of relevance, although testicular volume, ultrasound appearances, and Doppler studies may also be of importance.[87]

Vasectomy

Following vasectomy, the epididymis has a characteristic appearance of dilatation, with an inhomogeneous appearance on ultrasound described as ectasia of the epididymis, appearances which are unrelated to symptoms (Fig. 11.**41**).[88]

Epididymal Calcification

Calcification within the epididymis is frequent and usually represents benign disease.[89] The tunica vaginalis may occasionally calcify, producing a plaque with acoustic shadowing (Fig. 11.**42**). Calcification in or adja-

172 11 Diseases of the Testis and Epididymis

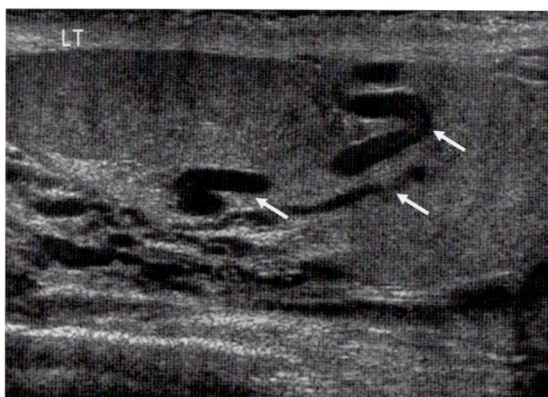

Fig. 11.39 **a** Serpiginous dilated (> 2 mm) veins at the lower aspect of the testis, with "tumbling echoes" present (arrows). A testicular varicocele

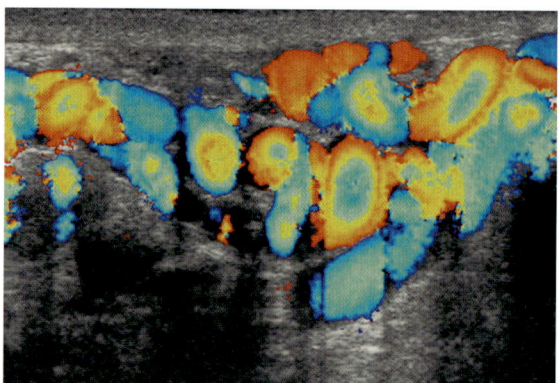

b The varicocele fills with color Doppler following the valsalva maneuver

Fig. 11.40 **a** Serpiginous dilated (> 2 mm) veins present within the testicular parenchyma (arrows). An intratesticular varicocele. **b** The varicocele fills with color Doppler following the valsalva maneuver

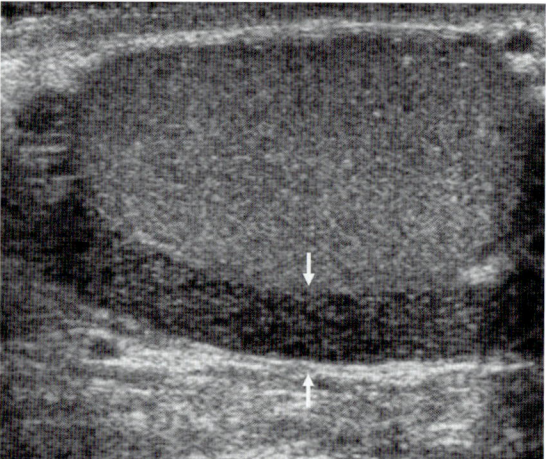

Fig. 11.41 The epididymis is dilated (arrows, > 4 mm) in a patient who has undergone a vasectomy, with a characteristic reflective pattern

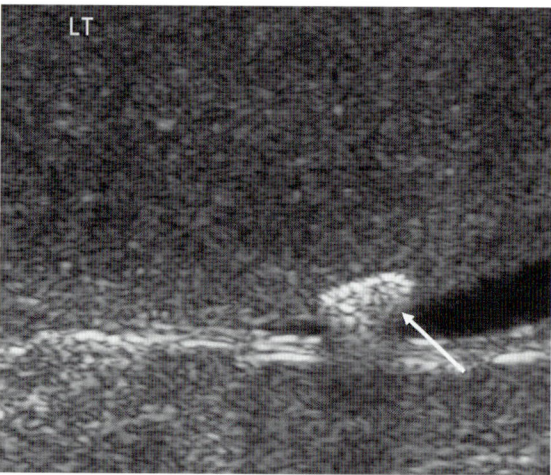

Fig. 11.42 A focus of high reflectivity adjacent to the outer border of the testis casting an acoustic shadow (arrow): Calcification within the tunica vaginalis

cent to the epididymis is a common finding and is usually due to chronic epididymitis. Hematoma and sperm granulomas (sperm extravasation with granuloma formation) may occur and produce a solitary high-reflective area within the epididymis. The appendix epididymis and appendix testis may calcify and are recognized by their characteristic position and shape.[60]

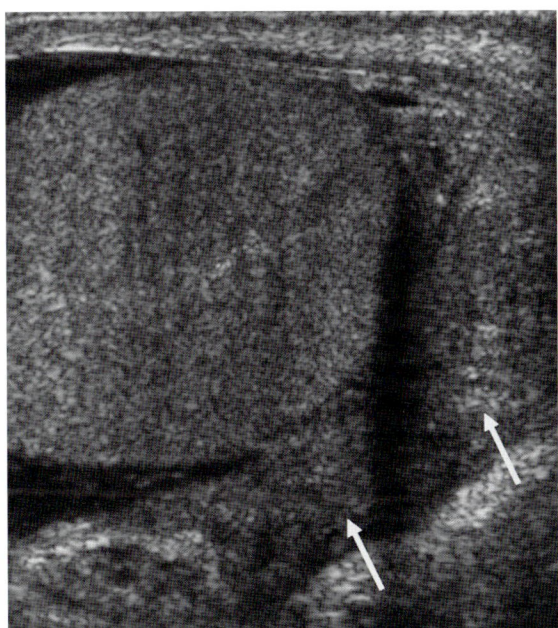
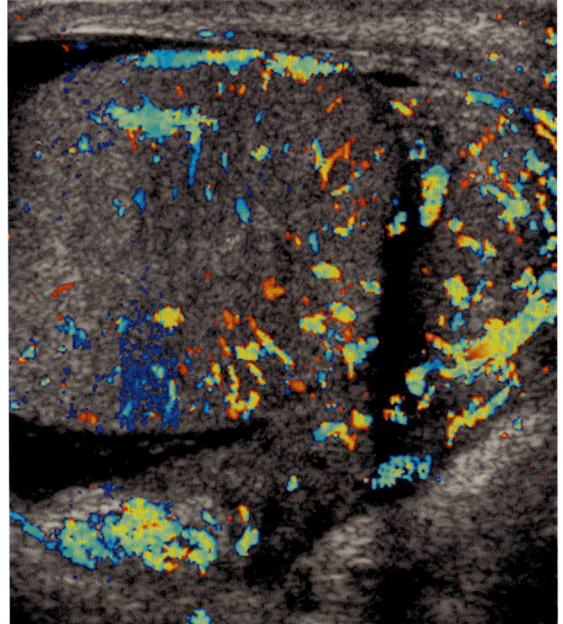

Fig. 11.**43 a** The epididymis is enlarged, of mixed reflectivity (arrows) with an accompanying hydrocele and changes in reflectivity of the adjacent testis. Acute epididymo-orchitis.

b There is marked increase in vascularity to the affected areas as demonstrated by color Doppler ultrasound; acute inflammatory changes of epididymo-orchitis

Inflammatory Disease

Epididymo-orchitis and Epididymitis

Epididymo-orchitis and epididymitis predominantly affect the sexually active male of less than age 40, the older patient with urological disease, and the prepubertal boy with an associated urogenital anomaly.[90] The main causative organisms in sexual transmitted diseases are *Chlamydia trachomatis* and *Neisseria gonorrhea*, whereas in prepubertal boys and in men over age 40, the organisms responsible are *E. coli* and *Proteus mirabilis*. Epididymitis causes acute scrotal pain of varying intensity, pyuria with fever, and at clinical examination the epididymis may be palpated as a thickened, tender structure separate from the testis.

On ultrasound, the epididymis may be involved in focal areas (often the lower is affected first) or in a global pattern, with enlargement, decreased reflectivity, and increased color Doppler flow (Fig. 11.**43**).[78,91] The presence of increased color Doppler to the inflamed epididymis is the hallmark for hyperemia and usefully aids the diagnosis of epididymitis and epididymo-orchitis. On spectral Doppler ultrasound, there is a high-flow, low-resistance pattern.[92] Reversal of flow during diastole may herald venous infarction.[81] There is often a reactive hydrocele, with septations if a pyocele develops, and scrotal wall thickening. The infection often spreads to the adjacent testis (epididymo-orchitis), seen as patchy areas of low reflectivity and increased color Doppler signal, an appearance that may persist for several months following treatment.[93]

Complications that may arise following acute epididymitis include testicular infarction following obstruction of the venous drainage (Fig. 11.**44**),[79] abscess formation (low-reflective area surrounded by increased color Doppler signal) (Fig. 11.**45**), pyocele, testicular atrophy, and chronic pain.

Summary points:
- Epididymo-orchitis presents with acute onset of pain
- Focal or diffuse enlargement of the epididymis
- Increased color Doppler flow to the affected areas
- Associated orchitis is a common occurrence
- Abscess is a complication

Chronic Epididymitis

Chronic epididymitis results in persistent pain and on ultrasound an enlarged epididymis with increased reflectivity is seen with areas of calcification present. Tuberculous epididymitis may present in a similar fashion to bacterial epididymitis but will not respond to standard antibiotic treatment.[94] Ultrasound features are not specific, although chronic disease with calcification and indolent abscess formation discharging onto the skin may be present (Fig. 11.**46**).[95,96]

11 Diseases of the Testis and Epididymis

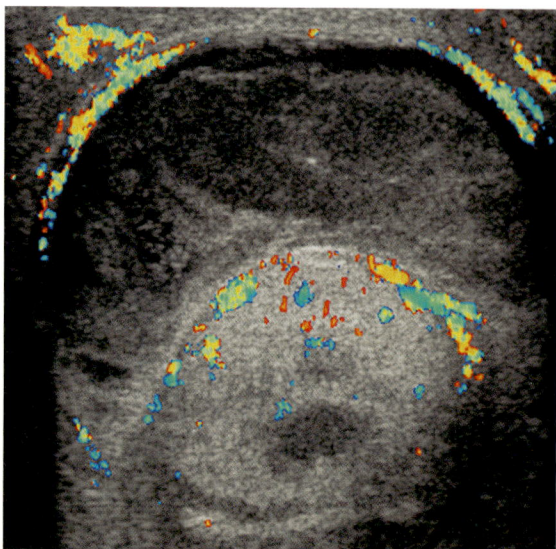

Fig. 11.**44 a** The epididymis is markedly dilated (long arrows) with a predominantly low-reflective appearance in a patient with severe epididymitis. Mixed reflectivity is present in the posterior aspect of the testis (arrowheads). **b** Color Doppler ultrasound demonstrates absence of flow signal in the epididymis and no color Doppler signal in the mixed-reflective region of the testis: Testicular venous infarction following severe acute epididymitis

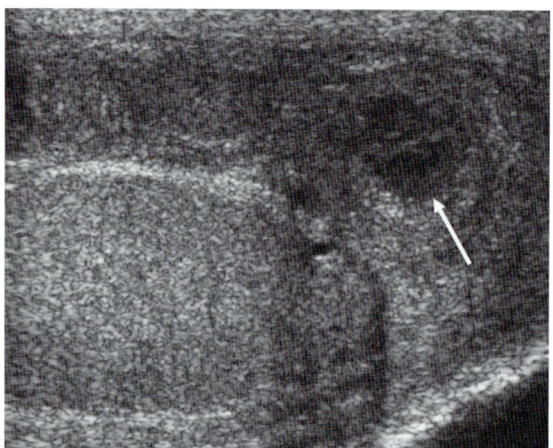

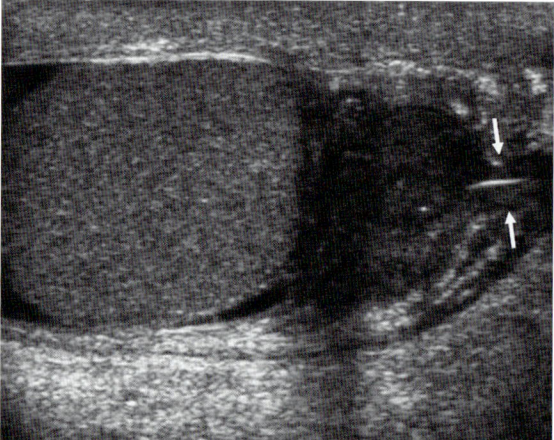

Fig. 11.**46** A low-reflective abnormality present at the lower aspect of the testis, contained within an enlarged epididymis, with a sinus tract (arrows) discharging pus onto the skin surface of the scrotal sac. An epididymal abscess secondary to chronic tuberculous epididymitis

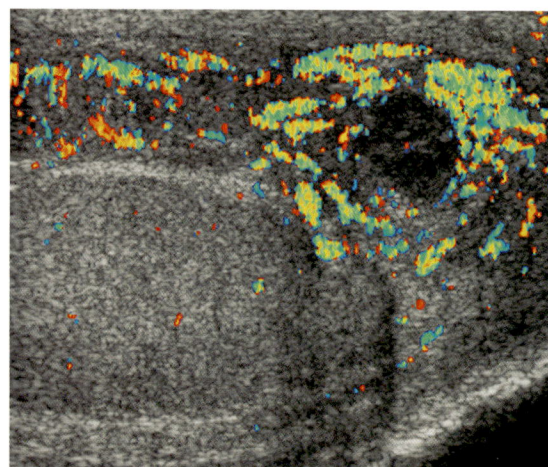

◁ Fig. 11.**45 a** There is a focal area of low reflectivity (arrow), containing debris, in the tail of the epididymis in a patient with acute epididymitis not responding to antibacterial therapy. **b** Color Doppler demonstrates increased color signal from around the low-reflective area, and absence of color Doppler signal within the lesion: An epididymal abscess

Extratesticular Focal Lesions

Extratesticular solid tumors are rare; the majority of extratesticular lesions are cystic abnormalities of the epididymis. Primary solid tumors of the extratesticular tissues are normally benign, although malignant lesions are seen. The reported prevalence of extratesticular solid tumors varies between 3% and 16% of all patients referred for scrotal ultrasound.[97,98] Metastases may also occur in the extratesticular space.

Epididymal Cysts and Spermatoceles

Extratesticular cysts are commonly found in the spermatic cord, epididymis (Fig. 11.47), tunica albuginea (Fig. 11.48), or tunica vaginalis. Epididymal cysts are most commonly found in the epididymal head, contain clear serous fluid, and on ultrasound demonstrate typical features of a cyst with posterior enhancement. A spermatocele consists of cystic dilatation of tubules of efferent ductules and occurs in the epididymal head (Fig. 11.49), often containing low-reflective debris representing spermatozoa.[99]

Sperm Granuloma

A sperm granuloma occurs secondary to inflammation, trauma, and vasectomy, thought to be a granulomatous reaction to extravasated sperm cells. On ultrasound a sperm granuloma is well-demarcated, of low reflectivity, and found in the epididymis, and often painful in the early stages.[100]

Benign Neoplasms (Table 11.2)

Lipoma
This is the most common benign tumor of the extratesticular space with a prevalence of 45%, commonly found in the spermatic cord.[101] Patients of all ages are affected, with the tumor manifesting as a nontender scrotal lump. At ultrasound a lipoma has a homogenous, high-reflective appearance, and varies in size. MR imaging will confirm the fat content of the lesion, prior to excision if necessary.

Adenomatoid Tumor
This is the most common tumor of the epididymis, accounting for 30% of all tumors of the extratesticular space. It is probably of a mesothelial origin. Adenomatoid tumors usually occur in the patient age 20 or older. They present as a painless mass, are slow growing, and arise in the tail of the epididymis (four times as common as the head) and are predominantly left-sided. The ultrasound appearance is nonspecific; the majority are isoreflective to the epididymis, well-defined, oval in

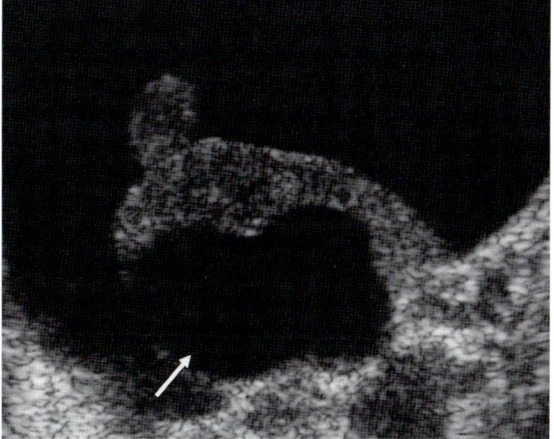

Fig. 11.47 A bilobulated epididymal head cyst (arrow)

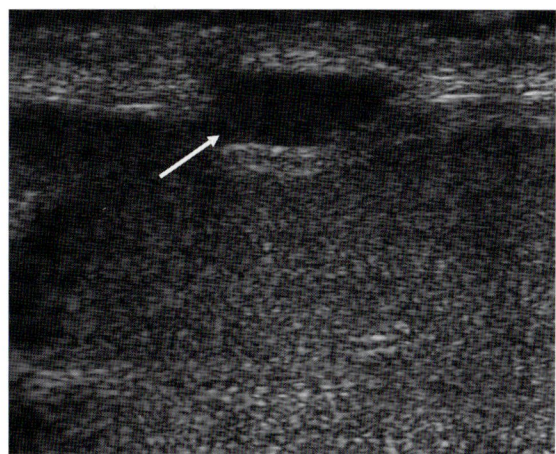

Fig. 11.48 A small tunica albuginea cyst (arrow)

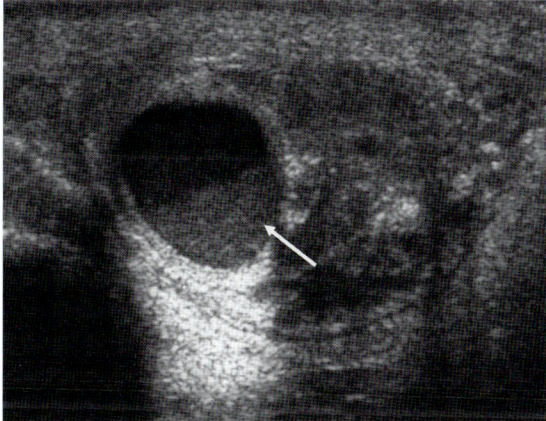

Fig. 11.49 A cyst in the epididymal head demonstrates debris (arrow) that is "layering" and produces posterior acoustic enhancement: A spermatocele

Table 11.2 Extratesticular neoplasms[106]

Benign
Adenomatoid tumor
Leiomyoma
Lipoma
Hemangioma
Cystadenoma
Fibrous pseudotumour
Sclerosing lipogranuloma

Malignant
Rhabdomyosarcoma
Liposarcoma
Leiomyosarcoma
Malignant schwannoma
Malignant fibrous histiocytoma
Pleomorphic hyalinizing angiectatic tumor

Metastases (in order of frequency)
Prostate
Kidney
Stomach
Colon
Ileum (carcinoid tumor)
Pancreas

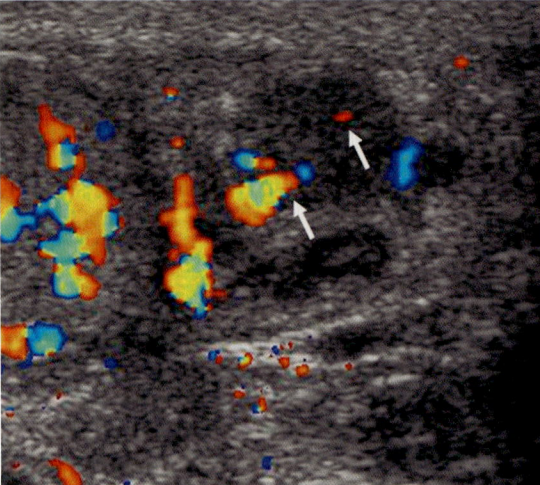

Fig. 11.50 **a** A focal, low-reflective mass (arrow) present in the tail of the epididymis. **b** On color Doppler ultrasound there is color signal to the central aspect of the mass (arrows), indicating the vascular solid nature of the lesion: An adenomatoid tumor of the epididymis

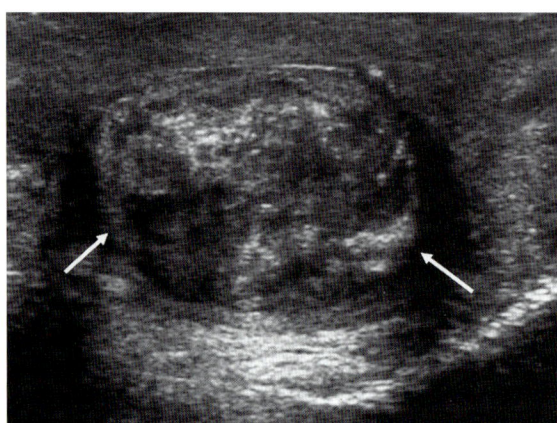

Fig. 11.51 **A fibrous pseudotumor of the epididymis**

shape, and may be cystic (Fig. 11.50).[102] Resection is normally curable, but will interfere with sperm ejaculation on the side of the resection.

Leiomyoma

This is the second commonest tumor of the epididymis, with a prevalence of 6%, commonly manifest in the fifth decade, frequently involving the epididymal head, and is often associated with a hydrocele. The patient presents with a slow-growing nontender mass. On ultrasound there are no specific features. A leiomyoma may be cystic or solid, and contain areas of calcification.[103]

Other rare benign tumors of the extratesticular space include hemangiomas, which may be indistinguishable from a varicocele, a cystadenoma associated with von Hippel–Lindau disease, appearing as a solid lesion with small cystic spaces in the head of the epididymis.[104] A fibrous pseudotumour (Fig. 11.51) may result from a prior history of trauma, hematocele, or from epididymo-orchitis.[105]

Malignant Neoplasms

Malignant lesions of the extratesticular space are rare, usually present as a mildly painful enlarging mass, and the vast majority are sarcomas.[106]

Rhabdomyosarcoma

This is the most common sarcoma of the spermatic cord (40% of extratesticular malignant lesions), peaking at age five and 16. The most common presentation is of an enlarging painless mass, but as an aggressive tumor may present with metastases. On ultrasound features are nonspecific; there is variable reflectivity with areas of necrosis and hemorrhage, and increased color Doppler flow of low resistance.[107]

Liposarcoma

This is very rare and usually arises from the spermatic cord, is of low-grade malignancy, spreading by local spread with patients presenting with a slow-growing fluctuant mass. Ultrasound demonstrates a high-reflective mass of varying size.

Other rare malignant lesions of the extratesticular space include leiomyosarcoma, which is seen as a predominantly low-reflective mass,[108] malignant schwannoma, and malignant fibrous histiocytoma. A mesothelioma may develop from the tunica vaginalis in patients exposed to asbestos.[109] Lastly, metastases to the extratesticular space occur from a testicular primary tumor, renal, prostate, and gastrointestinal tumors.

Scrotal Wall Abnormalities

Scrotal wall edema may occur in many conditions, including heart failure, liver failure, lymphatic obstruction, and venous obstruction. Lymph edema of the scrotal wall is classically described in filiarial worm infestations (Fig. 11.52).[110] Cellulite and Fournier gangrene are inflammatory causes of scrotal wall edema, where gas may be identified in the scrotal wall on ultrasound.[111]

> **Summary points:**
> - Extra-testicular lesions are nearly all benign abnormalities
> - The majority are epididymal head cysts
> - Lipomas occur commonly
> - Adenomatoid lesions are the commonest in the epididymis
> - Rhabdomyosarcoma occurs between age five and 16 yrs

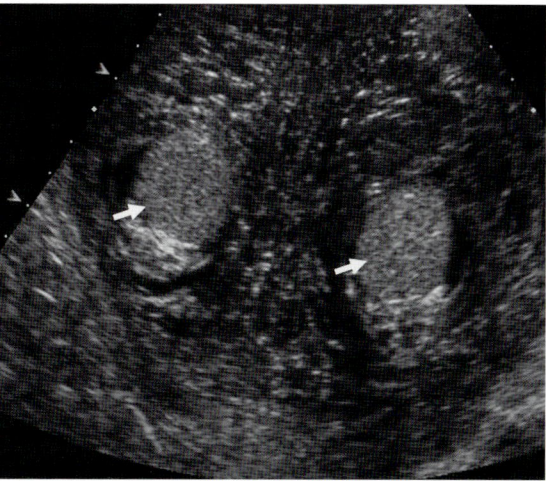

Fig. 11.**52 Gross edema of the scrotal sac surrounding the testes** (arrows)

References

1. Langman J. Genital system. Medical embryology. Baltimore: Williams and Wilkins: 1975:175–200.
2. The reproductive organs of the male. In: Williams PL, Warwick R, Dyson M, Bannister LH, eds. Gray's Anatomy. London: Churchill Livingstone: 1989:1424–1434.
3. Paltiel HJ, Diamond DA, Di Canzio J, Zurakowski D, Borer JG, Atala A. Testicular volume: comparison of orchidometer and US measurements in dogs. Radiology 2002;222: 114–119.
4. Ingram S, Hollman AS. Colour Doppler sonography of the normal paediatric testis. Clin Radiol 1994;49: 266–267.
5. Sellars MEK, Sidhu PS. Pictorial review: ultrasound appearances of the rete testis. Eur J Ultrasound 2001;14:115–120.
6. Sellars MEK, Sidhu PS. Utrasound appearances of the testicular appendages: pictorial review. Eur Radiol 2003;13: 127–135.
7. Keener TS, Winter TC, Nghiem HV, Schmiedl UP. Normal adult epididymis: evaluation with color Doppler ultrasound. Radiology 1997;202:712–714.
8. Rolnick D, Kawanoue S, Szanto P, Bush IM. Anatomical incidence of testicular appendages. J Urol 1968;100: 755–756.
9. Leung ML, Gooding GAW, Williams RD. High-resolution sonography of scrotal contents in asymptomatic subjects. AJR Am J Roentgenol 1984;143:161–164.
10. Middleton WD, Meredith MW. Analysis of intratesticular arterial anatomy with emphasis on transmediastinal arteries. Radiology 1993;189:157–160.
11. Nicolaou S, Cooperberg PL. The two-tone testis due to refractive shadowing of the intratesticular artery. J Ultrasound Med 1995;14:963–965.
12. Bustos-Obregon E, Holstein AF. The rete testis in man: ultrastructural aspects. Cell Tissue Research 1976;175: 1–15.
13. Rolinck D, Kawanove S, Szanto P. Anatomical incidence of testicular appendages. J Urol 1968;100: 755–756.
14. Johnson KA, Dewbury KC. Ultrasound imaging of the appendix testis and appendix epididymis. Clin Radiol 1996;51:335–337.

15. Strauss S, Faingold R, Manor H. Torsion of the testicular appendages: sonographic appearance. J Ultrasound Med 1997;16:189–192.
16. Rifkin MD, Kurtz AB, Pasto ME, Goldberg BB. Polyorchidism diagnosed preoperatively by ultrasonography. J Ultrasound Med 1983;2:93–94.
17. Amodio JB, Maybody M, Slowotsky C, Fried K, Foresto C. Polyorchidism: Report of 3 Cases and Review of the Literature. J Ultrasound Med 2004;23:951–957.
18. Chung TJ, Yao WJ. Sonographic features of polyorchidism. J Clin Ultrasound 2002;30:106–108.
19. Greenlee RT, Hill-Harmon MB, Murray T, Thun M. Cancer statistics. 2001. CA Cancer J Clin 2001;51:15–36.
20. Grantham JG, Charboneau JW, James EM, Kirschling RJ, Kvols LK, Segura JW, et al. Testicular neoplasms: 29 tumors studied by high-resolution US. Radiology 1985;157: 775–780.
21. Horstman WG, Melson GL, Middleton WD, Andriole GL. Testicular tumours: Findings with color Doppler US. Radiology 1992;185:733–737.
22. Bushby LH, Sriprasad S, Hopster D, Muir G, Clarke JL, Sidhu PS. High-frequency colour Doppler US of focal testicular lesions: crossing vessels criss-cross pattern. identifies primary malignant tumours. Radiology 2001;221:449.
23. Sidhu PS, Sriprasad S, Bushby LH, Sellars ME, Muir GH. Impalpable testis cancer. BJU Int 2004;93:888.
24. Woodward PJ, Schwab CM, Sesterhenn IA. Extratesticular scrotal masses: radiologic-pathologic correlation. Radiographics 2003;231:215–240.
25. Heiken JP. Tumors of the testis and testicular adenexa. In: Pollack HM, McClennan BL, eds. Clinical urography. Philadelphia: Saunders: 2000:1716–1741.
26. Mostofi FK, Sesterhenn IA, Davis CJ. Immunopathology of germ cell tumours of the testis. Semin Diag Pathol 1987;4:320–341.
27. Atchley JTM, Dewbury KC. Ultrasound appearances of testicular epidermoid cysts. Clin Radiol 2000;55: 493–502.
28. Shapeero LG, Vordermark JS. Epidermoid cysts of testes and role of sonography. Urology 1993;41:75–79.
29. Comiter CV, Renshaw AA, Benson CB, Loughlin KR. Burned-out primary testicular cancer: sonographic and pathological characteristics. J Urol 1996;156:85–88.
30. Avery GR, Peakman DJ, Young JR. Unusual hyperechoic ultrasound appearance of testicular Leydig cell tumour. Clin Radiol 1991;43:260–261.
31. Maizlin ZV, Belenky A, Kunichezky M, Sandbank J, Strauss S. Leydig cell tumors of the testis: gray scale and color Doppler sonographic appearance. J Ultrasound Med 2004;23:959–964.
32. Mazzu D, Jeffrey RB, Ralls PW. Lymphoma and leukaemia involving the testicles: findings on gray-scale and color Doppler sonography. AJR Am J Roentgenol 1995;164: 645–647.
33. Rayor RA, Scheible W, Brock WA, Leopold GR. High-resolution ultrasonography in the diagnosis of testicular relapse in patients with acute lymphoblastic leukaemia. J Urol 1982;128:602–603.
34. Garcia-Gonzalez R, Pinto J, Val-Bernal JF. Testicular metastases from solid tumours: an autopsy study. Ann Diagn Pathol 2000;4:397–400.
35. Carragher AM. One hundred years of splenogonad fusion. Urology 1990;35:471–475.
36. Putschar WGJ, Manion WC. Splenic-gonad fusion. Am J Pathol 1955;32:15–33.
37. Kalomenopoulou M, Katsimba D, Arvaniti M, Chakkas J, Sinopidis X, Kotakidou R, et al. Male splenic-gonald fusion of the continous type: sonographic findings. Eur Radiol 2002;12:374–377.
38. Henderson RG, Henderson DC, Reid IN, Atkinson PM. Case report: splenic-gonald fusion. The ultrasound appearances. Clin Radiol 1991;44:117–118.
39. Stewart VR, Sellars ME, Somers S, Muir GH, Sidhu PS. Splenogonadal fusion: B-mode and color Doppler sonographic appearances. J Ultrasound Med 2004;23:1087–1090.
40. Seidenwurm D, Smathers RL, Kan P, Hoffman A. Intratesticular adrenal rests diagnosed by ultrasound. Radiology 1985;155:479–481.
41. Avila NA, Premkumar A, Shawker TH, Jones JV, Laue L, Cutler GB. Testicular adrenal rest tissue in congenital adrenal hyperplasia:findings at gray-scale and color Doppler US. Radiology 1996;198:99–104.
42. Sidhu PS. Clinical and imaging features of testicular torsion: role of ultrasound. Clin Radiol 1999;54: 343–352.
43. Costa M, Calleja R, Ball RY, Burgess N. Segmental testicular infarction. BJU Int 1999;83:525.
44. Sriprasad SI, Kooiman GG, Muir GH, Sidhu PS. Acute sgmental testicular infarction: differentiation from tumour using high frequency colour Doppler ultrasound. Br J Radiol 2001;74:965–967.
45. Flanagan JJ, Fowler RC. Testicular infarction mimicking tumour on scrotal ultrasound: a potential pitfall. Clin Radiol 1995;50:49–50.
46. Gofrit ON, Rund D, Shapiro A, Pappo O, Landau EH, Pode D. Segmental testicular infarction due to sickle cell disease. J Ultrasound Med 1998;160:835–836.
47. Kramolowsky EV, Beauchamp RA, Milby WP. Color Doppler ultrasound for the diagnosis of segmental testicular infarction. J Urol 1993;150:972–973.
48. Ledwidge ME, Lee DK, Winter TC, III., Uehling DT, Mitchell CC, Lee FT, Jr. Sonographic diagnosis of superior hemispheric testicular infarction. AJR Am J Roentgenol 2002;1793: 775–776.
49. Salmeron I, Ramirez-Escobar MA, Puertas F, Marcos R, Garcia-Marcos F, Sanchez R. Granulomatous epididymo-orchitis: sonographic features and clinical outcome in brucellosis, tuberculosis and idiopathic granulomatous epididymo-orchitis. J Urol 1998;159:1954–1957.
50. Burke BJ, Parker SH, Pienkos EJ. The ultrasonographic appearance of coexistant epididymal and testicular sarcoidosis. J Clin Ultrasound 1990;18:522–526.
51. Hamm B, Fobbe F, Loy V. Testicular cysts: differentiation with US and clinical findings. Radiology 1988;168:19–23.
52. Harris RD, Chouteau C, Patrick M, Schned A. Prevalence and significance of heterogeneous testes revealed on sonography: ex vivo sonographic-pathologic correlation. AJR Am J Roentgenol 2000;175:347–352.
53. Subramanyan BR, Horri SC, Hilton S. Diffuse testicular disease: sonographic features and significance. AJR Am J Roentgenol 1985;145:1221–1224.
54. Mevorach RA, Lerner RM, Dvoretsky PM, Rabinowitz R. Testicular abscess: diagnosis by ultrasonography. J Urol 1986;136:1213–1216.
55. Backus ML, Mack LA, Middleton WD, King BF, Winter TC, True LD. Testicular microlithiasis: imaging appearances and pathologic correlation. Radiology 1994;192:781–785.
56. Woodward PJ, Sohaey R, O'Donoghue MJ, Green DE. Tumors and tumorlike lesions of the testis: radiologic-pathologic correlation. Radiographics 2002;22:189–216.

57. Ganem JP, Workman KR, Shaban SF. Testicular microlithiasis is associated with testicular pathology. Urology 1999;53:209–213.
58. Skakkebaek NE, Berthelsen JG, Giwercman A, Muller J. Carcinoma-in-situ of the testis: possible origin from gonocytes and precusor of all types of germ cell tumours except spermatocytoma. Int J Androl 1987;10:19–28.
59. Miller FNAC, Sidhu PS. Does testicular microlithiasis matter? A review. Clin Radiol 2002;57:883–890.
60. Bushby LH, Miller FNAC, Rosairo S, Clarke JL, Sidhu PS. Scrotal calcification: ultrasound appearances, distribution and aetiology. Br J Radiol 2002;75:283–288.
61. Miller FNAC, Rosairo S, Clarke JL, Sidhu PS. Testicular calcification: appearances, anatomical distribution and association with primary intratesticular malignancy in 2924 patients. Radiology 2000;217:S366.
62. Bhandary P, Abbit PL, Watson L. Ultrasound diagnosis of traumatic testicular rupture. J Clin Ultrasound 1992;20:346–348.
63. Herbener TE. Ultrasound in the assessment of the acute scrotum. J Clin Ultrasound 1996;24:405–421.
64. Gooding GA, Leonhardt WC, Marshall G, Seltzer MA, Presti JC. Cholesterol crystals in hydrocoeles; sonographic detection and possible significance. AJR Am J Roentgenol 1997;169:527–529.
65. Aziz ZA, Satchithananda K, Kham M, Sidhu PS. High frequency color Doppler ultrasonography of the spermatic cord arteries: resistive index in a cohort of 51 healthy men. J Ultrasound Med 2005;24:905–909.
66. Muschat M. The pathological anatomy of testicular torsion: explanation of its mechanism. Surg Gynae Obst 1932;54:758–763.
67. Corriere JN. Horizontal lie of the testicle: a diagnostic sign and torsion of the testis. J Urol 1972;107:616–617.
68. Blackhouse KM. Embryology of testicular descent and maldescent. Urol. Clin. Am 1982;9:315.
69. Zafaranolo S, Gerard PS, Wise G. Bilateral neonatal testicular torsion: ultrasonographic evaluation. J Urol 1986;135:589–590.
70. Caesar RE, Kaplan GW. Incidence of bell-clapper deformity in an autopsy series. Ped Urol 1994;441:114–116.
71. Rencken RK, DuPlessis DJ, DeHaas LS. Venous infarction of the testes - a cause of non-response to conservative therapy in epididymo-orchitis: a case report. SAfrMJ 1990;78:337–338.
72. Luker GD, Siegel MJ. Color Doppler sonography of the scrotum in children. AJR Am J Roentgenol 1994;163:649–655.
73. Williamson RCN. Torsion of the testis and allied conditions. Br J Surg 1976;63:465–476.
74. Cass AS, Cass BP, Veeraraghawan K. Immediate exploration of the unilateral acute scrotum in young male subjects. J Urol 1980;124:829–832.
75. Hricak H, Lue TF, Filly RA, Alpers CE, Zeineh SJ, Tanagho EA. Experimental study of the sonographic diagnosis of testicular torsion. J Ultrasound Med 1983;2:349–356.
76. van Dijk R, Karthaus HFM. Ultrasonography of the spermatic cord in testicular torsion. Eur J Radiol 1994;18:220–223.
77. Lerner RG, Mevorach RA, Hulbert WC, Rabinowitz R. Color Doppler US in the evaluation of acute scrotal disease. Radiology 1990;176:355–358.
78. Horstman WG, Middleton WD, Melson GL. Scrotal inflammatory disease: Color Doppler US findings. Radiology 1991;179:55–59.
79. Eisner DJ, Goldman SM, Petronis J, Millmond SH. Bilateral testicular infarction caused by epididymitis. AJR Am J Roentgenol 1991;157:517–519.
80. Dogra VS, Rubens DJ, Gottlieb RH, Bhatt S. Torsion and beyond: new twists in spectral Doppler evaluation of the scrotum. J Ultrasound Med 2004;23:1077–1085.
81. Sanders LM, Haber S, Dembner A, Aquino A. Significance of reversal of diastolic flow in the acute scrotum. J Ultrasound Med 1994;13:137–139.
82. McCombe AW, Scobie WG. Torsion of scrotal contents in children. Br J Urol 1988;61:148–150.
83. Linkowski GD, Avellone A, Gooding GA. Scrotal calculi: sonographic detection. Radiology 1985;156:484.
84. Meacham RB, Townsend RR, Rademacher D, Drose JA. The incidence of varicoceles in the general population when evaluated by physical examination, gray scale sonography and color Doppler sonography. J Urol 1994;151:1535–1538.
85. Dogra VS, Gottlieb RH, Oka M, Rubens DJ. Sonography of the scrotum. Radiology 2003;227:18–36.
86. Mehta AL, Dogra VS. Intratesticular varicocele. J Clin Ultrasound 1998;26:49–51.
87. Gordon SJ, Otite U, Maheshkumar P, Cannon P, Nargund VH. The use of scrotal ultrasonography in male infertility. BJU Int 2001;87:417.
88. Jarvis LJ, Dubbins PA. Changes in the epididymis after vasectomy: sonographic findings. AJR Am J Roentgenol 1989;152:531–534.
89. Martin B, Tubiana JM. Significance of scrotal calcification detected by sonography. J Clin Ultrasound 1988;16:545–552.
90. Siegal A, Snyder H, Duckett JW. Epididymitis in infants and boys: underlying anomalies and efficacy of imaging modalities. J Urol 1987;138:1100–1103.
91. Fitzgerald SW, Erickson SJ, Dewire DM, Foley WD, Lawson TL, Begun FP et al. Color sonography in the evaluation of the adult acute scrotum. J Ultrasound Med 1992;11:543–548.
92. Brown JM, Hammers LW, Barton JW, Holland CK, Scoutt LM, Pellerito JS, et al. Quantitative Doppler assessment of acute scrotal inflammation. Radiology 1995;197:427–431.
93. Cook JL, Dewbury K. The changes seen on high-resolution ultrasound in orchitis. Clin Radiol 2000;55:13–18.
94. Yang DM, Yoon MH, Kim HS, Jin W, Hwang HY, Kim HS, et al. Comparison of tuberculous and pyogenic epididymal abscesses: clinical, gray-scale sonographic and color Doppler sonographic features. AJR Am J Roentgenol 2001;177:1131–1135.
95. Kim SH, Pollack HM, Cho KS, Pollack MS, Han MC. Tuberculous epididymitis and epididymo-orchitis: sonographic findings. J Urol 1993;150:80–84.
96. Drudi FM, Laghi A, Iannicelli E, Di Nardo R, Occhiato R, Poggi R, et al. Tubercular epididymitis and orchitis: US patterns. Eur J Radiol 1997;7:1076–1078.
97. Beccia DJ, Krane RJ, Olsson CA. Clinical management of non-testicular intrascrotal tumors. J Urol 1976;116:476–479.
98. Frates MC, Benson CB, DiSalvo DN, Brown DL, Laing FC, Doubilet PM. Solid extratesticular masses evaluated with sonography: Pathologic correlation. Radiology 1997;204:43–46.

99. Rifkin MD, Kurtz AB, Goldberg BB. Epididymis examined by ultrasound: correlation with pathology. Radiology 1984;151:187–190.
100. Ramanathan K, Yaghoobian J, Pinck RL. Sperm granuloma. J Clin Ultrasound 1986;14:155–156.
101. Lioe TF, Biggart JD. Tumours of the spermatic cord and paratesticular tissue. A clinicopathological study. Br J Urol 1993;71:600–606.
102. Makarainen HP, Tammela TL, Karttunen TJ, Mattila SI, Hellstrom PA, Kontturi MJ. Intrascrotal adenomatoid tumors and their ultrasound findings. J Clin Ultrasound 1993;21:33–37.
103. Hertzberg BS, Kliewer MA, Hertzberg MA, Distell BM. Epididymal leiomyoma: sonographic features. J Ultrasound Med 1996;15:797–799.
104. Choyke PL, Glen GM, Wagner JP, Lubensky IA, Thakore K, Zbar B, et al. Epididymal cystadenomas in von Hippel-Lindau disease. Urology 1997;49:926–931.
105. Sajjad SM, Azizi MR, Llamas L. Fibrous pseudotumor of testicular tunic. Urology 1982;19:86–88.
106. Akbar SA, Sayyed TA, Jafri SZH, Hasteh F, Neill JSA. Multimodality imaging of paratesticular neoplasms and their rare mimics. Radiographics 2003;23:1461–1476.
107. Wood A, Dewbury KC. Case report: paratesticular rhabdomyosarcoma - colour Doppler appearances. Clin Radiol 1995;50:130–131.
108. Stein A, Kaplun A, Sova Y, Zivan I, Laver B, Lurie M, et al. Leiomyosarcoma of the spermatic cord: report of two cases and review of the literature. World J Urol 1996;14:59–61.
109. Kuwabara H, Uda H, Sakamoto H, Sato A. Malignant mesothelioma of the tunica vaginalis testis. Report of a case and review of the literature. Acta Pathol Jpn 1991;41:857–863.
110. Grainger AJ, Hide IG, Elliot ST. The ultrasound appearances of scrotal oedema. Eur J Ultrasound 1998;8:33–37.
111. Dogra VS, Smeltzer JS, Poblette J. Sonographic diagnosis of Fournier's gangrene. J Clin Ultrasound 1994;22:571–572.

12 Diseases of the Penis with Functional Evaluation

C. J. Wilkins, P. S. Sidhu

Introduction

The penis is well-suited for high-resolution ultrasound assessment; it is a superficial soft-tissue organ with no acoustic obstructions in the form of bone or gas. The role of ultrasound in the investigation of penile pathology, especially impotence, is well-established.[1] Conditions such as priapism, Peyronie disease, penile mass lesions, and the penile urethra may be usefully assessed by ultrasound. High-resolution gray-scale imaging, at frequencies from 7–13 MHz, alone or in combination with color and spectral Doppler, forms the basis of ultrasound evaluation. The addition of a pharmacological stimulant to produce an erection is established practice for evaluation of vascular causes of erectile dysfunction. This chapter will illustrate the techniques, normal and abnormal findings, and some of the pitfalls of penile ultrasonography with specific emphasis on the investigation of erectile dysfunction.

Normal Anatomy and Ultrasound Appearances

The penis is comprised of three cylindrical structures of erectile tissue: two dorsal corpora cavernosa and a ventral corpus spongiosum containing the penile urethra. The spongiosum is smaller proximally but expands distally to form the glans penis. The cavernosa are markedly distensible and are filled with sinusoidal tissue, which is essential to the erectile process. A tough, nondistensible fibrous capsule, the tunica albuginea, invests the corpora cavernosa with a much thinner layer covering the corpus spongiosum. The normal arterial supply to the penis is via the internal pudendal artery (a branch of the anterior division of the internal iliac artery), which divides into terminal branches: The dorsal penile artery (supplying the glans penis), the cavernosal artery (supplying the corpora cavernosa), and the bulbar artery (supplying the bulb and the corpus spongiosum). The cavernosal arteries give the main contribution to erectile function but anatomical variations are not uncommon. Emissary veins pierce the tunica albuginea and drain into the deep dorsal vein via the spongiosal, circumflex, and cavernosal veins (Fig. 12.1).[2]

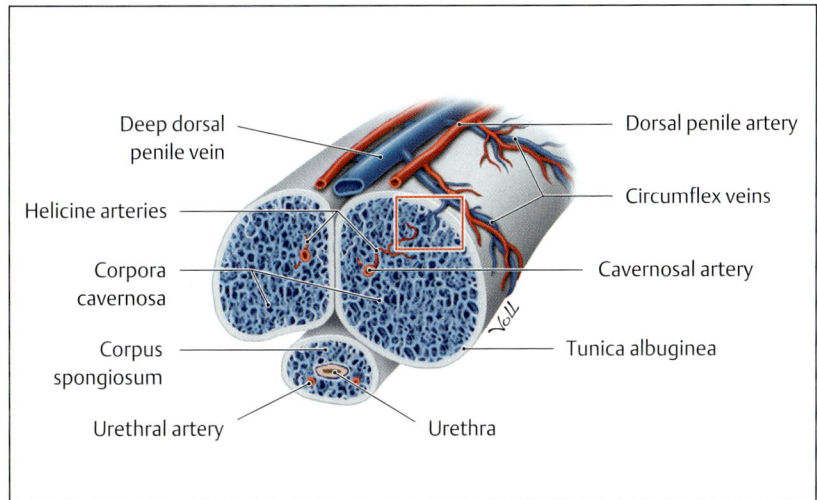

Fig. 12.1 Diagram of the anatomy of the penis

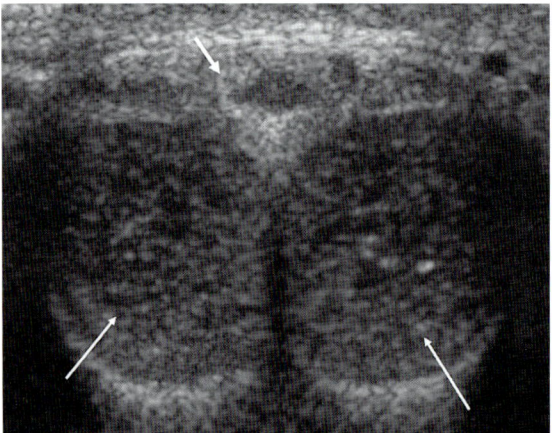

Fig. 12.2 **Transverse dorsal image of the flaccid penis,** demonstrating the paired corpora cavernosa (long arrows) and the higher reflectivity corpus spongiosum (short arrow)

Ultrasound identifies the paired corpora cavernosa, the cavernosal arteries, the tunica albuginea, and the corpus spongiosum. The corpora cavernosa are of uniform low reflectivity and the tunica can be seen as a thin high-reflective envelope (< 2 mm thick) surrounding the corpora. The corpus spongiosum is of slightly higher reflectivity. The reflective walls of the cavernosal arteries are usually clearly identified at the base of the penis and can often be identified as two parallel, high-reflective lines (Fig. 12.2).[3] The normal urethra is not identified.

Summary points:
- Ventral, high-reflective corpus spongiosum expands to form glans penis
- Dorsal paired low-reflective corpora cavernosa
  - Enveloped by the thin, highly reflective tunica albuginea
  - Distensible sinusoidal tissue essential for erectile function
- Internal pudendal artery divides into
  - Dorsal penile artery
  - Bulbar artery
  - Cavernosal arteries
- Venous drainage via the superficial and deep dorsal veins
  - Emissary veins pierce the tunica albuginea, draining into dorsal veins via cavernosal, spongiosal, and circumflex veins
  - The emissary vein/tunica region is the site of the veno-occlusive mechanism

Erectile Dysfunction

Erectile dysfunction is a common problem, affecting 20–30 million men in the United States.[4] The cause of impotence is multifactorial, but exclusion of an arterial and/or a venous cause is frequently required. Color and spectral Doppler ultrasound is the ideal, minimally-invasive technique for delineation of vascular abnormalities. A trial of sildenafil is often the first diagnostic test in patients likely to have an arteriogenic component to their erectile dysfunction; only nonresponders undergo further evaluation with color and spectral Doppler ultrasound. A reduction in requirements for Doppler ultrasound assessment of erectile dysfunction has resulted as sildenafil also serves as a therapeutic option for responders. There remains, however, a specific subset of usually younger patients in whom venogenic impotence is more likely. These patients form the bulk of current practice with a specific protocol designed to exclude a "false" venous leak in order to avoid the use of cavernosography in the majority of these patients.

Following formal clinical evaluation in an erectile dysfunction (ED) clinic, Doppler ultrasound assessment is conducted in a private setting. An attending urologist with a special interest in ED is ideally present. In general, the urologist undertakes intracavernosal injections, assesses the grade of erection, and counsels the patient regarding the risk of priapism. Several combinations of agents have been used for pharmacological induction of erection, either alone or in combination.[5,6] Current practice is to use prostaglandin E1 (PGE1) with or without the addition of intracavernosal phentolamine.

Baseline Imaging

A high-frequency linear "small parts" probe with a small footprint should be used. The penis is held in the anatomical position by the patient and baseline B-mode ultrasound imaging is performed in longitudinal and transverse planes. High-resolution gray-scale imaging should always be performed prior to assessment of vascular status. Important abnormalities include fibrotic plaque disease, focal cavernosal fibrosis or calcification, and tunica disruption. Baseline imaging allows optimum identification of injection sites and location of the cavernosal arteries; anatomical variants are common. Additionally, if baseline imaging is omitted, a spurious diagnosis of calcification/fibrosis of the corpora may be raised following inadvertent intracavernosal injection of air bubbles.

Stimulated Color Doppler Ultrasound

Current practice is to use PGE1 at a dose of 20 μg.[7] In the setting of maximal stimulation following this dose of PGE1 there is a risk of priapism with a reported incidence as high as 11%.[8] On ultrasound, absence of cavernosal artery flow or a resistive index (RI) > 1.00 (absent diastolic flow) is thought to be highly specific in predicting priapism; if seen during the poststimulation ultrasound examination, either immediate treatment or "in-hospital" observation is recommended.[9] However, experience suggests that absence of diastolic flow is a frequent occurrence in the "normal" responder, and is not a sinister finding leading to priapism. The alternative is to use a two-step method of sequential doses of PGE1 10 μg if the response to the first dose is suboptimal, but the examination is significantly shortened with the single-dose method. An expectant "wait and see" approach with patients given direct access to on-site urological opinion if their erection persists for more than four hours is a suggested policy.

Ultrasound Imaging Protocol

The right or left cavernosal artery may be interrogated with ultrasound; the normal diameter ranges from 0.2 to 1.0 mm and a variable increase in dimension is seen following pharmacological stimulation. However, the increase in the baseline diameter following pharmacological stimulation does not correlate with either the measured peak systolic velocity (PSV) or clinical grading of erection and it is not routine to measure arterial diameters.[10] It is normal practice to document a baseline angle-corrected PSV of the cavernosal artery selected for interrogation and to sample the same area on subsequent measurements. It has been suggested that spectral Doppler ultrasound analysis of the cavernosal artery in the flaccid penis provides a completely noninvasive method for assessment of arterial impotence.[11,12] However, the normal velocity criteria have not been established and no data regarding venous abnormalities can be obtained without pharmacostimulation.[12]

A customary response to pharmacostimulation allows color Doppler ultrasound depiction of the cavernosal arteries and the helicine branches (Fig. 12.3). Decreasing reflectivity of the corpora cavernosa from the periarterial region outward is seen as sinusoidal dilatation progresses (Fig. 12.4). Power, color, and spectral Doppler ultrasound all yield useful information regarding vascular anomalies and normal variants. Abnormal venous flow may also be directly visualized but cannot be measured objectively.

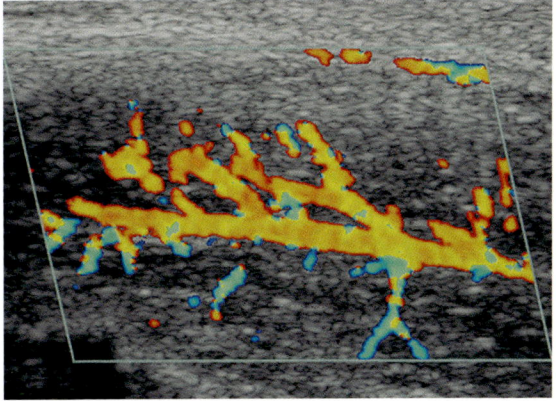

Fig. 12.3 Following pharmacostimulation, a longitudinal image through the corpora cavernosum demonstrates the cavernosal artery and helicine branches

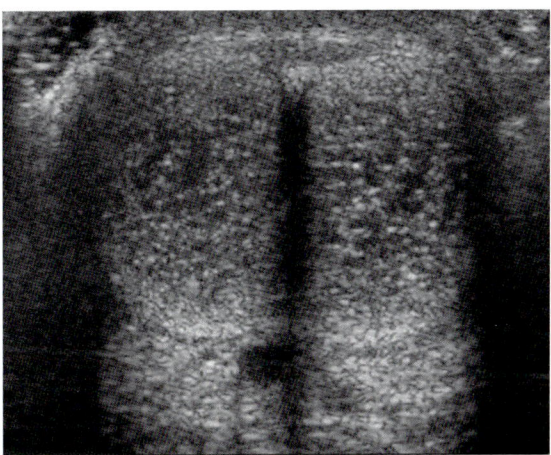

Fig. 12.4 **Transverse ventral image of the poststimulation penis,** demonstrating the paired corpora cavernosa filling with pockets of low-reflective blood as the penis becomes engorged

Assessment of Arterial Impotence

Following the pharmacological induction of an erection, dynamic assessment of the spectral Doppler waveform is performed. Color mapping of the vessels allows accurate spectral assessment by enabling consistent Doppler gate placement and angle correction.[13] Variations in the vascular supply are common[8,14] and include duplication of the cavernosal artery and cross communications between left and right cavernosal arteries (Fig. 12.5). If there is definite asymmetry, this should be documented and both arteries sampled during the course of the assessment. Additionally, color Doppler ultrasound allows visual recognition of high-velocity "jets" and damped pulsatility secondary to a proximal arterial stenosis, allowing specific interrogation with accurate spectral gate placement.

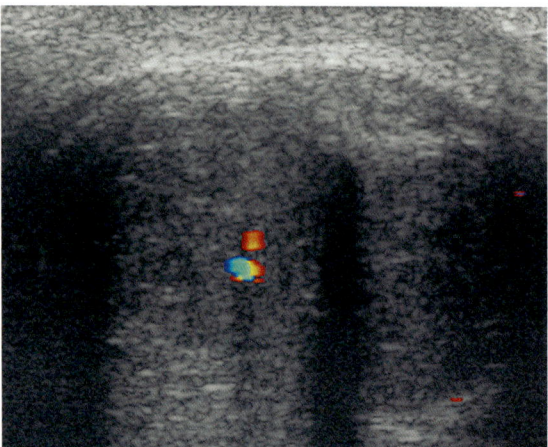

Fig. 12.**5 Transverse ventral image of the poststimulation penis,** demonstrating the paired corpora cavernosa with two arteries present on the right

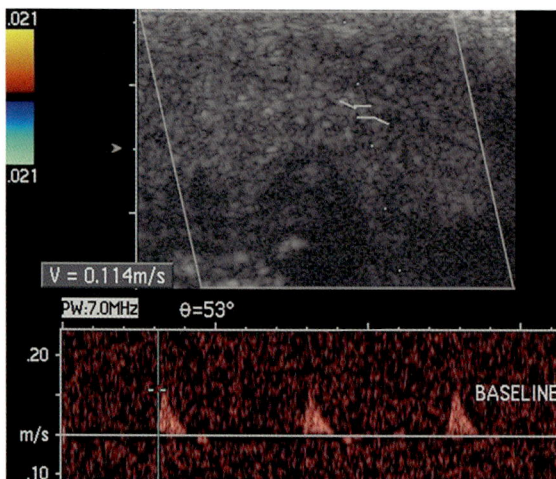

Fig. 12.**6 Baseline prestimulation assessment of the right cavernosal artery,** demonstrating the expected spectral Doppler waveform of the artery with a PSV measured at 11.4 cm/s. The baseline artery may be difficult to locate and often does not return a Doppler signal sufficient to obtain a spectral Doppler waveform

The cavernosal artery should be sampled at the base of the penis (Fig. 12.**6**). At this site, more consistent velocity readings are obtained, it is possible to achieve the optimal angle of insonation and the effect of distal arterial variants is reduced.[13] The PSV and end diastolic velocity (EDV) are assessed every five minutes after the administration of PGE1[15] and the clinical response documented every 15 minutes according to an accepted grading system.[16] Self-stimulation has been advocated as an adjunct to pharmacological stimulation in order to obtain a maximal response.[17]

Following pharmacostimulation there is a variable temporal response. A characteristic sequence of changes in the spectral Doppler waveform, with increasing penile rigidity, has been described. There is increased systolic and diastolic flow early in tumescence. Diastolic flow then decreases and there is eventually minimal or reversed diastolic flow as veno-occlusion and maximal rigidity occur.[18] Forward systolic flow often decreases at full rigidity prior to the detumescent phase when diastolic flow returns. Assessment over 30 minutes is occasionally required to ensure that the maximal effect has been attained, although 20 minutes is normally sufficient.[19] The accepted "normal" lower limits for the PSV range from 25 to 35 cm/s. A PSV of 35 cm/s or greater indicates definite arterial sufficiency following adequate pharmacological stimulation (Fig. 12.**7**), whereas a PSV < 25 cm/s is diagnostic of arterial insufficiency as the cause of ED (Fig. 12.**8**). Intermediate values are not specific and in this group sildenafil is often used as some will have mild to moderate arterial insufficiency and may benefit.[20]

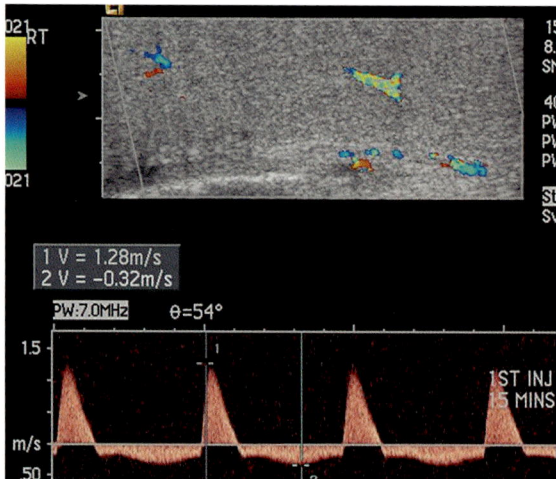

Fig. 12.**7 Normal response demonstrated on spectral Doppler ultrasound 15 minutes after administration of 10 μg of PGE1.** The PSV is 128 cm/s and the EDV is −32 cm/s, accompanied by full tumescence. The patient has an intact arteriovenous mechanism and another cause for ED should be sought

Assessment of Venogenic Impotence

There is continuing debate about the utility of color Doppler ultrasound in the diagnosis of venogenic impotence.[21,22] Cavernosography with cavernosometry remains the diagnostic reference standard, as this technique measures outflow resistance without the need for adequate arterial inflow.[23] The advantage of ultrasound lies in the minimally-invasive nature of the procedure and the ability to screen patients to identify a normal

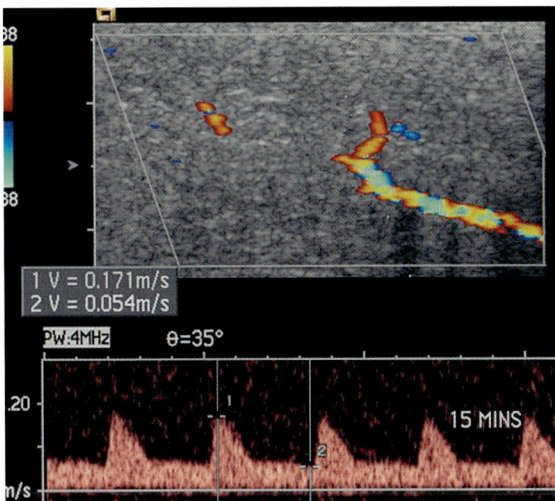

Fig. 12.8 **Arterial insufficiency demonstrated on spectral Doppler ultrasound, 15 minutes after administration of 20 μg of PGE1.** The PSV is 17.1 cm/s and the EDV is 5.4 cm/s, accompanied by incomplete tumescence. In the presence of inadequate arterial input, a diagnosis of venous leak cannot be made

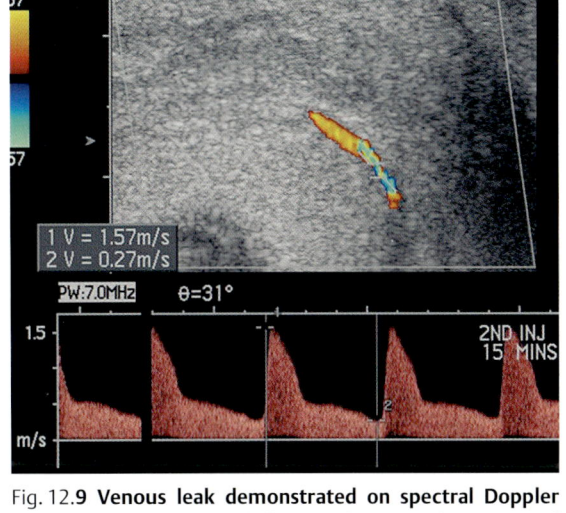

Fig. 12.9 **Venous leak demonstrated on spectral Doppler ultrasound, 15 minutes following the second injection of 10 μg of PGE1.** The PSV is 157 cm/s and the EDV is 27 cm/s, accompanied by incomplete tumescence. In the presence of adequate arterial input, there is a sustained high forward flow in diastole: features of failure of the mechanism of venous closure

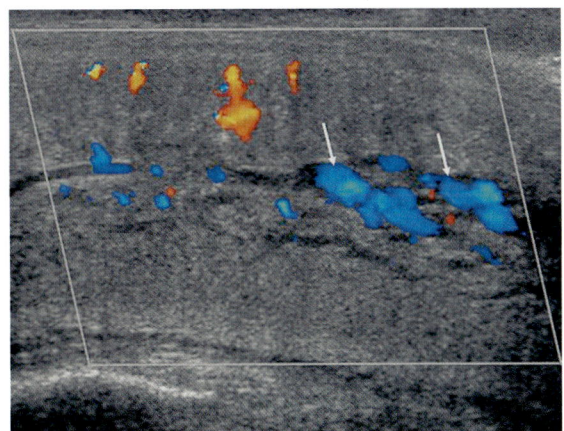

Fig. 12.10 **a** Poststimulation longitudinal image through the right corpora cavernosum, demonstrating venous channels (arrows) separate from the right cavernosal artery.

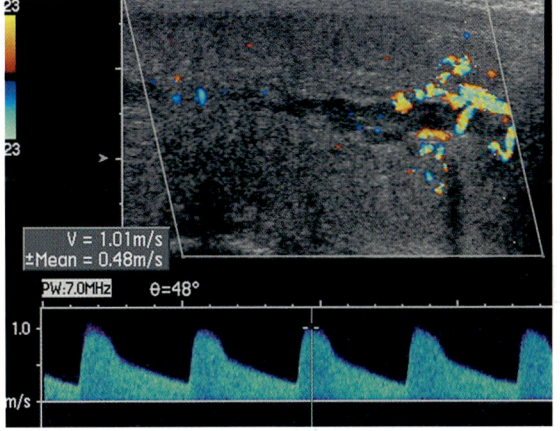

b Doppler interrogation of the right cavernosal artery confirms a waveform pattern of a venous leak (PSV of 101 cm/s and continuing high forward flow in diastole)

erectile response. Following a positive color Doppler ultrasound for a venous leak, cavernosography is generally still required for anatomical delineation of the draining veins if surgical or endovascular therapy is being contemplated.[24,25]

Having established a normal arterial response with a PSV > 35 cm/s, an EDV of > 5 cm/s is usually accepted as the level above which a venous leak is present (Fig. 12.9).[21,22] In practice in young patients with good arterial input, reversal of EDV should normally be seen and it may be appropriate to lower the EDV threshold in this group. As well as forward diastolic flow in the cavernosal artery, continuous flow in the dorsal vein or other abnormal draining veins may also be seen, but is not a requisite for the diagnosis (Fig. 12.10).

False Positive Venous Leak

In young patients, a suboptimal response to pharmacological stimulation with PGE1 may occur and manifests as continued forward flow in diastole. This results from inadequate relaxation of sinusoidal smooth muscle and consequent failure of veno-occlusion due to high anxiety levels and increased sympathetic drive. Phentolamine, an alpha-adrenergic antagonist, attenuates the effect of this increased sympathetic tone, resulting in

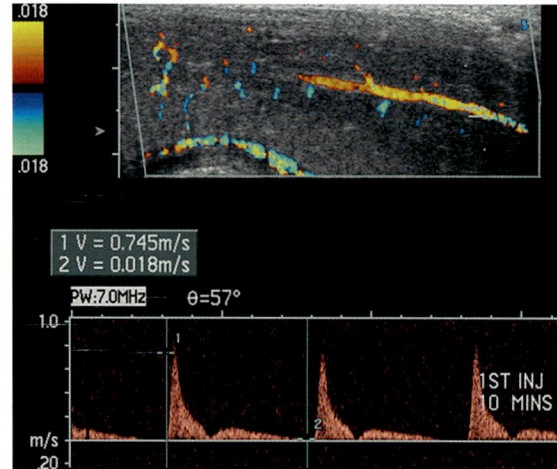

Fig. 12.**11 a** Ten minutes following the second injection of 10 μg of PGE1, the PSV is 74.5 cm/s and the EDV is 1.8 cm/s, accompanied by incomplete tumescence. The EDV remained above baseline at 20 minutes, with incomplete tumescence.

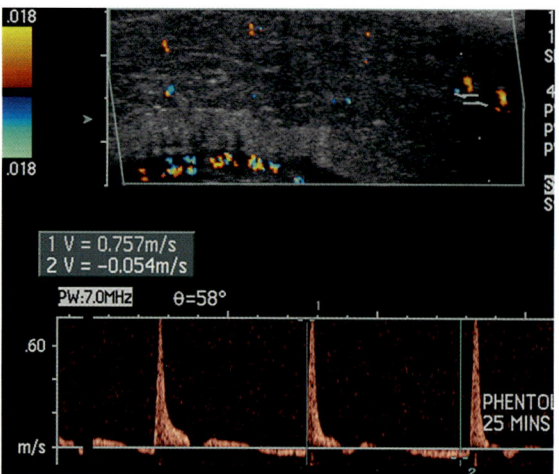

b Addition of 2 mg of phentolamine after continuing elevation of the EDV 25 minutes following the administration of 20 μg of PGE1. The PSV is 75.7 cm/s and the EDV is –5.4 cm/s, accompanied by complete tumescence, excluding venous leak. There has been narrowing of the spectral Doppler trace in comparison to the previous image

better sinusoidal relaxation.[26] When an apparent venous leak is identified in such patients, we supplement the examination with administration of 2 mg of intracavernosal phentolamine. Following phentolamine, many of these patients exhibit statistically significant increases in the grade of erection and PSV, and a decrease in EDV, often with abolition of the apparent venous leak diagnosed by conventional color and spectral Doppler ultrasound criteria (Fig. 12.**11**).[27]

Administration of phentolamine following an initial dose of PGE1 is safe and has increased diagnostic sensitivity when compared with a repeat dose of PGE1 alone.[28] The use of intracavernosal phentolamine would therefore seem necessary before a venous leak can be diagnosed by dynamic ultrasound assessment in the younger patient. Of greater importance, phentolamine, as an oral preparation, may offer a therapeutic approach in this very specific group of patients.[29,30] Venous leak not reversed by phentolamine is highly predictive of a structurally-based abnormality and cavernosometry with a view to surgical repair might then be recommended.

Summary points:
Stimulated Color Doppler Ultrasound Technique
- Patient explanation and consent for risk of priapism
- High-frequency small parts transducer (7–14 MHz)
- Baseline imaging for fibrosis, plaque, and arterial identification
- Arterial interrogation should be as proximal as possible at the base of the penis with color flow to direct spectral Doppler gate placement
- If significant asymmetry is noted (> 10 cm/s between sides), mapping of anatomical variants should be performed; this may also indicate unilateral arterial disease, e.g. following trauma

Hemodynamic Parameters for Stimulated Color Doppler Ultrasound Technique
- Adequate arterial inflow if PSV > 35 cm/s
- Borderline arterial inflow if PSV < 35 cm/s but > 25 cm/s
- Arterial insufficiency if PSV < 25 cm/s
- Given PSV > 35 cm/s venous leak is diagnosed if EDV < 0 cm/s
- Reversal of end diastolic flow is expected in younger patients with an adequate arterial inflow
- Phentolamine may be required in young patients to avoid spurious diagnosis of venous leak secondary to anxiety-induced adrenergic drive

Vascular Pathology

Priapism

Priapism is divided into "high-flow" and "low-flow" states.[31] In high-flow priapism, for example from a posttraumatic arteriovenous fistula (AVF), abnormally high arterial inflow cannot be fully compensated by increased venous outflow and leads to persistent tumescence but rarely full rigidity. B-mode ultrasound imaging usually reveals engorgement of the corpora with periarterial hypoechogenicity in association with an elevated cavernosal artery PSV and high forward diastolic flow at spectral Doppler ultrasound examination (Fig. 12.**12**). The draining veins are often prominent and may exhibit arterialized waveforms. In long-standing cases, penile edema may be a prominent feature (Fig. 12.**13**). Clinically there is usually painless tumescence with arterial oxygenated blood in the corpora cavernosa.[32] Selective arterial embolization of the internal pudendal or cavernosal artery is often the first line management of high-flow arterial priapism.[33,34] The site of an AVF may be imaged directly and allow selective embolization of the ipsilateral cavernosal artery alone.

Low-flow priapism occurs following veno-occlusive problems, for example in sickle cell patients, with a full and often painful erection; there is deoxygenated blood on corporal aspiration.[35,36] Ultrasound may be helpful in the acute stage in those patients who do not respond to simple measures such as evacuation of the corpora or alpha-adrenergic agonist injection (usually phenylephrine). Findings are of low or absent diastolic flow with variable, but usually not high, arterial inflow consistent with a high-resistance vascular bed. Low-flow priapism requires prompt early treatment as there is relative hypoxia and in resistant cases a surgical shunt (corporospongiosal or corporovenous) may be required to prevent subsequent cavernosal fibrosis.[37]

In the long term, ultrasound is used to assess fibrosis and erectile dysfunction secondary to hypoxic damage from chronic priapism. In addition, the return of flow following recanalization of previously embolized arteries can be demonstrated and indicates a favorable outcome.[38,39]

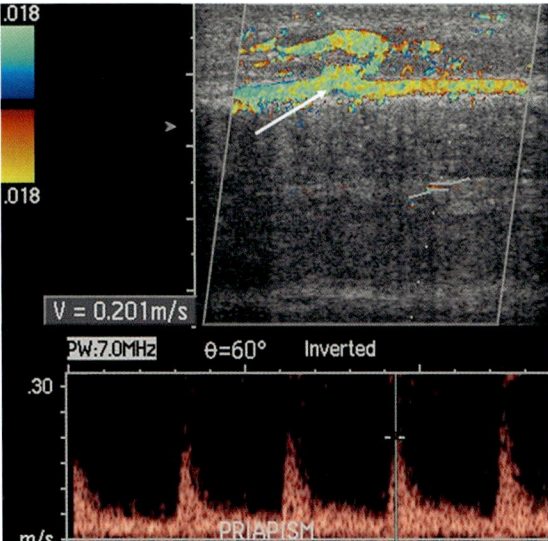

Fig. 12.**12** "High-flow" priapism with an elevated PSV in the right cavernosal artery of 20.1 cm/s with increased flow in the veins (arrow). The spectral Doppler waveform is of a low-resistance pattern, suggesting patency of the draining veins

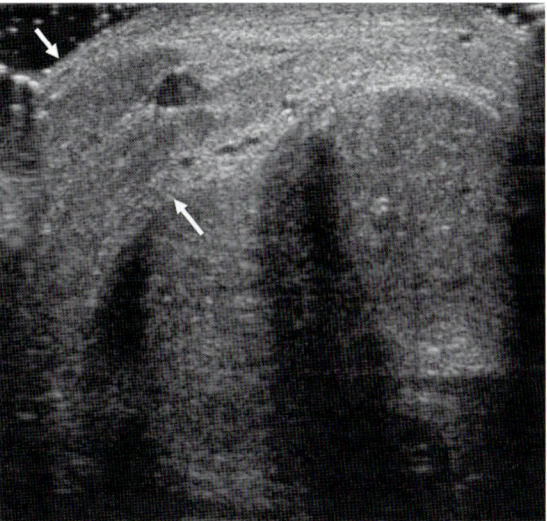

Fig. 12.**13** "High-flow" priapism with marked edema of the skin (arrows) and dilated corpora cavernosa

> **Summary points:**
> High-flow priapism
> - Oxygenated corporal blood on aspiration
> - Spectral Doppler waveforms show continuous increased systolic and diastolic flow with a low-resistance pattern
> - In the posttraumatic patient an AVF may be identified and can guide therapy
>
> Low-flow priapism
> - Deoxygenated corporal blood on aspiration
> - Spectral Doppler waveforms show low or no diastolic flow with a high resistance pattern
> - Edema
>
> Differentiation is necessary as a low-flow priapism requires urgent treatment

Structural Pathology

Penile Fibrosis

Peyronie Disease

Peyronie disease is characterized by the formation of plaques in the tunica albuginea of the penis, resulting in pain and curvature of the erect penis. The occurrence is highest in the 40–60-year-old group, where the incidence is estimated at 0.4–1.0%. The cause of Peyronie disease is poorly understood. Factors associated with Peyronie disease include trauma, vascular, disease, diabetes mellitus, and there is also a genetic component. The clinical diagnosis is based on the presence of pain, plaque formation, and angulation on erection. The plaques occur most often on the dorsal shaft of the penis and are readily palpated.

On ultrasound the plaques of Peyronie disease may be of low or high reflectivity,[40] and, if long-standing, often contain calcification (Fig. 12.**14**).[41] These lie between the corpora cavernosa and may be difficult to demonstrate on ultrasound if not calcified, but are nearly always palpable. Focal or diffuse thickening of the tunica (which becomes more apparent following pharmacological stimulation) may be the only ultrasound feature.[42] Ultrasound imaging at the site of maximal penile deviation, if present, or at the site of a palpable lesion, will invariably demonstrate an abnormality. In patients with Peyronie's disease there is not only a higher incidence of venous impotence, secondary to distortion of the tunica albuginea, but also an increased incidence of arterial and mixed vascular abnormalities.[43] B-mode assessment of calcification allows patient selection for lithotripsy therapy, and color Doppler ultrasound examination is important prior to possible corrective surgery to ascertain the course of the cavernosal arteries in relation to plaques.[44]

Iatrogenic Fibrosis

In patients treated with intracavernosal stimulation therapy for ED, in particular with papaverine, areas of penile fibrosis may develop.[45] This may be severe enough to require cessation of treatment, and ultrasound examination can delineate areas of fibrosis allowing follow-up and guiding decisions on therapy.[46] In some patients there may be intracorporal calcification without any associated plaque and this is thought to result from regions of focal fibrosis or possibly previous trauma (Fig. 12.**15**).[3]

> **Summary points:**
> - In Peyronie disease, plaques may or may not be calcified
> - In the flaccid state plaques can be difficult to visualize, but may become apparent during tumescence; image at the site of maximal curvature
> - Both arterial and venous diseases are more common in Peyronie disease—mixed cause is often present requiring careful assessment to guide therapy
> - Plaques and/or fibrosis may occur following treatment with PGE1 and can necessitate cessation of treatment

Tunica Albuginea Defect

Congenital or acquired tunica albuginea defects may be visualized. A focal weakness in the tunica may lead to herniation of the corpora cavernosa with attendant venous leak due to failure of compression of the emissary veins (Fig. 12.**16**).[47]

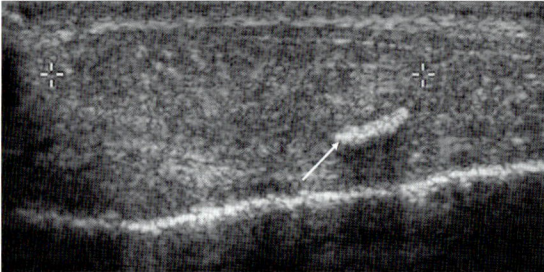

Fig. 12.**14** Plaque of fibrosis (between cursors) with a calcified focus (arrow), causing an acoustic shadow typical of Peyronie disease, demonstrated on a longitudinal image of the corpora cavernosum

Penile Fracture

Penile fracture usually presents acutely with a history of pain, swelling, and sudden loss of erection during intercourse.[48] Ultrasound can be useful both in the acute and chronic phases. Acute hematoma, secondary to simple superficial vessel rupture, or more importantly, a tunica albuginea defect (which usually requires immediate surgical management) can often be identified (Fig. 12.17). Ultrasound aids diagnosis in cases where the history or clinical findings are atypical. Documentation of the site and extent of fracture is relevant since the results of early surgical repair are favorable.[49,50] Complications of penile fracture include corporal fibrosis with or without plaque formation, disruption of the tunica albuginea, and rarely urethral disruption. Impotence due to impairment of the veno-occlusive mechanism may also occur. Ultrasound may be used both to guide initial management and for long-term follow-up of these patients.[51]

Penile Masses

Differentiation of a variety of penile masses on ultrasound is possible; these include hematoma, cavernosal herniation, and Peyronie's plaques. Penile hematoma is usually secondary to trauma to the erect penis and has a variable appearance depending the time of imaging and the stage of evolution. Acutely it may be of high reflectivity and, as resolution occurs, decreased reflectivity with or without cystic regions is often seen. Cavernosal herniation is usually easily diagnosed by visualization of the tunica defect, isoreflective corporal tissue seen in continuity, and, if large, color or power Doppler visualization of vascular continuity with the corpora proper.

In addition, penile carcinoma and, rarely, metastatic tumor deposits may be visualized. Penile carcinoma is usually identified as a superficial, low-reflective mass involving the glans penis and, although ultrasound is not particularly useful in local staging, it may be helpful in defining the anatomical relationships of larger tumors and assessing invasion of the tunica albuginea and corpora.[52] Penile carcinoma primarily involving the corpora cavernosa is rare but may be identified on ultrasound as an irregular mixed, low-reflective region within the corpora with areas of increased color flow (Fig. 12.18). Occasionally the penis may be the site of secondary deposits and, although secondary deposits are often better defined on ultrasound examination, the appearances are broadly similar to those of primary penile cancer involving the corpora.[53] A further unusual "mass" which may be encountered is a penile prosthesis, easily identifiable by parallel high-reflective walls and symmetrical structure.

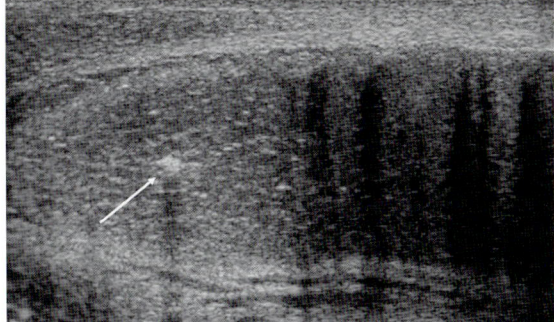

Fig. 12.15 Longitudinal image of the glans penis, demonstrating a reflective focus causing acoustic shadowing (arrow), which is likely to represent an area of focal fibrosis/calcification

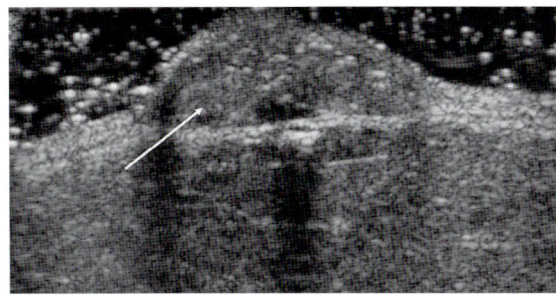

Fig. 12.16 Following PGE1 stimulation, a longitudinal image demonstrates a tunica albuginea defect, with associated herniation of corpora cavernosa tissue, of unknown cause (arrow)

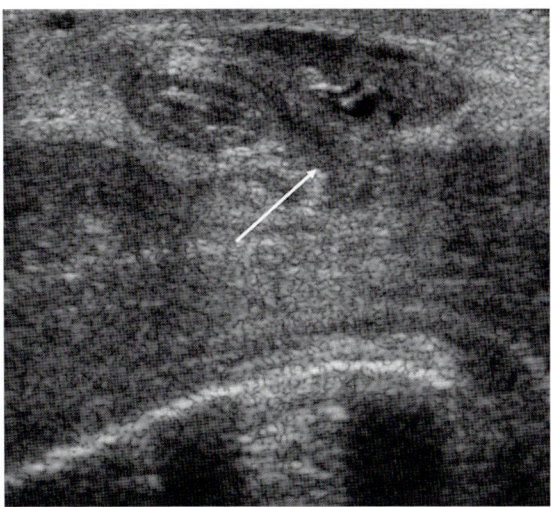

Fig. 12.17 A longitudinal image of a penile fracture with the defect in the reflective tunica albuginea being clearly identifiable. Hematoma formation has occurred (arrow)

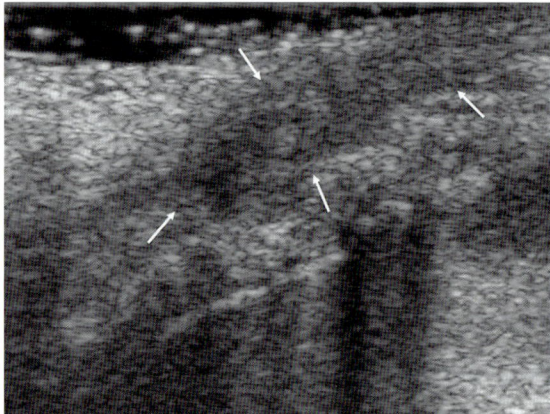

Fig. 12.18 A mixed-reflective intracorporeal lesion (arrows), which is relatively poorly defined and demonstrates features of malignancy

Other masses occurring in the penis include those found in the skin and subcutaneous tissues elsewhere, including cysts, lipomas, and neurofibromata, and are imaged in the same manner as those found at other sites.

Urethral Ultrasound

A combination of contrast urethrography and urethroscopy is utilized for the investigation of urethral pathology, and the practice of urethral ultrasound is limited to a few enthusiasts.[54]

The normal urethra is only visualized on ultrasound when distended with fluid. This may be achieved by instilling lignocaine gel or normal saline in a retrograde direction via the urethral meatus in a manner analogous to conventional urethrography. Alternatively, antegrade passage of urine with constriction of outflow at the glans by means of a clamp or the patients hand during the ultrasound examination may be utilized. Imaging is performed in longitudinal and transverse planes.

The normal urethra distends to approximately 6 mm with smooth, highly reflective walls. Strictures, intraluminal masses, and calculi are well-visualized. The main disadvantage compared to contrast urethrography is that the posterior urethra cannot be imaged. The strengths of the technique are that the periurethral tissues are identified and the degree of fibrosis outside a stricture can be demonstrated; if this is prolific then simple urethrotomy is less likely to succeed and open repair may be considered. Similar information may also be gained from intraurethral ultrasound using scope-mounted scanners. Follow-up of strictures is possible without any ionizing radiation burden. This technique has also been successfully employed in hypospadias, a condition more difficult to image using conventional techniques.[55]

References

1. King BF. The penis. In: Rumack CM, Wilson SR, Charboneau JW, eds. Diagnostic ultrasound. St. Louis: Mosby Year Book: 1997:823–842.
2. Williams PL, Warwick R, Dyson M, Bannister LH. Splanchnology. In: Williams PL, Warwick R, Dyson M, Bannister LH, eds. Gray's Anatomy. London: Churchill Livingstone: 1989: 1432–1433.
3. Doubilet PM, Benson CB, Silverman SG, Gluck CD. The penis. Sem Ultrasound, CT, MRI 1991;12:157–175.
4. Benet AE, Melman A. The epidemiology of erectile dysfunction. Urol Clin North Am 1995;22:699–709.
5. Eardley I, Sethia K. Intracorporal injection therapy. In: Eardley I, Sethia K, eds. Erectile dysfunction. Current investigation and management. London: Mosby-Wolfe: 1998:77–88.
6. van Halen H, Peskar BA, Sticht G, Hertfelder HJ. Pharmacokinetics of vasoactive substances administered into the human corpus cavernosum. J Urol 1994;151:1227–1230.
7. Kim SC, Seo KK, Park BD, Lee SW. Risk factors for an early increase in dose of vasoactive agents for intracavernous pharmacotherapy. Urol Int 2000;65:204–207.
8. Patel U, Amin Z, Friedman E, Vale J, Kirby RW, Lees WR. Colour flow and spectral Doppler imaging after papaverine-induced penile erection in 220 impotent men: study of temporal patterns and the importance of repeated sampling, velocity asymmetry and vascular anomalies. Clin Radiol 1993;48:18–24.
9. Cormio L, Bettocchi C, Ricapito V, Zizzi V, Traficante A, Selvaggi FP. Resistive index as a prognostic factor for prolonged erection after penile dynamic colour Doppler ultrasonography. Eur Urol 1998;33:94–97.
10. Patel U, Lees WR. Penile sonography. In: Solibiati L, Rizzatto G, eds. Ultrasound of superficial structures. London: Churchill Livingstone: 1995:229–242.
11. Roy C, Saussine C, Tuchmann C, Castel E, Lang H, Jacqmin D. Duplex Doppler sonography of the flaccid penis: potential role in the evaluation of impotence. J Clin Ultrasound 2000;28:290–294.
12. Mancini M, Bartolini M, Maggi M, Innocenti P, Villari N, Forti G. Duplex ultrasound evaluation of cavernosal peak systolic velocity and waveform acceleration in the penile flaccid state: clinical significance in the assessment of the arterial supply in patients with erectile dysfunction. Int J Androl 2000;23:199–204.
13. Kim SH, Paick JS, Lee SE, Choi BI, Yeon KM, Han MC. Doppler sonography of deep cavernosal artery of the penis: variation of peak systolic velocity according to sampling location. J Ultrasound Med 1994;13:591–594.
14. Mancini M, Bartolini M, Maggi M, Innocenti P, Forti G. The presence of arterial anatomical variations can affect the results of duplex sonographic evaluation of penile vessels in impotent patients. J Urol 1996;155:1919–1923.
15. Govier FE, Asase D, Hefty TR, McClure RD, Pritchett TR, Weissman RM. Timing of penile color flow duplex ultrasonography using a triple drug mixture. J Urol 1995;153: 1472–1475.

16. Virag R, Frydman D, Legman M, Virag H. Intracavernous injection of papaverine as diagnostic and therapeutic method in erectile failure. Angiology 1984;35:79–83.
17. Montorsi F, Guazzoni G, Barbieri L, Galli L, Rigatti P, Pizzini G, et al. The effect of intracorporeal injection plus genital and audiovisual sexual stimulation versus second injection on penile color Doppler sonography parameters. J Urol 1996;155:536–540.
18. Lue TF. Erectile dysfunction. N Engl J Med 2000;342: 1802–1813.
19. Chiou RK, Alberts GL, Pomeroy BD, Anderson JC, Carlson LK, Anderson JR, et al. Study of cavernosal arterial anatomy using color and power Doppler sonography: impact on hemodynamic parameter measurement. J Urol 1999; 162: 358–360.
20. Benson CB, Aruny JE, Vickers MA. Correlation of duplex sonography with arteriography in patients with erectile dysfunction. AJR Am J Roentgenol 1993;160:71–73.
21. Quam JP, King BF, James EM, Lewis RW, Brakke DM, Ilstrup DM, et al. Duplex and color Doppler sonographic evaluation of vasculogenic impotence. AJR Am J Roentgenol 1989;153:1141–1147.
22. Bassiouny HS, Levine LA. Penile duplex sonography in the diagnosis of venogenic impotence. J Vasc Surg 1991;13: 75–82.
23. Lue TF, Hricak H, Schmidt RA, Tanagho EA. Functional evaluation of penile veins by cavernosography in papaverine-induced erection. J Urol 1986;135:479–482.
24. Frust G, Muller-Mattheis V, Cohnen M, Trautner C, Haastert B, Saleh A, et al. Venous incompetence in erectile dysfunction: evaluation with color-coded duplex sonography and cavernosometery/-graphy. Euro Radiol 1999;9:35–41.
25. Fowlis GA, Sidhu PS, Jager HR, Agarwal S, Jackson JE, Zafar F, et al. Preliminary report: Combined surgical and radiological penile vein occlusion for the management of impotence caused by venous-sinusoidal incompetence. Br J Urol 1994;74:492–496.
26. Aversa A, Rocchietti-March M, Caprio M, Giannini D, Isidori A, Fabbri A. Anxiety-induced failure in erectile response to intracorporeal prostaglandin-E1 in non-organic male impotence: a new diagnostic approach. Int J Androl 1996;19: 307–313.
27. Gontero P, Sriprasad S, Wilkins CJ, Donaldson N, Muir GH, Sidhu PS. Phentolamine re-dosing during penile dynamic colour Doppler ultrasound: a practical method to abolish a false diagnosis of venous leakage in patients with erectile dysfunction. Br J Radiol 2004;77:922–926.
28. Aversa A, Bonifacio V, Moretti C, Frajese G, Fabbri A. Redosing of prostaglandin-E1 versus prostaglandin-E1 plus phentolamine in male erectile dysfunction: a dynamic color power Doppler study. Int J Impot Res 2000;12:33–40.
29. Goldstein I. Oral phentolamine: an alpha-1, alpha-2 adrenergic antagonist for the treatment of erectile dysfunction. Int J Impot Res 2000;12:75–80.
30. Wespes E, Rondeux C, Schulmann CC. Effect of phentolamine on venous return in human erection. Br J Urol 1989;63:95–97.
31. Harmon WJ, Nehra A. Priapism: diagnosis and management. Mayo Clin Proc 1997;72:350–355.
32. Bastuba MD, Saenz de Tejada I, Dinlenc CZ, Sarazen A, Krane RJ, Goldstein I. Arterial priapism: diagnosis, treatment and long-term follow-up. J Urol 1994;151: 1231–1237.
33. Walker TG, Grant PW, Goldstein I, Krane RJ, Greenfield AJ. "High-flow" priapism: treatment with superselective transcatheter embolization. Radiology 1990;174:1053–1054.
34. Kang BC, Lee DY, Byun JY, Baek SY, Lee SW, Kim KW. Posttraumatic arterial priapism: colour Doppler examination and superselective arterial embolization. Clin Radiol 1998; 53:830–834.
35. Hamre MR, Harmon EP, Kirkpatrick DV, Stern MJ, Humbert JR. Priapism as a complication of sickle cell disease. J Urol 1991;145:1–5.
36. Fowler JE, Koshy M, Strub M, Chinn SK. Priapism associated with sickle cell haemoglobinopthies: prevalence, natural history and sequelae. J Urol 1991;145:65–68.
37. Carter RG, Thomas CE, Tomskey GC. Cavernospongiosum shunts in the treatment of priapism. Urology 1976;7: 292–295.
38. Bastuba MD, Saenz dT, I, Dinlenc CZ, Sarazen A, Krane RJ, Goldstein I. Arterial priapism: diagnosis, treatment and long-term follow-up. J Urol 1994;151:1231–1237.
39. Goto T, Yagi S, Matsushita S, Uchida Y, Kawahara M, Ohi Y. Diagnosis and treatment of priapism: experience with 5 cases. Urology 1999;53:1019–1023.
40. Tunuguntla HS. Management of Peyronie's disease: a review. World J Urol 2001;19:244–250.
41. Chou YH, Tiu CM, Pan HB, Lin SN, Hsu CC, Wu CC, et al. High-resolution real-time ultrasound in Peyronie's disease. J Ultrasound Med 1987;6:67–70.
42. Brock G, Hsu GL, Nunes L, von Heyden B, Lue TF. The anatomy of the tunica albuginea in the normal penis and Peyronie's disease. J Urol 1997;157:276–281.
43. Kadioglu A, Tefekli A, Erol H, Cayan S, Kandirali E. Color Doppler ultrasound assessment of penile vascular system in men with Peyronie's disease. Int J Impotence Res 2000;12:263–267.
44. Levine LA, Coogan CL. Penile vascular assessment using color duplex sonography in men with Peyronie's disease. J Urol 1996;155:1270–1273.
45. Pery M, Rosenberger A, Kaftori JK, Vardi Y. Intracorporeal calcifications after self-injection of papaverine. Radiology 1990;176:81–83.
46. Chew KK, Stuckey BG, Earle CM, Dhaliwal SS, Keogh EJ. Penile fibrosis in intracavernosal prostaglandin E1 injection therapy for erectile dysfunction. Int J Impot Res 1997;9:225–229.
47. Mondaini N, Sriprasad S, Hopster D, Sidhu PS, Muir GH. Congenital herniation of cavernous tissue through the tunica albuginea with osseous metaplasia of the penis. Br J Urol Int 2002;89:971.
48. Zargooshi J. Penile fracture in Kermanshah, Iran: report of 172 cases. J Urology 2000;164:364–366.
49. Asgari MA, Hosseini SY, Safarinejad MR, Samdzadeh B, Bardideh AR. Penile fractures: evaluation, therapeutic approaches and long-term results. J Urology 1996;155: 148–149.
50. El Bahnasawy MS, Gomha MA. Penile fractures: the successful outcome of immediate surgical intervention. Int J Impot Res 2000;12:273–277.
51. Gontero P, Sidhu PS, Muir GH. Penile fracture repair: assessment of early results and complications using color Doppler ultrasound. Int J Impot Res 2000;12:125–129.
52. Horenblas S, Kroger R, Gallee MP, Newling DW, van Tinteren H. Ultrasound in squamous cell carcinoma of the penis;

a useful addition to clinical staging? A comparison of ultrasound with histopathology. Urology 1994;43:702–707.
53. Vapnek JM, Hricak H, Carroll PR. Recent advances in imaging studies for staging of penile and urethral carcinoma. Urol Clin North Am 1992;19:257–266.
54. Berman LH, Bearcroft PW, Spector S. Ultrasound of the male anterior urethra. Ultrasound Q 2002;18:123–133.
55. Toms AP, Bullock KN, Berman LH. Descending urethral ultrasound of the native and reconstructed urethra in patients with hypospadias. Br J Radiol 2003;76:260–263.

13 Oncological Management of Tumors of the Urogenital Tract

D. Dodds, V. Hughes

The treatment of all tumors affecting the entire urogenital tract is an extensive subject and cannot be covered in a relatively short chapter such as this.

We have therefore limited the discussion to the treatment of the four most common neoplasms, i.e., prostate, bladder, kidney, and testis. Increasingly, such neoplasms are treated in purpose-designed multidisciplinary clinics where patients can benefit from the expertise of specialist urological surgeons, as well as clinical and medical oncologists with a special interest in the treatment of genitourinary tumors. In addition, specialist urological nurses have an increasing role in patient management, providing information and support to patients and their families at what can be a difficult and stressful time. Discussion of the pathological features and radiological findings is an essential aspect of overall patient management and should ideally be undertaken in every patient diagnosed with a genitourinary neoplasm.

Treatment of Bladder Cancer

For the purpose of discussion, bladder cancer treatment is best divided into the treatment of superficial and muscle-invasive disease. Superficial disease includes those tumors which are noninvasive or invade only subepithelial tissue. In the United Kingdom, this disease is usually treated by urologists. Tumors invading into bladder-wall muscle and beyond are usually treated by oncologists (Fig. 13.1).

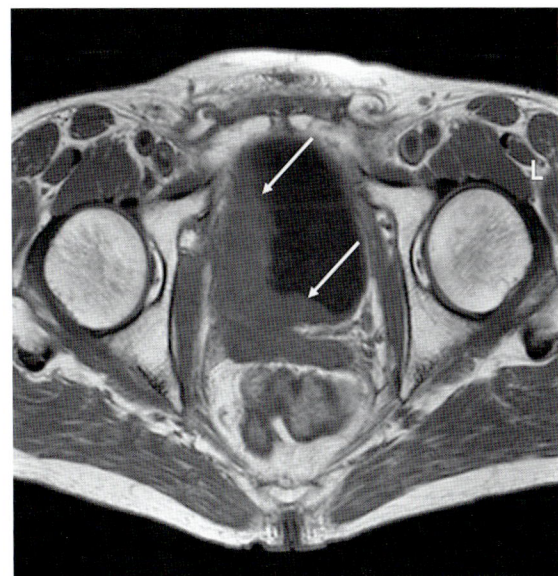

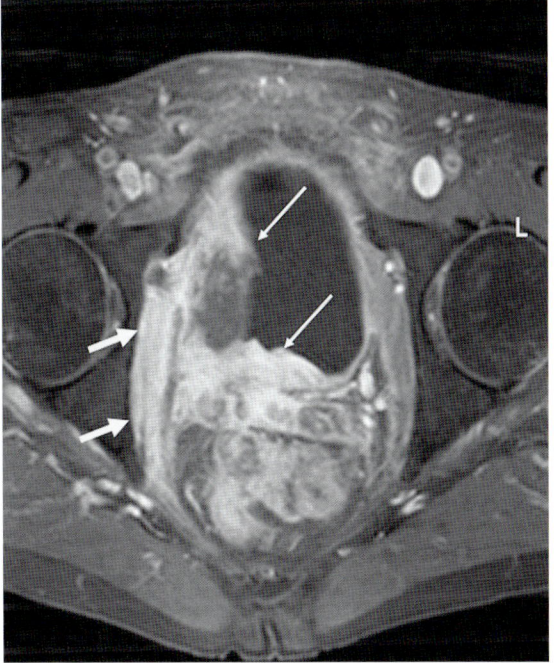

Fig. 13.1 **a** Axial T1-weighted magnetic resonance imaging (MRI) scan showing an extensive bladder tumor (arrows) involving the posterior and right lateral wall of the bladder with clear evidence of extravesical extension into the perivesical tissues. **b** Gadolinium-enhanced image of the same area showing the extensive primary lesion (arrows) with an area of central tumor necrosis. In addition, however, there is better delineation of the extravesical extension and marked contrast enhancement of the right obturator internus muscle (thick arrows) indicative of tumor involvement

Treatment of Superficial Disease

There are a number of prognostic factors associated with superficial disease, including the total number of tumors, histological grade, tumor size, and recurrence at three-month cystoscopy.[1,2] Low-grade papillary tumors can be treated by transurethral resection (TUR) alone or by thermocoagulation with a neodymium laser. Random biopsies of apparently healthy mucosa are also taken, as there can be a field change affecting the entire urothelium.

Intravesical Therapy

This therapy is given in order to either prevent recurrence following endoscopic resection or as definitive local therapy for unresectable superficial disease. A number of agents are available, including adriamycin, epirubicin, and mitomycin C. There is little to choose between these drugs in terms of efficacy and toxicity. A meta-analysis of randomized trials using this treatment showed that the disease-free interval could be prolonged with intravesical chemotherapy, but there was no impact on progression-free or overall survival.[3] Patients with adverse prognostic factors are usually advised to undergo a course of treatment although the most effective regimen is still undecided. Even a single installation given in the immediate postresection phase can be effective.[4] A common regimen is to prescribe mitomycin C or epirubicin weekly for six weeks and then reassess. There is little or no systemic toxicity with such treatment, but 6–40% of patients will develop symptoms secondary to chemical cystitis.

Prognosis

Patients with papillary noninvasive lesions can expect a five-year survival of 90%. This falls to 75% for T1 lesions. Superficial tumors of high grade are a distinct pathological entity with progress to muscle invasion in 50% of cases.[5]

Carcinoma in situ (CIS) also has an aggressive course and is treated in a similar way to high-grade superficial disease. Intravesical therapy is usually given first, with radical cystectomy reserved for chemotherapy failure. There is no effect on overall survival treating in this way.[6] A course of bacille Calmette–Guérin (BCG) therapy is given in these cases, often weekly for six weeks followed by reassessment. The mechanism of action of BCG is largely unknown but it is known to have immunomodulatory effects and also induces a major inflammatory reaction within the bladder mucosa. The response rate to this treatment is 70%. However, only about 30% remain tumor-free at 10 years.[7]

Treatment of Muscle-Invasive Disease

Following staging investigations to exclude distant metastases, patients considered to have localized bladder cancer can be offered either radical cystectomy or nonsurgical treatment with radiation or chemoradiation. Distant metastases are sought by means of chest x-ray (CXR), computed tomography (CT) of the abdomen and pelvis, magnetic resonance imaging (MRI) of the pelvis, and bone scanning if appropriate.

Factors to be considered in guiding patients in their decision include the following:
- The local extent of the tumor as indicated by cystoscopy and bimanual examination
- The local appearances on CT or MR imaging
- The presence of pelvic lymphadenopathy
- The general medical condition of the patient
- The presence of poor prognostic factors, e.g., anemia or hydronephrosis
- The wishes of the patient
- The pathological features, e.g. adenocarcinoma responds poorly to radiation
- The presence of CIS in random bladder biopsies

Radical cystectomy involves complete removal of bladder, prostate, and seminal vesicles in the male. In females, the corresponding operation involves removal of the bladder, cervix, uterus, fallopian tubes, and anterior vaginal wall.

Urine is then diverted into one of three reservoirs:
- Ileal conduit where both ureters are implanted into the terminal ileum and brought out as an incontinent stoma
- A continent reservoir where an intra-abdominal reservoir is fashioned from the stomach or bowel and urine drained by regular catheterization[8]
- Orthotopic bladder substitution where a similar reservoir is reanastamosed to the urethra[9]

The urethra should not be spared if the tumor involves the bladder neck or posterior urethra or in the presence of CIS.

The five-year survival rate for patients treated by cystectomy alone is between 15 and 80%, depending on staging. Retrospective surgical results are generally better than for radiation alone, but when allowance is made for confounding factors such as selection bias, stage migration, i.e., clinical versus pathological staging and prognostic factors, there is little difference in overall results and certainly no survival benefit. Cystectomy can also be offered in the event of local failure following radiotherapy, again with no effect on overall survival.

Nonsurgical options for localized or locally advanced disease include radiation alone, neoadjuvant and adjuvant chemotherapy, and concomitant chemoradiation.

Modern radiotherapy techniques utilize planning CT scans and carefully fractionated regimens to minimize toxicity and avoid the chances of a geographical miss on the tumor. Prior to treatment the bladder is emptied to decrease the volume. Treatment is usually given in small daily fractions for four to six weeks to a total dose of 52–60 Gray (Gy). The side effects of radical radiotherapy include radiation cystitis, proctitis, and lethargy. In the longer term urinary function may deteriorate due to bladder fibrosis, although this is not common.

Combined Modality Therapy

Attempts have been made to improve the results of local treatments by the integration of chemotherapy. The recognition that a significant number of patients die of metastatic disease without local failure made the introduction of systemic therapy attractive in this setting.

There have been a number of trials of chemotherapy given in a neoadjuvant setting, i.e., before definitive local therapy. The largest study reported to date is the MRC/EORTC Trial which examined the effect of three pulses of cisplatin-based chemotherapy before either cystectomy or radiation therapy. The survival benefit reported did not reach statistical significance, nor did the improvement in local control.[10] However, a recently published meta-analysis of neoadjuvant chemotherapy in bladder cancer has shown a 5% overall survival benefit for the use of multiagent cisplatin-based therapy irrespective of the type of local treatment.[11]

Chemotherapy given after surgery or radiation, i.e. in the adjuvant setting, has been less well-studied and no definite conclusions can be drawn at this time.

Concomitant Chemotherapy/Radiation

Chemotherapy agents can be utilized as radiation sensitizes and has direct cytotoxic activity. There have been a large number of phase II studies showing the safety and apparent efficacy of this approach.[12,13] The most commonly used agent is cisplatin, often combined with other drugs such as fluorouracil (5FU) and gemcitabine. In addition to which drugs are best to use, there are also questions concerning optimal timing of drug delivery in relation to radiation treatment, as well as the potential for induction chemotherapy. Most of the published data also points to the importance of maximal TUR of tumor before consideration is given to any form of bladder-sparing treatment. There is currently a large phase III trial recruiting in the United Kingdom using both 5FU and mitomycin C in combination with external beam radiation therapy.

Metastatic Disease

Despite improvements in local control, about 50% of patients with muscle-invasive disease will eventually die with widespread metastatic disease. Untreated, the mean survival of patients with metastatic disease is three to six months.[14] With modern multiagent chemotherapy this figure rises to about one year.[14] It is now well-established that multiagent, cisplatin-based regimens offer the best chance of response and survival benefit.[15] Until recently the combination of methotrexate, vinblastine, adriamycin (doxorubicin) and cisplatin (MVAC) was the gold standard. A randomized phase III trial was published in 2000 which examined the combination of cisplatin and gemcitabine against MVAC. This trial showed similar response rates (49% vs. 46%), but with significantly less toxicity in those treated with cisplatin/gemcitabine.[16]

The combination of cisplatin, gemcitabine, and paclitaxel is now being investigated against the new gold standard of cisplatin/gemcitabine in an attempt to further improve results.

> **Summary points:**
> - Intravesical chemotherapy can prevent recurrence of superficial bladder cancer but does not affect progression-free or overall survival
> - Localized, muscle-invasive bladder cancer can be treated by either primary radical cystectomy or radical radiotherapy with cystectomy reserved for radiation failures
> - Multimodality therapy is emerging as a useful option with maximal transurethral resection of bladder tumor (TURBT) followed by concomitant chemotherapy/radiation
> - Metastatic bladder cancer has a poor prognosis, with a median survival of 12 months with modern multiagent chemotherapy
> - Newer regimens, e.g. cisplatin/gemcitabine, are less toxic but equally efficacious

Treatment of Prostate Cancer

The incidence of prostate cancer is rising and it is now the second most commonly diagnosed cancer in men.

It has been recognized for some time that many men diagnosed as suffering from prostate cancer will die of some unrelated cause.[17] In view of this and also the potential toxicity of treatment, some patients are advised to avoid specific therapy. Typically this applies to patients with poor life expectancy and with low-grade, good-prognosis tumors, especially if asymptomatic.

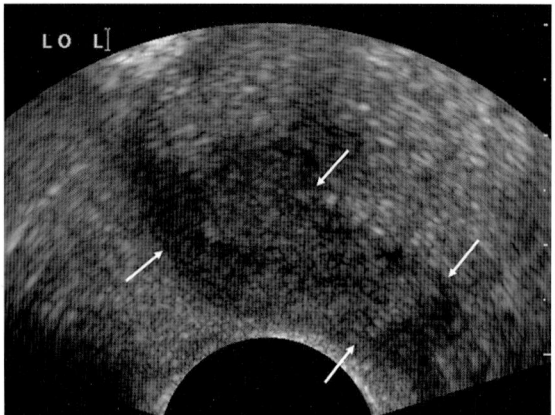 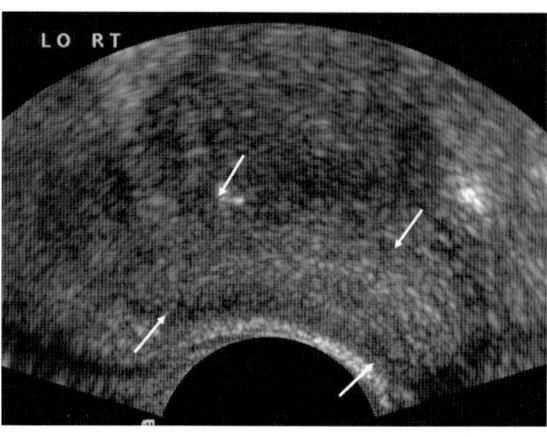

Fig. 13.2 **a** Saggital ultrasound scan of the left lobe of the prostate showing a very hypoechoic peripheral zone lesion (arrows) consistent with prostatic carcinoma. **b** A similar saggital scan in the same patient of the normal right lobe for comparison. The peripheral zone is uniform and echogenic (arrows)

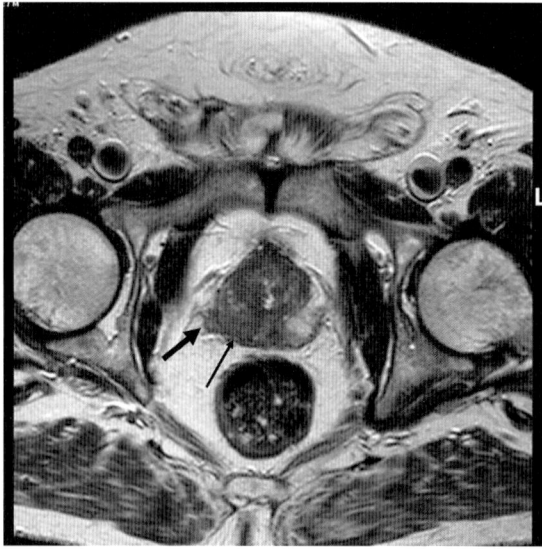

Fig. 13.3 **Axial T2-weighted scan of the prostate showing extensive low signal change** (arrow) **throughout the right peripheral zone of the gland.** The appearances are those of carcinoma. Tumor extension is noted into the right neurovascular bundle (thick arrow)

For purposes of description, the treatment of prostate cancer can most conveniently be divided into:
- Treatment of intracapsular disease (Fig. 13.2)
- Treatment of localized disease extending outside the capsule, often referred to as locally advanced disease (Fig. 13.3)
- Treatment of metastatic disease (Figs. 13.4, 13.5)

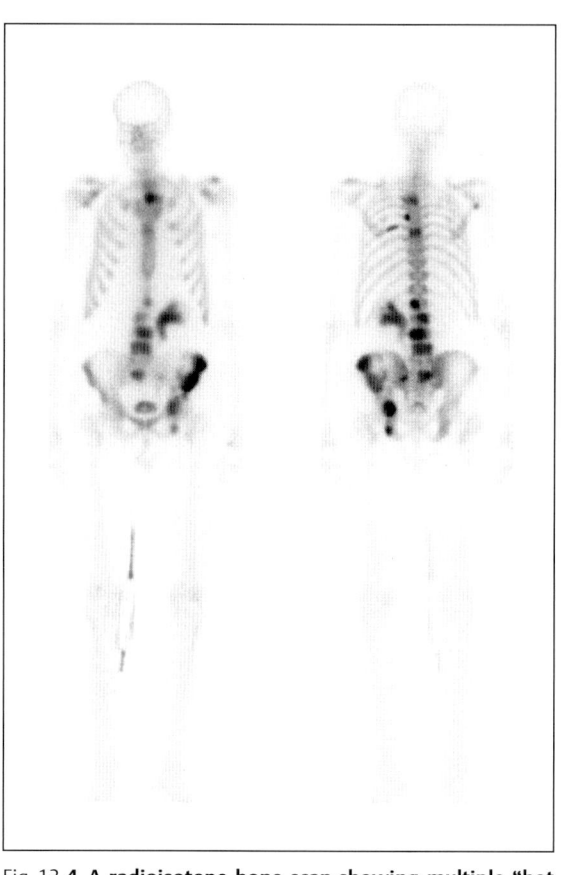

Fig. 13.4 **A radioisotope bone scan showing multiple "hot spots" in the spine, pelvis, and one of the ribs on the left.** The features are those of metastatic disease. The patient was known to have a prostatic primary. Left-sided hydronephrosis is also noted and the patient is catheterized

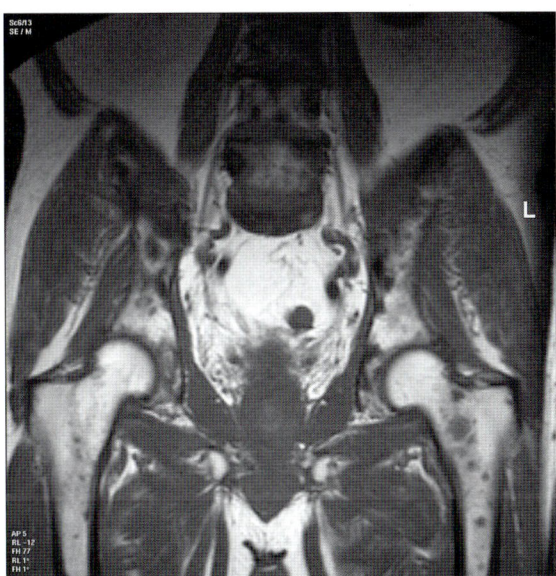

Fig.13.5 **Coronal T1-weighted MRI scan performed as part of a prostate tumor staging scan.** This shows multiple, focal, low-signal lesions throughout both femora, pelvis, and lumbar spine consistent with metastatic disease

Treatment of Intracapsular Disease

This is an area of considerable controversy. The main options of active surveillance, radical prostatectomy, external beam radiation therapy, and interstitial therapy have never been compared in a prospective manner. One study has shown no evidence of survival benefit for active therapy over an age-matched control.[18] Radical prostatectomy can be performed by the retropubic, perineal, or laparoscopic route with similar results.[19] Pelvic lymphadenectomy is performed initially and if frozen section analysis shows tumor involvement, further surgery is abandoned. Nerve-sparing radical prostatectomy is said to result in improved rates of urinary incontinence and impotence. The best results in terms of operative mortality and morbidity come from single-institution centers, but the operation is still regarded as having considerable long-term morbidity; the mortality is 1–1.5%. Total urinary incontinence is rare, but some control difficulties are reported in up to 30% of cases.[20] The risk of impotence after radical prostatectomy is variously reported as between 24 and 89%. This risk is increased with age and poor pretreatment function.

In addition to impotence, attention is also now being paid to overall quality of sexual function after radical prostate cancer treatment but there is little data at present.

An alternative treatment for patients with intracapsular disease is a radioisotope implant procedure. Prostate brachytherapy involves the introduction of radioactive isotopes directly into the gland. This is usually performed with the aid of transrectal ultrasound (TRUS) guidance and the radioisotope is delivered through the perineum via a template grid system. Iodine[125] and palladium[103] are the most commonly-used isotopes. The side effects are similar to external beam therapy, but there is usually slightly greater urinary irritation. The use of prostate brachytherapy has increased dramatically in the last 10 years in tandem with improvements in technology. The main advantage of this form of therapy is its convenience. The procedure involves a maximum of two hospital visits of relatively short duration. The efficacy and toxicity compare favorably to external beam therapy and radical prostatectomy.[21]

External beam radiation therapy can be used as monotherapy in the treatment of good-prognosis intracapsular disease. Megavoltage beams are used to cover the prostate with a small margin and treatment is usually given daily to a total dose of 64–78 Gy. Escalating radiation dose has been shown to be an independent factor in improving local control and decreasing prostate-specific antigen (PSA) failure, especially in higher-risk patients.[22]

There have been a number of technological developments over the last 10 years or so which have resulted in improvements in the ability to plan and deliver high doses of radiation to the prostate gland in a consistent and reproducible manner. These include three-dimensional (3-D) treatment-planning systems and computer-controlled delivery systems allowing conformal shaping of radiation beams. It is now possible to vary the beam intensity or fluence of each portal and by so doing the radiation dose distribution can be shaped accurately to the contours of the prostate. This is known as intensity-modulated radiation therapy (IMRT). By using such techniques, doses of up to 81 Gy can be delivered without excessive toxicity.[23]

Patients with good-prognosis intracapsular disease are given treatment options such as radical prostatectomy, radical external beam radiotherapy, and implantation. A recently published retrospective trial by D'Amico et al.[24] examined the PSA failure rate in patients treated by external beam (866 patients), radical prostatectomy (888 patients), or implantation (218 patients).There was no difference in outcome for low-risk patients defined as PSA < 10 ng/mL, stage T2a or less, and Gleason score 6 or less.

Treatment of Locally Advanced Disease

Whilst some patients with good-prognosis, early-stage disease can undoubtedly be cured by high doses of carefully fractionated external beam radiation, patients who have extracapsular disease, i.e. T3/T4 disease, PSA > 20, Gleason score 8–10, and/or pelvic lymph node involvement, are likely to fail radiation therapy alone. For such high-risk patients the combination of androgen ablation and radiation therapy is often prescribed. Several trials have shown benefit in these situations with regard to biochemical and local control.[25,26] A survival benefit has also been demonstrated especially when androgen ablation is continued in an adjuvant fashion after definitive local therapy.[27] However, the exact timing and duration of hormone treatment is not yet fully characterized.

Treatment of Metastatic Disease

Hormonal therapy for metastatic prostate cancer can be spectacularly successful in palliating symptoms and in gaining biochemical control. The response rate is 80–90% in previously untreated patients. The problem is that the emergence of hormone-resistant disease is inevitable with a median duration of response of 12–18 months.

The timing of introduction of hormonal therapy has been debated for some time, with the major question being whether or not to actively treat an asymptomatic man with metastatic disease. For some time it was assumed that treatment could be deferred until symptoms developed as there was no survival benefit from treatment and significant drug-induced toxicity. However, a more rigorous examination of the original Veterans Administration studies has shown that more patients suffer disease complications and die of prostate cancer in the deferred treatment group.[28] These findings were confirmed in the Medical Research Council trial reported in 1997.[29]

Hormonal therapy in prostate cancer can either block the production of androgens or act in competition with androgens at target-organ receptor sites. Castrate levels of testosterone can be achieved by surgical or medical castration. Bilateral orchidectomy was originally described by Huggins and Hodges in 1941.[30]

Medical castration is performed by the luteinizing hormone, releasing hormone (LHRH) group of drugs such as goserelin and leuprorelin. These have an initial stimulatory effect on the pituitary gonadotrophins, follicle-stimulating hormone (FSH), and luteinizing hormone (LH). The resulting testosterone surge then elicits a negative feedback effect on the hypothalamus and pituitary with resultant desensitization. Castrate levels of testosterone are accomplished in about four weeks. An oral antiandrogen drug such as cyproterone acetate is usually prescribed during any potential period of testosterone surge.

LHRH analogues are given by subcutaneous injection on a monthly or three-monthly basis. Side effects of either form of castration are predictable due to very low levels of circulating androgens and include loss of libido, hot flushes, tiredness, and loss of muscle tone.

Responses to second-line hormone therapies such as antiandrogens, low-dose estrogens, and progestational agents are usually minor and of short duration.[31]

Treatment of Hormone-Refractory Prostate Cancer

The development of hormone-refractory prostate cancer (HRPC) portends a poor prognosis with a median survival of 9–12 months. Optimal therapy for this diverse group of patients has yet to be determined, but due to the myriad of clinical scenarios treatment must be individualized. Until recently no specific treatment had been shown to prolong survival.

Chemotherapy treatment has emerged as a useful tool in the treatment of hormone-refractory disease in the last decade. Two trials published in 1996 showed the palliative benefit of the combination of mitoxantrone and corticosteroids along with a reasonable toxicity profile.[32,33] Although no survival benefit was demonstrated there was an improvement in pain control and quality of life in both trials. This treatment (mitoxantrone and corticosteroid) was until recently considered standard first-line chemotherapy treatment for fit patients with hormone-refractory disease.

Recently, interest has focussed on the potential of the taxane group of drugs and especially docetaxel (Taxotere) either alone or in combination with drugs such as estramustine[34] and vinorelbine. Docetaxel can be given on a weekly basis, which is sometimes useful in frail, heavily-pretreated patients. The results of two phase III trials comparing standard mitoxantrone/steroid treatment with Taxotere have now been published. In the TAX 327 trial mitoxantrone was compared with two different schedules of Taxotere, given either weekly or three-weekly along with corticosteroids. There was a significant survival benefit in the three-weekly Taxotere arm. In addition, Taxotere-treated patients, showed improved pain control and quality of life and had improved PSA responses.[35]

The SWOG trial compared Taxotere/estramustine with mitoxantrone/prednisone and also showed a small but statistically significant survival benefit for the Taxotere-treated patients.[36]

Palliative radiotherapy is useful for painful bone metastases, as well as for symptomatic soft-tissue disease. Systemic radiotherapy with strontium 89 injection can also be useful especially for widespread flitting bone pain. Recently the introduction of bisphosphonate therapy with zoledronic acid, given as a monthly 15-minute infusion, has shown benefit in reducing skeletal complications in hormone-refractory disease.[37]

> **Summary points:**
> - Prostate cancer is now the second most commonly diagnosed malignancy in men
> - Intracapsular disease can be treated by active surveillance, radical prostatectomy, interstitial implantation, or external beam radiotherapy with similar long-term results
> - Locally advanced disease and poor-prognosis disease is managed by the combination of hormonal therapy and external beam radiotherapy
> - Metastatic disease responds well to hormone therapy initially but the emergence of drug resistance is inevitable after a mean of 12–18 months
> - Treatment of hormone-refractory disease with taxane-based chemotherapy has been shown to palliate symptoms and improve survival
> - Options for treatment of hormone-refractory disease include palliative radiotherapy, intravenous chemotherapy, strontium[89], zoledronic acid, and corticosteroids

Treatment of Testicular Tumors

Germ cell tumors of the testis are the commonest malignancies in men aged 20–40. Peak incidence is around age 25–35, and the incidence appears to be rising.

Possible causes include exposure to estrogenic materials prenatally, testicular maldescent, and a familial predisposition. Abnormalities in chromosome 12 are seen in almost all cases of testicular cancer.

Over 95% of patients will be cured, but issues such as fertility and long-term toxicity must be borne in mind, and most patients will opt to have sperm samples stored prior to any treatment, with the possible exception of para-aortic radiation in stage I seminoma.

The classical presentation is with a painless lump, however, most will have symptoms of pain or swelling. Patients with advanced disease can present with symptoms attributable to their metastases.

The initial investigation should be testicular ultrasound, ideally within two weeks of presentation. (Fig. 13.6) This helps to exclude pathologies such as epididymo-orchitis.

Definitive diagnosis of a testicular tumor and review of its pathology and prognostic information therein is achieved by inguinal orchiectomy. Even in those patients who clearly have more advanced disease, the procedure should be undertaken at some point, as che-

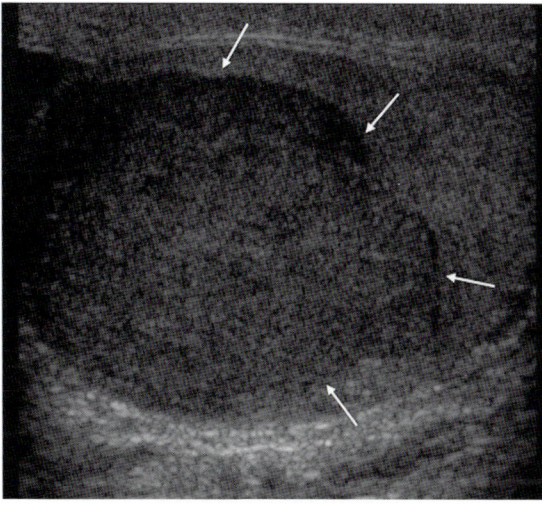

Fig. 13.6 **Ultrasound scan of the right testicle in a young man presenting with a painless scrotal mass.** Ultrasound scan confirmed the presence of a large hypoechoic solid mass (arrows) within the testis consistent with tumor. Histology showed a teratoma

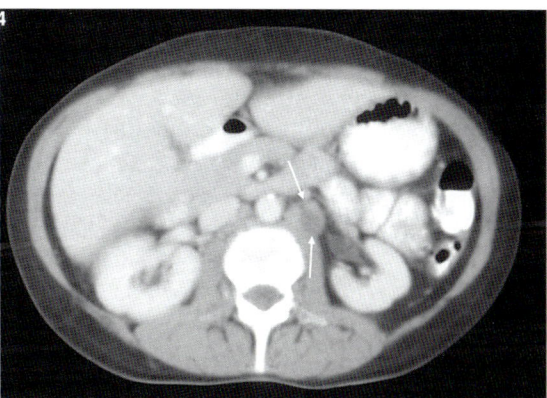

Fig. 13.7 **Axial CT scan of a patient with a left-sided testicular teratoma at renal level showing the presence of a left-sided para-aortic lymph node measuring just over 2 cm in diameter** (arrows). There is slight prominence of the left renal pelvis

motherapy is inadequate to sterilize the primary tumor (Fig. 13.7). In addition to this, preoperative tumor markers including alpha-fetoprotein (AFP), human beta-chorionic gonadotropin (beta-HCG), and lactate dehydrogenase (LDH) should be checked, and if raised, should be monitored until they become normal postoperatively. AFP levels are raised in about 70% of teratomas, but never in seminomas. About 50% of teratomas will have an elevated human chorionic gonadotropin (HCG) level and seminomas can also show a modest elevation.

There are a number of histological classifications, including World Health Organization (WHO) and the British Testicular Tumors Panel. Tumors are divided

Table 13.1 The Royal Marsden staging system for testicular tumors

Stage		
I	No metastasis	
IM	Rising serum markers with no other evidence of metastasis	
II	Abdominal node metastasis:	
	A ≤ 2 cm in diameter	
	B 2–5 cm in diameter	
	C ≥ 5 cm in diameter	
III	Supradiaphragmatic nodal metastasis:	
	M mediastinal	
	N supraclavicular, cervical, or axillary	
	O No abdominal node metastasis	
	ABC Node stage as defined in stage II	
IV	Extralymphatic metastasis lung:	
	L1 ≤ 3 metastases	
	L2 ≥ 3 metastases, all ≤ 2 cm diameter	
	L3 ≥ 3 metastases, 1 or more > 2 cm diameter.	
	L+, Br+, Bo+—liver, brain or bone metastases.	

into seminoma and nonseminoma. Seminomas are classical or spermatocytic. Nonseminomas generally include multiple cell types. All pathological samples should be reviewed by an expert pathologist.

Both the tumor, node, metastasis (TNM) and Royal Marsden systems are in use to assign patients a clinical stage.

The Royal Marsden staging is shown in Table 13.1

Seminoma

Around 75% of seminomas are stage I. The standard treatment is adjuvant radiotherapy to the para-aortic nodes. There has been some evidence to suggest standard radiotherapy schedules can be shortened, although this remains under discussion.[38] Other options include surveillance and adjuvant chemotherapy, neither of which is currently accepted as standard treatment.

Surveillance can be problematic in what is usually a nonmarker secreting tumor; it requires intensive follow-up in terms of cost, time, and radiological investigation. Also, on surveillance around 15–20% of patients will relapse, and although they can almost all be salvaged,[39,40] this has a psychological cost attached to it. Adjuvant chemotherapy for seminoma is still regarded as experimental whilst the results of a large MRC trial looking at this issue are awaited (TE19).

A very small proportion of patients will relapse after standard radiotherapy (2–3%) and these can be salvaged with chemotherapy.[41]

The role of retroperitoneal lymph node dissection in both seminoma and nonseminoma varies geographically. It is rarely practiced in the United Kingdom, but plays a very prominent part in treatment in the United States.

Stage IIA and IIB seminoma may be treated with radiotherapy alone to the affected and at-risk nodes; cure rates of over 90% can be achieved. Patients with more bulky disease should be offered platinum-based combination chemotherapy along similar lines to the treatment of metastatic nonseminoma.

Non-seminoma Germ Cell Tumor

Patients with stage I nonseminoma have a management strategy defined according to the pathological characteristics of their tumor. Those 50% of men who have vascular invasion in their tumor are at higher risk of relapse than those without (48% against 15%),[42] and therefore should be offered chemotherapy in the form of two cycles of platinum-based chemotherapy. Those without are generally offered surveillance protocols, which involve frequent clinic assessments, chest radiology, tumor markers, and CT scans frequently in the first two years, a requirement which is being examined in a current MRC trial.

The introduction of platinum-based chemotherapy was a major step toward vastly improved cure rates, and has evolved over the years. A regime in common use today involves the combination of cisplatin, etoposide and bleomycin (BEP). However, the high cure rate and significant toxicity has resulted in efforts to identify those patients who are more or less likely to be cured by standard chemotherapy. The International Germ Cell Cancer Collaborative Group was formed in 1991 and from a database of over 6000 patients generated a very useful staging system for metastatic disease based on prognostic factors.[43] The "good" prognosis group would be expected to have cure rates of around 90%, intermediate 80%, and poor 45%.

It is now generally accepted that good-prognosis patients can be treated with shorter schedules than previously, with equivalent results, in an attempt to reduce toxicity.[44]

Those patients in other prognostic groups are less numerous and therefore there is a relative paucity of randomized data looking at alternatives. An EORTC phase II/III study is in progress (TE21).

Following completion of chemotherapy, consideration should be given to resection of residual masses. Around 50% of masses in patients treated for teratoma may contain viable germ cell tumor or teratoma, and further chemotherapy may be of benefit, but this is controversial. The picture is even less clear for patients with treated seminoma, but generally masses are not considered for resection unless bulky. Optimal timing of both clinical and radiological review is unclear and is being investigated, but should aim to detect relapse at an early stage and monitor long-term toxicity from treatment.

> **Summary points:**
> - Incidence of testicular tumors is increasing
> - Cure rates are high and emphasis is on reducing long-term toxicity
> - Stage I and nonbulky stage II seminoma are treated with radiotherapy
> - Bulky stage II seminoma and the majority of non-seminomas are managed with platinum-based chemotherapy with curative intent
> - Following chemotherapy patients with residual tumor masses should be considered for surgical excision

Treatment of Renal Cell Carcinoma

Renal cell carcinoma (RCC) is a relatively rare condition, accounting for only 2–3% of all cancers worldwide. However, the incidence is rising. The median age at diagnosis is 62, and the male to female ratio is 2:1. Possible risk factors include cigarette smoking, obesity, diet, and occupational exposures to materials such as asbestos, end-stage renal disease (ESRD), and some congenital disorders such as von Hippel–Lindau disease, tuberous sclerosis, and polycystic kidney disease. Abnormalities of chromosome 3p are present in the majority of sporadic and hereditary renal cancers.

The classical presentation is with flank pain, hematuria, and a palpable abdominal mass. However, with the advent of more sophisticated imaging the diagnosis is made incidentally in more than 50% of patients.

Five-year survival is 55–60% and has improved in recent years.
Approximately 85% of all RCCs are adenocarcinomas—either clear cell or papillary tumors, the remainder being made up of transitional cell carcinomas of the renal pelvis.

The staging of RCC is outlined in Table 13.**2**.

Investigation

Most patients have cross-sectional imaging preoperatively with CT being the gold standard (Fig. 13.**8**). Despite this, up to 17% of patients with a preoperative radiological diagnosis of RCC are found to have other pathologies such as sarcoma, metastases, and cysts.[45] One classification system has been introduced in an attempt to differentiate between cysts and RCC.[46]

Table 13.**2 Staging of renal cell carcinoma (TNM 2002)**

T1	≤ 7 cm; limited to the kidney
T1a	≤ 4 cm
T1b	> 4 cm
T2	> 7 cm; limited to the kidney
T3	Adrenal or perinephric invasion; major veins
T3a	Adrenal or perinephric invasion
T3b	Renal vein(s), vena cava below diaphragm
T3c	Vena cava above diaphragm
T4	Beyond Gerota fascia
N1	Single
N2	More than one

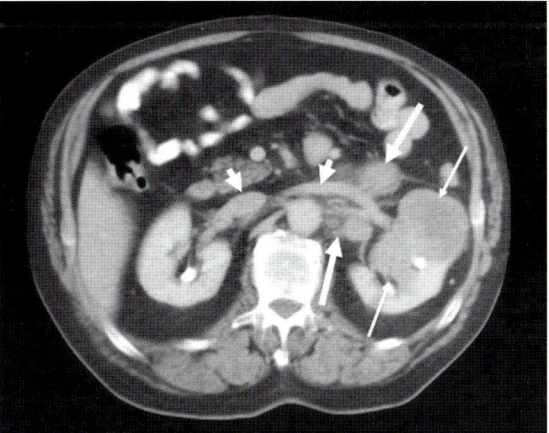

Fig. 13.**8 Axial CT scan showing a large, thick-walled renal tumor of the left kidney** (thin arrows) **with a large amount of central necrosis.** Marked local hilar adenopathy (thick arrows) is present. The left renal vein and inferior vena cava (arrowheads) are patent

There may, therefore, be a role for percutaneous biopsy. However, whilst relatively sensitive, it appears to be poor at adequately excluding renal malignancy. It is worthwhile, where a nonrenal malignancy is suspected, for example lymphoma or a metastatic lesion.

Prognosis can be variable, and therefore a staging system based on TNM stage, histological grade, and performance status amongst other data has been devised by the University of California at Los Angeles group (UCLA Integrated Staging System).[47] This system has been further developed and is now used in algorithm form to stratify patients postoperatively.[48]

Surgical Treatment

Surgical resection is the standard treatment of localized RCC, usually in the form of radical nephrectomy. This involves ligation of the renal artery and subsequently of the renal vein prior to removal of the kidney, perirenal fat, and Gerota fascia, with the aim of avoiding tumor dissemination. The value of lymphadenectomy is controversial. As RCC can metastasize by blood-borne and lymphatic routes; it seems logical that therapeutic lymphadenectomy would be beneficial. However, the extent of dissection required and effect on morbidity remains uncertain. The EORTC study 30881 has looked at this question and it appears that there is no increase in mortality or morbidity with lymphadenectomy. However, the follow-up is not yet long enough to make any definitive comment on survival.[49]

The complication rate of radical nephrectomy is 3% and the death rate 1%.[50]

More recently nephron-sparing surgery and partial nephrectomy have gained in popularity. Such procedures seem to be equivalent to radical surgery in tumors < 4 cm in size.[51]

Adrenalectomy remains of uncertain benefit. A normal adrenal gland on CT has a 100% negative predictive value in one recent study.[52] It therefore seems reasonable to omit adrenalectomy in the face of a normal CT.

Nephrectomy in metastatic disease is a controversial issue. Although not curative, there is now data from two randomized trials to suggest a survival benefit in selected patients. The first shows a survival benefit of three months,[53] and the second 10 months.[54]

There is scanty evidence to support the theory that spontaneous regression of metastases follows nephrectomy in any significant number of patients. Palliative benefits may include reduction of hematuria and pain. However, these ends can sometimes be achieved with the judicious use of other modalities, such as embolization. The psychological benefit to a patient receiving surgery to "remove the cancer" cannot be overestimated. Clearly, to opt for or against nephrectomy is a complex decision to make, on an individual patient basis, along with the patient and their family. It has been shown, however, that only around 20% of patients with metastatic RCC in one case series were offered nephrectomy because of unresectability or poor performance status.[55]

Nonsurgical Treatment

In patients not suitable for surgery, external beam radiation can offer some palliative benefit. There is an uncertain role for postoperative radiation, with most studies being negative.[56,57]

As metastatic renal cancer often has a long natural history, there can be an argument made for radical treatment of isolated metastases. One series of patients treated with a "curative metastectomy" recorded a five-year survival of 44%.[58] Favorable features were a disease-free interval of more than one year, solitary metastasis and age < 60. One further advance in treatment is in stereotactic radiosurgery for isolated brain metastasis with one series showing a median survival of 11 months with no immediate mortality, suggesting this may be a viable alternative to surgery.[59]

Responses to chemotherapy rarely exceed 10%, and for this reason chemotherapy is not advocated in patients with metastatic renal cancer not in the context of a clinical trial.

The natural history of renal cancer and reports of occasional spontaneous regression suggest an immunological role. This provides a rationale for the use of biological therapies. Immunotherapy with interferon-α-2 has become the cornerstone of medical management for metastatic renal cancer. There are now a number of randomized trials supporting the use of interferon, the largest being an MRC trial.[60] This showed a statistically significant survival advantage for the use of interferon as against the use of medroxyprogesterone acetate (MPA) in patients with metastatic RCC, with a reduction in the odds of death of 28% (Fig. 13.9).

The standard treatment for metastatic RCC has therefore become subcutaneous interferon-α-2, 10 megaunits, three times per week. This treatment is not without toxicity, however, with around 70% of patients suffering side effects which included influenza-like symptoms, depression, anorexia, and fatigue. 24% of patients receiving interferon had a dose reduction versus 7% on MPA.

However, at the end of the treatment period (12 weeks) there were minimal differences in reported toxicities, other than reduced appetite, suggesting patients can tolerate this treatment.

Current trials are evaluating the role of the additional interleukin 2 and 5FU (MRC RE04).

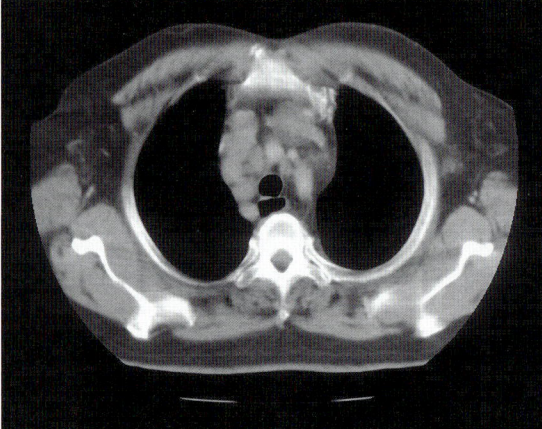

Fig. 13.9 Axial CT scan of the mediastinum showing widespread mediastinal lymphadenopathy

Summary points:
- RCC is commonly now an incidental diagnosis
- Radical nephrectomy is the mainstay of treatment in localized disease
- There is only a limited role for radiotherapy and chemotherapy in all stages of the disease
- There is an established role for immunotherapy with interferon-α in metastatic disease, possibly in combination with IL-2 and 5FU

References

1. Parmar MK, Freedman LS, Hargreave TB, Tolley DA. Prognostic factors for recurrence and follow up policies in the treatment of superficial bladder cancer. J Urology 1989; 2:284–8.
2. Kurch KH, Denis L, Bouffioux C, et al. Factors affecting recurrence and progression in superficial bladder tumours. Eur J Cancer 1995;31:1840–6.
3. Pawinski A, Sylvester R, Kurch KH. A combined analysis of EORTC and MRC randomised clinical trials for the prophylactic treatment of stage Ta and T1 bladder cancer. J Urology 1996;156:1934–40.
4. Tolley DA, Parmer MK, Grigor K. The effect of intravesical mitomycin C on recurrence of newly diagnosed superficial bladder cancer. J Urology 1996;155:1233–8.
5. Herr HW. Tumour progression and survival of patients with high grade non-invasive transitional cell carcinoma. J Urology 2000;1:60–1.
6. Lamm DL, Blumenstein BA, Crawford ED, et al. A randomized trial of intravesical doxorubicin and immunotherapy with BCG for transitional cell carcinoma of the bladder. N Eng J Med 1991;325:1205–9.
7. Herr HW. Transurethral resection in regionally advanced bladder cancer. Urol Clin North Am 1992;19:695–700.
8. Koch NG, Hulten L, Myrvold HE. Ileo-anal anastomosis with interposition of the ileal Koch pouch. Dis Colon Rectum 1989;32:1050–4.
9. Koch NG, Ghonein MA, Lycke KG, Mahran MR. Replacement of the bladder by the urethral Koch pouch. J Urol 1989;141:1111–16.
10. Trialists. Neoadjuvant cisplatin, methotrextate and vinblastine chemotherapy for muscle-invasive bladder cancer: a randomised controlled trial. Lancet 1999;354: 533–40.
11. Advanced Bladder Cancer (ABC) Meta-Analysis Collaboration. Neo-adjuvant chemotherapy in invasive bladder cancer: a systematic review and meta-analysis. Lancet 2003;361:1927–34.
12. Housset M, Manland C, Chrietien Y. Combined radiation and chemotherapy for invasive transitional cell carcinoma of the bladder. J Clin Oncol 1993;11;2150–7.
13. Coppin CM, Gospodarowicz M-K, James K, et al. Improved local control of invasive bladder carcinoma by concurrent cisplatin and preoperative or definitive radiation. J Clin Oncol 1996;14:2901–7.
14. Loehrer PJ, Sr, DeMulder P. Management of metastatic bladder cancer. In: Raghavan D, Scher HI, Leibel S, et al., eds. Principles and practice of genitourinary oncology. Philadelphia, PA: Lippincott-Raven: 1997: 299–305.
15. Sternberg CN, Yagoda A, Scher HI, et al. Methotrexate, vinblastine, adriamycin, cisplatin for advanced transitional cell carcinoma of the urothelium. Cancer 1989;64: 2448–58.
16. Von der Maase H, Hansen SW, Roberts JT, et al. Gemcitabine and Cisplatin versus MVAC in advanced or metastatic bladder cancer. Results of a large, randomized, multinational, multicenter, phase III study. J Clin Oncol 2000;18: 3068–3077.
17. Parker SL, Tong T, Bolden S, Wingo PA. Cancer Statistics. Ca Cancer J Clin 1997;47:5–27.
18. Chodak GA, Thisted RA, Gerber GS. Et al. Results of conservative management of clinically localised prostate cancer. N Eng J Med 1994;330:242–248.
19. Sullivan LD, Weir MJ, Kinahan JE, Taylor DL. A comparison of the relative merits of radical perineal and retropubic prostatectomy. Br J Urol 2000;85:95–100.
20. Fowler FJ, Barry MJ. Patient-reported complications and follow-up treatment after radical prostatectomy. Urology 1993;42:622–628.
21. Ragde H, Elgamal A, Snow P, et al. Ten-year disease-free survival after transperineal sonography-guided iodine-125 brachytherapy with or without 45 gray external beam radiotherapy in the treatment of patients with clinically localised low to high gleason grade prostate cancer. Cancer 1998;83:989–1001.
22. Pollack A, Zagers GK, Smith LG. Preliminary results of a randomised radiotherapy dose escalation study comparing 70 Gy with 78 Gy for prostate cancer. J Clin Oncol 2000; 18:3904.
23. Leibel SA, Zelefsky MJ, Kutcher GJ, et al. Conformal radiation therapy in localised carcinoma of the prostate. A phase I dose escalation study. J Urology 1994;269:2650.
24. D'Amico AV, Whittington R, Malkowicz SB, et al. Biochemical outcome after radical prostatectomy, external beam radiation or interstitial radiation therapy for clinically localised prostate cancer. J Am Med Assoc 1998;280: 969–974.
25. Pilipich MV, Kral JM, Al-Sarraf M. Androgen deprivation with radiation therapy compared with radiation therapy alone for locally advanced prostatic carcinoma: a randomised comparative trial of the Radiation Therapy Oncology Group. Urology 1995;45:616.
26. Zelefsky MJ, Leibel SA, Burman CM, et al. Neo-adjuvant hormone therapy improved the therapeutic ratio in patients with bulky prostatic cancer treated with 3-dimensional conformal tadiation therapy. Int J Radiat Oncol Biol Phys 1994;29:755.
27. Bolla M, Gonzalez D, Warde P, et al. Improved survival in pateints with locally advanced prostate cancer treated with radiotherapy and goserelin. N Eng J Med 1997; 337:295.
28. Sarosy MF. Do we have a national treatment plan for stage D1 carcinoma of the prostate? World J Urol 1990;8:27–31.
29. The Medical Research Council Prostate Cancer Working Party Investigators Group. Immediate versus deferred treatment for advanced prostatic cancer: initial results of the Medical Research Council Trial. Br J Urol 1997;79: 235–246.
30. Huggins MA, Stevens RE, Hodges CV. Studies on prostate cancer, effects of castration on advanced carcinoma of the prostate. J Urol 1944;46:997–1006.

31. Smith DC. Secondary hormone therapy. Semin Urol Oncol 1997;15:3–12.
32. Tannock IF, Osoba D, Murphy K. et al. Chemotherapy with mitoxantrone plus prednisone or prednisone alone of symptomatic hormone resistant prostate cancer. J Clin Oncol 1996;14:1556–1564.
33. Kantoff PW, Conaway M, Winer E, et al. Hydrocortisone with or without mitoxantrone in patients with hormone-refractory prostate cancer; preliminary results from a prospective randomised cancer and leukaemia group B study comparing chemotherapy to best supportive care. J Clin Oncol 1996;15(Suppl):25.
34. Sinibaldi V, Carducci M, Moore-Cooper S, et al. Phase II evaluation of docetaxel plus 1 day oral estramustine phosphate in the treatment of patients with androgen-independent prostate carcinoma. Cancer 2002;94:1457–1465.
35. Tannock I, deWit R, Berry W, et al . Docetaxel plus prednisone or mitoxantrone plus prednisone for advanced prostate cancer. N Engl J Med 2004;351:1502–1512.
36. Petrylak DP, Tangen CM, Hussain MHA, et al. Docetaxel and estramustine compared with mitoxantrone and prednisone for advanced refractory prostate cancer. N Engl J Med 2004;351:1513–1520.
37. Saad F, Gleason DM, Murray RA, et al. Randomised, placebo-controlled trial of zoledronic acid in patients with hormone-refractory metastatic prostate cancer. J Natl Cancer Inst 2002;94:1458–1468.
38. Fossa S, Jones WG, Stenning SP for the TE18 Collaborator, MRC Clinical Trials Unit, London, UK. Quality of life (QL) after radiotherapy for stage I seminoma: results from a randomised trial of two RT schedules (MRC TE18). Proc Am Soc Clin Oncol 2002;21:750a.
39. G Read, Stenning SP, Cullen MH, et al. Medical Research Council prospective study of surveillance for stage I testicular teratoma. J Clin Oncol 1992;10:1762–68.
40. Warde P, Gospodarowicz MK, Panzarella T, et al. Long-term outcome and cost in the management of stage I testicular seminoma. Can J Urol 2000;7:967–72.
41. Zagars GK. Management of stage I seminoma: radiotherapy. In: Horwich A, ed. Testicular cancer—investigation and management. 2nd ed. London: Chapman and Hall: 1996: 99–122.
42. Dearnaley DP, Stenning SP. Management of clinical stage 1 nonseminomatous germ cell tumours (NSGCT): influence of prognostic factors on choice of treatment. In: Jones WG, Appleyard I, Harnden P, eds. Germ Cell Tumours IV. London: John Libbey: 1998;187–188.
43. International Germ Cell Cancer Collaborative Group. International germ cell consensus classification; a prognostic factor-based staging system for metastatic germ cell cancers. J Clin Oncol 1997;15:594–603.
44. de Wit R, Roberts JT, Wilkinson PM, et al. Equivalence of three or four cycles of bleomycin, etoposide, and cisplatin chemotherapy and of a 3 or 5-day schedule in good-prognosis germ cell cancer: a randomized study of the European Organization for Research and Treatment of Cancer Genitourinary Tract Cancer Cooperative Group and the Medical Research Council. J Clin Oncol 2001;19:1629–40.
45. Silver DA, Morash C, Brenner P, et al. Pathologic findings at the time of nephrectomy for renal mass. Ann Surg Oncol 1997;4:570.
46. Bosniak MA. The current radiological approach to renal cysts. Radiology 1986;158:1–10.
47. Zisman A, Pantuck AJ, Dorey F, et al. Improved prognostication of renal cell carcinoma using an integrated staging system. J ClinOncol 2001;19:1649–1657.
48. Zisman A, Pantuck AJ, Wieder J, et al. Risk group assessment and clinical outcome algorithm to predict the natural history of patients with surgically resected renal cell carcinoma. J Clin Oncol 2002;20:4559–4566.
49. Blom JHM, van Poppel H, Marechal JM, et al and members of the EORTC-GU Group. Radical nephrectomy with and without lymph node dissection: preliminary results of the EORTC randomised phase III protocol 30881. Eur Urol 1999;89:570–5.
50. Ljungberg B, Alamdari FI, Holmberg G, et al. Radical nephrectomy is still preferable in the treatment of localised renal cell carcinoma. A long-term follow-up study. Eur Urol 1998;33;79–85.
51. Hafez KS, Fergany AF, Novick AC. Nephron sparing surgery for localised renal cell carcinoma: impact of tumour size on patient survival, tumour recurrence and TNM staging. J Urol 1999;162:1930–33.
52. Sawai Y, Kinouchi T, Mano M, et al. Ipsilateral adrenal involvement from renal cell carcinoma: retrospective study of the predictive value of CT. Urology 2002;59:28–31.
53. Flanigan RC, Salmon SE, Blumerstein BA, et al. Nephrectomy followed by interferon-alfa-2b compared with interferon-alfa-2b alone for metastatic renal cell carcinoma. N Engl J Med 2001;345:1655–59.
54. Mikisch GH, Garin A, van Poppel H, et al. Radical nephrectomy plus interferon-alfa based immunotherapy compared with interferon-alfa alone in metastatic renal-cell carcinoma: a randomised trial. Lancet 2001;358:966–970.
55. Bromwich E, Hendry D, Aitchison M. Cytoreductive nephrectomy: is it a realistic option in patients with renal cancer? BJU International 2002;89:523–525.
56. Kjaer M, Iversen P, Hvidt V, et al. A randomised trial of postoperative radiotherapy versus observation in stage II and III renal adenocarcinoma. Scand J Urol Nephrol 1997;21:285–289.
57. Aref I, Bociek R, Salhani D. Is post-operative radiation for renal cell carcinoma justified? Radiother Oncol 1997;43: 155–157.
58. Kavolius JP, Mastorakos DP, Pavlovich C, et al. Resection of metastatic renal cell carcinoma. J Clin Oncol 1998;16: 2261–2266.
59. Mori Y, Kondziolka D, Flickinger JC, et al. Stereotactic radiosurgery for brain metastasis from renal cell carcinoma. Cancer 1998;83:344–353.
60. Medical Research Council Renal Cancer Collaborators. Interferon and survival in metastatic renal carcinoma: early results of a randomised controlled trial. Lancet 1999;353: 4–17.

Section 3

The Urogenital Tract in the Child

14 Ultrasound of the Pediatric Urogenital Tract   **207**

14 Ultrasound of the Pediatric Urogenital Tract

M. E. K. Sellars

Introduction

Ultrasound is the initial imaging investigation for examination of the urinary tract in children and infants, providing precise anatomical information. Ultrasound is robust in the face of a "moving" target, allows repeated examinations without any radiation hazard, and is viewed by the patient as a "friendly" procedure with the examiner close at hand. The ability to image in real-time is an asset, although one disadvantage of ultrasound is the poor appreciation of the capabilities of the technique by clinicians. Imaging findings on ultrasound together with clinical presentation will determine which further investigations, if any, are needed. Ultrasound of the urogenital tract in children and infants should always precede any other type of imaging investigation.

Ultrasound Imaging Techniques

No preparation is required for imaging the urogenital tract in the pediatric population. Ultrasound of the kidneys is performed with the patient lying in a supine and/or a prone position following the application of warmed gel. An assortment of transducers may be necessary to optimize visualization depending on patient age and size. These include curvilinear and phased-array or linear transducers with a frequency ranging between 3 and 7.5 MHz.

Longitudinal and transverse images are obtained of the kidney and bladder and the testes where required, with the bladder routinely examined first. Often the bladder is emptied during the examination. Visualization of the bladder allows bladder volume to be calculated, as well as to give an estimation of any exaggeration of distal ureteric and renal pelvic measurements in the presence of a distended bladder. In an unobstructed system, these appearances should resolve following micturition. Bladder volume assessment in children referred following a urinary tract infection (UTI), in those with neurological problems, or distal urinary tract obstruction is particularly important.[1]

The adrenal glands may be visualized with the patient lying supine (right adrenal gland) and in a right decubitus position (left adrenal gland) using the liver, spleen, and left kidney as an acoustic window, respectively. The testes are readily examined using a linear high-frequency transducer.

Normal Anatomy

Kidney

The normal neonatal kidney, up to about age 12 weeks, has a cortex of high reflectivity, prominent low-reflective pyramids, and a nondilated collecting system (Fig. 14.1).[2] Unlike the adult kidney there is less renal sinus or perirenal fat. The kidney often has a lobulated appearance with the indentations present between the renal pyramids. Renal length is the most commonly used measurement of renal size.[3] Renal length is best measured with the highly mobile infant or young child lying in the prone position, preventing foreshortening of the coronal or sagittal views. Normal standards exist for comparing renal length with age and height; any deviation in length from the proposed normal values would imply the presence of renal disease.[4] In 80% of children the left kidney is the same size or slightly longer than the right kidney.[5] A difference in length of > 1 cm between the kidneys would imply an underlying abnormality, either due to scarring producing a small kidney or due to pathological processes such as pyelonephritis producing renal enlargement.[6]

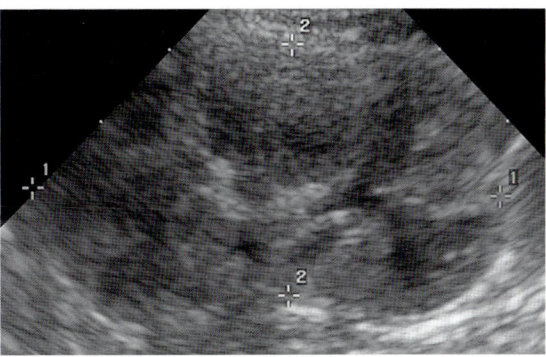

Fig. 14.1 **Normal kidney.** The normal neonatal kidney (between cursors) has a cortex of high reflectivity, prominent low-reflective pyramids, and a nondilated collecting system

Bladder

The distended bladder is of smooth outline with a wall thickness of < 3 mm. On transverse imaging the distal ureters may be seen lying posterior to the bladder with an anterior–posterior diameter < 2 mm.[7] This distal ureteric diameter may be exaggerated in the presence of a distended bladder and must therefore be reassessed following micturition.

Testis

The testis should always be present in the scrotal sac, but occasionally, if retractile, are found at the external inguinal ring area. Ultrasound is a useful initial investigation for an undescended testis, often present within the inguinal canal. The normal testis is of medium-level reflectivity, with the epididymis seen as a separate entity. The tunica albuginea appears as a thin, high-reflective line surrounding the testis. Color Doppler flow is not always present in the normal infant testis, and is more reliably detected as the testicular volume increases at puberty.[8,9] Fluid within the scrotal sac is readily appreciated.[5]

> **Summary points:**
> - Transducers with a frequency ranging between 3 and 7.5 MHz give the best overall assessment of the urogenital tract
> - Renal length is best measured with the child lying in the prone position
> - Distal ureteric diameter may be exaggerated in the presence of a distended bladder
> - The normal testis is of medium reflectivity surrounded by a thin, highly reflective tunica albuginea

Congenital Anomalies Affecting Renal Position and Number

Renal Fusion

Horseshoe Kidney

This is the most common form of renal fusion, affecting approximately one in 600 births. The medially orientated lower renal poles are joined by an isthmus, either of functioning renal tissue or of a fibrous band which crosses anterior to the aorta and inferior vena cava (IVC).[10] On ultrasound a horseshoe kidney is best imaged in the coronal plane, although ultrasound diagnosis may be difficult. The lower poles may be tapered,

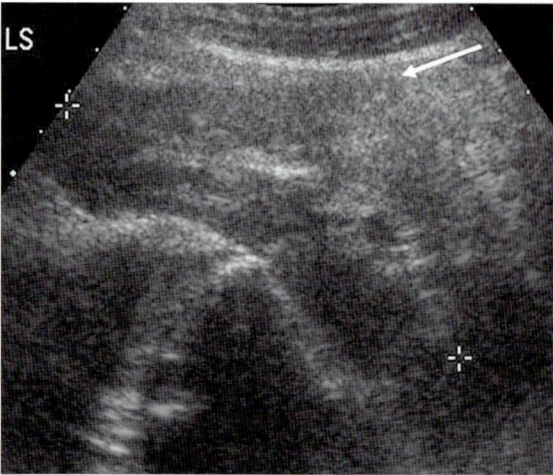
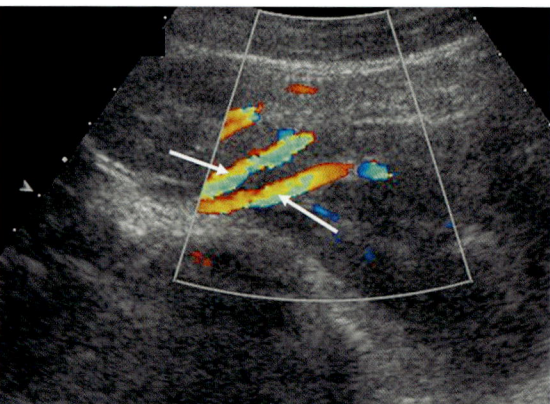

Fig. 14.2 **Crossed-fused ectopia. a** B-mode image of crossfused ectopia (between cursors) with an anterior notch present (arrow). No renal tissue was identified in the contralateral renal fossa. **b** On the color Doppler ultrasound image, two renal arteries (arrows) are seen supplying the superior and inferior kidneys

elongated, and poorly defined; often directed medially. The fused kidneys are susceptible to infection, trauma, calculus, and tumor formation, which may be either a Wilms tumor or an adenocarcinoma.

Cross-Fused Ectopia

Here, both kidneys are located on the same side of the abdomen. The lower pole of one kidney is fused with the superior pole of the inferiorly placed kidney (Fig. 14.2). A characteristic anterior and/or posterior notch provides a major clue to the correct diagnosis. The ureters enter each side of the bladder in their normal position.[11]

Renal Ectopia

The embryonic kidney originates in the pelvis. As the fetal spine elongates and the kidneys become fixed to

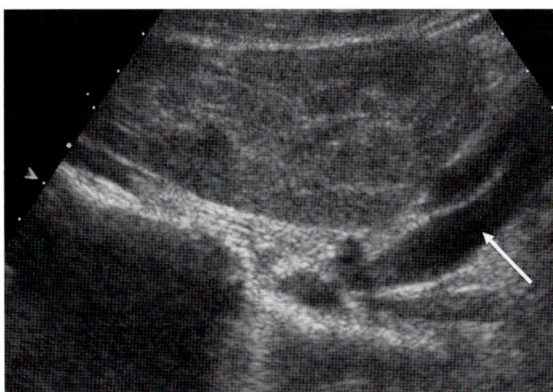 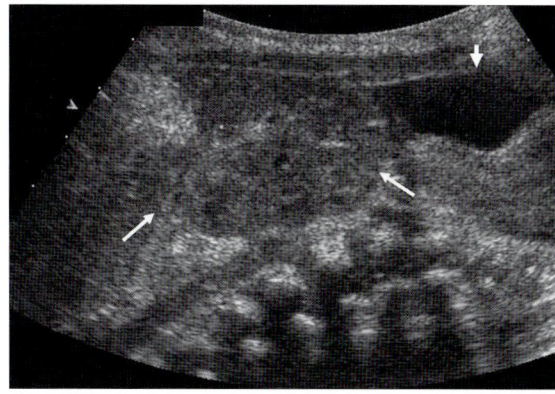

Fig. 14.3 **Pelvic kidney. a** Pelvic kidney in a pediatric patient close to the iliac vessels (arrow). **b** Pelvic kidney (between arrows) in a newborn child with the bladder (short arrow) adjacent to the lower aspect of the pelvic kidney

the retroperitoneum, the kidneys migrate cranially.[12] Ectopic kidneys can be found anywhere along their migratory path but are most commonly found in the pelvis and are usually malrotated. Although patients may present with a mass, most pelvic kidneys are asymptomatic (Fig. 14.3). There is an associated increased risk of infection and hydronephrosis in these abnormally placed kidneys. The ectopic kidney may be difficult to locate on ultrasound and, in the presence of an empty renal fossa, further imaging should be performed to locate the ectopic kidney; a ^{99m}Tc-dimercaptosuccinic acid (^{99m}Tc-DMSA) scan is normally performed to locate the ectopic kidney.[13]

Renal Agenesis and Hypoplasia

Renal agenesis may be unilateral or bilateral. The latter is incompatible with life, and neonates with this condition tend to die from chronic renal failure toward the end of the first week of life.

Duplication Anomalies

Renal duplication is the most common renal anomaly.[14] Renal duplication is thought to be due to early division of the ureteral bud, resulting in separation of the renal pelvis into two moieties.[12] More commonly a unilateral phenomenon, bilateral duplication does occur. The changes of duplication may be partial or complete with the development of two ureters and ectopic insertion of the ureters into the bladder. The ureter from the upper moiety, often associated with a ureterocele, enters the bladder inferior to the lower-pole ureter, an inverse relationship known as the "Weigert–Meyer" rule. Due to the shorter course through the bladder wall, the ureter draining the lower renal moiety is susceptible to vesicoureteric reflux (VUR). The upper-pole moiety, in turn, is susceptible to obstruction. Pelviureteric junction (PUJ) obstruction of the lower moiety may also be seen.

Constant leakage of urine in the presence of a normal voiding pattern may be seen in girls due to ectopic insertion of the ureter anywhere along the lower urogenital tract, including the vagina and perineum. In boys, the ectopic ureter terminates above the external sphincter and this problem does not occur.[15] Although ultrasound will detect most duplex systems and their associated complications, the examination may be entirely normal. Further imaging in the form of cystography and ^{99m}Tc-DMSA studies are needed for further evaluation.

> **Summary points:**
> - Horseshoe kidney is best imaged in the coronal plane
> - In cross-fused ectopia the ureters enter the bladder in their normal position
> - Renal duplication is the commonest renal anomaly
> - Ectopic kidneys are most commonly found in the pelvis

Hydronephrosis

Hydronephrosis is the most commonly detected antenatal abnormality and a common indication for postnatal imaging.[5,15] Ultrasound is sensitive in detecting hydronephrosis and is able to assess dilatation involving the renal tract along its entire length from the renal calyces down to the vesicoureteric junction (VUJ).[15,16] Hydronephrosis may be discovered incidentally or be found in patients presenting for investigation of a UTI, abdominal pain, renal failure, or hypertension (Fig. 14.4). When assessing the neonate referred with an antenatal diagnosis of hydronephrosis, early imaging may under-

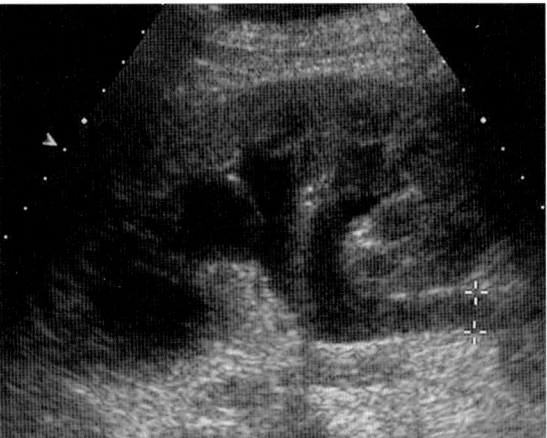

Fig. 14.4 **Hydronephrosis.** A moderate degree of hydronephrosis with dilatation of the upper ureter (between cursors)

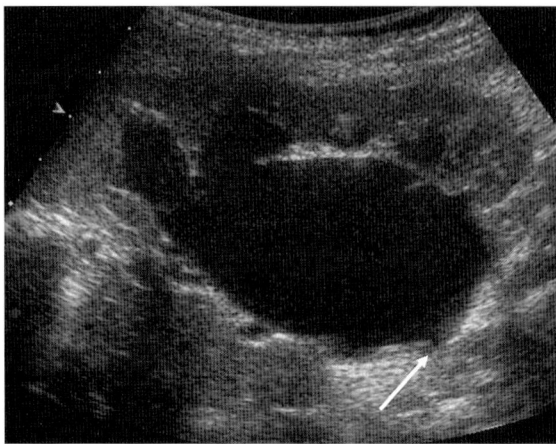

Fig. 14.5 **PUJ obstruction.** A dilated pelvis and thinning of the renal parenchyma in a long-standing PUJ obstruction. The expected PUJ is indicated by the arrow

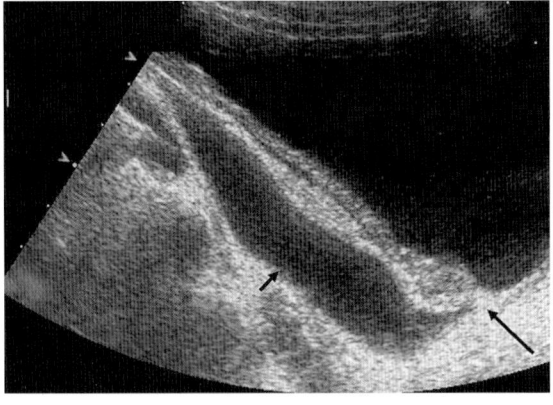

a

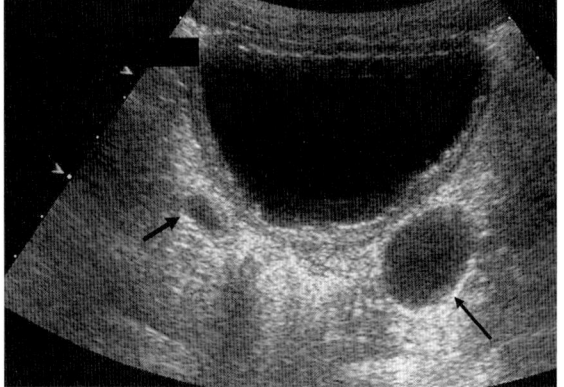

b

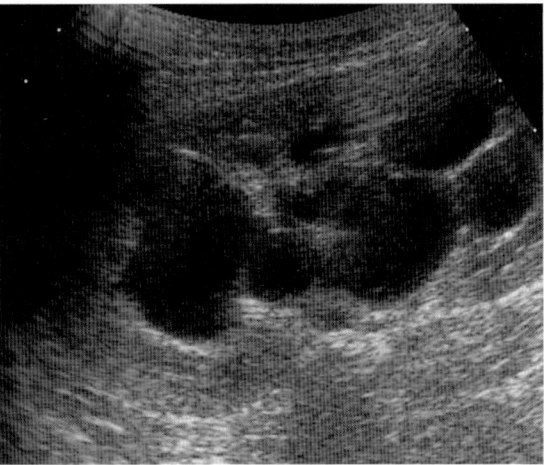

c

Fig. 14.6 **VUJ obstruction. a** Narrowing at the VUJ (arrow), with dilatation of the distal ureter (short arrow). **b** Transverse image through the bladder, with marked dilatation of the left ureter (long arrow) and prominence of the right ureter (short arrow). **c** Resulting hydronephrosis of the left kidney

estimate the degree of hydronephrosis, as physiological dehydration secondary to poor feeding may be present.[17] Furthermore, a reduced glomerular filtration rate (GFR) in the first few days of life is often present.[18] As many as 18–30% of antenatally diagnosed hydronephrosis resolve in the postnatal period and are probably due to atony of the collecting system in the presence of maternal progesterone.[19]

Hydronephrosis may be divided into two groups: obstructive and nonobstructive causes. Obstructive causes include PUJ obstruction (Fig. 14.5), VUJ obstruction (Fig. 14.6), posterior urethral valves (Fig. 14.7), and other causes of bladder outlet obstruction. Causes of nonobstructive hydronephrosis are predominantly congenital in origin.

Obstructive Hydronephrosis

Pelviureteric Junction Obstruction
This is the most common congenital obstruction of the urinary tract but may be acquired following extrinsic compression of the PUJ by an anomalous blood vessel, band, or adhesion or due to presence of a calculus or blood clot.[15] It occurs more commonly in male infants and is reported to involve the left kidney more than the right.[20] The diagnosis can be made following antenatal ultrasound or may be detected in the child presenting with pain, hematuria, infection, or an upper abdominal mass. Classically, ultrasound demonstrates pelvicalyceal dilatation without ureteral dilatation (Fig. 14.**5**). Appearances may be bilateral and asymmetrical. Further imaging to confirm the ultrasound diagnosis and assess renal function includes scintigraphy and cystography to exclude the presence of coexistent reflux which may be seen in the contralateral kidney.

Vesicoureteric Junction Obstruction
Vesicoureteric junction (VUJ) obstruction is due to dysmotility of the distal ureter. Other causes of distal ureteric obstruction include congenital stenosis, distal ureteric calculi or intraluminal blood clot, a neurogenic bladder, or extrinsic compression on the ureter from a pelvic mass. Ultrasound demonstrates a dilated distal ureter lying posterior to the bladder and varying upper tract dilatation, although there may be no associated hydronephrosis (Fig. 14.**6**). Further imaging would include scintigraphy and cystography.

Posterior Urethral Valve
During the seventh week of fetal development, the urogenital membrane ruptures and incomplete disintegration of this membrane may lead to the development of a posterior urethral valve (PUV).[21,22] PUV is the most common congenital cause of lower urinary tract obstruction in the male infant, producing acute obstruction in the infant, although milder cases may not present until later in childhood (Fig. 14.**7**). Although familial occurrence is rare, cases have been reported amongst siblings and identical twins.[23] Diagnosis may be made on antenatal imaging with typical ultrasound findings of a thick-walled trabeculated bladder, bilateral hydroureter, and bilateral hydronephrosis, although a normal upper tract is seen in up to 10% of cases.[22]

An elongated dilated posterior urethra may be seen inferior to a dilated bladder neck, probably best demonstrated on a postnatal transperineal ultrasound

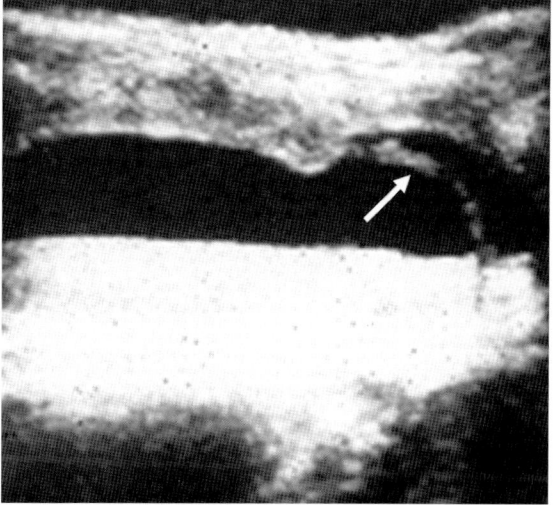

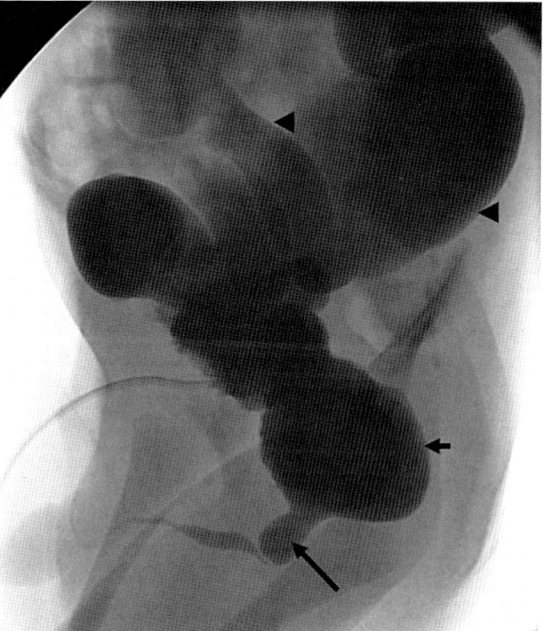

Fig. 14.**7 Posterior urethral valves. a** Longitudinal image of the posterior urethra demonstrating a posterior urethral valve (arrow). (Courtesy of Dr. U. Patel and Dr. D. Rickards, London, UK) **b** Image from micturating cystourography in a male infant, demonstrating bilateral dilated ureters (arrowheads), the bladder (short arrow), and a distended posterior urethra (long arrow). These appearances have arisen due to the presence of posterior urethral values. (Courtesy of Dr. G. Irwin, Glasgow, UK)

where highly reflective valve leaflets traversing the dilated posterior urethra are visualized.[23] The ultrasound examination is best performed with the infant lying supine with the legs slightly elevated and placing the transducer beneath the scrotum to reveal the dilated posterior urethra lying anteriorly.[22]

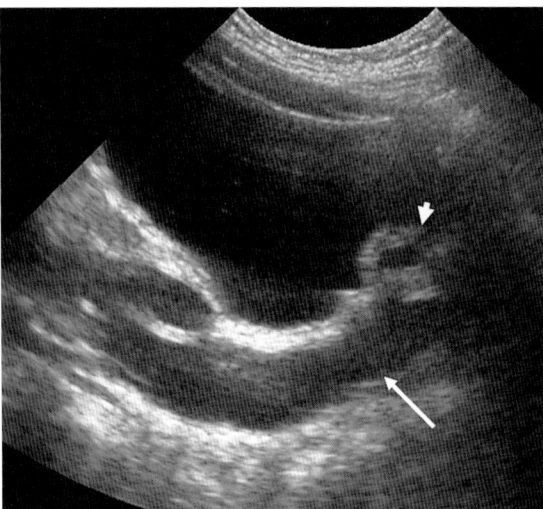

Fig. 14.**8 Ureterocele.** Longitudinal image of the bladder, demonstrating a thick-walled ureterocele (short arrow) with dilatation of the corresponding ureter (long arrow). (Courtesy of Dr. G. Irwin, Glasgow, UK)

Severe renal tract obstruction may produce renal dysplasia. The kidneys are highly reflective and contain multiple cortical cysts. Rarely due to back-pressure from the dilated system, does urine escape from a ruptured calyceal fornix, renal parenchymal tear, or even from a distended bladder, protecting against renal failure. This has been reported to occur in utero and is associated with the presence of contained urinomas and ascites.[24]

Ureteroceles

Ureteroceles are congenital abnormalities seen in approximately one in 500 births, occurring more commonly in female infants (Fig. 14.**8**).[23,25] The distal intravesical ureter undergoes cystic dilatation and may be orthotopic or ectopic in location, the latter associated with a duplex renal system.[22] Orthotopic ureteroceles are less common, tend to be smaller, narrower, and may prolapse into the urethra producing bladder outlet obstruction.[25] The ectopic ureterocele is associated with hydronephrosis of the upper renal moiety of a duplex system, and is situated inferomedial to the bladder trigone near the bladder neck.[26] Ultrasound reveals a dilated ureter from the kidney down to the bladder, where it ends in a round anechoic intravesicular thin-walled cystic structure of variable size and shape. The ureterocele may expand and collapse with ureteral contraction, appearing solid when collapsed. The ectopic ureterocele may become large enough to obstruct the ipsilateral lower pole ureter or contralateral ureter and may be associated with reflux and recurrent UTIs.

Nonobstructive Hydronephrosis

Vesicoureteric Reflux

Vesicoureteric reflux (VUR) occurs due to incompetence of the VUJ, either as a result of immaturity or maldevelopment, occurring in up to 50% of children who present with a UTI and in 0.5% of asymptomatic patients.[27] Although ultrasound is not the primary diagnostic procedure for detecting VUR, it is the first-line investigation for assessing the renal tract. Ultrasound indicators of VUR are nonspecific and include ureteric and pelvicalyceal dilatation, renal pelvic or ureteral wall thickening, loss of corticomedullary differentiation, and signs of renal dysplasia.[28] A normal ultrasound does not exclude VUR; even imaging during micturition does not improve the sensitivity of VUR detection. Use of microbubble ultrasound contrast agents may be helpful in assessing VUR.[29] Following catheterization of the bladder and instillation of microbubble contrast, all grades of reflux have been detected in children with VUR, by observing the movement of the microbubbles in the ureter and pelvicalyceal system. The use of microbubble contrast agents in children is currently not licensed. The urethra is not examined during the microbubble contrast study which concentrates on the upper renal tracts; a micturating cystogram would still have to be performed in boys to exclude the presence of a PUV. Most neonatal hydronephrosis, proved to be due to VUR, resolve spontaneously by approximately age five years.[30] However, it has been reported that up to 25% of infants with prenatal hydronephrosis and a normal postnatal ultrasound have VUR, which would suggest that a micturating cystogram needs to be performed on all infants with an antenatal diagnosis of hydronephrosis.

Megaureters

Primary megaureter is described as the ureteral equivalent of Hirschsprung disease, occurring more commonly in male infants.[31] The distal segment of the ureter does not demonstrate peristalsis, resulting in relative obstruction and dilatation of the more proximal renal tract. Ultrasound demonstrates the presence of a tortuous dilated hyperperistaltic ureter proximal to a narrowed atonic segment.[32] These appearances may be detected on antenatal imaging with minimal or no associated pelvicalyceal dilatation (Fig. 14.**9**).

Megacalycosis

Megacalycosis is a rare congenital anomaly and is usually an incidental finding on ultrasound. Features include dilatation and an increase in the number of calyces without dilatation of the renal pelvis or ureter, or evidence of renal scarring.

Urinary Tract Infections

Urinary tract infections (UTIs) are one of the most common clinical problems seen in the pediatric population, with a tendency to affect girls more often. The importance of imaging is to identify any underlying anatomical abnormality that may predispose the child to pyelonephritis, as well as to exclude renal obstruction and VUR. Ultimately, the long-term aim is to prevent the development of renal scarring with the associated complications of renal failure and hypertension.[5,15] VUR is reported to occur in up to 50% of children with a documented UTI; a combination that leads to renal scarring.[33] Age is an important determinant, as in the older child with normal kidneys scarring rarely develops. Infants under age one year are most at risk of renal parenchyma damage due to VUR in the presence of infected urine.

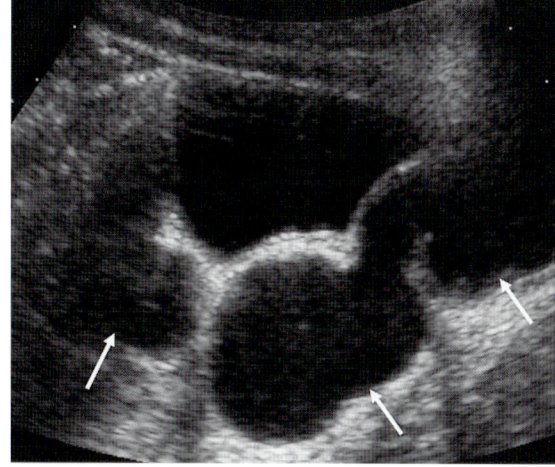

Fig. 14.**9 Megaureter.** A markedly dilated ureter, folded on itself several times (arrows)

Acute Pyelonephritis

Acute pyelonephritis is often difficult to diagnose in children and ultrasound is a poor technique for identifying disease; findings on ultrasound are nonspecific and may be normal. The affected kidney may be enlarged, of relatively high reflectivity, with an associated loss of the normal corticomedullary differentiation and mild hydronephrosis due either to atony of the collecting system, VUR, or PUJ obstruction.[34] Focal, low-reflective areas may be seen on gray-scale imaging with color Doppler imaging demonstrating triangular vascular defects which resolve with antibiotic therapy (Fig. 14.**10**).[35]

Chronic Pyelonephritis (Reflux Nephropathy)

In chronic pyelonephritis the kidneys are classically small and highly reflective, with dilatation of the collecting systems and loss of the normal corticomedullary differentiation (Fig. 14.**11**). These findings on ultrasound are nonspecific and may be seen in the end-stages of a number of renal diseases. Renal scarring is most marked at the renal poles, areas most often associated with VUR.

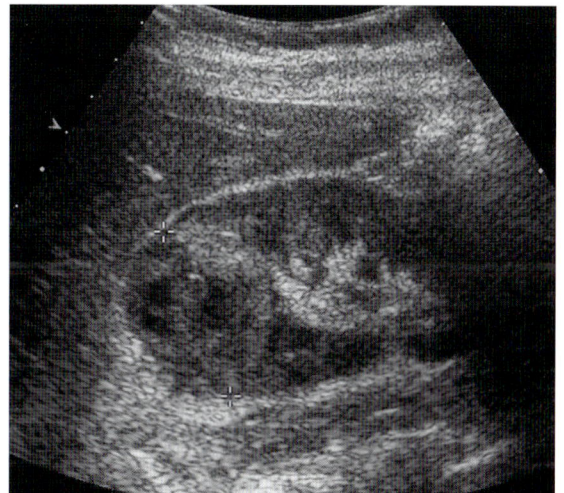

a

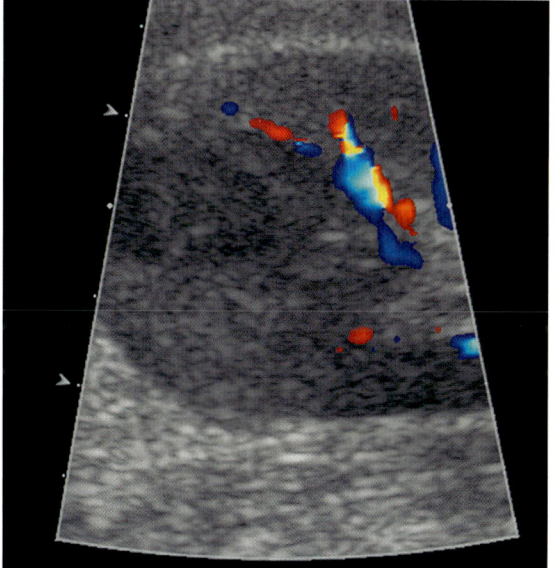

b

Fig. 14.**10 Acute focal pyelonephritis. a** Focal area of mixed reflectivity in the upper aspect of the kidney, representing a focal area of pyelonephritis (between cursors). No color Doppler flow to the focal infected area is demonstrated. (Courtesy of Dr. N. Sathanathan, Dartford, UK)

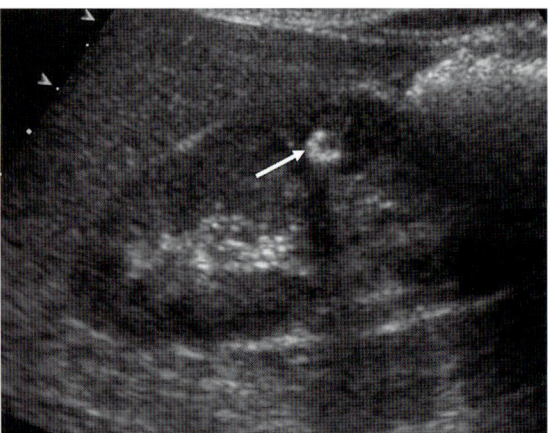

Fig. 14.**16 Angiomyolipoma.** A focal lesion in the renal cortex of high reflectivity in keeping with an angiomyolipoma (arrow)

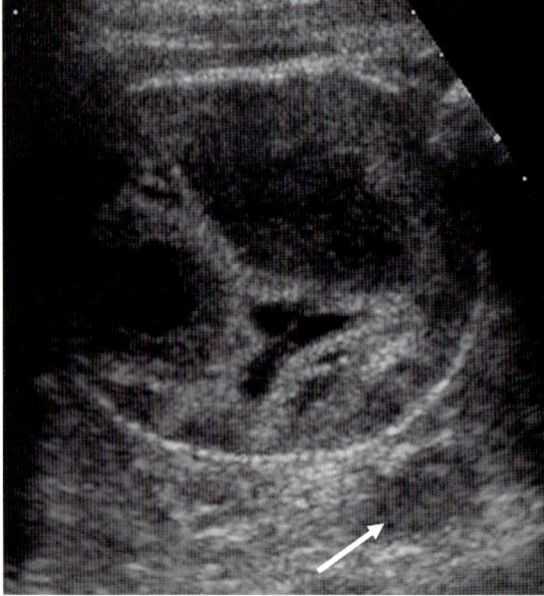

Fig. 14.**17 Multilocular cystic nephroma.** A multiseptated mass at the upper aspect of the left kidney (arrow) in keeping with a multilocular cystic nephroma

■ Nongenetic Disease

Simple Cysts

Simple renal cysts are rare, incidental findings in the pediatric population. These cortical lesions are usually thin-walled, anechoic, and well-defined on ultrasound, demonstrating characteristic posterior acoustic enhancement without communication with the collecting system. No vascular flow is present within these cysts or the cyst wall, although reflective material within the cyst may represent infection or past hemorrhage.

Cystic Dysplasia

Cystic dysplasia is a congenital abnormality that arises following abnormal metanephric development, resulting in the persistence of immature renal tissue with subsequent poor renal function. The kidney is shrunken and of high reflectivity, containing small subcentimeter cortical cysts. These appearances may be bilateral. Cystic dysplasia is associated with renal duplication, PUVs, crossed-fused ectopia, horseshoe kidney, and pelvic kidneys.[39]

Multicystic Renal Dysplasia

Multicystic renal dysplasia is the second most common cause of an abdominal mass in the newborn. Multicystic renal dysplasia occurs following failure of the ureteric bud to form a connection with the metanephric mesoderm, resulting in the arrest of development of the definitive fetal kidney.

On ultrasound the kidney is replaced by anechoic cysts of varying sizes which characteristically do not communicate with each other. There is no visible renal cortex or central renal pelvis.[43] These appearances usually involve the entire kidney but may involve the upper pole of a duplex system. The contralateral kidney is hypertrophied and further examination of this kidney is important as there is a 30% incidence of associated VUR, PUJ obstruction, and ureteric stenosis.[39] Over time the kidney may involute and not be identified on ultrasound. However, if the multicystic renal dysplasia remains unchanged or even increases in size, this predisposes the patient to hypertension and possible risk of malignancy, a controversial issue.[47]

Multilocular Cystic Nephroma

This is a rare benign lesion, which is uncommon under age two years. The lesion appears as a multiloculated cyst, which is difficult to distinguish from a cystic Wilms tumor.[48,49] Ultrasound demonstrates a well-circumscribed, multiloculated cystic mass with septations (Fig. 14.**17**).

Acquired Cystic Renal Disease

Cysts may be seen on ultrasound following infection, especially tuberculosis, and trauma, or be associated with a necrotic tumor. Patients with chronic renal disease and those on dialysis are also prone to cyst development.[16]

> **Summary points:**
> - Enlarged kidneys of increased reflectivity are classically seen in a ARPKD
> - Cysts may be seen in children with ADPKD
> - Simple renal cysts are rare
> - Medullary cystic disease of the kidney may involve the upper pole of a duplex system

Renal Tumors

Ultrasound is normally the first imaging investigation to assess the child who presents with an abdominal mass.

Benign Renal Tumors

Mesoblastic Nephroma

Mesoblastic nephroma is the most common cause of a renal mass seen in the neonate and may be detected on antenatal ultrasound imaging. Patients usually present with a nontender palpable mass and, on occasion, hypertension. On ultrasound a mesoblastic nephroma is a solid lesion of variable appearance, either homogenous or heterogonous, depending on the presence of necrosis or hemorrhage. Although a mesoblastic nephroma is often termed a "congenital Wilms tumor," it has no malignant potential.[50]

Angiomyolipoma

Although not common in the pediatric population, these hamartomas may be seen on ultrasound in those children with tuberous sclerosis. These small, highly reflective lesions are usually multiple, bilateral, and associated with the presence of renal cysts, with a tendency to develop and grow during adolescence.

Malignant Renal Tumors

Wilms Tumor

A Wilms tumor is the most common malignant renal tumor seen in children under age five years with a peak incidence at age three. There is an increased incidence in children with hemihypertrophy, Beckwith–Wiedeman syndrome, nephroblastoma, horseshoe kidney, and sporadic aniridia, where the tumor tends to occur earlier in life. Typical presentation is with an asymptomatic abdominal mass.[51]

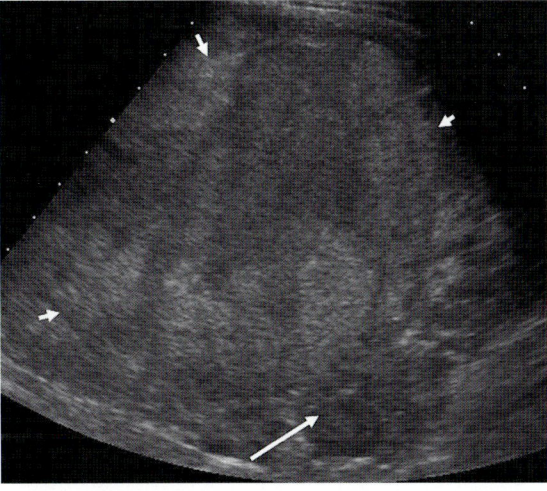
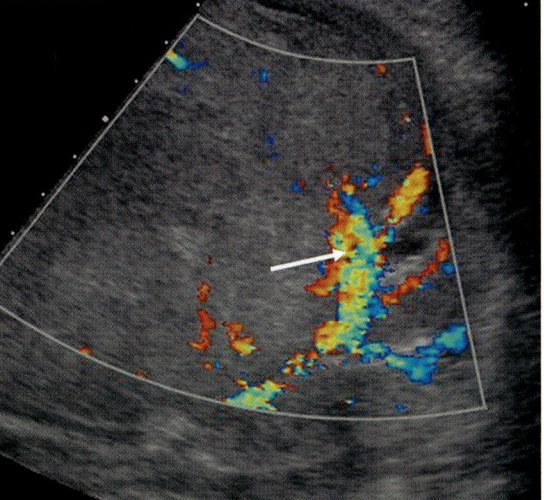

Fig. 14.**18 Wilms tumor. a** A large heterogeneous irregular mass (short arrows) arises from the upper aspect of the kidney (arrow). **b** The heterogeneous mass demonstrates a variable amount of color Doppler signal, with displacement of the renal vessels (arrow)

On ultrasound a Wilms tumor is well-defined, often with a heterogeneous appearance due to the presence of necrosis, hemorrhage, and calcification (Fig. 14.**18**).[52] As the tumor increases in size, displacement of the surrounding retroperitoneal structures and extension into both the renal vein and IVC occurs. Ascites, lymphadenopathy, and low-reflective liver metastases may be seen. The importance of assessing the contralateral kidney both at presentation and on follow-up is important as 5% of cases are bilateral. Following the initial ultrasound examination, further imaging includes computed tomography (CT) of the chest and abdomen and magnetic resonance (MR) angiography to assess vascular involvement.

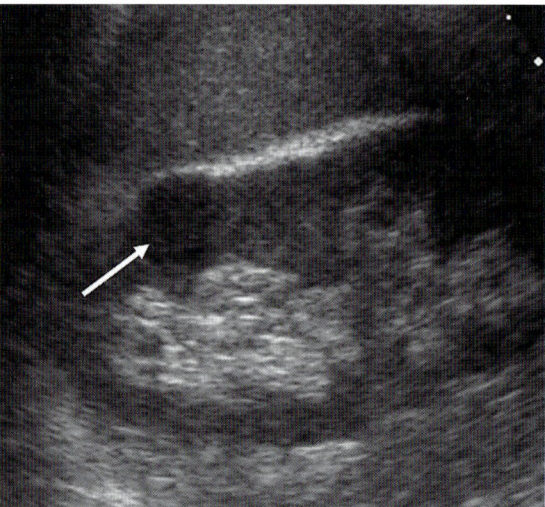

Fig. 14.**19 Renal lymphoma.** A low-reflective, solid lesion (arrow) in the kidney, representing posttransplant lymphoproliferative disease (PTLD), in a pediatric patient following liver transplantation

Renal Cell Carcinoma

Renal cell carcinoma (RCC) is a rare tumor in the pediatric age group and tends to occur in an older age group with a peak incidence at age nine. Unfortunately, an RCC carries a poor prognosis. On ultrasound, the tumor resembles that of a Wilms tumor, although calcification tends to be commoner.

Lymphoma

Primary involvement of the kidneys with lymphoma is rare. On ultrasound the kidneys are enlarged and may either contain discrete anechoic or low-reflective masses or be diffusely low-reflective due to infiltration (Fig. 14.**19**).[53]

Leukemia

On ultrasound, kidneys involved with leukemia are symmetrically enlarged and of normal to increased reflectivity. There may be hydronephrosis secondary to retroperitoneal lymphadenopathy.

Summary points:
- Mesoblastic nephroma is the commonest renal mass seen in the neonate
- Highly reflective angiomyolipoma may be seen in children with tuberous sclerosis
- Wilms tumor is a well-defined, heterogeneous mass on ultrasound
- RCC is rare in children and carries a poor prognosis

Renal Trauma

Renal injury is usually caused by blunt abdominal trauma, in many cases resulting from a hyperflexion fall or a motor vehicle accident.[54] Ultrasound is not normally the first-line investigation but is routinely used to monitor resolution of the renal injuries.[55] Hematoma has a variable appearance on ultrasound and may appear complex, becoming low-reflective with resolution. Renal lacerations present either as low- or high-reflective defects with associated cortical irregularity. Ultrasound is also useful in the follow-up of perinephric collections, mainly hematomas and urinomas, which may also be seen as a complication of renal biopsy, a form of iatrogenic renal injury.[56]

Renal Calcification

Nephrolithiasis

In the pediatric population renal calculi are usually seen following infection or in children with metabolic abnormalities. Classically renal calculi are of high reflectivity and may cast an acoustic shadow depending on size and matrix composition. There may be associated hydronephrosis.

Nephrocalcinosis

Nephrocalcinosis arises from the deposition of calcium salts within the renal parenchyma, commonly within the pyramids, seen on ultrasound as a highly reflective kidney with reversal of the normal pattern of corticomedullary differentiation (Fig. 14.**20**). Appearances are more commonly bilateral, although unilateral disease does occur. In the neonate, nephrocalcinosis most commonly occurs following treatment with the diuretic frusemide. Other causes of nephrocalcinosis include renal tubular acidosis, medullary sponge kidney, and a variety of metabolic disorders. There are four patterns of calcium deposition within the kidney (patterns A–D), demonstrating a general progression of severity of disease.[57]

Vascular Anomalies

Renal Vein Thrombosis

A renal vein thrombosis most often occurs following hypovolemia in the pediatric population but is also described as a complication of a Wilms tumor. On ultrasound the kidney may be enlarged with associated loss of corticomedullary differentiation in the acute phase, although this is reversible. In chronic renal vein thrombosis the kidneys are small with normal corticomedullary differentiation.[58]

Renal Transplant

Ultrasound provides the clinicians with useful information regarding the transplant kidney in the immediate postoperative period, as well as in the long term; ultrasound is the best method for evaluating renal morphology. Good-quality images are generally obtained due to the superficial position of the transplanted pelvic kidney. The pyramids and corticomedullary junction can be easily identified using a high-frequency transducer.[59] Color and spectral Doppler imaging are used to assess arterial and venous blood flow within the kidney.[60]

In acute rejection, ultrasound findings are nonspecific; there is swelling of the kidney with loss of the normal corticomedullary differentiation and an increase in the arterial resistance index (RI) on spectral Doppler imaging.[61] Renal biopsy remains the reference standard for diagnosis of rejection. Hydronephrosis of the transplant kidney may be present, which may follow either from edema at the site of anastomosis of the ureter to the bladder or following vascular ischemia with stricture formation. VUR is a common consequence following transplantation and a further cause for dilatation of the collecting system.

Fluid collections are commonly seen on ultrasound following renal transplantation. Lymphoceles are the most common and tend to resolve spontaneously. Urinomas are associated with an anastomotic leak and tend to present as a clear perinephric collection. Large collections may produce extrinsic ureteric compression with consequent hydronephrosis. Ultrasound may be used to guide aspiration or drain placement within these collections.[62] Vascular complications such as renal artery thrombosis, stenosis, or pseudoaneurysm may be visualized with color and spectral Doppler ultrasound (Fig. 14.21).

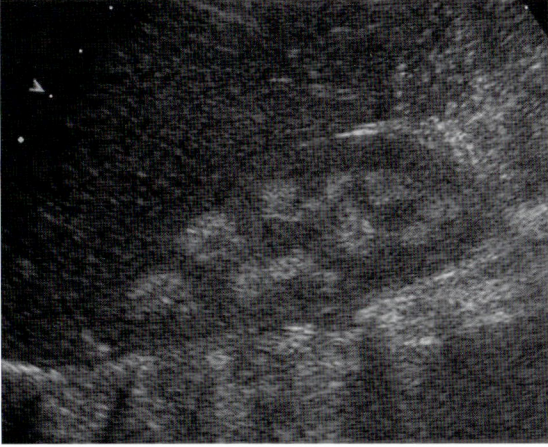

Fig. 14.20 **Nephrocalcinosis.** A "Type C" pattern of nephrocalcinosis, with the renal pyramids full of calcium deposits, giving the appearance of reversal of the normal corticomedullary differentiation

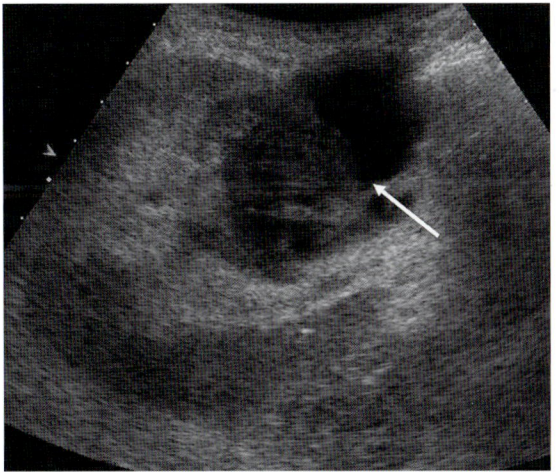

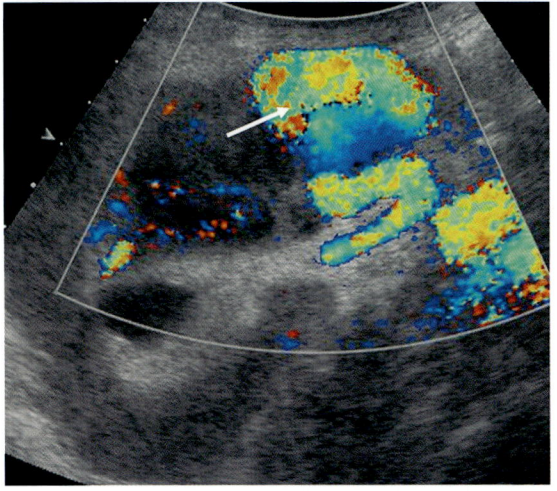

Fig. 14.21 **Renal transplant pseudoaneurysm. a** A low-reflective area adjacent to the hilum of the transplant kidney (arrow) with high-reflective hematoma in the posterior aspect. **b** Color Doppler ultrasound confirms the arterial vascular nature of the lesion; a transplant renal artery pseudoaneurysm, demonstrating the "yin–yang" sign (arrow)

> **Summary points:**
> - Ultrasound is useful in the follow-up of perinephric collections following blunt abdominal trauma
> - Nephrocalcinosis is commonly a bilateral disease with four patterns of calcium deposition
> - Changes seen on ultrasound in acute renal vein thrombosis are reversible
> - Ultrasound findings of acute rejection are nonspecific
> - Reflux is a common complication following transplantation

Abnormalities of the Bladder and Distal Urinary Tract

Bladder Exstrophy

In bladder exstrophy, which occurs more commonly in boys, the bladder is located outside the abdomen due to abnormal development of the anterior abdominal wall and anterior wall of the bladder.[25] The upper renal tracts are normal and urine flows directly from the bladder out onto the anterior abdominal wall. Other associated urological abnormalities include an incomplete external urethral sphincter and a hypospadias.

Urachal Anomalies

There are four different urachal anomalies that arise due to the persistence of the embryonic connection between the bladder and umbilicus, which should normally close at birth.[63] The most obvious is the patent urachus, with urine discharging from the umbilicus. The other types of urachal anomaly may only be detected in later life.[25] The most common abnormality is the urachal diverticulum, which arises in an anterior position from the bladder apex and may be associated with prune belly syndrome or a PUV. The urachal cyst is a blind-ending pouch which lies in a suprapubic location and does not communicate with the bladder or umbilicus. On ultrasound this abnormality is of low reflectivity but may become infected or contain hemorrhage following trauma. The urachal sinus extends distally from the umbilicus (Fig. 14.22).

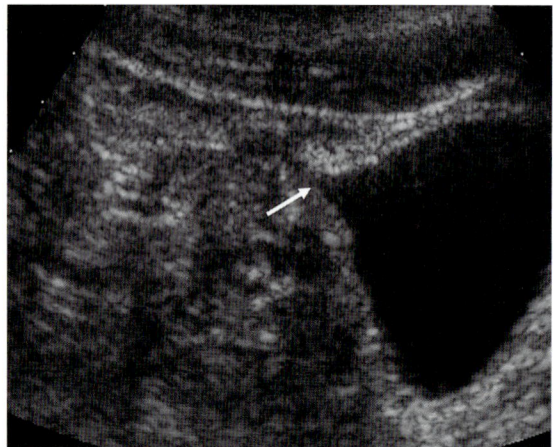

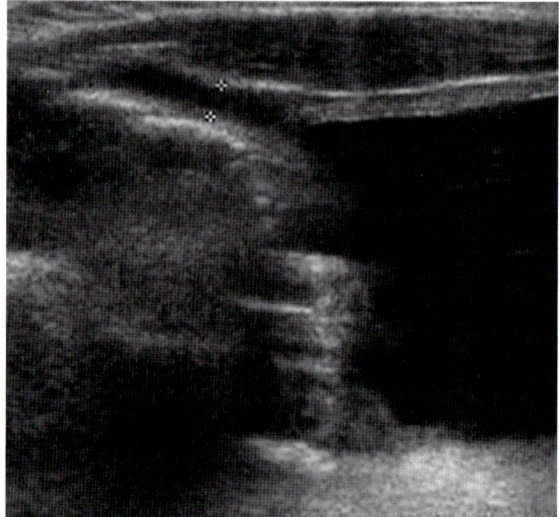

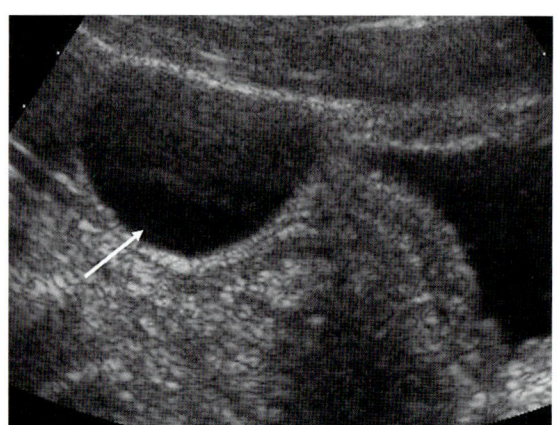

Fig. 14.22 **Persistent urachus. a** A small urachal remnant diverticulum (arrow) is present at the upper aspect of the bladder. **b** A persistent urachal sinus (between cursors) is present at the upper aspect of the bladder. **c** A persistent urachal cyst remnant (arrow) is present at the upper aspect of the bladder

Bladder Diverticula

Bladder diverticula are common and are often an incidental finding on ultrasound, presenting as anechoic fluid-filled structures projecting from the bladder wall. Bladder diverticula may be associated with infection, stone formation, VUR, and bladder outlet obstruction.[25] A diverticulum at the VUJ, the "Hutch diverticulum," is associated with ipsilateral VUR in approximately 50% of cases.[64]

Prune Belly Syndrome (Eagle–Barrett Syndrome)

Prune belly syndrome (or abdominal muscle deficiency syndrome) is seen predominantly in boys and presents with a triad of hypoplastic abdominal muscles, cryptorchidism, and abnormalities of the urinary tract (dilated tortuous ureters, large bladder, patent urachus, dilated prostatic urethra). There is a spectrum of urinary tract abnormalities with the most severely affected patients presenting with renal dysplasia, gross dilatation of the collecting systems, and hydroureter.[65]

Infection

Ultrasound may reveal uniform or focal bladder-wall thickening. Debris and calculi may also be seen.

Bladder Tumors

Bladder tumors are rare; rhabdomyosarcoma is the most common bladder tumor in the pediatric group. Rhabdomyosarcoma is the most common malignant sarcoma in children presenting in the first three years of life, more commonly in boys. On ultrasound, the mass is homogenous and multilobulated, resembling a bunch of grapes. There may be associated hydronephrosis due to bladder-wall thickening at the VUJ or bladder outlet obstruction.[25] Other bladder tumors include transitional cell carcinoma (TCC), neurofibroma, pheochromocytoma, and the cavernous hemangioma.

Neuropathic Bladder

A neuropathic bladder may be congenital, associated with sacral agenesis, the presence of a myelomeningocele, or secondary to trauma, spinal cord tumors, or cerebral palsy. Ultrasound appearances are variable and may be subtle and nonspecific. The bladder may be thick-walled, trabeculated (muscle fibers give an

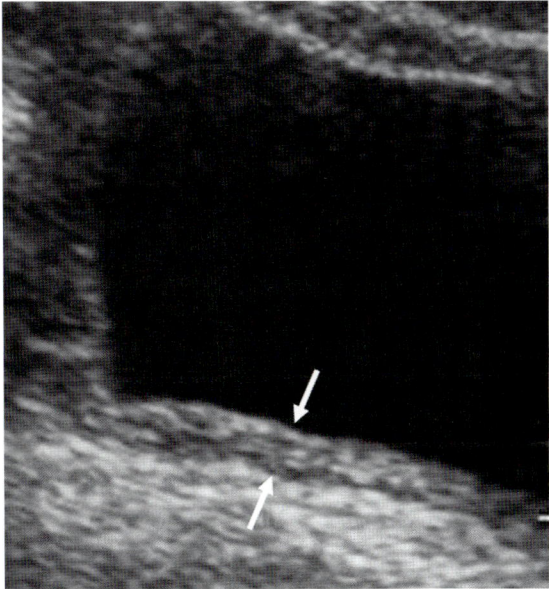

Fig. 14.23 **Thickened bladder wall.** The bladder wall is thickened in a patient with a neuropathic bladder (between arrows)

irregular outline to the inner bladder wall), with a large postmicturition volume and dilatation of the upper renal tracts (Fig. 14.23).

Bladder Trauma

In children the bladder lies predominantly within the abdomen and is vulnerable to injury.[56] Extraperitoneal rupture of the bladder occurs at the bladder neck and is associated with pelvic fractures. Extraperitoneal rupture is more common than intraperitoneal rupture and usually follows blunt abdominal trauma in the presence of a distended bladder.[54] Ultrasound is not routinely used to assess the injured child but may reveal free fluid within the pelvis and abdomen, occasionally demonstrating a defect within the bladder wall. The bladder is best assessed with CT cystography. Urethral injuries tend to occur in boys and are less common than bladder injuries. Ultrasound has no role in assessing urethral trauma.

> **Summary points:**
> - In bladder exstrophy the upper renal tracts are normal
> - The most common urachal anomaly is the urachal diverticulum
> - Bladder diverticula are common
> - The most severely affected patients with prune belly syndrome present with renal dysplasia, gross dilatation of the collecting systems, and hydrourethra

Adrenal Glands

Anatomy

The normal adrenal gland has a characteristic V- or Y-shape. In the neonate the gland has a low-reflective cortex and a central high-reflective medulla (Fig. 14.24). This appearance gradually changes and by age one year the adrenal glands resemble those of the adult, with loss of differentiation between the cortex and medulla.[66]

Congenital Anomalies

Adrenal gland anomalies are rare and usually associated with renal anomalies.

Congenital Adrenal Hyperplasia

Congenital adrenal hyperplasia is an autosomal recessive disorder that manifests in newborns with ambiguous genitalia or virilism in newborn girls. Ultrasound reveals an enlarged adrenal gland which has an irregular surface, the "cerebriform" pattern.[67]

Adrenal Agenesis

Adrenal agenesis is a rare finding associated with agenesis of the ipsilateral kidney and occurs early during fetal development.

Adrenal Hypoplasia

Adrenal hypoplasia occurs in anencephalic infants and may be associated with hypoplasia of the thyroid gland and gonads.[68]

Adrenal Ectopia

In adrenal ectopia, the adrenal gland lies in its normal suprarenal position but lies beneath the capsule of the kidney or liver.[68]

Adrenal Fusion

Adrenal fusion results in the horseshoe (circumrenal) adrenal gland which is produced when the limbs of the two glands fuse. Adrenal fusion may be associated with a horseshoe kidney or other congenital renal anomalies. A circular adrenal gland is formed when the two wings fuse completely.[68]

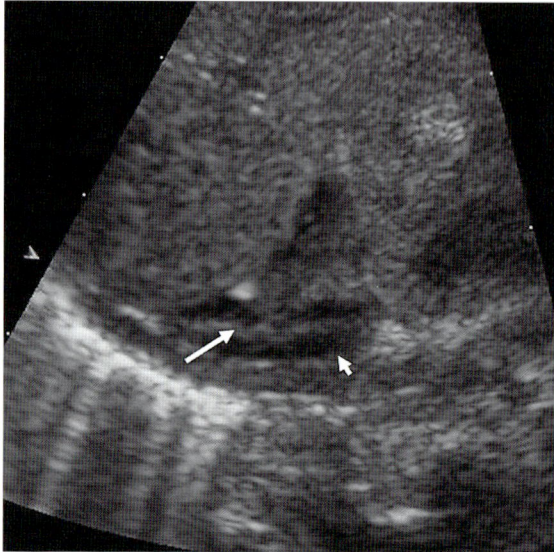

Fig. 14.24 **Normal adrenal gland.** The normal Y-shaped adrenal gland; the high-reflective central area (long arrow), represents the adrenal medulla, and a low-reflective peripheral area represents the adrenal cortex (short arrow)

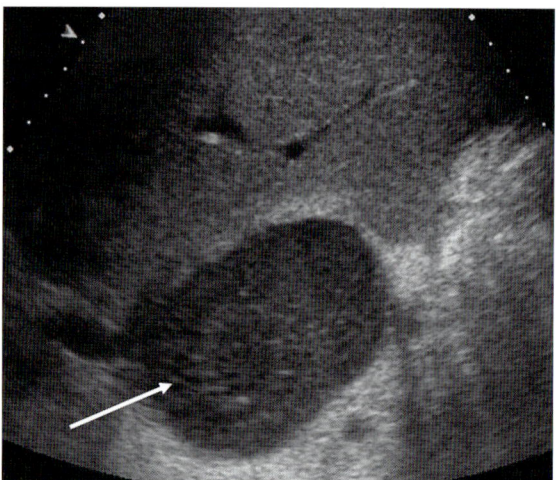

Fig. 14.25 **Adrenal hemorrhage.** A mixed-reflective area of hemorrhage into the left adrenal gland (arrow)

Adrenal Hemorrhage

Adrenal hemorrhage occurs in approximately two in 1000 births and is the most common cause of an adrenal mass in the neonate.[69] Hemorrhage is associated with birth trauma, septicemia, and hypoxia and is often right-sided. In the older child it may be seen following trauma and meningitis. On ultrasound, adrenal hemorrhage may be of low reflectivity or present as a high-reflective mass, depending on the age of the hemorrhage (Fig. 14.25). The mass decreases in size and reflectivity over time, becoming cystic and may eventually calcify.[70]

Adrenal Cysts

The adrenal cyst is usually seen on antenatal imaging and is typically well-defined and anechoic. These cysts may be seen in Beckwith–Wiedemann syndrome and hemihypertrophy.

Adrenal Tumors

Neuroblastoma

A neuroblastoma is a malignant tumor of neural crest cells that arises primarily in the adrenal gland and is the most common adrenal tumor in children, usually occurring in children under age four years.[71] Spread is early and wide; most children will have metastases at presentation. On ultrasound, a neuroblastoma is a solid, poorly defined, heterogeneous mass with foci of calcification (Fig. 14.26). Characteristically a neuroblastoma encases as well as displaces vessels and adjacent retroperitoneal structures. The kidney may be displaced inferiorly and the aorta and IVC anteriorly.[72] Lymph node spread of tumor is usually present but difficult to visualize on ultrasound. Imaging of the liver may reveal metastases. Staging of the disease requires further imaging with CT or MR.

Pheochromocytoma

A pheochromocytoma is a rare tumor usually associated with neurocutaneous syndromes and is normally diagnosed on biochemical investigations. The tumor is normally well-defined on ultrasound with a highly reflective texture.

> **Summary points:**
> - In congenital adrenal hyperplasia the enlarged adrenal gland has an irregular surface on the ultrasound
> - Adrenal hemorrhage may be of reduced or increased reflectivity
> - Neuroblastoma characteristically encases vessels and adjacent retroperitoneal structures

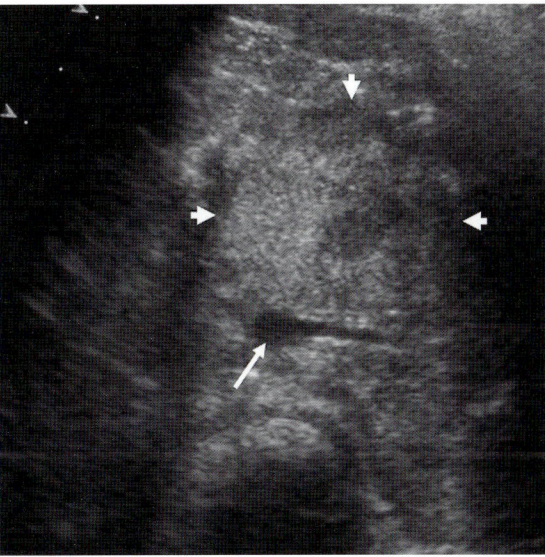

Fig. 14.26 **Neuroblastoma.** A transverse image of the upper abdomen, demonstrating a large, poorly defined heterogeneous mass (short arrows), a neuroblastoma, lying anterior to the confluence of the portal vein and splenic vein (arrow)

Testis

Congenital Anomalies

Cryptorchidism

During the seventh month of intrauterine life, the testes normally descend through the inguinal canal into the scrotal sac. Failure of this process is a common problem in male infants, which manifests as a unilateral or bilateral empty scrotum.[73] The ectopic testis may lie anywhere along the line of the ureter or vas deferens, and in 10% of cases both testes are affected (Fig. 14.27). Complications that arise following this abnormality of migration include testicular atrophy, infertility, and an increased incidence of malignant change. Ultrasound may be used to search for the ectopic testis, particularly so for locating the testis lying at or near the inguinal canal but less successful in locating an intra-abdominal testis.[74] MR imaging should be used for localizing intra-abdominal testis.[75] The kidneys should also routinely be imaged to assess for associated urological anomalies.

Congenital Torsion

Prenatal torsion of the testis is rare and not considered a surgical emergency. On ultrasound, the affected testis may be small and highly reflective or enlarged and of low reflectivity, containing multiple cystic spaces.[23] There may be an associated simple anechoic or complex, mixed-reflective hydrocele. An inguinal hernia is invariably present. Increased blood flow is seen within

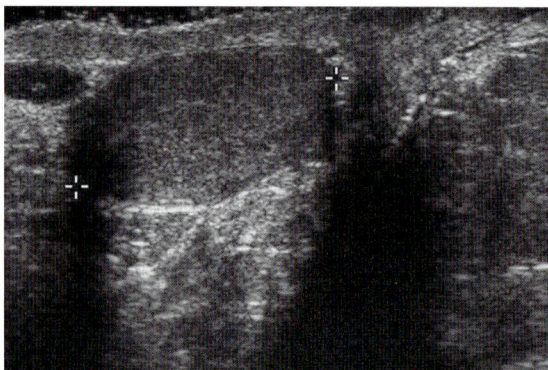

Fig. 14.**27 Inguinal testis.** A midlevel-echo undescended testis (between cursors) lying in the left inguinal canal

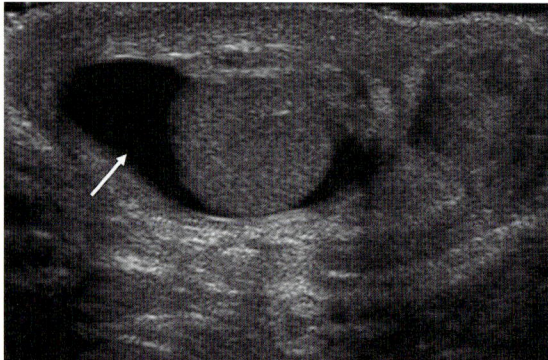

Fig. 14.**28 Hydrocele.** The right testis is outlined by anechoic fluid (arrow), representing a hydrocele

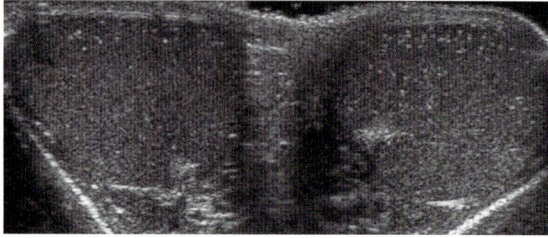

Fig. 14.**29 Testicular microlithiasis.** Bilateral testicular microlithiasis seen as foci of high reflectivity without the presence of acoustic shadowing

the periphery of the scrotum, with no flow demonstrated in the testis on color Doppler ultrasound.

Cystic Dysplasia

Cystic dysplasia is a rare congenital anomaly. Multiple irregular anechoic cystic spaces can be seen along the mediastinum testis on ultrasound.[76,77] As with most congenital testicular disorders, the renal tracts must be examined. Cystic dysplasia is associated with ipsilateral renal agenesis, renal duplication, and multicystic dysplastic kidney.[23]

Hydrocele

This is the most common cause of a scrotal mass in an infant; it may be either congenital or acquired, and unilateral or bilateral (Fig. 14.**28**). At closure of the processus vaginalis, a variable amount of fluid may be trapped within the tunica vaginalis forming a stable hydrocele. If there is a persistent patent processus vaginalis, the hydrocele may vary in size. Surgery is required to close the patent processus vaginalis, whereas the stable hydrocele usually reabsorbs. Acquired hydrocele are often secondary to inflammation, trauma, torsion, or tumor. The testis is surrounded by fluid, which if multiloculated suggests inflammatory change. In rare cases, a painful hydrocele may be the presenting symptom of appendicitis if there is a persistent patent processus vaginalis.[78]

Testicular Microlithiasis

Testicular microlithiasis is asymptomatic and is an incidental finding on ultrasound (Fig. 14.**29**). There is an association of testicular microlithiasis with primary malignancy of the testis, and ultrasound surveillance has been suggested.[79]

■ Scrotal Inflammation

Ultrasound of the scrotal sac and its contents can be extremely difficult in the child presenting with inflammatory disease. The asymptomatic side should be examined first to obtain the child's confidence and a baseline image for comparison with the affected side.

Epididymitis

Inflammation of the epididymis is primarily the consequence of infection, but may also arise following trauma or reactive to torsion of the testis or one of the testicular appendages.[80] The epididymis is enlarged and of high reflectivity on ultrasound (Fig. 14.**30**). Epididymo-orchitis following bacterial infection in sexually active boys, if florid and untreated, may be complicated by abscess formation and testicular infarction. Renal anomalies such as a duplex collecting system with insertion of the ectopic ureter into the vas deferens or seminal vesicles must be excluded.[15]

■ Testicular Torsion

Testicular torsion occurs most commonly in infants and adolescents. The testis rotates like a "bell-clapper" due to a narrow mesenteric attachment extending from the

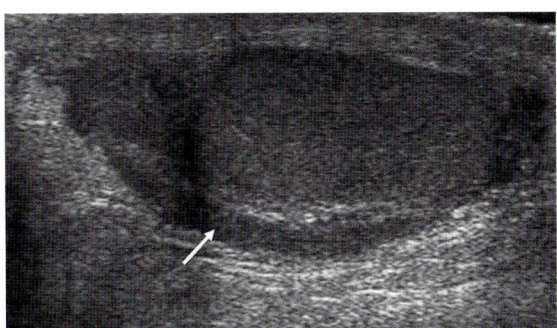

Fig. 14.**30 Acute epididymitis. a** On the B-mode ultrasound image the epididymis (arrow) is thickened with prominence of the epididymal head. **b** On the color Doppler ultrasound image there is increased color signal present in the epididymal (arrow) in keeping with acute epididymitis. (Courtesy of Dr. P.S. Sidhu, London, UK)

spermatic cord to the testis and epididymis.[81] An estimated 30% of boys who present with acute scrotal pain will have testicular torsion as a cause for the symptoms and need surgical intervention. However, most pediatric urologists would prefer to explore an acute scrotum early rather than rely on imaging to differentiate between testicular torsion and other causes of acute scrotal inflammation.[82] Ultrasound appearances are variable depending on the duration of symptoms. In the early phase, < 24 hours, the epididymis and testis are enlarged and blood flow within the affected testicle may be absent or reduced. After 24 hours, no blood flow is seen on color Doppler ultrasound and the testis becomes of high reflectivity and heterogeneous due to hemorrhage and infarction.

In the pediatric population the ultrasound diagnosis of testicular torsion is even more problematic than in the adult patient.[83] There is often asymmetry in the blood flow through the small testes normally and comparison with the unaffected side may not help.[8,9] Intermittent torsion and incomplete torsion may produce normal, increased, or decreased blood flow on Doppler ultrasound (Fig. 14.**31**). Ultrasound is not, therefore, always reliable in diagnosing testicular torsion and care must be taken in dismissing the diagnosis in the child who presents with an acutely painful scrotum and has a normal ultrasound.[81]

Torsion of the Testicular Appendix

The appendix testis lies at the upper pole of the testis in the groove between the testis and head of the epididymis and is best seen in the presence of a hydrocele (Fig. 14.**32**). The appendix measures between 1 and 7 mm in length and is of similar reflectivity to the epididymal head.[84] Torsion of the testicular appendix is more common than testicular torsion, occurring in boys between ages three and 13.[85] In torsion of the appendix, ultrasound of the testis is normal, with

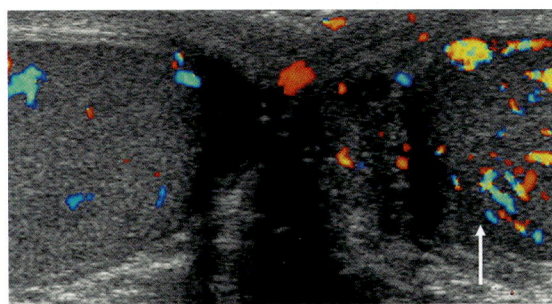

Fig. 14.**31 Spontaneous testicular detorsion.** There is marked increase in color Doppler flow to the left testis (arrow) in comparison to the flow in the right. These appearances are associated with spontaneous testicular detorsion and may be misinterpreted as excluding torsion as the cause of testicular pain. (Courtesy of Dr. P.S. Sidhu, London, UK)

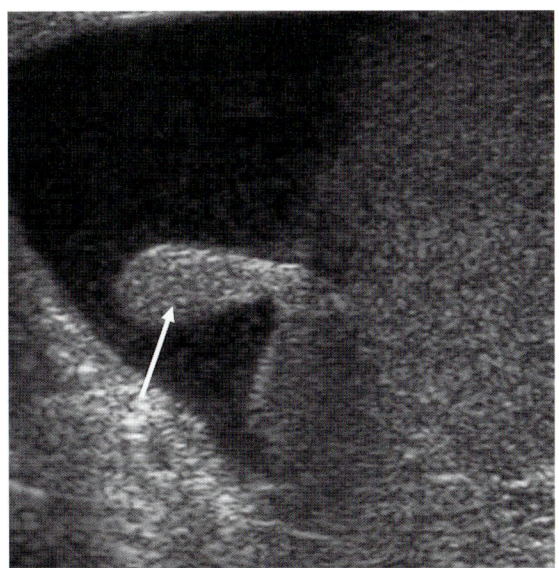

Fig. 14.**32 Torsion of an appendix testis.** A high-reflective appendix testis (arrow) surrounded by fluid: Torsion of the appendix testis

Testicular Tumors

Germ Cell Tumors

Germ cell tumors, divided into seminomatous and nonseminomatous, are the commonest primary testicular tumors. Seminomatous tumors are rare in children, whereas 80% of nonseminomatous tumors present in children under age two years.[88] Most of these nonseminomatous are malignant and present as a painless mass.[89] A yolk sac tumor (infantile embryonal carcinoma) produces alpha-fetoprotein (AFP) exclusively. On ultrasound, the testis may be enlarged or the tumor may appear as a focal low- or high-reflective mass (Fig. 14.33). Focal or diffuse areas of increased vascularity may also be seen.[90]

Stromal Tumors

Leydig cell tumors are the most common stromal tumor. The peak age for presentation is four years and these children tend to present with precocious puberty. Sertoli cell tumors usually present around 18 months and tend to be benign.

Rhabdomyosarcoma

A rhabdomyosarcoma is a malignant tumor which may involve the spermatic cord, epididymis, or testis.

Lymphoma and Leukemia

Less than 10% of testicular tumors are metastatic deposits, most commonly from lymphoma or leukemia. The testes are enlarged, although imaging is usually nonspecific.

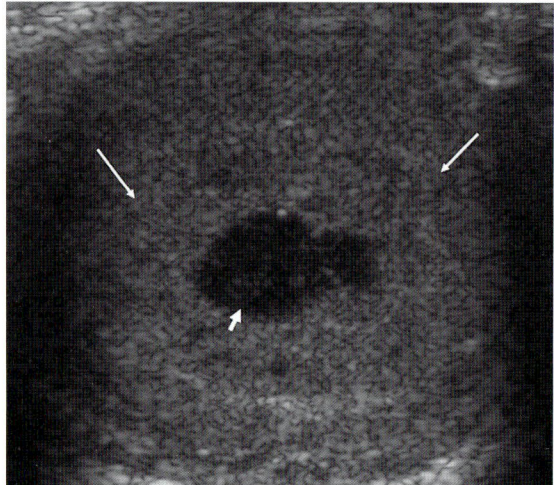
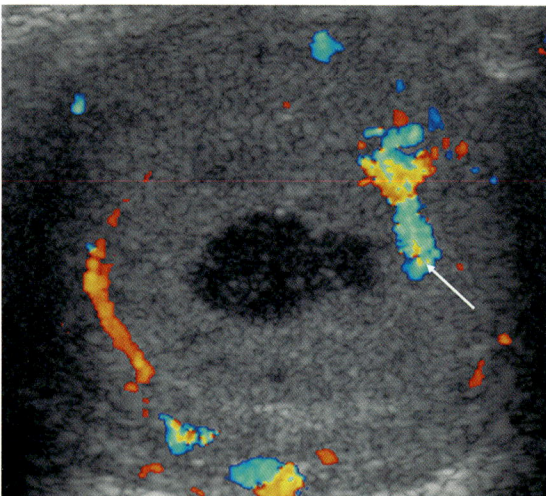

Fig. 14.33 Testicular tumor. a A focal testicular lesion (arrows) in the lower aspect of the testis with an area of low reflectivity (short arrow), representing a yolk sac tumor. b Color Doppler ultrasound image of the yolk sac tumor demonstrating intralesional color signal (arrow). (Courtesy of Dr. P. S. Sidhu, London, UK)

low-resistance arterial blood flow on Doppler ultrasound. Often there is an inflammatory reaction in the epididymis, which is enlarged and hyperemic.[86] The appendix itself tends to be of higher reflectivity, although 30% are of reduced reflectivity.

Testicular Trauma

Following a direct blow to the testis, ultrasound may reveal a high-reflective or a low-reflective intratesticular hematoma often associated with a complex heterogeneous hematocele.[87]

> **Summary points:**
> - Ultrasound is not successful in locating the intra-abdominal testis
> - Hydrocele is the commonest cause of a scrotal mass in the infant
> - Ultrasound diagnosis of testicular torsion is difficult in the pediatric population
> - Torsion of the testicular appendix is more common than testicular torsion
> - Germ cell tumors may present at ultrasound with a focal mass or a diffusely enlarged testis

References

1. Bis KG, Slovis TL. Accuracy of bladder volume measurement in children. Pediatr Radiol 1990;20:457–460.
2. Haller JO, Berdon WE, Friedman AP. Increased renal cortical echogenicity: a normal finding in neonates and infants. Radiology 1982;142:173–174.
3. Holloway H, Jones TB, Robinson AE, Harpen MD, Wiseman AJ. Sonographic determination of renal volumes in normal neonates. Pediatr Radiol 1983;13:212–214.
4. De Sanctis J, Connolly SA, Bramson RT. Effect of patient position on sonographically measured renal length in neonates, infants and children. AJR Am J Roentgenol 1998;170:1381–1383.
5. Kraus SJ. Genitourinary imaging in children. Pediatr Clin North Am 2001;48:1381–1424.
6. Donnolly LF. Genitourinary tract. In: Donnolly LF, ed. Fundamentals of paediatric radiology. Pennsylvania: WB Saunders Company: 2001:141–170.
7. Jequier S, Rousseau O. Sonographic measurements of the normal bladder in children. AJR Am J Roentgenol 1987;149:563–566.
8. Ingram S, Hollman AS. Colour Doppler sonography of the normal paediatric testis. Clin Radiol 1994;49:266–267.
9. Albrecht T, Lotzof K, Hussain HK, Shedden D, Cosgrove DO, de Bruyn R. Power Doppler US of the normal prepubertal testis: does it live up to its promises? Radiology 1997;203:227–231.
10. Strauss S, Dushnitsky T, Peer A, Manor H, Libson E, Lebensart PD. Sonographic features of horseshoe kidney: review of 34 patients. J Ultrasound Med 2000;19:27–31.
11. McCarthy S, Rosenfield AT. Ultrasonography in crossed renal ectopia. J Ultrasound Med 1984;3:107–112.
12. Langman J. Genital system. Medical embryology. Baltimore: Williams and Wilkins: 1975:175–200.
13. Gordon I. Paediatric uroradiology. In: Grainger RG, Allison DJ, eds. Grainger and Allison's Diagnostic Radiology. New York: Churchill Livingstone: 1997:1513–1549.
14. Schaffer SA, Shih YH, Becker JA. Sonographic identification of collecting system duplications. J Clin Ultrasound 1983;11:309–312.
15. Shalaby-Rana E, Lowe LH, Blask AN, Majid M. Imaging in paediatric urology. Pediatr Clin North Am 1997;44:1065–1089.
16. Haddad MC, Birawi GA, Hemadeh MS, Melhem RE, Al-Kutoubi AM. The gamut of abdominal and pelvic cystic masses in children. Eur Radiol 2001;11:148–166.
17. Fernbach SK, Maizels M, Conway JJ. Ultrasound grading of hydronephrosis: introduction to the system used by the Society for Fetal Urology. Pediatr Radiol 1993;23:478–480.
18. Docimo S, Silver RI. Renal ultrasonography in newborns with prenatally hydronephrosis: why wait? J Urol 1997;157:1387–1389.
19. Zerin JM, Ritchey ML, Chang AC. Incidental vesicoureteral reflux in neonates with antenatally detected hydronephrosis and other renal abnormalities. Radiology 1993;187:157–160.
20. Brown T, Mandell J, Lebowitz RL. Neonatal hydronephrosis in the era of sonography. AJR Am J Roentgenol 1987;148:959–963.
21. Dinneen MD, Dhillon HK, Ward HC, Duffy PG, Ransley PG. Antenatal diagnosis of posterior urethral valve. Br J Urol 1993;72:364–369.
22. Cremin BJ. A review of the ultrasonic appearances of posterior urethral valves and ureterococeles. Pediatr Radiol 1986;16:357–364.
23. Blews DE. Sonography of the neonatal genitourinary tract. Radiol Clin North Am 1999;37:1199–1208.
24. Chen CP, Shih SL, Liu FF, Jan SW, Tsai TC, Chang PY, et al. In utero urinary bladder perforation, urinary ascites and bilateral contained urinomas secondary to posterior urethral valves: clinical and imaging findings. Pediatr Radiol 1997;27:3–5.
25. Fernbach SK, Feinstein KA. Abnormalities of the bladder in children: imaging findings. AJR Am J Roentgenol 1994;162:1143–1150.
26. Keesling CA, O'Hara SM, Charez DR, King LR. Sonographic appearance of the bladder after endoscopic incision of ureteroceles. AJR Am J Roentgenol 1998;170:759–763.
27. Wood BP, Ben-Ami T, Teele RL, Rabinowitz R. Ureterovesical obstruction and megaloureter: diagnosis by real-time US. Radiology 1985;156:79–81.
28. Hiraoka M, Hashimoto G, Hori C, Tsukahara H, Konishi Y, Sudo M. Use of ultrasonography in the detection of ureteric reflux in children suspected of having urinary infection. J Clin Ultrasound 1997;25:195–199.
29. Mentzel HJ, Vogt S, Patzer L, Schubert R, John U, Misselwitz J, et al. Contrast-enhanced sonography of vesicoureterorenal reflux in children: preliminary results. AJR Am J Roentgenol 1999;173:737–740.
30. Belman BA. A perspective on vesicoureteral reflux. Urol Clin North Am 1995;22:139–150.
31. Meyer JS, Lebowitz RL. Primary megaureter in infants and children: a review. Urol Radiol 1992;14:296–305.
32. Berrocal T, Lopez-Pereira P, Arjonilla A, Gutierrez J. Anomalies of the distal ureter, bladder, and urethra in children: embryologic, radiologic, and pathologic features. Radiographics 2002;22:1139–1164.
33. Gordon I. Urinary tract infection in paediatrics: the role of diagnostic imaging. Br J Radiol 1990;63:507–511.
34. Talner LB, Davidson AJ, Lebowitz RL, Dalla-Palma L, Goldman SM. Acute pyelonephritis: can we agree on terminology? Radiology 1994;192:297–305.
35. Dacher JN, Pfister C, Monroc M, Eurin D, Le Dossour P. Power Doppler sonographic pattern of acute pyelonephritis in children: comparison with CT. AJR Am J Roentgenol 1996;166:1451–1455.
36. Robinson PJ, Pocock RD, Frank JD. The management of obstructive renal candidiasis in the neonate. Br J Urol 1987;59:380–382.
37. Tiu CM, Chou YH, Chiou HJ, Lo CB, Yang JY, Chen KK, et al. Sonographic features of xanthogranulomatous pyelonephritis. J Clin Ultrasound 2001;29:279–285.
38. Kim J. Ultrasonographic features of focal xanthogranulomatous pyelonephritis. J Ultrasound Med 2004;23:409–416.
39. de Bruyn R, Gordon I. Imaging in cystic renal disease. Arch Dis Child 2000;83:401–407.
40. Melson GL, Shackelford GD, Cole BR, McClennan BL. The spectrum of sonographic findings in infantile polycystic kidney disease with urographic and clinical correlations. J Clin Ultrasound 1985;13:113–119.
41. Premkumar A, Berdon WE, Levy J, Amodio J, Abrahamson SJ, Newhouse JH. The emergence of hepatic fibrosis and portal hypertension in infants and children with autosomal renal polycystic kidney disease. Initial and follow-up sono-

graphic and radiographic findings. Pediatr Radiol 1988;18: 123–129.
42. Blickman JG, Bramson RT, Herrin JT. Autosomal renal polycystic kidney disease: long-term sonographic findings in patients surviving the neonatal period. AJR Am J Roentgenol 1995;164:1247–1250.
43. Grossman H, Rosenberg ER, Bowie JD, Ram P, Merten DF. Sonographic diagnosis of renal cystic diseases. AJR Am J Roentgenol 1983;140:81–85.
44. Boal DK, Teele RL. Sonography of infantile polycystic kidney disease. AJR Am J Roentgenol 1980;135:575–580.
45. Walker FC, Loney LC, Root ER, Melson GL, McAlister WH, Cole BR. Diagnostic evaluation of adult polycystic kidney disease in childhood. AJR Am J Roentgenol 1984;142: 1273–1277.
46. Casper KA, Donnelly LF, Chen B, Bissler JJ. Tuberous sclerosis complex: renal imaging findings. Radiology 2002; 225:451–456.
47. Stuck KJ, Koff SA, Silver TM. Ultrasonic features of multicystic dysplastic kidney: expanded diagnostic criteria. Radiology 1982;143:217–221.
48. McAlister WH, Siegel MJ, Askin FB, Kissane JM, Shackelford GD. Multilocular renal cysts. Urol Radiol 1979;1:89–92.
49. Madewell JE, Goldman SM, Davis CJ, Hartman DS, Feigen DS, Lichtenstein JE. Multilocular cystic nephroma: a radiographic-pathologic correlation of 58 patients. Radiology 1983;146:309–321.
50. Hartman DS, Lesar MS, Madewell JE, Lichtenstein JE, Davis CJ. Mesoblastic nephroma: radiologic-pathologic correlation of 20 cases. AJR Am J Roentgenol 1981;136:69–74.
51. Lowe LH, Isuani BH, Heller RM, Stein SM, Johnson JE, Navarro OM, et al. Pediatric renal masses: Wilms tumor and beyond. Radiographics 2000;20:1585–1603.
52. De Campo JF. Ultrasound of Wilms' tumor. Pediatr Radiol 1986;16:21–24.
53. Hartman DS, David CJ, Goldman SM, Friedman AC, Fritzsche P. Renal lymphoma: radiologic-pathologic correlation of 21 cases. Radiology 1982;144:759–766.
54. Sandler CM, Corl FM, West OC, Tamm EP, Fishman EK, Goldman SM. Imaging of renal trauma: a comprehensive review. Radiographics 2001;21:557–574.
55. McKenney KL, Nunez DB, McKenney MG, Asher J, Zelnick K, Shipshak D. Sonography as the primary screening technique for blunt abdominal trauma: experience with 899 patients. AJR Am J Roentgenol 1998;170:979–985.
56. Pollack HM, Wein AJ. Imaging of renal trauma. Radiology 1989;174:896–897.
57. Patriquin H, Robitaille P. Renal calcium deposition in children: sonographic demonstration of the Anderson-Carr progression. AJR Am J Roentgenol 1986;146:1253–1256.
58. Rosenfield AT, Zeman RK, Cronan JJ, Taylor KJ. Ultrasound in experimental and clinical renal vein thrombosis. Radiology 1980;137:735–741.
59. Pozniak MA, Dodd GD, Kelcz F. Ultrasonographic evaluation of renal transplantation. Radiol Clin North Am 1992;30:1053–1066.
60. Mutze S, Turk I, Schonberger B, Filimonow SI, Bollow M, Petersein J, et al. Colour-coded duplex sonography in the diagnostic assessment of vascular complications after kidney transplantation in children. Pediatr Radiol 1997;27: 898–902.
61. Pozniak MA, Kelcz F, D'Alessandro A, Oberley T, Stratta R. Sonography of renal transplants in dogs: the effect of acute tubular necrosis, cyclosporine nephrotoxicity, and acute rejection on resistive index and renal length. AJR Am J Roentgenol 1992;158:791–797.
62. Silver TM, Campbell D, Wicks JD, Lorber MI, Surace P, Turcotte J. Peritransplant fluid collections. Ultrasound evaluation and clinical significance. Radiology 1981;138: 145–151.
63. Robert Y, Hennequin-Delerue C, Chaillet D, Dubrulle F, Biserte J, Lemaitre L. Urachal remnants: sonographic assessment. J Clin Ultrasound 1996;24:339–344.
64. Blane CE, Zerin JM, Bloom DA. Bladder diverticula in children. Radiology 1994;190:695–697.
65. Salihu HM, Tchuinguem G, Aliyu MH, Kouam L. Prune belly syndrome and associated malformations. A 13-year experience from a developing country. West Indian Med J 2003;52:281–284.
66. Oppenheimer DA, Carroll BA, Yousem S. Sonography of the normal neonatal adrenal gland. Radiology 1983;146: 157–160.
67. Avni EF, Rypens F, Smet MH, Galetty E. Sonographic demonstration of congenital adrenal hyperplasia in the neonate: the cerebriform pattern. Pediatr Radiol 1993;23: 88–90.
68. Burton EM, Strange ME, Edmonds DB. Sonography of the circumrenal and horseshoe adrenal gland in the newborn. Pediatr Radiol 1993;23:362–364.
69. Heij HA, Taets van Amerongen AH, Ekkelkamp S, Vos A. Diagnosis and management of neonatal adrenal haemorrhage. Pediatr Radiol 1989;19:391–394.
70. Mittelstaedt CA, Volberg FM, Merten DF, Brill PW. The sonographic diagnosis of neonatal adrenal hemorrhage. Radiology 1979;131:453–457.
71. Hugosson C, Nyman R, Jorulf H, McDonald P, Rifai A, Kofide A, et al. Imaging of abdominal neuroblastoma in children. Acta Radiol 1999;40:534–542.
72. Hiorns MP, Owens CM. Radiology of neuroblastoma in children. Eur Radiol 2001;11:2071–2081.
73. Friedland GW, Chang P. The role of imaging in the management of the impalpable undescended testis. AJR Am J Roentgenol 1988;151:1107–1111.
74. Gersovich EO. High-resolution ultrasound in the diagnosis of scrotal pathology. Normal scrotum and benign disease. J Clin Ultrasound 1993;21:355–373.
75. Siemer S, Humke U, Uder M, Hildebrandt U, Karadiakos N, Ziegler Mm. Diagnosis of nonpalpable testes in childhood: comparison of magnetic resonance imaging and laparoscopy in a prospective study. Eur J Pediatr Surg 2000;10: 114–118.
76. Jimenez-Lopez M, Ramirez-Garrido F, de D Lopez-Gonzalez Garrido J, Mantas-Avilla J, Nogueras-Ocana M, Jimenez-Verdejo A, et al. Dilatation of the rete testis: ultrasound study. Euro Radiol 1999;9:1327–1329.
77. Sellars MEK, Sidhu PS. Pictorial review: ultrasound appearances of the rete testis. Euro J Ultrasound 2001;14: 115–120.
78. Satchithananda K, Beese RC, Sidhu PS. Acute appendicitis presenting with a testicular mass: ultrasound appearances. Br J Radiol 2000;73:780–782.
79. Miller FNAC, Sidhu PS. Does testicular microlithiasis matter? A review. Clin Radiol 2002;57:883–890.
80. Hollman AS, Ingram S, Carachu R, Davis C. Colour Doppler imaging of the acute paediatric scrotum. Pediatr Radiol 1993;23:83–87.
81. Sidhu PS. Clinical and imaging features of testicular torsion: role of ultrasound. Clin Radiol 1999;54:343–352.

82. Lindsey D. Boys with acute testicular pain should be presumed to have a torsion until proved otherwise. J Emerg Med 1994;12:531.
83. Wallace AD, Hollman AS. Colour Doppler ultrasound of the paediatric scrotum. Imaging 1996;8:324–334.
84. Sahni D, Jit I, Joshi K, Sanjeev S. Incidence and structure of the appendices of the testis and epididymis. Anatomy 1996;189:341–348.
85. Sellars MEK, Sidhu PS. Utrasound appearances of the testicular appendages: pictorial review. Eur Radiol 2003;13:127–135.
86. Strauss S, Faingold R, Manor H. Torsion of the testicular appendages: sonographic appearance. J Ultrasound Med 1997;16:189–192.
87. Hricak H, Jeffrey RB. Sonography of acute scrotal abnormalities. Radiol Clin North Am 1983;21:595–603.
88. Barth RA, Teele RL, Colodny A, Retik A, Bauer S. Asymptomatic scrotal masses in children. Radiology 1984;152:65–68.
89. Luker GD, Siegel MJ. Asymptomatic scrotal masses in children. Radiology 1994;191:561–564.
90. Sidhu PS, Sriprasad S, Bushby LH, Sellars ME, Muir GH. Impalpable testis cancer. BJU Int 2004;93:888.

Section 4

Other Imaging Modalities in the Urogenital Tract

15 Non-Ultrasound Imaging of the Urogenital Tract 233

15 Non-Ultrasound Imaging of the Urogenital Tract

S. D. Heenan, U. Patel

Introduction

Ultrasound has an important role in the investigation of the urinary tract. However, other imaging modalities are needed when ultrasound is not conclusive. The aim of the present chapter is to summarize and discuss these other imaging modalities in the context of diagnostic pathways for certain diseases, particularly in a complimentary role to ultrasound.

Plain Abdominal Radiograph

Prior to the introduction of ultrasound, the plain abdominal radiograph followed by an intravenous or excretory urogram (IVU) was the mainstay of urinary tract imaging, staples which still maintain an important role in current clinical practice. The plain radiograph will demonstrate the presence or absence of calcification or calculi related to the urogenital tract. It is important to ensure the entire urogenital tract is imaged adequately from the upper poles of the kidneys to the bladder base. Additional views may be necessary; oblique views or tomography may improve visualization of the upper tracts if bowel gas or feces obscure the relevant areas. Radiographs in both inspiration and expiration will determine whether calcification is intrarenal or extrarenal. On plain radiographs, it is often possible to determine the renal contour and the outline of the normal psoas muscle due to the differential density of kidney and adjacent perinephric fat. Despite this, renal outlines are better demonstrated following administration of intravenous contrast at IVU or, ideally, with ultrasound. Absence of the psoas muscle outline may suggest retroperitoneal disease, but the psoas muscle outline is not present in up to 25% of "normal" radiographic examinations. The lower ribs, lumbar spine, and pelvis should be scrutinized for congenital vertebral anomalies, such as spina bifida in children and destructive lesions in adults that might indicate metastatic disease.

Intravenous Urogram

Excretory urography was first introduced into radiological practice in the mid-1900s and the technique has changed little over the intervening years. Although an IVU remains an important source of information regarding the upper tract anatomy including the ureters and gives some indication of renal function, an IVU rarely stands alone. Increasingly, bowel preparation (administration of laxatives) is not required, although the patient should be well-hydrated, particularly if there is a history of renal impairment, diabetes mellitus, or multiple myeloma. An IVU is contraindicated in the presence of iodine allergy, previous allergic reaction, and care needs to be taken in those with severe asthma.

Following a control radiograph, a nonionic, low-osmolar contrast medium is injected as an intravenous bolus. A standard radiographic sequence is detailed in Table 15.1. However, this will be subject to local guidelines and the clinical indication for the study (Table 15.2). Oblique, prone, and delayed images may all be helpful in maximizing the information obtained from the study.

The early images will allow for assessment of renal size, shape, contour, and position, as well as perfusion.

Table 15.**1 Standard radiographic sequence for excretory urography**

Immediate coned renal area ± tomography
Coned renal area 5 mins after contrast injection
Abdominal compression (if no obstruction/recent surgery/aortic aneurysm)
Coned renal area 10 mins after contrast injection
Full-length release at 15 mins to include kidneys/ureters/bladder
Full-length or coned after micturition

Table 15.**2 Indications for excretory urography**

Calculus disease
Obstruction
Mucosal lesions in the investigation of hematuria
Developmental anomalies
Papillary necrosis
Medullary sponge kidney
Tuberculosis

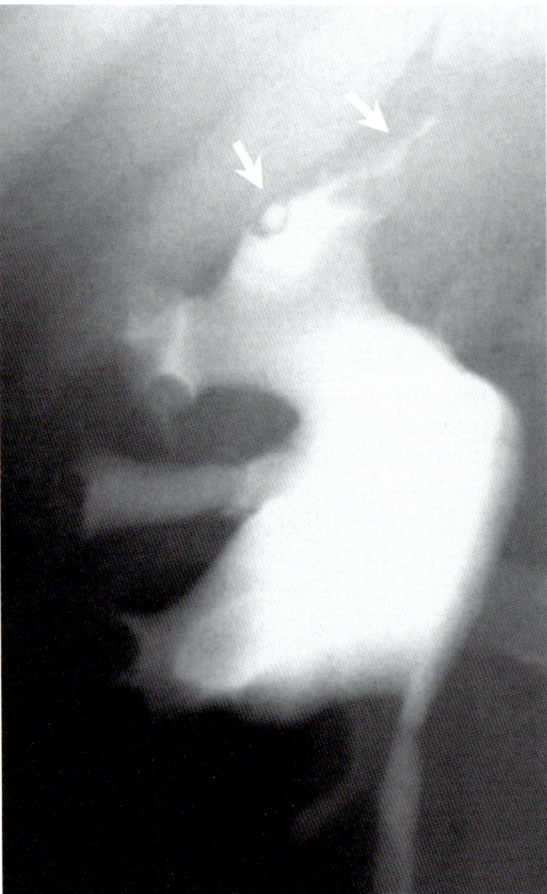

Fig. 15.1 An intravenous urography image of the right kidney, demonstrating the fine linear tracks (arrows) of early papillary necrosis in an otherwise normal pelvicalyceal system. These appearances would not be seen with ultrasound

Later radiographs will demonstrate the morphology of the papillae and calyces and also indicate the degree of renal excretion. These images should be interpreted in the context of the pattern of normal variants, which include complex and unusually large or small calyces, papillary blushes, and vascular impressions. Developmental anomalies, such as a horseshoe, duplex, or pelvic kidney should be readily demonstrated. A dilated pelvicalyceal system as a result of obstruction secondary to calculi, tumor, or bladder outflow obstruction is well-documented. However, one of the most important indications for an IVU is the investigation of hematuria and medical renal disease; an IVU is the only noninvasive imaging modality that can demonstrate calyceal and ureteric abnormalities with high resolution. Abnormalities including papillary necrosis (Fig. 15.1), medullary sponge kidney, renal tuberculosis, and small transitional cell carcinomas may only be seen at IVU.

Micturating Cystourethrography and Other Contrast Studies

The micturating cystourethrogram (MCU) is an invasive examination requiring direct catheterization of the urinary bladder, primarily utilized for the investigation of pediatric urinary tract infections (UTIs) and reflux nephropathy. Using an aseptic technique and following catheterization, dilute water-soluble iodinated contrast medium is instilled into the bladder to full capacity. Once the patient is in the erect position, the catheter is removed and the patient empties their bladder whilst concurrent fluoroscopic imaging documents any vesicoureteric reflux (VUR). Oblique films are necessary to show the posterior urethra, which is important in boys to demonstrate the presence of posterior urethral valves.

The principal method for imaging of the male urethra is contrast urethrography, either descending, as above, or ascending. Once fully distended with contrast medium, oblique images will show the full length of urethra from fossa naviculare to sphincter. The urethra can then be assessed for strictures and mucosal lesions, the commonest abnormalities. Following pelvic trauma, contrast urethrography may be combined with a cystogram and descending examination to demonstrate the integrity of the entire urethra (Fig. 15.2). There is no ideal method for imaging the female urethra, and ultrasound (either transvaginal or a transrectal approach), MCU, and magnetic resonance (MR) imaging may be useful (Fig. 15.3).

Retrograde contrast examination of the ureters after direct catherization, usually under a general anaesthetic, may be the only method of demonstrating small mucosal abnormalities if the IVU is inconclusive. Similarly, with ileal conduits it is often difficult to demonstrate the site of ureteric anastomosis at IVU, and direct introduction of contrast medium into the ileal loop, a "loopogram," with reflux into ureters may delineate this region.

Computed Tomography

The combination of ultrasound and an IVU may resolve many of the clinical conundrums arising in renal and urological medicine. However, cross-sectional imaging in the form of computed tomography (CT) and MR imaging are vital complementary diagnostic tools. Newer and constantly evolving technology has led to an increase in the use of CT and MR imaging. For example, unenhanced helical CT has largely replaced an IVU for evaluation of presumed calculi-induced renal colic. Table 15.3 lists important applications for the use of CT imaging.

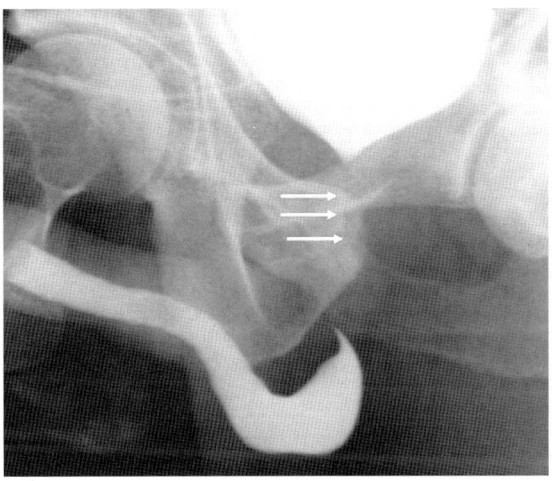
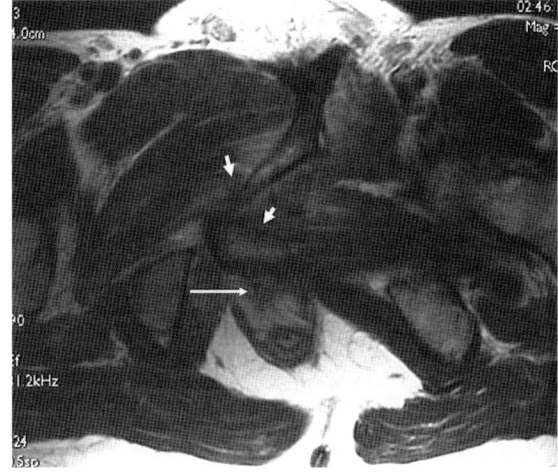
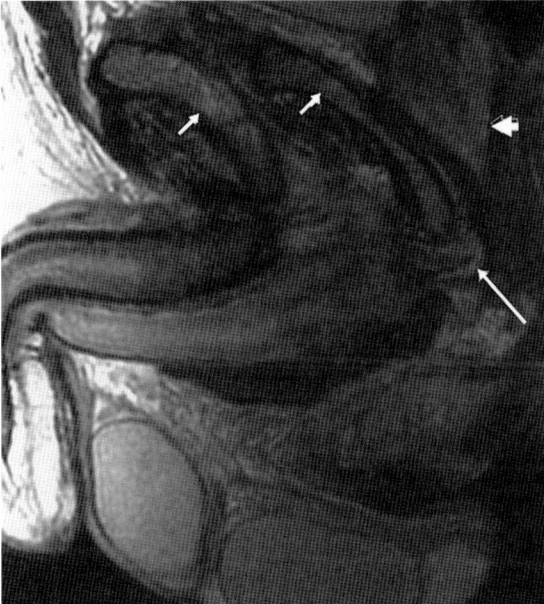

Fig. 15.**2 a** Cystography combined with an ascending urethrogram following a "closed-book" fracture, demonstrating an obstructed proximal urethra (arrows). **b** Axial T2-weighted MR image, demonstrating compression of proximal urethra (long arrow) by overriding pubic rami (short arrows). **c** Sagittal T2-weighted MR image, demonstrating compression of proximal urethra (long arrow) by overriding pubic rami (short arrows). The prostate is not involved (arrowhead)

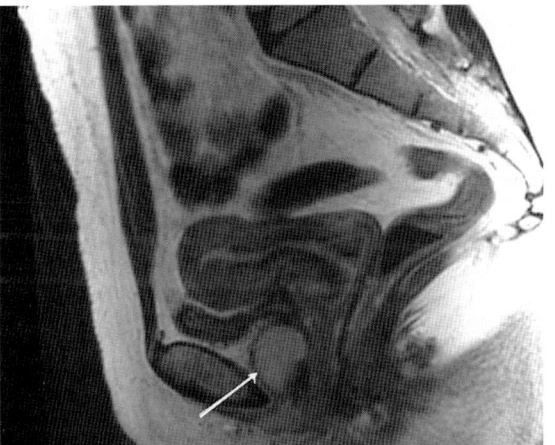

Fig. 15.**3** Urethral diverticulum on sagittal T2-weighted MR image (arrow)

Table 15.**3 Main indications for CT imaging**

Characterization of renal cysts/masses when ultrasound is equivocal
Staging of malignant disease (renal, bladder, prostate, testicular)
Assessment of renal calculi (particularly with acute colic)
Renal trauma
Evaluation of the retroperitoneum
CT angiography

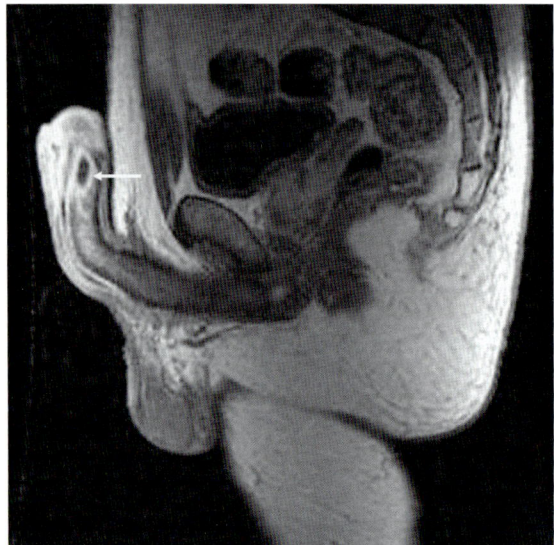

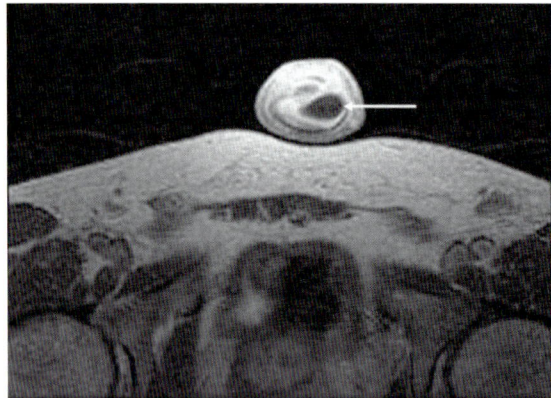

Fig. 15.4 **a** Squamous cell carcinoma of distal urethra complicated by abscess formation (arrow) in the corpus cavernosum on postgadolinium contrast T1-weighted MR image in the sagittal plane. **b** Postgadolinium contrast T1-weighted MR image in the axial plane, demonstrating the abscess (arrow) complicating a squamous cell carcinoma

The CT machine comprises multiple x-ray tubes aligned with opposing x-ray detectors, which are arranged in a ring within a gantry. As the patient passes through the scanner, x-ray photons pass through the patient with varying degrees of ease, are then detected and reconstructed to build up an image of differing tissue densities. "Slip-ring" technology and the subsequent arrival of helical then multislice CT scanners in the late 1990s has meant that the abdomen and pelvis can now be rapidly imaged in a single breath-hold, reducing artifact and allowing for fine collimation. In conjunction with advances in software, the resulting images can be reconstructed in multiple planes or as three-dimensional reconstructions. Enthusiasm for the new possibilities that these changes have brought to CT imaging must be tempered by the knowledge that there is an increase in radiation burden and large contrast load to the kidneys in enhanced studies; this is not to be dismissed lightly.

Magnetic Resonance Imaging

MR imaging relies on the spinning hydrogen ions (or protons) present in body water to obtain cross-sectional images. These ions have a positive charge and when placed in a very strong magnetic field align themselves along the axis of the field. By applying radio waves, the protons alter the way they spin and gain energy. When the radio waves are stopped, energy is released as the protons "relax" back to their original state. The energy can then be converted to produce a representative image as different tissues relax at different rates. MR imaging is not suitable for everyone, particularly the claustrophobic patient, although new "open" magnets may partially solve this problem. Contraindications include cardiac pacemakers, intracranial aneurysm clips, and intraorbital metal fragments.

Previously relatively long imaging times proved problematic in MR examinations. However, rapid changes in MR imaging technology allows for faster imaging with less movement artifact, improved image quality, and image resolution (Fig. 15.4). Breath-hold imaging techniques allow for the performance of gadolinium-enhanced MR angiography and venography; this is of particular use in the investigation of renal artery stenosis (RAS) and for evaluation of venous involvement of renal tumors. Although CT is able to show renal calculi more accurately, MR urography using rapidly acquired heavily T2-weighted coronal images can demonstrate dilated pelvicalyceal systems and ureters down to the level of obstruction (Fig. 15.5). Advantages of MR imaging include both the lack of ionizing radiation and use of non-nephrotoxic contrast media; this is of particular advantage in pregnancy and renal failure. Clinical indications for MR imaging have been increasing over the past decade and MR imaging is now the standard imaging modality in staging pelvic cancers, including prostate carcinoma (Table 15.4). Whilst functional MR imaging has been accepted for routine use in neurological disorders, it has not yet been fully explored in nephrourological disease, but has the capacity to challenge nuclear medicine techniques.

Radionuclide Imaging

While the previously described imaging methods contribute primarily anatomical and structural information, radionuclide imaging provides complementary functional and quantitative data. The imaging agents are radiopharmaceuticals, which comprise a radionuclide combined with a biological molecule. These radiopharmaceuticals are administered, usually intravenously, to target a specific organ or system. The radionuclide component emits gamma rays, which are detected using a gamma camera. Anatomical resolution is poor, but unique physiological data is obtained. Table 15.5 summarizes some of the commonly used radionuclides and the indications for their use.

Glomerular Filtration Rate

Glomerular filtration rate (GFR) is ideally measured using an agent that is not protein bound, is completely filtered by the glomerulus, undergoes no resorption or secretion, and is only excreted by the kidneys; in clinical practice ^{51}Cr-ethylene diamine tetraacetic acid (^{51}Cr-EDTA) is the most convenient radiopharmaceutical to fit these properties. To calculate the GFR, a plasma clearance method is used, which is defined as the notional volume of plasma cleared of ^{51}Cr-EDTA in a given time. A single injection method is used with varying timing of subsequent blood samples, from one to several taken three to five hours after injection but up to 24 hours if the GFR is expected to be < 15 mL/min.

Static Renal Imaging

The commonest indication for a ^{99m}Tc-dimercaptosuccinic acid (^{99m}Tc-DMSA) examination is to assess the kidneys for scarring, usually associated with reflux nephropathy in children, and to provide an accurate measure of divided renal function. While roughly 15% of the static renal imaging agent is excreted in the urine, the majority of ^{99m}Tc-DMSA is fixed in the proximal tubules of functioning renal parenchyma. Images are acquired two to three hours following intravenous injection, maximizing the best target-to-background ratio, although delayed views may be necessary with reduced renal function. Anterior, posterior, and posterior–oblique views are routinely acquired, whilst pelvic views should be obtained if there is any possibility of an ectopic kidney. Focal cortical defects usually indicate the presence of renal scarring (Fig. 15.6). Divided renal function is calculated by measuring the number of "counts" within regions of interest (ROI) drawn around the kidneys on both anterior and posterior views to provide a geometric mean that is independent of renal depth.

Dynamic Renal Imaging

Both ^{99m}Tc-diethylene triamine pentaacetic acid (^{99m}Tc-DTPA) and ^{99m}Tc-mercaptoacetyltriglycine (^{99m}Tc-MAG3) can be used to perform dynamic isotope

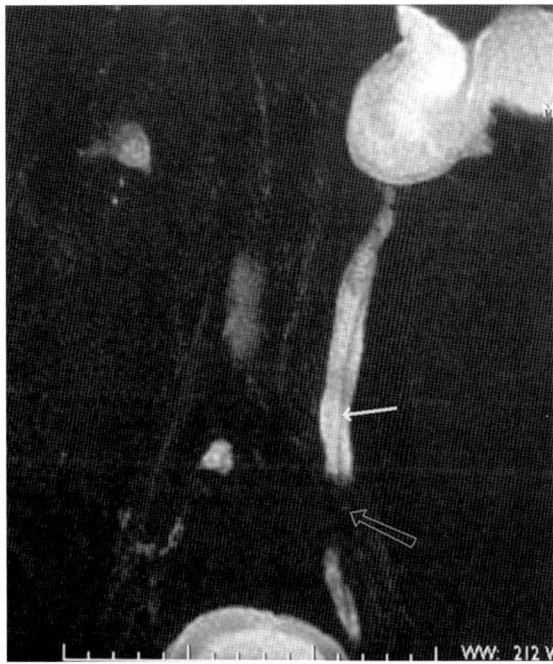

Fig. 15.5 **A heavily T2-weighted coronal MR image, demonstrating a dilated renal pelvis and ureter to the level of an obstructing transitional cell carcinoma (TCC) of the distal ureter in a nonfunctioning left kidney** (open arrow). A ureteric stent (solid arrow) is present in the left ureter

Table 15.4 **Indications for MR imaging**

Staging of pelvic cancers
Characterization of renal masses when CT and ultrasound are equivocal
MR urography
MR angiography
Long-term follow-up of renal masses in von Hippel–Lindau and tuberous sclerosis
Detection of undescended testes
Urethral diverticulum

Table 15.5 **Radionuclide techniques in the urogenital tract**

Total renal function	GFR using ^{51}Cr-EDTA
Divided renal and intrarenal distribution of function	Static ^{99m}Tc-DMSA scan
Perfusion, transit time, and outflow kinetics	Dynamic ^{99m}Tc-DTPA or ^{99m}Tc-MAG3 scan ± frusemide
Renovascular hypertension	Dynamic ^{99m}Tc-DTPA or ^{99m}Tc-MAG3 scan before and after captopril
VUR	Dynamic ^{99m}Tc-DTPA or ^{99m}Tc-MAG3 scan followed by indirect cystography or ^{99m}Tc-pertechnetate direct cystogram
Bone imaging, e.g. for bone metastases	^{99m}Tc-methylene diphosphonate

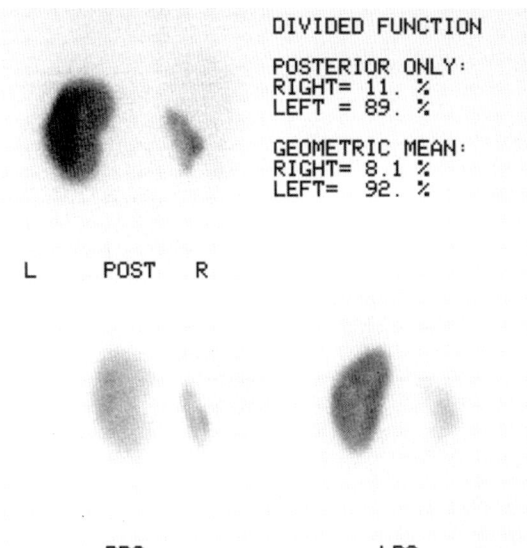

Fig. 15.6 A ^{99m}Tc-DMSA examination demonstrating a small, scarred right kidney and normal left kidney

renography. Whilst ^{99m}Tc-DTPA is solely filtered by the kidney, ^{99m}Tc-MAG3 has a more complex interaction but is predominantly excreted by tubular secretion. ^{99m}Tc-MAG3 may also be excreted by the hepatobiliary system in renal failure, with advantages over ^{99m}Tc-DTPA due to a lower radiation dose and better images both in children and in renal failure.

The appropriate radioisotope is injected as an intravenous bolus and posterior images are acquired dynamically over 20–40 minutes (anterior images are obtained in renal transplant patients). An ROI is drawn around the renal outlines and after background correction, a time-activity curve or renogram is generated with "counts" in the ROI plotted against time. The renogram is divided into three phases: The first two to three minutes represent the vascular phase, followed by the secretory and excretory phases. By examining the different components of the curves, a picture of renal perfusion, excretion, and drainage may be obtained.

As renal uptake or function is proportional to renal blood flow, divided renal function may also be calculated by assessing the relative heights or rate of rise of the curves in the first two to three minutes before any radioisotope has left the kidneys. Individual relative function is expressed as a percentage.

Diuresis Renography

Urinary flow rate can influence the appearance of the renogram. If the kidney demonstrates pelvicalyceal dilatation, it may be necessary to challenge the kidney with significantly raised flow rates by administering a diuretic, such as frusemide (furosemide). The diuresis will promote washout of tracer in a nonobstructed system depicted by a fall in the time-activity curve. If the pelvicalyceal system is truly obstructed, diuresis will increase the dilatation with a continued rise in the slope of the time-activity curve. Different protocols for diuretic administration have been described with the original account specifying injection 20 minutes after the radioisotope to allow for assessment of the unmodified upper tracts and alleviate the need for diuretic administration if normal. If pelvicalyceal dilatation is present, maximal flow rates will be required and injection 15 minutes prior to radionuclide administration (F-15 protocol) is more appropriate, allowing dynamic imaging to commence at peak diuresis.

Captopril Renography

Following the initial description in 1983 by Majd et al., renograms performed before and after administration of 25–50 mg of captopril may be used to demonstrate RAS.[1] This relies on the presence of high levels of angiotensin II in renovascular hypertension. Angiotensin-converting enzyme (ACE) inhibitors block the vasoconstricting effect that maintains GFR in RAS and the second time-activity curve will show a reduction in perfusion and a delay to peak. A change in split function can also be seen. Sensitivities and specificities vary according to the study population, but a prospective multicenter trial evaluated 380 hypertensive patients, who had a ^{99m}Tc-DTPA examination before and after administration of captopril; 125 of the study group subsequently had a significant RAS at renal angiography.[2] Overall RAS of > 70% was detected with a sensitivity of 83% and specificity of 93% if renal function was normal. The performance of the test decreased in impaired renal function.

Direct and Indirect Cystography

As an adjunct to renography, a voiding study may subsequently be performed in toilet-trained children. The child sits with their back against the gamma camera head with the kidneys and bladder in the field of view and voids while fast frames are acquired dynamically. VUR can be seen as an increase in "counts" over the kidney or ureters (Fig. 15.7). Direct cystography is more invasive, requiring catheterization of the bladder and instillation of ^{99m}Tc-pertechnetate with a further disadvantage of the lack of visualization of the posterior urethra in males. However, direct ^{99m}Tc-pertechnetate cystography gives a lower radiation dose than a MCU and can be useful in the follow-up of children under age three.

Bone Scintigraphy

Radiolabeled diphosphonates are absorbed onto the crystalline bony matrix and, at sites of increased osteoblastic activity, there is more marked uptake of tracer. This technique can therefore be used to demonstrate and follow up bony metastases in malignancies of the urinary tract, such as prostate cancer (Fig. 15.**8**). Bone scans are very sensitive but not very specific and although patterns of extensive metastatic disease are fairly characteristic, other diagnoses, including trauma, Paget disease, and arthropathies, may have to be considered.

Angiography and Interventional Techniques

Although Doppler ultrasound, with or without microbubble ultrasound contrast media, has allowed the study of tissue vascularity (e.g., renal vascularity, renal and testicular masses, varicocele assessment, and erectile studies), more direct angiography is still used, either catheter (or conventional) angiography or less invasive methods such as CT and MR angiography. Catheter angiography is an invasive technique requiring arterial cannulation and intra-arterial contrast injection but remains the reference investigation for renovascular disease, particularly cases of acute, severe renal hemorrhage. CT or MR angiography are carried out after peripheral intravenous contrast injection, and the study parameters are set to visualize the vessels at the moment of peak contrast opacification, with the results further manipulated to enhance the vascular tree. CT and MR angiography compete with Doppler ultrasound as screening investigations, at the expense of cost and availability but with better accuracy in many situations. Further invasive diagnostic techniques are the study of upper or lower tract urodynamics or pyeloureterography.

Problem-Solving

Other imaging modalities supplement ultrasound findings and in this section radiological imaging strategies will be discussed in the context of common clinical problems, highlighting the strengths and weaknesses of the various investigations.

Renal Masses

The vast majority (99%) of renal masses are accounted for by simple renal cysts, with the ultrasound examination being fully diagnostic and further imaging unnecessary. The remaining 1% of masses need to be further evaluated by CT or MR imaging, supported by ultrasound correlation (Fig. 15.**9**). High-reflective masses on ultrasound are not always angiomyolipoma,

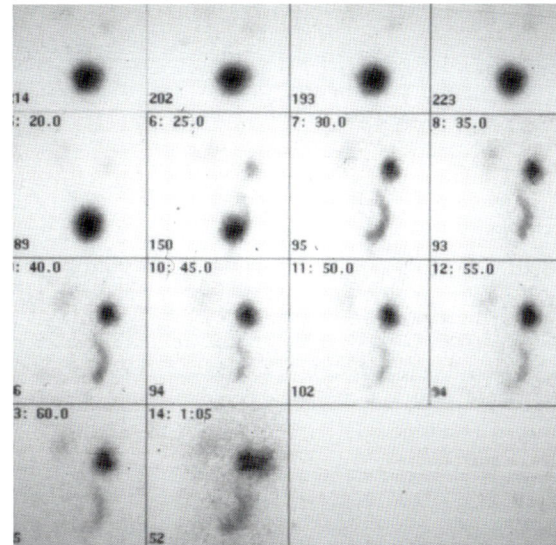

Fig. 15.**7** A ^{99m}Tc-DTPA indirect cystography examination, demonstrating activity refluxing into right renal collecting system on micturition, which is indicative of VUR (posterior view)

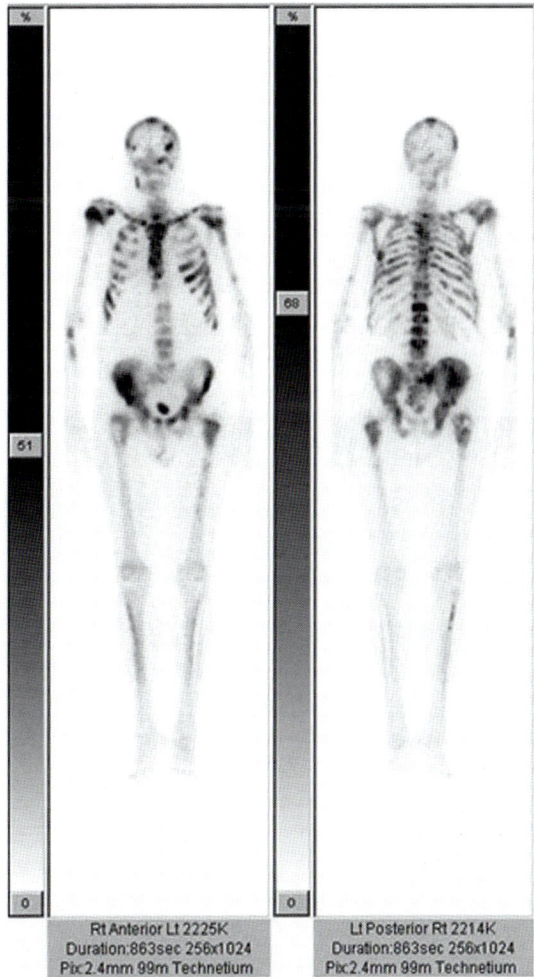

Fig. 15.**8** Multiple bony metastases from prostate carcinoma as the primary tumor demonstrated in the skull, spine, ribs, proximal femora, and right humerus

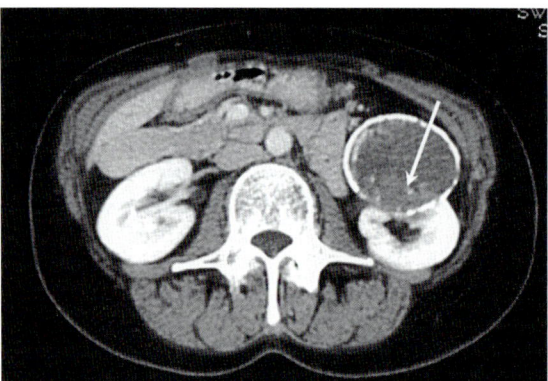

Fig. 15.**9** A renal cell carcinoma (RCC) demonstrated on CT imaging as a large, solid left renal mass with peripheral rim calcification (arrow)

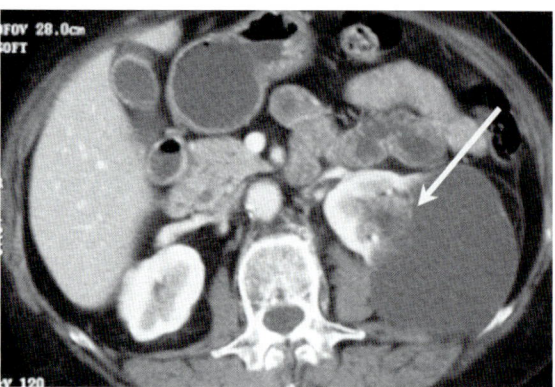

Fig. 15.**10** CT examination of a left renal cyst, demonstrating subtle contrast enhancement of solid elements within the cyst (arrow), raising the possibility of malignancy

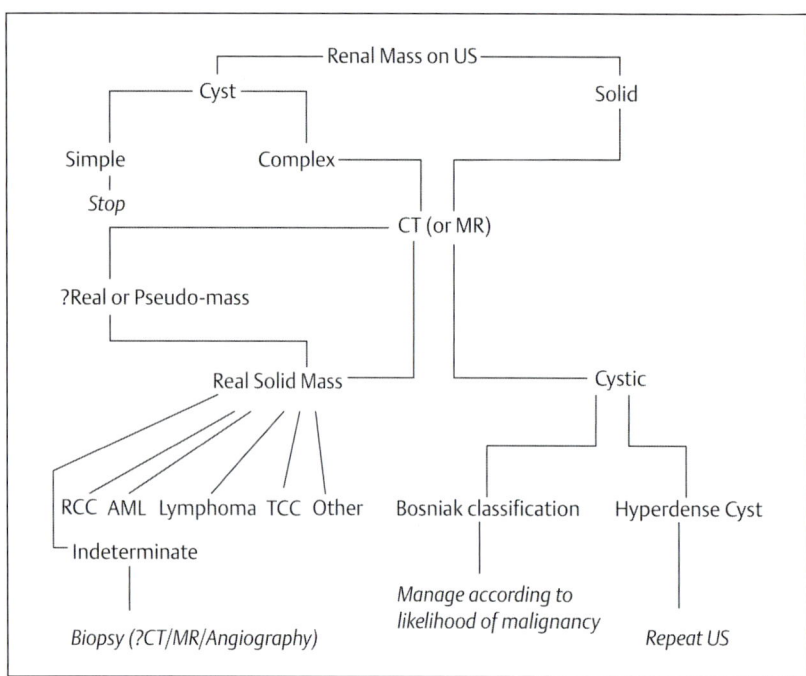

Fig. 15.**11** Imaging algorithm for analysis of a renal mass discovered on ultrasound (RCC: Renal Cell Carcinoma; AML: Angiomyolipoma; TCC: Transitional Cell Carcinoma).

and in one study up to one third of small renal cell carcinomas were of high reflectivity on ultrasound.[3] Tissue enhancement is vitally important information for determining the likelihood of malignancy, and subtle enhancement can only be measured on CT or MR imaging (Fig. 15.10). This particularly applies to small (< 3 cm) renal masses, documented in a study where the false negative rate for ultrasound in assessing small renal masses was 75% compared to 40% for CT in exclusion of renal cancer.[4] A suggested diagnostic algorithm may be used for all solid and complex cystic masses found on an ultrasound examination (Fig. 15.11).

Staging of Malignant Disease

Renal Cell Carcinoma

A renal mass which turns out to be a renal cell carcinoma (RCC) is often found incidentally on ultrasound or CT imaging. Tumor staging is usually performed with CT, with assessment of the size, position, and extent of the tumor dictating whether a radical or partial nephrectomy or adjuvant therapy will be required. The presence of lymphadenopathy, adrenal gland, renal vein, or inferior vena cava (IVC) involvement and tumor

Table 15.6 **TNM staging of renal cell carcinoma**

Tx		Tumor cannot be assessed
T0		No evidence of primary tumor
T1		Tumor ≤ 7 cm in greatest dimension limited to kidney
T2		Tumor > 7 cm in greatest dimension limited to kidney
T3		
	T3a	Invasion of ipsilateral adrenal gland or perinephric tissue but confined by Gerota's fascia
	T3b	Extension into renal vein or IVC below diaphragm
	T3c	Extension into renal vein or IVC above diaphragm
T4		Invasion through Gerota's fascia
N0		No lymph node metastases
N1		Single ipsilateral lymph node
N2		Multiple regional, contralateral, or bilateral lymph nodes
N3		Fixed regional lymph nodes
N4		Juxtaregional lymph nodes involved
M0		No distant metastases
M1		Distant metastases

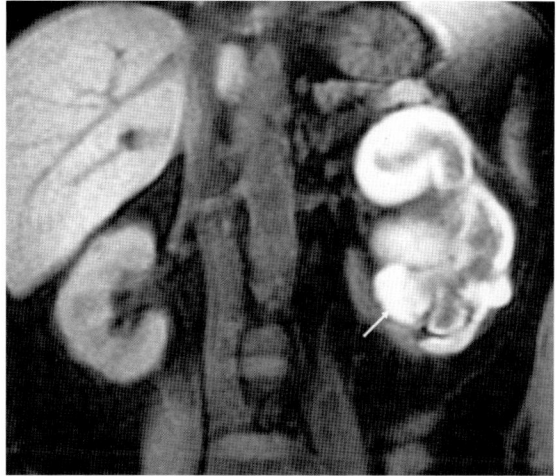

Fig. 15.**12** Coronal fat-suppressed T1-weighted MR image of a hemorrhagic left RCC (arrow)

invasion through Gerota's fascia are all important staging and prognostic indicators (Table 15.**6**).

Metastases from an RCC commonly involve lung and liver; therefore a chest radiograph, at least, is required for complete staging. Ultrasound or CT imaging of the liver for metastases and the contralateral kidney for a synchronous tumor, which occurs in 2% of patients, will be performed at the same time as assessment of the primary tumor. MR imaging is a useful problem-solving tool; it is helpful in evaluating renal vein or IVC involvement, using a combination of imaging planes and, if necessary, MR venogaphy (Figs. 15.**12**, 15.**13**). The multiplanar capabilities of MR imaging may also be useful in revealing the extent of bulky tumors with possible invasion of adjacent organs, but tends to be less discerning than CT when lesions are < 3 cm. Occasionally renal angiography may be necessary in preparation for nephron-sparing surgery in solitary kidneys.

Bladder Carcinoma

A transitional cell carcinoma (TCC) of the bladder will usually present with hematuria, as do most tumors of the urogenital tract. There is limited data on the role of different imaging techniques in the diagnosis of bladder cancer. Normally in any patient with hematuria, a cystoscopy and imaging of the upper renal tracts is necessary. The choice of imaging of the upper renal tracts depends on local departmental guidelines but will include an ultrasound, plain abdominal radiograph, and an IVU. A bladder tumor is often seen as a filling defect on an IVU and when the bladder is well-distended,

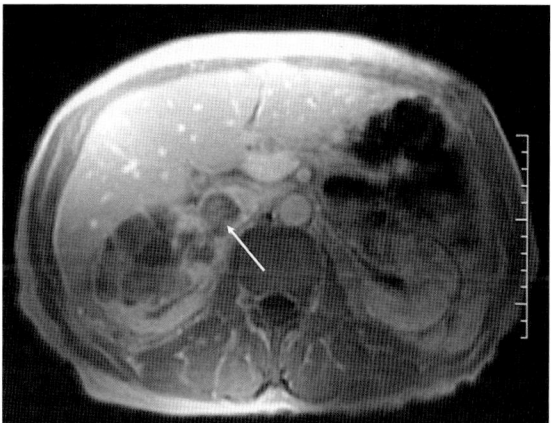

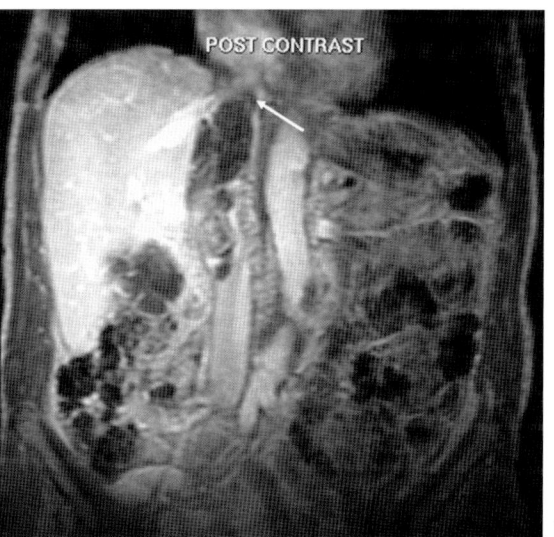

Fig. 15.**13 a** Axial postgadolinium-enhanced T1-weighted MR image of a right renal cell carcinoma invading the IVC (arrow). **b** Coronal postgadolinium-enhanced T1-weighted MR image, demonstrating the superior extent of tumor thrombus within the IVC to the level of the diaphragm (arrow)

Table 15.7 **TNM staging of bladder cancer**

Tis		In situ disease
Ta		Papillary tumor confined to epithelium (mucosa)
T1		Invasion to lamina propria
T2		
	T2a	Invasion into superficial muscle (inner half)
	T2b	Invasion into deep muscle (outer half)
T3		
	T3a	Microscopic invasion into perivesical fat
	T3b	Macroscopic invasion into perivesical fat
T4		
	T4a	Invasion into prostate, uterus, vagina
	T4b	Invasion into pelvic or abdominal walls
N0		No regional lymph node metastases
N1		Metastasis in single lymph node ≤ 2 cm
N2		Single > 2 ≤ 5 cm, multiple ≤ 5 cm
N3		Single > 5 cm
M0		No distant metastases
M1		Distant metastases

ultrasound will demonstrate a soft-tissue papillary or sessile mass arising from the bladder wall. Once a bladder tumor has been demonstrated on ultrasound, it is necessary to perform an IVU to exclude a coexisting mucosal abnormality of the renal collecting system and ureters. An ultrasound will be more discerning at demonstrating concurrent RCC. Although an IVU has always been considered the "gold standard" for imaging upper renal tracts, CT has a role in demonstrating renal pelvic and ureteral tumors. There may be a role for a combination of CT and ultrasound, in the future, to replace an IVU in this scenario.

The histology of the resected tumor, usually performed at cystoscopy, determines depth of tumor invasion. The majority of bladder carcinomas are superficial and a transurethral resection (TUR) is both a staging procedure as well as treatment. These Ta and T1 bladder tumors are followed up regularly with a cystoscopy and treated with either further TUR or intravesical therapy, with no further role for imaging.

For invasive bladder carcinoma, the prognosis is firmly dependent on the depth of tumor invasion and, as with other urogenital tumors, staging is according to the tumor, node, metastasis (TNM) classification (Table 15.7).

Stage T2 tumors and above appear to have a more aggressive natural history and 20–30% of patients with pT2 and pT3a organ-confined disease have regional lymph node metastases.[5] Hydronephrosis, in the context of invasive bladder carcinoma, also gives a poorer prognosis. Although radiology has a limited role in diagnosis, the extent of local and systemic disease needs to be assessed and for this both CT and MR imaging can be used. As in imaging of prostate cancer, neither CT nor MR can demonstrate microscopic disease and both are unable to distinguish superficial from muscle-invasive tumors. The main role of CT and MR imaging is to differentiate organ-confined disease from extravesical disease. It is important to try to image patients prior to TUR of a bladder carcinoma, as post-surgical change (bladder-wall fibrosis and edema) may mimic disease and result in overstaging of disease. CT and conventional MR imaging have a similar sensitivity and specificity for bladder carcinoma detection, ranging from 60–100%.[6] Breath-hold contrast-enhanced dynamic T1-weighted MR images will improve accuracy to 85% over conventional MR imaging.[7] Staging accuracy for lymph node involvement is similar as that for carcinoma of the prostate.

Metastatic disease to regional lymph nodes, liver, lung, and bone can be evaluated by a combination of studies, for example CT for abdomen and pelvis, chest radiograph for lung involvement, and a radioisotope bone scan if there is a possibility of bone-marrow metastases.

Prostate Carcinoma

Once the diagnosis of prostate cancer has been made using transrectal ultrasound (TRUS) and biopsy, the subsequent clinical management depends on the histological grade of the tumor, level of prostate-specific antigen (PSA) and stage of disease. To be considered potentially curable, disease staging has to indicate local disease and then imaging is required to evaluate the presence of extracapsular spread (Table 15.8). The role of TRUS is detailed in the chapter on prostate ultrasound. The use of MR imaging in staging prostate cancer is not established and as such is not advocated for routine use. At present CT and MR imaging are probably comparable in accuracy for lymph node assessment, but MR imaging is better for local staging and bone-marrow metastases (due to the ability to manipulate imaging parameters with resultant superior soft-tissue characterization and multiplanar capabilities).

T1-weighted MR images demonstrate the normal prostate and seminal vesicles as uniform intermediate signal surrounded by high-signal periprostatic fat. With T2-weighting, the normal prostate has a high-signal peripheral zone and lower, heterogeneous signal central gland. The seminal vesicles are shown as high-signal multilocular cystic structures. Seventy-five percent of tumors arise from the peripheral zone and are of low signal intensity, but prostatitis, infarction, and calcification may mimic this appearance. Postbiopsy hemorrhage may also show as low signal intensity within the gland on T2-weighted images. Differentiation of hemorrhage from tumor may be achieved by detection of high signal intensity representing hemorrhage on T1-weighted images. Hemorrhagic changes may result in overestimation of tumor extent and MR imaging should probably be delayed for three weeks following a TRUS biopsy.

Extracapsular spread is demonstrated by a focal bulge, loss of a well-defined capsule or low-signal soft-tissue infiltrating through the capsule into the periprostatic fat or superiorly into the seminal vesicles. As only 25% of prostate carcinoma arise from the central gland, MR imaging will struggle to detect a carcinoma given the variable signal returned from the central gland affected with the more common benign prostatic hyperplasia (BPH). To complete the examination, surface coil images should be obtained to assess the whole pelvis for lymphadenopathy with T1-weighted sagittal sequences through the lumbosacral spine to determine the presence of bony metastases (Fig. 15.**14**).

Studies in the late 1980s showed rather disappointing results with MR imaging in prostate carcinoma.[8,9] However, the introduction of new coils (the pelvic phased-array and endorectal coils), use of orthogonal planes, and increasingly experienced observers have shown an apparent improvement in accuracy. Despite some encouraging reports, it is recognized that it is not possible to detect microscopic extracapsular extension. The use of MR imaging remains controversial, with contradictory studies showing widely divergent accuracy for prostate carcinoma detection ranging from 58 to 90%.[10] For example, a study from 1996 showed a reduction in understaging from 42% to 22% and a specificity for extracapsular invasion of 96% using the endorectal coil.[11] In the same year another group suggested that staging with an endorectal coil overstaged 21% of patients, denying the patients a potentially curative procedure, advising against routine use of MR imaging in prostate carcinoma staging.[12] Other centers have reported significant artifacts with the endorectal coil that have degraded images resulting in nondiagnostic studies in 20% of patients.[13] Whilst the controversy continues, accuracy for demonstrating seminal vesicle invasion, particularly with the combined endorectal and pelvic phased-array coil, appears to be consistently high, up to 96% (Fig. 15.**15**).[14]

Further new developments with faster MR imaging techniques have allowed dynamic postcontrast image acquisition following a rapid bolus of intravenous gadolinium.[15] Early intense enhancement followed by rapid washout of contrast implies the presence of malignant angiogenic neovasculature and may improve accuracy. MR spectroscopy uses similar technology to

Table 15.**8** TNM staging of prostate cancer

Tx		Primary tumor cannot be assessed
T0		No evidence of primary tumor
Tis		Carcinoma in situ
T1		Tumor not apparent clinically or radiologically
	T1a	Tumor found by chance in less than 5% resected tissue
	T1b	Tumor found by chance in over 5% resected tissue
	T1c	Tumor found at needle biopsy only
T2		Confined to the prostate
	T2a	Involves less than half of one lobe
	T2b	Involves more than half of one lobe
	T2c	Both lobes
T3		Through prostatic capsule
	T3a	Unilateral extracapsular spread
	T3b	Bilateral extracapsular spread
	T3c	Involving seminal vesicles
T4		Invasion of adjacent organs and structures (other than seminal vesicles)
N0		No lymph node involvement
N1		Single lymph node involvement ≤ 2 cm
N2		Single lymph node ivolvement > 2 cm, or multiple nodes
M0		No metastases
M1a		Nonregional lymph nodes
M1b		Bone metastases
M1c		Other sites

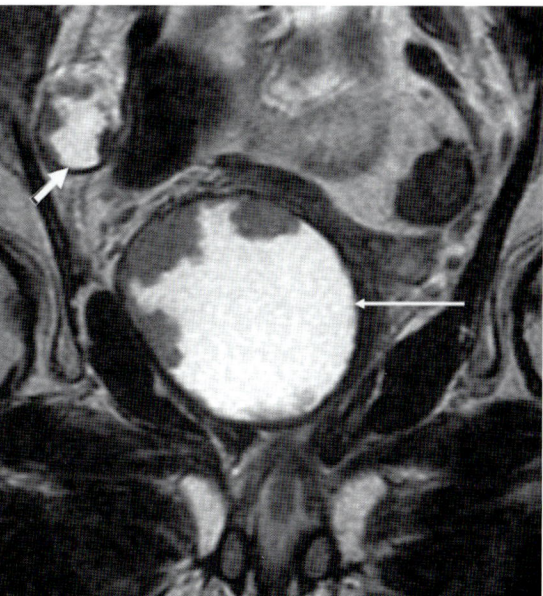

Fig. 15.**14** Coronal T2-weighted MR image of a large cystic adenocarcinoma of the prostate (long arrow) with right external iliac node involvement (thick arrow)

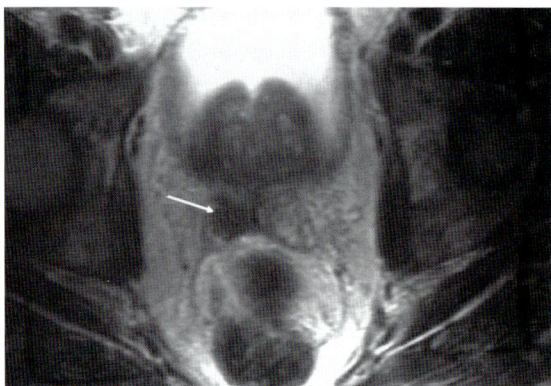

Fig. 15.15 Axial T2-weighted MR image, demonstrating a T3b prostate cancer with right seminal vesicle invasion (arrow)

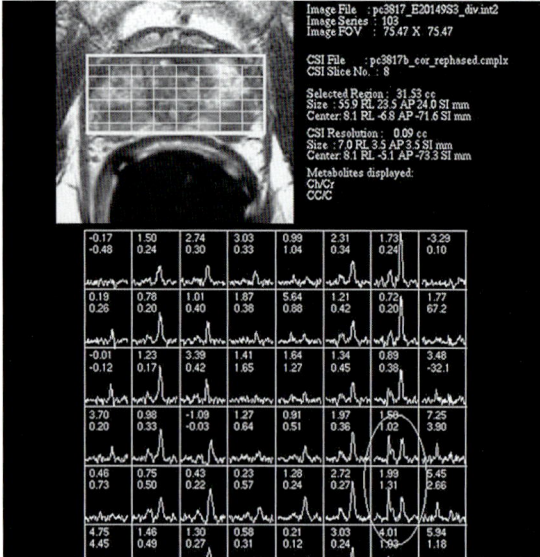

Fig. 15.16 MR spectroscopy superimposed on conventional T2-weighted MR image through the prostate confirming carcinoma in left midzone with raised choline peak on left relative to citrate peak on right (circled), compared to the spectra obtained elsewhere

conventional MR imaging but, rather than anatomical images, provides functional information by showing the relative concentrations of various metabolites contained within the structure under investigation. Spectra are produced which show peaks and troughs, with the area under the curve corresponding to concentration of metabolite. In the case of prostate carcinoma, three metabolites—citrate, creatine, and choline—are measured. Prostate carcinoma has significantly higher choline and lower citrate levels compared to normal tissue and BPH. Tumor tissue can, therefore, be identified by demonstrating an increased choline/citrate ratio and correlating this with conventional T2-weighted images (Fig. 15.16). Work is underway to determine whether these ratios reflect histological grade of disease and how helpful this might be in directing intensity-modulated radiation therapy. It seems that not only may MR spectroscopy be of use when combined with MR imaging in preoperative staging and localization of prostate cancer but may also prove useful in treatment follow-up.[16]

Generally, if the PSA is > 10 ng/mL or if the patient has bone pain, then a bone scan using ^{99m}Tc-labeled diphosphonate is performed. This evaluates the whole skeleton for bony metastatic disease. Any indeterminate regions may be evaluated with MR imaging.

Testicular Tumors

Scrotal ultrasound is the imaging investigation of choice in the diagnosis of testicular tumors. Ultrasound is able to differentiate intratesticular from extratesticular lesions and can resolve lesions down to 1 mm in diameter. Other imaging modalities are used once the diagnosis has been made to stage the disease. This is usually CT for evaluation of the retroperitoneum and a chest radiograph for demonstration of metastases to the lungs.

Calculus Disease

Ultrasound is limited in the assessment of both acute and chronic urolithiasis, particularly compared to CT or a plain abdominal radiograph and provides incomplete pelvicalyceal anatomical information.[17,18] With acute calculi, reported sensitivities for ultrasound range from 37–64% for calculus detection and 74–85% for detection of acute obstruction.[19–21] However, the accuracy varies considerably; a further study reported a sensitivity of only 24% with a specificity of 90%.[22] Ultrasound may "miss" calculi smaller than 5 mm in the pelvicalyceal system, ureter, or renal pelvis.[23] In all patients with acute ureteric colic, the ultrasound examination should be supported by a plain abdominal radiograph. If symptoms persist, a negative ultrasound examination in these patients should be followed by an IVU or CT. Many centers employ CT as the initial diagnostic study for acute ureteric colic; over 99% of renal calculi will be seen on CT.[24] Examples of nonvisualized calculi are matrix or struvite calculi, or those calculi due to indinavir therapy. CT has the highest diagnostic accuracy of any imaging modality (95% compared to 80% for IVU) in acute ureteric colic; this is an important consideration when a patient may be labeled as a "stone-former" on the basis of a radiological finding. In the initial landmark study, a calculus was confidently seen in 11 out of 12 patients on CT compared with only five patients on the corresponding IVU.[26] All subsequent reports have confirmed this impressive diagnostic performance.

For management of a patient with chronic or known urinary tract calculi, size may be measured readily on ultrasound, but the precise intrarenal location, an important consideration in management therapy, can be difficult to resolve. An IVU is always necessary prior to extracorporeal shock-wave lithotripsy (ESWL) or percutaneous nephrolithotomy to confirm location (Fig. 15.17) and define the pelvicalyceal anatomy.[17,18] The position of pelvicalyceal calculi are demonstrated with more precise detail on three-dimensional (3-D) CT, performed on the new multichannel CT scanners (Fig. 15.18). Pelvicalyceal anatomy cannot be confidently delineated on ultrasound unless there is pelvicalyceal system dilatation, but in the future 3-D ultrasound may provide as much anatomical information as an IVU. Further limitations of ultrasound for follow-up of chronic calculi include reproducibility of size measurements and assessment of fragmentation after lithotripsy. Orthogonal planes are used in ultrasound, unlike the fixed planes for plain radiography or CT, and this introduces an interobserver variation in size estimation. This was demonstrated in one study where ultrasound and CT measurements were concordant in only 79% of patients.[22] Satisfactory fragmentation after therapy is also difficult to assess on ultrasound compared to the plain abdominal radiograph, as fragments are usually resolved as a single mass by the poorer spatial resolution of ultrasound. Fowler et al. found that ultrasound could identify only 39% of patients with multiple calculi.[22] For ureteric calculi, the plain abdominal radiograph is also preferred as the calculi are more reliably visualized whilst awaiting calculus passage or the decision to intervene. Therefore the role of ultrasound in the long-term management of calculi may be restricted to those with asymptomatic calculi who are not undergoing active management. In all other patients the ultrasound needs to be supplemented with a plain abdominal radiograph or IVU.

The contribution of MR urography is limited to patients in whom irradiating investigations are contraindicated: The pregnant woman with a dilated kidney on ultrasound but no calculus seen (Fig. 15.19).[27] Nuclear medicine is useful in selected cases, such as in determining the function of a calculus-bearing kidney with poor cortical preservation on ultrasound. There is no defined threshold, but < 10% preserved function (after treatment of associated obstruction/sepsis) may not be worth treating and nephrectomy may be indicated.

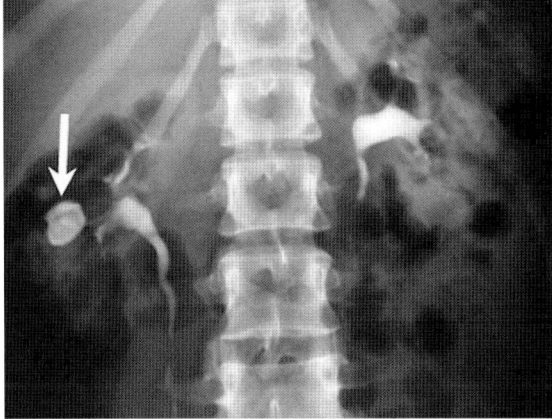

Fig. 15.**17** An IVU showing a calculus in a calyceal diverticulum (arrow). Although ultrasound demonstrated the calculus, the intracalyceal location is better demonstrated with an IVU. Knowledge of intracalyceal anatomy has a bearing on treatment

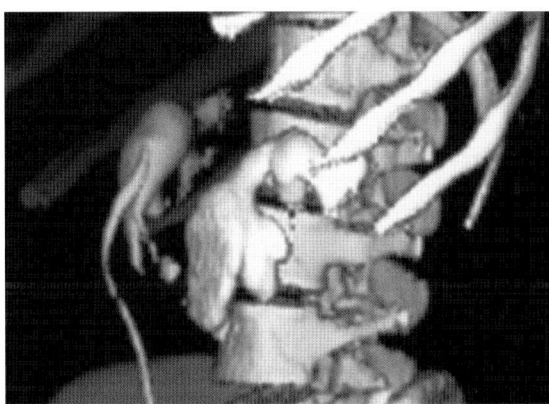

Fig. 15.**18** A 3-D CT reconstruction, demonstrating the relationships of the calyces and renal pelvis

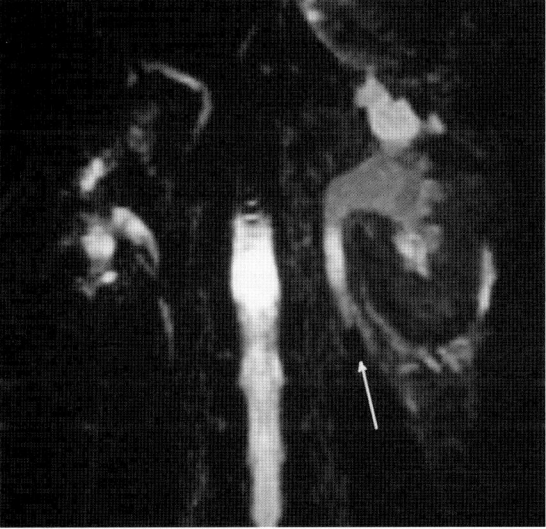

Fig. 15.**19** MR urography, demonstrating an obstructing calculus in proximal left ureter (arrow) with swollen, edematous left kidney in a pregnant patient

Renal Outflow Obstruction

Renal outflow obstruction is a common clinical problem, with an incidence of approximately 4% at postmortem in adults. Renal outflow obstruction has a significant morbidity, which includes infection, renal parenchymal loss, and renal failure, but if detected early enough is a potentially reversible condition. It is vital that renal outflow obstruction is recognized before irreversible damage causes renal impairment.

The cause of renal obstruction is varied and may present acutely, as with calculus disease. However, it may have a more insidious and silent onset, which makes early detection problematic. Renal obstruction is defined as a proved increase in resistance to the flow of urine and may be acute or chronic, unilateral or bilateral. Not all patients with renal obstruction have a defined "anatomical" site of obstruction despite having increased pressures more proximally, for example in bladder-neck dysfunction and primary megaureter. In a number of patients renal obstruction may be equivocal, where a combination of functional and dynamic studies may be necessary to make an assessment.

The diagnosis of renal obstruction is made most often on either ultrasound or IVU depending on the clinical indication and departmental guidelines. Ultrasound relies on the demonstration of a dilated pelvicalyceal system. The use of resistance index (RI) and ureteric "jets" may provide additional physiological information. In acute obstruction, an IVU will show a characteristic delayed, dense nephrogram with dilated renal pelvis and the anatomical level of obstruction, although sometimes delayed films may be required. CT will show similar features and may be useful in determining the cause of obstruction by an extrinsic compression. In acute obstruction, MR and radionuclide imaging do not have an established role unless the patient is pregnant or has an iodinated contrast medium allergy. However, a nuclear medicine renogram with diuretic administered 15 minutes prior to the examination is often required in equivocal cases, where the renal pelvis is dilated and it is uncertain whether this is truly obstructed (Fig. 15.**20**). A nuclear medicine renogram may also be required to measure divided renal function; often used to follow-up postsurgical patients, particularly those with complicated calculus disease and pelviureteric junction (PUJ) obstruction.

Rarely, it may be necessary to perform perfusion pressure flow studies, as originally described by Whitaker.[28] This is an invasive technique requiring percutaneous direct puncture of the renal collecting system. The needle is used to instill a combination of saline and iodinated contrast media at a rate of 10 mL/min until contrast fills the pelvis and overflows into the bladder. At the same time a catheter is introduced into the bladder to measure intravesical pressure. A differential pressure between the two systems of > 22 cm of water indicates a significant obstruction requiring intervention; if < 12 cm of water, renal obstruction is unlikely.

Similarly urodynamics of the lower urinary tract combined with fluoroscopy can be used to assess bladder function, particularly in the investigation of probable bladder outflow obstruction, urinary incontinence, and a neuropathic bladder. The procedure is similar to that of MCU but it is necessary to catheterize the bladder with two tubes, one for filling and one for pressure measurements. Urodynamics also requires a further catheter in the rectum to measure total abdominal pressure. Intrinsic bladder pressure is calculated by subtracting total abdominal pressure from total bladder pressure. Voided volumes and flow rates can also be measured.

Renal Artery Stenosis

Doppler ultrasound may be used as an initial screening investigation for suspected renal artery stenosis (RAS), but any abnormalities need to be confirmed by conventional catheter angiography, CT, or MR angiography (Fig. 15.**21**).[29] Even at catheter angiography, full confirmation of the presence of a RAS may need to be supplemented with intra-arterial pressure measurements to assess the hemodynamic significance of any renal artery narrowing. MR angiography is reported to be 97% sensitive compared to 69% for captopril-enhanced Doppler ultrasound for the diagnosis of RAS.[30]

Renal Transplantation

The use of ultrasound, first-line imaging for the monitoring of renal transplantation has been described in Chapter 5. Nuclear renography may be a useful adjunct in a number of circumstances, for example with surgical complications (Fig. 15.**22**). If the collecting system is dilated, functional imaging with MAG3 renography can determine whether the collecting system is obstructed. Although the role of MR angiography still requires further clarification, it may be used to exclude a transplant RAS if Doppler ultrasound is noncontributory or technically difficult.

Urinary Tract Trauma

In the patient with major abdominal trauma, ultrasound is often used for initial assessment, to assess for a renal hematoma, collections in the renal bed (in-

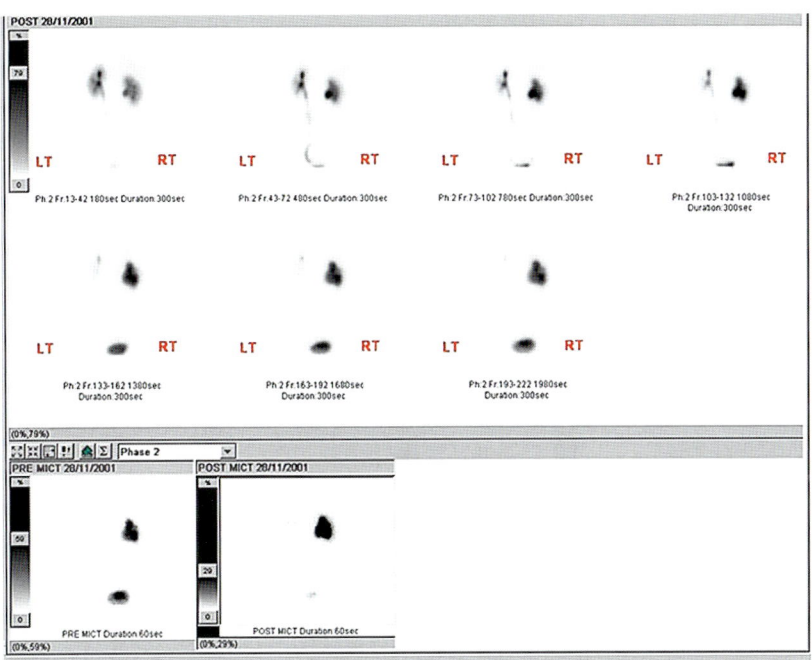

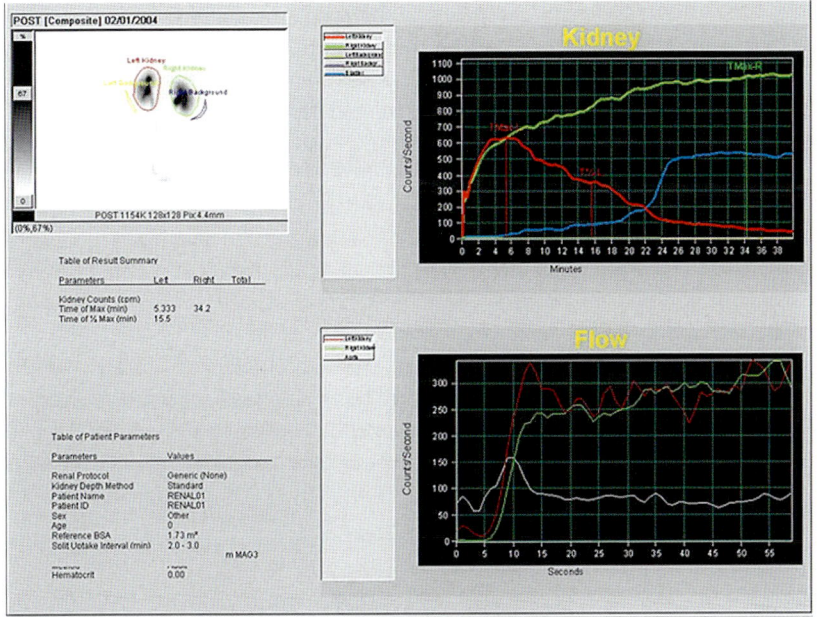

Fig. 15.**20 a** F-15 MAG3 renogram demonstrates a dilated right pelvicalyceal system with hold-up of isotope over 300 seconds which persists following micturation. **b** F-15 MAG3 renography time–activity curves for the right and left kidneys demonstrate a rising time–activity curve (green line) on the right to confirm right PUJ obstruction. Note normal pattern of uptake, drainage, and fall in time–activity curve within the left kidney (red line)

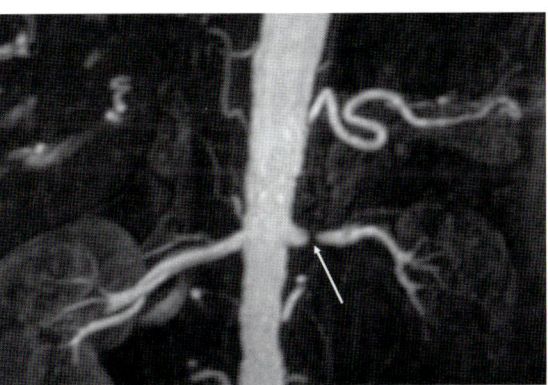

Fig. 15.**21 MR** angiography, demonstrating a left RAS (arrow)

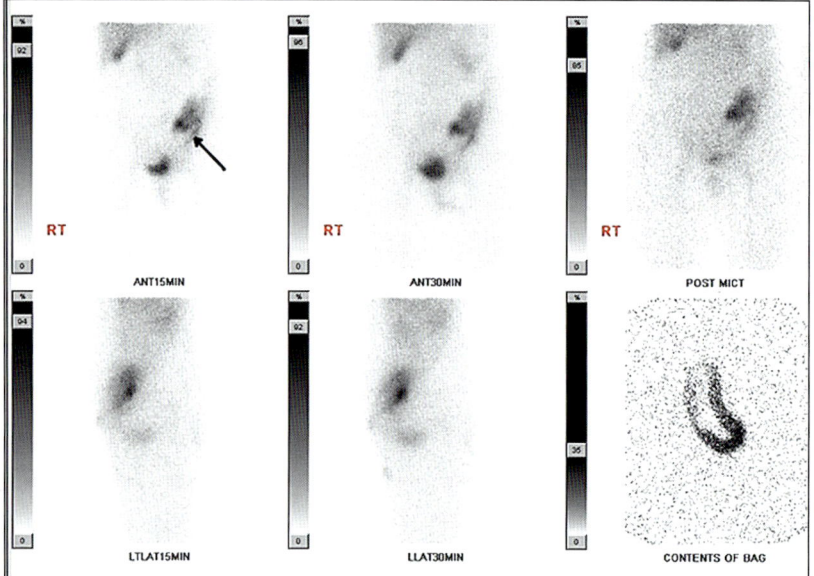

Fig. 15.**22 A MAG3 renogram showing a renal transplant in the left iliac fossa.** Activity is seen to extend beyond the confines of the transplant kidney and ureter (arrow) consistent with a urinary leak. Urinary activity is also demonstrated in the drainage bag that was overlying the wound, confirming presence of a leak. Note the activity within the gallbladder due to hepatobiliary excretion that occurs in renal impairment with MAG3 renography

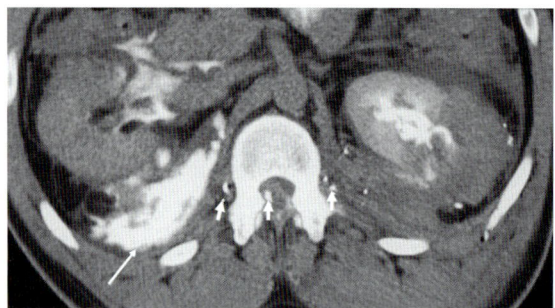

Fig. 15.**23 A contrast-enhanced CT, demonstrating major bilateral renal trauma following a gun-shot injury with active extravasation of contrast on the right** (arrow). The path of the bullet can be traced through the spinal canal (short arrows)

dicating either vascular or collecting system injury), or in the pelvis (if the ureter, bladder, or urethra is damaged). With urinary tract trauma, the main concern is damage to the renal vasculature, renal parenchyma, ureteric injury (often iatrogenic), bladder, or urethra.[31] Rarely the site of active bleeding may be seen with Doppler ultrasound. If any abnormality is seen on ultrasound or if the patient is unstable despite a normal ultrasound examination, further imaging is necessary to identify the area of injury and quantify the degree of injury. The kidneys are best assessed by contrast-enhanced CT (Fig. 15.23)[31] or an IVU if subtle collecting system injury is suspected. Similar considerations apply to the ureter, which is best assessed with an IVU (or coronal reformats with CT). For suspected bladder and urethral injuries cystourethrography should be performed.

Summary points:

Investigations	Most common indications	Advantages	Disadvantages
Plain radiographs	• Calcifications • Bony abnormalities	• Simple • Cheap	• Ionizing radiation
Intravenous urography (IVU)	• Imaging of upper tracts in hematuria • Calculus disease • Urinary obstruction • Anatomy of congenital anomalies	• Good anatomy and resolution of upper tracts and ureters	• Ionizing radiation • Contrast media required; allergic reactions and nephrotoxicity
Micturating cyto-urethrography (MCU)	• Imaging of ureters, bladder, and urethra predominantly in children	• Good resolution • Good anatomical definition • Complete, one-stage lower-tract imaging	• Ionizing radiation • Invasive
Investigations	**Most common indications**	**Advantages**	**Disadvantages**
Computed tomography (CT)	• Calculus disease • Hematuria • Urinary obstruction • Characterization of renal masses • Staging of malignant disease • Trauma	• Now readily available • Calculi/hemorrhage well-demonstrated • Subtle enhancement well seen • 3-D CT becoming a reality	• Ionizing radiation • Contrast media (see IVU)
Magnetic resonance (MR) imaging	• Problem-solving of renal masses • Renal artery stenosis (RAS) • Renal vein/inferior vena cava (IVC) thrombus in malignant disease • Staging pelvic malignancies	• No ionizing radiation • Multiplanar capabilities • Good soft-tissue characterization • Contrast medium is not nephrotoxic • Useful in renal failure and pregnancy	• Expensive • Not as readily accessible • Difficult in claustrophobic patients • No pacemakers/aneurysm clips, etc.
Radionuclide imaging	• Assessment of drainage in hydronephrotic kidney • Evaluation of vesicoureteric reflux (VUR) in children • Demonstration of scarring in reflux nephropathy • Accurate divided function in surgical planning and follow-up • Assessment of perfusion in RAS • Staging bone scans	• Both functional and anatomical information • Usually noninvasive • Lower dose in children cf. MCU	• Ionizing radiation • Not available in all institutions
Renal angiography	• RAS	• Good resolution ("gold standard")	• Invasive • Nephrotoxic contrast media may be required but CO_2 can be used

References

1. Majd M, Potter BM, Guzzetta PC, et al. Effect of captopril on efficacy of renal scintigraphy in detection of renal artery stenosis. J Nucl Med 1983;24:23.
2. Fommei E, Ghione S, Hilson AJ, et al. Captopril radionuclide test in renovascular hypertension: a European multicentre study. European Multicentre Study Group. Eur J Nuc Med 1993;20:617–623.
3. Forman HP, Middleton WD, Melson GL, et al. Hyperechoic renal cell carcinomas: increase in detection at US. Radiology 1993;188;431–434.
4. Jamis-Dow CA, Choyle PL, Jennings SB, et al. Small renal masses: detection with CT versus US and pathologic correlation. Radiology 1996;198:785–788.
5. Pressler LB, Petrylak DP, Olsson CA. Invasive transitional cell carcinoma of the bladder: prognosis and management. In: Oesterling JE, Richie JP, eds. Urologic oncology. Philadelphia: WB Saunders: 1997:275–295.
6. Nishimura K, Hida S, Nishio Y, et al. The validity of magnetic resonance imaging in the staging of bladder cancer: comparison with computed tomography and transurethral ultrasonography. Jpn J Clin Oncol 1988;18:217–226.
7. Tanimoto A, Yuasa Y, Imai Y, et al. Bladder tumour staging: comparison of conventional and gadolinium-enhanced dynamic MR staging and CT. Radiology 1992;185:741–747.

8. Sciebler ML, Tomaszewski JE, Bezzi M, et al. Prostatic carcinoma and benign prostatic hyperplasia: correlation of high-resolution MR and histopathologic findingc. Radiology 1989;172:131–137.
9. Mukamel E, Hannah J, Barbaric Z, DeKernion JB. The value of computerised tomography scan and magnetic resonance imaging in staging prostatic carcinoma: comparison with the clinical and histological staging. J Urol 1986;136:1231–1233.
10. Engelbrecht MRW, Barentsz JO, Jager GJ, et al. Prostate cancer staging using imaging. Br J Urol Intl 2000;86:1.
11. Cornud F, Belin X, Flam T, et al. Local staging of prostate cancer by endorectal MRI using fast spin-echo sequences: prospective correlation with pathological findings after radical prostatectomy. Br J Urol 1996;77:843–50.
12. Perrotti M, Kaufman R, Jennings TA, et al. Endorectal coil magnetic resonance imaging in clinically localised prostate cancer: is it accurate? J Urol 1996;156:106–109.
13. Husband JE, Padhani AR, Macvicar AD, Revell P. Magnetic resonance imaging of prostate cancer: comparison of image quality using endorectal and pelvic phased array coils. Clin Radiol 1998;53:673–681.
14. Hricak H, White S, Vigneron D, et al. Carcinoma of the prostate gland: MR Imaging with pelvic phased-array coils versus integrated endorectal-pelvic phased-array coils. Radiology 1994;193:703–709.
15. Brown G, Macvicar DA, Ayton V, Husband JE. The role of intravenous contrast enhancement in magnetic resonance imaging of the prostatic carcinoma. Clin Radiol 1995;50:601–606.
16. Scheidler J, Hricak H, Vigneron DB, et al. Prostate cancer: localisation with 3-D proton MR spectroscopic imaging—clinicopathologic study. Radiology 1999;213:473–480.
17. Sandhu C, Anson KA, Patel U. Urinary tract stones—part 1: role of radiological imaging in diagnosis and treatment planning. Clin Radiol 2003;58:415–421.
18. Sandhu C, Anson KA, Patel U. Urinary tract stones—part 2: current status of treatment. Clin Radiol 2003;58:422–433.
19. Sinclair D, Wilson S, Toi A, Greenspan L. The evaluation of suspected renal colic: ultrasound scan versus excretory urography. Ann Emerg Med 1989;18:556–559.
20. Aslaksen A, Gothlin JH. Ultrasonic diagnosis of ureteral calculi in patients with acute flank pain. Eur J Radiol 1990;11:87–90.
21. Deyoe LA, Cronan JJ, Breslaw BH, Ridlen MS. New techniques of ultrasound and color Doppler in the prospective evaluation of acute renal obstruction. Do they replace the intravenous urogram? Abdo Imaging 1995;20:58–63.
22. Fowler KA, Locken JA, Duchesne JH, Williamson MR. US for detecting renal calculi with non-enhanced CT as a reference standard. Radiology 2002;222:109–113.
23. Juul N, Holm-Bentzen M, Rygaard H, Holm HH. Ultrasonographic diagnosis of renal stones. Scand J Urol Nephrol 1987;21:135–137.
24. Smith RC, Coll DM. Helical computed tomography in the diagnosis of ureteric colic. BJU Int 2000;86 (Suppl 1):33–41.
25. Bruce RG, Munch LC, Hoven AD, Jerauld RS, Greenburg R, Porter WH, et al. Urolithiasis associated with the protease inhibitor indinavir. Urology 1997;50:513–518.
26. Smith RC, Choe KA, et al. Acute flank pain: Comparison of non-contrast-enhanced CT and intravenous urography. Radiology 1995;194:789–794.
27. Rothpearl A, Frager D, Subramanian A, Bashist B, Baer J, Kay C, et al. MR urography: technique and application. Radiology 1995;194:125–130.
28. Whitaker RH. Methods of assessing obstruction in dilated ureters. Br J Urol 1973;45:15–22.
29. Urban BA, Ratner LE, Fishman EK. Three-dimensional volume-rendered CT angiography of the renal arteries and veins: normal anatomy, variants, and clinical applications. Radiographics 2001;21:373–386.
30. Qanadli SD, Soulez G, Therasse E, et al. Detection of renal artery stenosis: prospective comparison of captopril-enhanced Doppler sonography, captopril-enhanced scintigraphy, and MR angiography. Am J Roentgenol 2001;177:1123–1129.
31. Smith JK, Kenney PJ. Imaging of renal trauma. Radiol Clin North Am 2003;41:1019–1035.

Section 5

New Developments: Ultrasound Contrast Agents

16 The Native Kidney 253
17 The Transplant Kidney 264

16 The Native Kidney
E. Leen

Introduction: Classes of Ultrasound Contrast Agents

The ideal ultrasound contrast agent for renal imaging should be safe, stable in the vascular system to survive pulmonary capillary circulation, and capable of modifying the acoustic properties of the regions of interest within the kidneys. Most of the current contrast agents satisfy these criteria to some degree. These agents consist of microbubbles which measure 2–10 μm in diameter and are well-recognized to be the most effective backscatterers (see below).[1–4]

Ultrasound contrast agents are sometimes labeled as first-, second-, or third-generation. First-generation agents (e.g., Levovist, Schering AG, Berlin) consist of those which trap air and have a short persistence time. Second-generation agents (e.g., SonoVue, Bracco spa, Milan) contain insoluble gases such as perfluorocarbons with prolonged longevity (Table 16.1). Stability of these microbubbles is provided in the form of a shell made of denatured albumin, lipid, or surfactant layers. In contrast, third-generation agents (e.g., Sonovist, Schering AG, Berlin) use polymer shells and contain either air or perfluorocarbons with a much longer persistence time.[5]

Earlier agents were primarily designed to be blood pool agents and have been shown to be highly effective in enhancing spectral/color/power Doppler signals

Table 16.1 Ultrasound contrast agents

Licensee	Trade name	Code name	Composition	Application/status
Acusphere	A1700		Polylactic-coglycolic, polycaprolactone, copolymers; perfluorocarbon gas	Myocardial perfusion, phase II/III
Point Biomedical	BiSphere	PB127	Double-walled gelatin/polymer spheres filled with air	Myocardial perfusion, phase II/III
Amersham Health	Optison	FS069	Perfluoropropane-filled albumin microspheres	Left ventricular opacification / endocardial border delineation. Marketed in Europe and United States
Schering AG	Imavist	AFO-150	Surfactant shell containing perfluorohexane vapor in nitrogen gas	Left ventricular opacification / endocardial border delineation. (NDA-filed in United States) Myocardial perfusion, phase II Noncardiac, phase II
Schering AG	Levovist*	SHU 508A	Suspension of galactose microparticles and palmitic acid in water	LVO/EBD and noncardiac. Marketed in Europe
Schering AG	Sonovist	SHU 563A	Polybutylcyanoacrylate microspheres containing air	Noncardiac, phase II. Marketed in Europe
Bracco Spa		BR14	Phospholipid shell containing perfluorobutane	Liver: phase I, II. Marketed in Europe
Bracco Spa	SonoVue	BR1	Phospholipid-stabilized SF6 gas	Noncardiac; marketed in Europe; phase II/III in United States LVO/EBD NDA-filed in United States and Europe. Myocardial perfusion, phase II
Bristol Myers Squibb Medical Imaging Inc.	Definity	MRX-115	Phospholipid-coated microbubbles of perfluoropropane/air with gas-filled lipid bilayers	LVO/EBD: Marketed in United States Noncardiac, phase II/III in United States
Amersham Health	Sonazoid	NC 100100	Perfluorobutane gas encapsulated in lipid shell	LVO/EBD, NDA-submitted in United States, Noncardiac, phase II/III

*Registered

within the macrovasculature on fundamental, i.e. conventional imaging modes, lasting up to seven minutes following an intravenous bolus administration and approximately up to 15–20 minutes after an infusion.[6,7] Agents such as SonoVue (Bracco Spa, Milan), Definity (Bristol Myers Squibb, Boston), Optison (Amersham, Oslo), and Imavist (Schering AG, Berlin), although primarily designed to be blood pool agents, have shown to be trapped or slowed in the hepatic sinusoids and spleen enhancing the parenchyma, which may last up to six minutes.[8] This characteristic is useful for both the detection and characterization of lesions deficient of sinusoids, for example metastasis. These, therefore, appear as a filling defect.[9]

Agents such as NC100100 (Amersham, Oslo), Levovist (Schering AG, Berlin), and SHU 563A (Schering AG, Berlin) have additional tissue-specific properties.[10–12] They are selectively taken up by the Kupffer cells of the reticuloendothelial system, after the vascular phase, and may enhance the normal hepatic and splenic parenchyma for up to an hour on either fundamental or harmonic, gray-scale, or Doppler modes, depending on the dosage used. The advantage of this property is that lesions which are deficient of Kupffer cells or associated with Kupffer cell dysfunction do not retain the contrast agent, thereby improving the lesion-to-tissue contrast ratio. However, none of these agents have been shown to be trapped in the kidneys.

In Europe and Asia, SonoVue and Levovist are currently commercially available for radiological clinical applications, whilst in North America only Definity is licensed for radiological applications. However, agents which are already licensed for cardiac imaging such as Optison or Definity in the United States can also be used off-labeled for abdominal imaging.

Summary points:
- Ultrasound contrast agents are very safe to use clinically
- There are different classes of agents based on different formulations and all can be used for renal imaging
- They are now commercially available in Europe, North America, Latin America, and Asia

Microbubble Behavior and Imaging Modes

The interaction between the insonating ultrasound beam and the microbubbles is very complex; a basic understanding of their behavior under various sound fields has been fundamental to the development of improved methods of visualizing and displaying the contrast agents. On insonation at low amplitude (0–100 kPa), microbubbles behave as linear backscatterers, alternatively contracting and expanding according to the positive and negative pressures of the sinusoidal sound waves. As the incident pressure increases (100 kPA–1 Mpa) they begin to show nonlinear characteristics with emission of harmonics (i.e., on the negative portion of the sound waves the bubbles can become quite large, but on the positive portion there is a limit to which they can contract) and this asymmetry is what constitutes the harmonic emissions. With a further increase in the peak pressure of the incident ultrasound field, the shell of the microbubble is disrupted; during this process a transient, strong, nonlinear echo is emitted (stimulated acoustic emission [SAE]/loss of correlation [LOC]) and the microbubbles are destroyed.[13] Fundamental color/power Doppler modes and the newer harmonic modes (tissue, pulse/phase inversion) use the microbubbles' nonlinear and transient scattering properties to enhance signals from the contrast agents over those of background tissue.

Ultrasound contrast agents are indeed very effective in enhancing fundamental spectral/color/power Doppler signals within the macrocirculation of the kidneys. However, blooming of the color/power Doppler signals and shadowing artifacts may obscure enhancement of the blood pool and further degradation may arise from the respiratory and cardiac motion artifacts on the fundamental modes. Adjustment of the color/power Doppler gain counteracts the benefit of using the contrast agents. Fortunately, the use of harmonic modes effectively displays the microbubble signals while suppressing the tissue motion artifacts.

Unlike computed tomography (CT) and magnetic resonance (MR) contrast agents, most ultrasound agents on fundamental gray-scale mode are not depicted in the microcirculation and do not enhance the renal parenchyma at clinical doses as the echo from the tissue is still far too strong compared with that from the small volume of contrast within the microcirculation of the tissue itself. The simplest method of displaying the signals from the microbubbles in the microcirculation, over those of tissue, is to destroy the microbubbles in the microcirculation at high ultrasound output (above a mechanical index [MI] of 1.0) by using fundamental color/power Doppler modes (SAE/LOC) imaging).[14,15] This method emits the strongest signals. Furthermore, Doppler modes are ideal because they are very sensitive. A mosaic of color Doppler signals and color enhancement are displayed on color/power Doppler mode respectively. Gray-scale enhancement is also achieved effectively as a result of the same destructive process, by using the harmonic imaging modes.

However, these fundamental Doppler and tissue-harmonic modes are inherently limited by poorer resolution and lack of penetration. Destruction of the microbubbles results in transience of the effect unless there is replenishment of the new microbubbles in the scan plane. Therefore, only microbubbles which can perfuse the imaging space between frames may be visible. In clinical practice the contrast enhancement is seen only on one frame (the first frame) because scanning is performed at a frame rate at which the interval between frames far exceeds the time for new microbubbles to perfuse the scanning plane. This forms the basis for interval delay imaging, or intermittent imaging. Short or long delay times can also be used to emphasize vascular or tissue contrast, respectively. More importantly, this technique can accentuate the differential perfusion kinetics between normal renal tissue and tumors, which may be used to improve tissue characterization.

This destructive technique is a highly effective method of displaying contrast in the microcirculation, irrespective of whether the microbubbles are in motion or not. But it is limited as it only produces transient displays of contrast and heterogeneous enhancement; transience may be partially resolved by using repeated or higher doses of contrast agents. However, shadowing artifacts from the larger vessels carrying higher concentrations of the contrast agents may be limiting.

Newer Nonlinear Imaging Modes

Methods such as pulse/phase inversion harmonic imaging have had quite an impact in displaying contrast enhancement of the parenchyma. In pulse inversion imaging, a sequence of two ultrasound pulses is transmitted instead of one single pulse. The first pulse is an in-phase pulse and the second is a mirror image of the first. For any linear target, the response to the second pulse is an inverted copy of the response from the first pulse. These are then summated and all linear echoes are cancelled. However, for a nonlinear target such as microbubbles, the responses to positive and negative pulse, are different and therefore do not cancel each other on summation. The fundamental components of the echo are cancelled whilst the even harmonic components are added, resulting in twice the harmonic level of a single pulse. They allow the use of broader transmit and receive bandwidths with improved resolution and increased sensitivity to contrast, thereby overcoming some of the limitations of the simple harmonic modes.[16,17] These advantages also permit the use of a much lower, nondestructive output power level for continuous imaging, thus obviating the need for intermittent/interval delay imaging; at such a low MI, the background tissue appears quite dark and this can to be compensated by increasing the gain setting. More recent improvements now allow adequate visualization of deep-seated lesions (10–15 cm) which were previously problematical.

Another method of displaying contrast agent signals over those of tissue, based on the nonlinear properties of the microbubbles, is known as power modulation. This is a multipulse technique with alteration of the acoustic amplitude of the transmitted pulses. It applies an initial pulse followed by a second pulse which is half the amplitude of the first. Since the reflections from tissues are linear, doubling the half-amplitude reflection results in a signal similar to the full-amplitude signal. Change in the transmit amplitude induces changes in the response of the microbubbles. Upon reception, echoes from the half-amplitude-transmitted pulse are adjusted in amplitude and subtracted from the full-amplitude echoes. This procedure removes most of the linear responses at the fundamental frequency and the remaining echoes contain mainly nonlinear signals from the microbubbles.[18,19] Power modulation is used in combination with low-frequency wideband transducers, enabling ultraharmonic imaging, which improves tissue-signal subtraction and, thereby, increases the contrast-to-tissue ratio.

Summary points:
- Some understanding of the complex interaction between microbubbles and the insonating ultrasound beam is important
- Microbubble responses vary at different mechanical indices
- Real-time imaging is now possible at low MI with nonlinear imaging techniques

Optimization of Equipment Settings and Practical Aspects

Irrespective of the equipment used, any of the nonlinear imaging modes (pulse inversion harmonic [PIH] or Power PIH for Philips; coherent contrast imaging [CCI]; or contrast pulse sequencing [CPS] for Acuson Sequoia, THI or ECI for Siemens Elegra, etc.) combined with a very low MI (0.1–0.2) scanning protocol using agents such as SonoVue, Definity, Optison, or Sonazoid are essential to enable real-time continuous imaging of the kidney. Only small volumes of contrast agent are required for a complete examination; this ranges between 0.5 mL for Definity to 2.4 mL for SonoVue. The MI and receiver gain can be adjusted according to the patient's body habitus, but the MI should be kept as low as possible. If, however, the image remains too dark despite receiver gain compensation and the anatomical landmarks are lost, it may be worth increasing the MI up to 0.35–0.4 and as soon as the arrival of the contrast agent is seen, it can be adjusted down to 0.2. The focal zone, if singular, should be set low down the screen (usually 4/5). Persistence setting, which refers to the temporal smoothing that the scanner performs in displaying images, should also be minimized. There are other parameters, such as dynamic range/compression and line density, which would also affect microbubble destruction and contrast display sensitivity, but these would already have been optimized by the equipment manufacturer and the user is best advised to adopt the default setting for the individual contrast agent.

Standardization of the scanning protocol is important to ensure coverage of the whole kidney. In our unit, sagittal sweeps followed by axial sweeps are first performed. This sequence of scanning is repeated systematically over and over throughout the vascular phase. The whole examination should be recorded on SVHS video or digitally on extended cine-loop archived on hard drive for further review. The first pass of the bolus is indeed very short and allows the assessment of the vascularity of the lesion. Irrespective of tumor vascularity, most lesions, if not all, should be detectable. It is important to understand the temporal changes in the echogenicity of the lesions relative to the adjacent renal parenchyma, which may occur during the vascular phase, for the purpose of characterization. Repeat injections are feasible for a more complete examination.

In the characterization of focal lesions, a standardized scanning protocol is also useful to evaluate the tumoral vascular morphology during the vascular phase. As it is now possible to scan at very low MI and visualize the temporal changes of lesional enhancement and its vascular morphology in real-time, there is in fact no need for any "interval delay scanning technique" to accentuate the differential vascularity between the lesion and the normal renal tissue. Following the administration of the contrast agent, gentle sweeps to cover the whole lesion are recommended instead of maintaining the same scanning plane continuously. Although there is minimal destruction when scanning at low MI, significant microbubble destruction still occurs when the probe is kept within the same scan plane. In addition, when sweeping through the lesion, a three-dimensional (3-D) perspective of the lesional vascular morphology is obtained. These sweeps can be repeated over the whole vascular phase.

However, the equipment settings and scanning protocols are different for agents such as Levovist and Sonovist as they are best displayed using nonlinear imaging modes set at high MI (> 1.0). Specific imaging modes, agent detection imaging (ADI) available on both Acuson and ATL5000, are specifically designed for using Levovist and are highly effective in displaying contrast using a color map with high resolution. However, at higher MI imaging, interval-delay imaging is necessary to enable visualization of the parenchymal enhancement.

Clinical Applications

Although ultrasound contrast agents have been under development for a long time, their clinical applications in the kidney have been limited to enhancing Doppler signals in difficult cases. However, recent improvements in nonlinear imaging modes combined with the introduction of second-generation contrast agents will undoubtedly broaden the scope of its diagnostic potential beyond simply rescuing failed Doppler examinations. There are indications from early reports to suggest that the use of contrast-enhanced ultrasound may be promising in various clinical perspectives.

Focal Renal Lesions (see Chapter 8)

Renal cysts are common incidental lesions found on all imaging modalities, and those which are simple are not clinically relevant. However, complex cysts may have malignant potential, depending upon the number and thickness of the septations, presence of mural nodules, and/or peripheral calcification.[20] The option of surgical resection relies on the demonstration of hypervascularity of these nodules or septations, which is usually based on contrast-enhanced CT or MR imaging. Previous studies using Levovist-enhanced power Doppler ultrasound have shown that the use of contrast improved the sonographic evaluation of the vascularity of the septations and nodules which was superior when compared with contrast-enhanced CT.[21] Contrast-enhanced ultrasound with the new nonlinear imaging modes, by virtue of the higher spatial resolution compared with power Doppler, may further improve its diagnostic accuracy (Figs. 16.**1**, 16.**2**).

Unenhanced ultrasound is well-known to be limited in the detection of small focal renal masses compared with an enhanced CT scan;[22] of lesions measuring < 5 mm, the detection rate for CT and ultrasound was 47% and 0%, respectively, and even for lesions measuring 15–20 mm, the detection rates were 100% and 58%, respectively. However, there were still a substantial proportion of lesions measuring < 1 cm which had not been detected by either modality. Whilst we can assume that contrast-enhanced ultrasound may improve the detection of small focal lesions, it remains to be seen whether it can match contrast-enhanced CT and

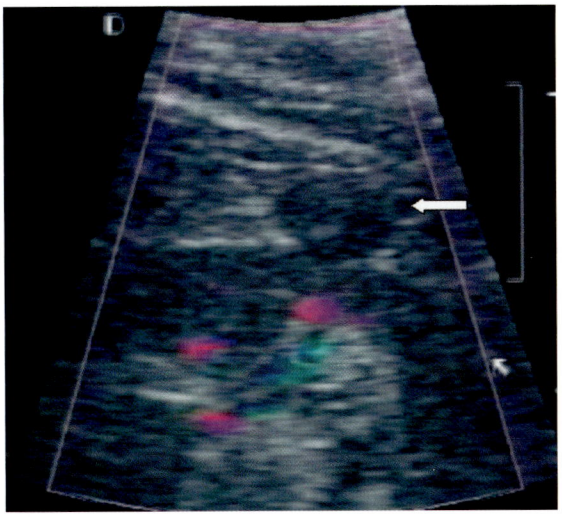
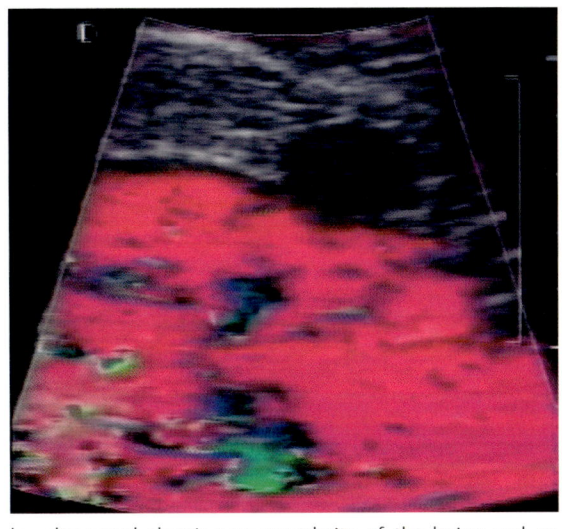

Fig. 16.1 **a** Baseline fundamental ultrasound showing apparent echoes inside a lesion at the lower pole of the kidney suggestive of a renal mass. (arrow). **b** Contrast-enhanced color Doppler ultrasound showing no vascularity of the lesion and no intralesional echoes confirming simple renal cyst. (Courtesy of R.G. Barr, Ph.D. M.D., Youngstown, Ohio, US)

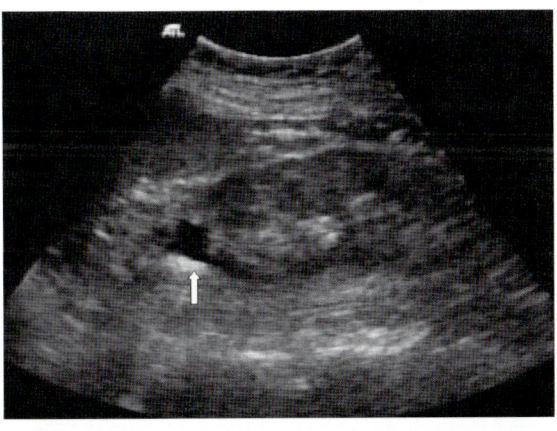
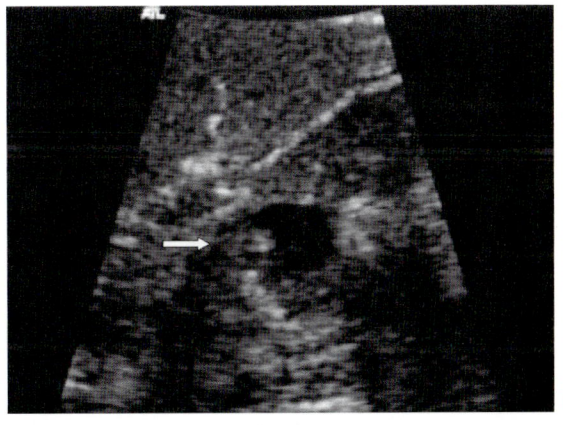
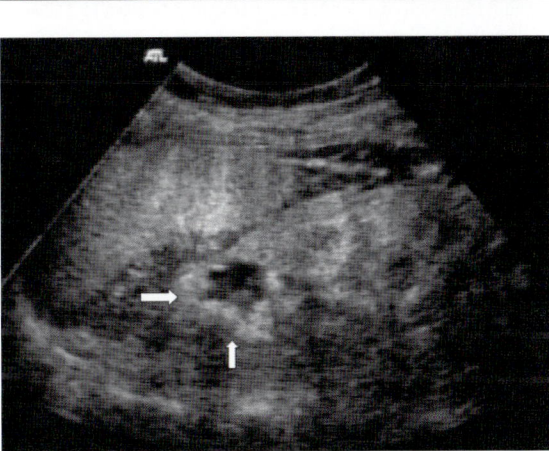
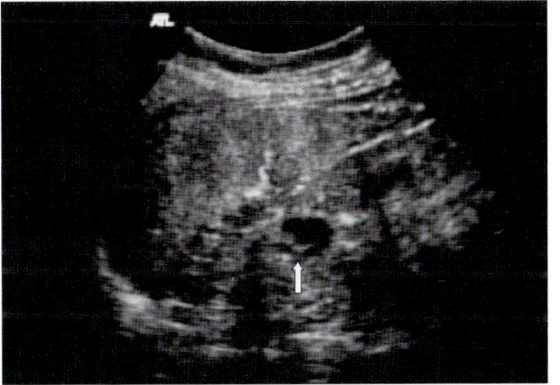

Fig. 16.2 **a** Baseline fundamental ultrasound showing a small cyst with some irregularity on the inner aspect of the capsule (arrow). **b** Contrast-enhanced nonlinear imaging ultrasound scan showing nodular enhancement inside the cyst (arrow). **c** Magnified view confirmed the nodular enhancement (arrows). **d** Delayed scan showing septal enhancement consistent with complex renal cyst (arrow) which was confirmed as malignant. (Courtesy of R.G. Barr, Ph.D. M.D., Youngstown, Ohio, US)

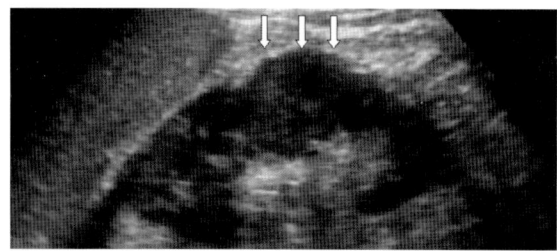
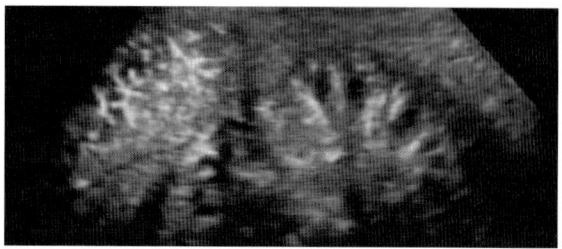
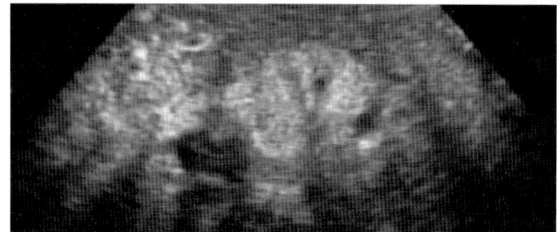

Fig. 16.3 a Baseline fundamental ultrasound showing distortion of the renal cortex by an apparent mass with altered echogenicity (arrows). b Contrast-enhanced nonlinear imaging ultrasound scan showing normal branching of the intrarenal arteries inside the apparent mass in the early vascular phase, confirming normal renal tissue instead of tumor. c Interval delay imaging showing similar enhancement of apparent lesion as with normal adjacent renal cortical tissue. Appearances were those of a splenic hump. (Courtesy of R.G. Barr, Ph.D. M.D., Youngstown, Ohio, US)

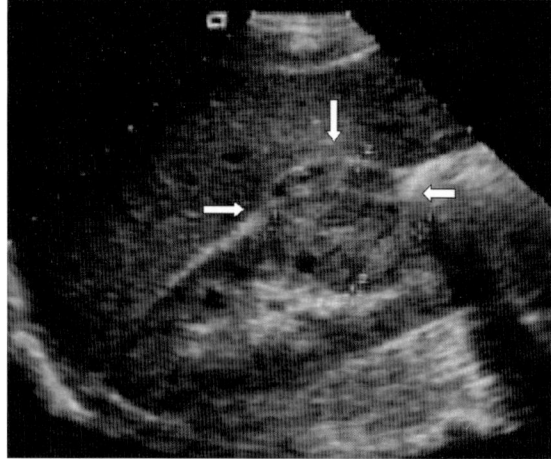
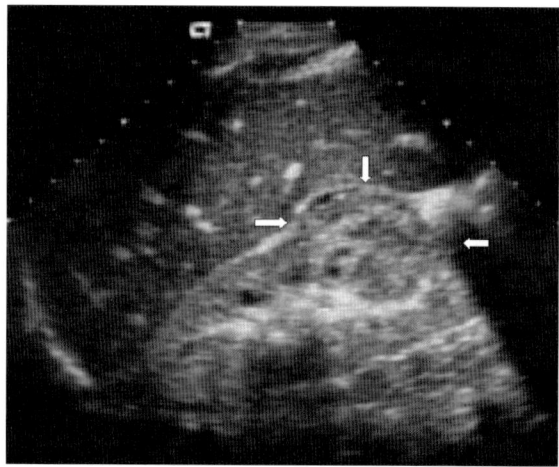

Fig. 16.4 a Baseline fundamental ultrasound showing deformity of the renal cortex by a mass of altered mixed echogenicity (arrows). b Contrast-enhanced nonlinear imaging ultrasound scan showing large abnormal vessels (arrows) inside the enhanced hypervascular mass in the early vascular phase, confirming renal cell carcinoma. (Courtesy of R.G. Barr, Ph.D. M.D., Youngstown, Ohio, US)

MR. In the same study the authors showed that CT and ultrasound correctly characterized 80% and 82%, respectively, of lesions measuring 10–35 mm. However, an early study with contrast-enhanced ultrasound has shown its limitation in the characterization of focal hyperechoic lesions, although it improved the differentiation between pseudotumor and neoplasm.[23]

Other focal renal lesions, including infarcts, infection, and laceration/hematoma, are also associated with reduced or lack of perfusion; these are easily depicted using contrast-enhanced ultrasound. Although there are only anecdotal reports and published abstracts to substantiate the efficacy of this new technique, intuitively one can assume contrast-enhanced ultrasound may have a role to play in the characterization of benign and malignant lesions, as well as in the guidance, monitoring, and follow-up of radiofrequency (RF) ablation of renal tumors (Figs. 16.3–5). Further prospective studies are still required to determine the true value of the technique in clinical practice.

Contrast-enhanced ultrasound with nonlinear imaging modes may potentially replace CT in the evaluation of these complex renal cystic lesions and their follow-up or as an adjunct in the evaluation of the indeterminate small renal lesion found on CT or MR imaging. It may be of particular value in the evaluation of patients at higher risk of CT contrast nephrotoxicity or those who are claustrophobic for MR imaging.

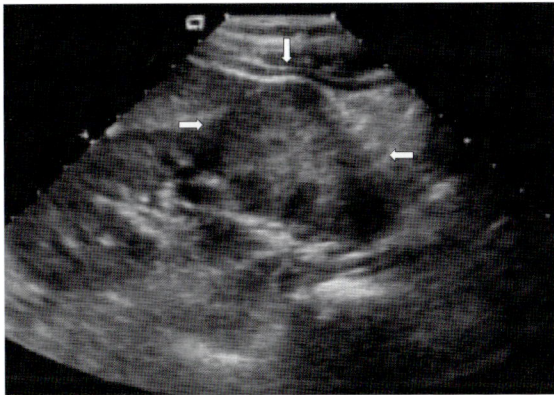
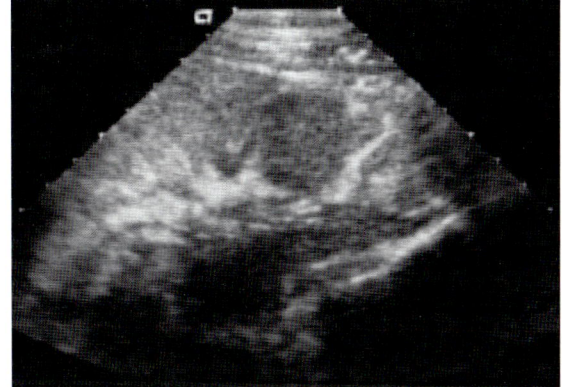
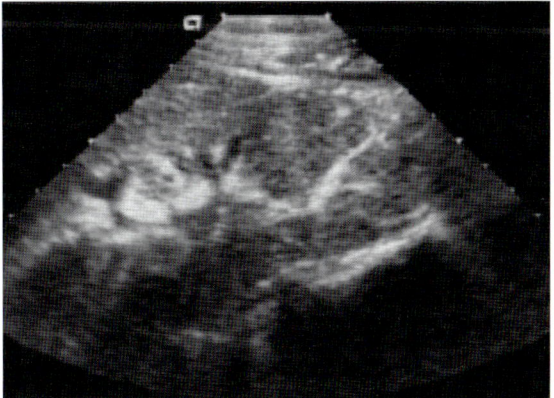

Fig. 16.**5 a** Baseline fundamental ultrasound showing renal mass which is poorly delineated (arrows). **b** Contrast-enhanced nonlinear imaging ultrasound scan showing small tumoral vessels permeating the periphery of the relatively hypovascular mass which is displacing the normal renal vessels. **c** Delayed contrast-enhanced nonlinear imaging ultrasound scan showing improved delineation of the tumor margin. (Courtesy of R. G. Barr, Ph.D. M.D., Youngstown, Ohio, US)

Renal Artery Stenosis (see Chapter 3)

Fundamental Doppler ultrasound remains one of the imaging modalities used in the assessment of renal artery stenosis (RAS), given its noninvasiveness and wide accessibility. However, the technique has not gained widespread support in clinical practice because of the lack of standardization of the technique and reports of differing accuracies.[24] There are obvious problems, such as difficulty in the visualization of the entire length of the artery to depict the stenosis, the presence of accessory arteries, which are difficult to identify, and poor spectral Doppler sampling because of respiratory movement and resultant inaccurate Doppler angle correction. When visualization of the proximal portion of the artery is impossible, the assessment of the downstream waveform alteration caused by a stenosis has been suggested as an adjunct examination, but such assessment has been marred by substantial measurement variability and lack of reproducibility.

There is evidence that contrast-enhanced Doppler ultrasound improves the visualization of the renal arteries and significantly reduces the number of equivocal examinations.[25] In a multicenter study of 191 patients, renal artery accessibility improved from 75% to 90% after contrast administration and the accuracy in detecting RAS also improved from 65% to 78% by using renal angiography as the reference standard (Fig. 16.**6**).[26] Contrast-enhanced harmonic imaging is also known to further improve renal artery visualization with sensitivities over 95%.[27]

However, improved visualization of the renal artery may not be clinically sufficient. The challenge lies in the identification of hemodynamically significant stenoses suitable for interventional therapy. There is some evidence that supplementary functional imaging using ultrasound contrast agent may be of value in the diagnosis of renal ischemia, analogous to other functional tests such as captopril scintigraphy. In a pilot study of 20 patients with suspected renovascular hypertension, analysis of the time-intensity renal enhancement curves using harmonic power Doppler imaging with SonoVue showed a significant increase in the area under the curve and maximum peak intensity parameters in patients with significant RAS compared with the normal renal artery or nonsignificant RAS.[28] Furthermore, the area under the curve apparently returned to the normal range once successful revascularization had

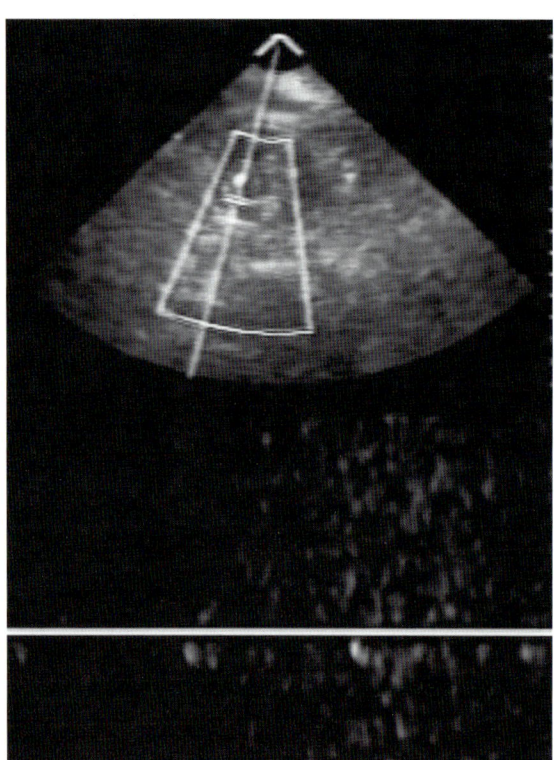

Fig. 16.6 a Unenhanced duplex color Doppler ultrasound assessment of the renal artery with poor signal acquisition in suspected RAS. b Contrast-enhanced scan improved the duplex color Doppler ultrasound assessment. High-velocity flow with blooming of the color Doppler signals and aliasing of the spectral Doppler signals were noted consistent with RAS. The PSV in the main renal artery was 2.4 m/s^{-1}. (Courtesy of R.G. Barr, Ph.D. M.D., Youngstown, Ohio, US)

been accomplished. Studies of a large patient population and evaluation of the technique following a captopril challenge are required.

Determination of the normal range for indices such as area under the curve, peak intensity, wash-in and wash-out gradients remain to be established and assessment is needed concerning the effect of body mass, sex, cardiac output, fasting status, etc. Comprehensive functional imaging studies in humans using newer nonlinear imaging modes remain necessary.

Acute Urinary Obstruction

Previous studies have shown that occlusion of the ureter is associated with reduction in global renal blood flow.[29] This vasoconstrictive response can be assessed with Doppler ultrasound through the measurement of the resistive index. There has been some skepticism regarding this method because some investigators have shown a relative lack of sensitivity for the diagnosis of acute obstruction.[30,31] Experimental studies have shown that functional imaging in the form of a time-intensity curve assessment by using contrast-enhanced gray-scale harmonic imaging may be complementary in depicting the renal hemodynamic changes associated with acute obstruction.[32] The area under the curve was significantly reduced during obstruction and correlated well with mean cortical blood flow. However, this index did not return to baseline values after relief of the obstruction; it was postulated to result from mild residual obstruction related to ureteric edema after prolonged instrumentation.

Summary points:
Current and potential roles of microbubble contrast agents include:
- Characterization of complex renal cysts
- Assessment of renal masses, trauma, infection, infarction, and obstruction
- Guidance of RF ablation and assessment of response
- Evaluation of renal artery stenosis
- Adjunct for patients at high risk of radiograph contrast nephrotoxicity and those claustrophobic for MR imaging

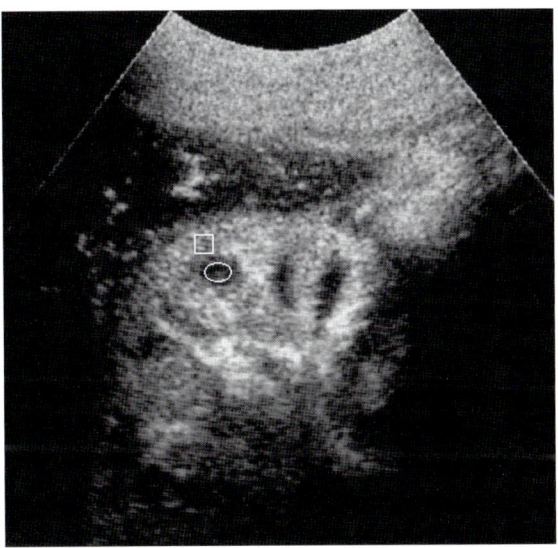

Fig. 16.7 SonoVue enhancement of the right native kidney. **a** Square region of interest assessing renal cortical enhancement. Oval region of interest assessing renal medullary enhancement. **b** Normal time–renal corticomedullary curves

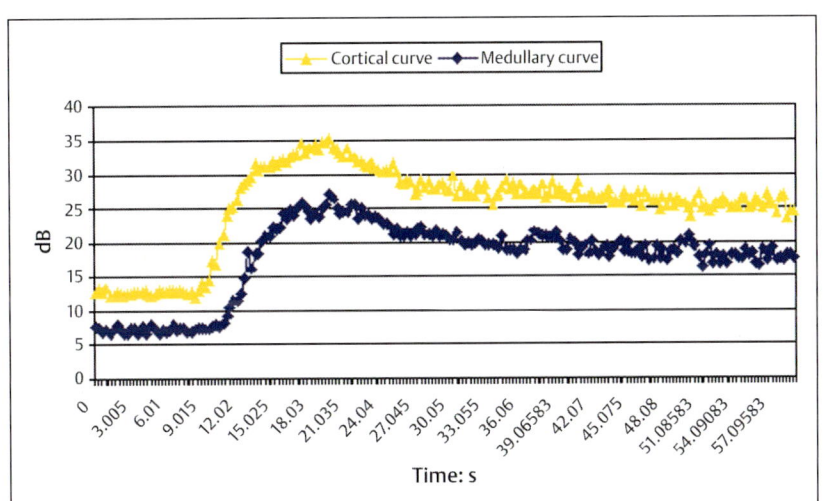

Functional Renal Imaging

Organ viability and functions are highly dependent upon organ blood flow and regional tissue perfusion; accurate measurement of the flow or perfusion changes may therefore be useful in the detection and characterization of vascular pathologies. Functional renal imaging with contrast agents is comparatively new, as novel sonographic techniques capable of evaluating microcirculation only became available recently.

Second-generation contrast agents such as SonoVue and Optison are ideally suited for assessment of renal blood flow, as the microbubbles are uniformly small, free-flowing, and remain entirely intravascular; they are therefore not affected by glomerular filtration or tubular transport. Repeated measurements can also be made sequentially, as the microbubbles may be cleared from the circulation fairly rapidly, especially when using small doses. However, there are inherent limitations as a result of the nonlinearity of the technique, microbubble attenuation, and destruction upon insonation.

Quantification of the relative concentration of the microbubbles can now be made by analysis of the "raw" RF data using the manufacturer-supported software such as Qlab (Philips, Bothell, US) or by videodensitometric analysis of the postprocessed screen-display data using the manufacturer's or independent off-the-shelf analysis software. The relationship between microbubble concentration and video intensity is known to be exponential, with a linear range occurring at lower contrast concentration;[33] therefore small doses of contrast agents should be used. Using nonlinear imaging modes at low MI, the time-intensity curves of the renal cortex and medulla can be obtained following a bolus intravenous injection of 1 mL of SonoVue (Fig. 16.7). Parameters such as contrast "arrival time," "peak enhancement," "in-flow gradient," and "area under the curve" can be measured for various regions of interest

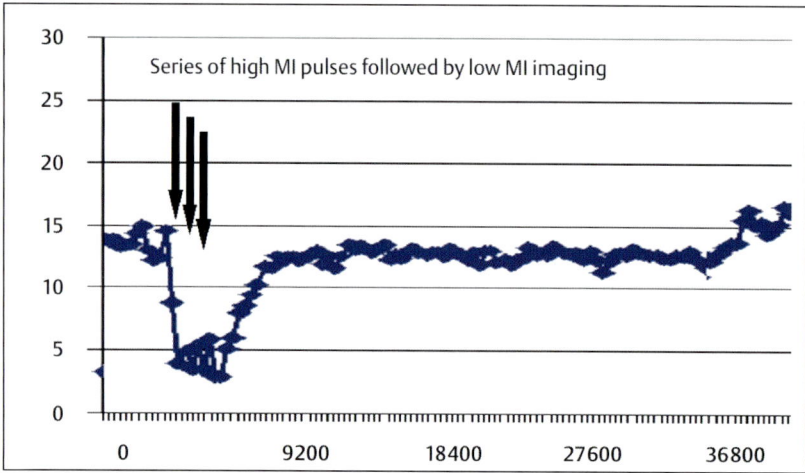

Fig. 16.**8 Destruction–reperfusion curve.** The arrows point to a series of high MI scan frames (Time axis scale (1/1000) seconds).

to evaluate relative to hemodynamic change. This method can be used to monitor sequentially the effect of therapy or disease progression. Other methods of quantification of renal regional blood flow and volume include the "destruction/reperfusion" techniques with constant infusion of microbubbles to maintain steady state. One method is simply based on initially destroying the microbubbles at high MI and subsequently observing the reperfusion kinetic profile at low MI imaging from which parameters such as "arrival time" and "wash-in gradient" can be calculated (Fig. 16.**8**). Wei et al. described another method using a high MI technique where the exponential relationship between increasing pulsing intervals and video intensity is derived.[34] Future studies are clearly required to assess the value of these techniques in clinical practice.

References

1. Burns PN, Hilpert P, Goldberg BB. Intravenous contrast agent for ultrasound Doppler: in vivo measurement of small tumour vessel dose-response. Proc IEEE Eng Med Biol Soc 1990:12;322–4.
2. Forsberg F, Wu Y Makin IRS, et al. Quantitative acoustic characterisation of a new surfactant based ultrasound contrast gent. Ultrasound Med Biol 1997;23:1201–8.
3. Hoff L, Christiansen C, Skotland T. Consideration about the contribution to acoustic backscatter from Albunex microspheres with different sizes. J Ultrasound Med 1994;13: 181–2.
4. Burns PN. Harmonic imaging with ultrasound contrast agents. Clin Radiol 1996; 51(Suppl1):50–5.
5. Leen E. Ultrasound contrast harmonic imaging of abdominal organs. Semin Ultrasound CT MR 2001 Feb;22: 11–24.
6. Leen E, Angerson WJ, Yarmenitis S, et al. Multicentre clinical study of Sonovue™ (BR1), a new ultrasound contrast agent in Doppler investigation of focal hepatic lesions: efficacy. Eur J Radiol 2002;41:200–6.
7. Correas JM, Burns PN, Lai X, Qi X. Infusion versus bolus of an ultrasound contrast agent: in vivo dose-response measurements of BR1. Invest Radiol 2000;35:72–9.
8. Kono Y, Steinbach GC, Peterson T, Schmid-Schonbein GW, Mattrey RF. Mechanism of parenchymal enhancement of the liver with a microbubble-based US contrast medium: an intravital microscopy study in rats. Radiology 2002;224: 253–7.
9. Leen E, Horgan P. Ultrasound contrast agents for hepatic imaging with nonlinear modes. Curr Probl Diagn Radiol 2003;32:66–87.
10. Albrecht T, Blomley MJ, Burns PN, Wilson S, Harvey CJ, Leen E, Claudon M, Calliada F, Correas JM, LaFortune M, Campani R, Hoffmann CW, Cosgrove DO, LeFevre F. Improved detection of hepatic metastases with pulse-inversion US during the liver-specific phase of SHU 508A: multicenter study. Radiology 2003;227:361–70.
11. Bauer A, Becher H, Blomley M, Borges A, Cosgrove D, Leen E, Schlief R, Tiemann K. Ultrasonic imaging of organ perfusion with SH U 563A. Acad Radiol 2002;9(Suppl 1):46–51.
12. Ramnarine KV, Kyriakopoulou K, Gordon P, McDicken NW, McArdle CS, Leen E. Improved characterisation of focal liver tumours: dynamic power Doppler imaging using NC100100 echo-enhancer. Eur J Ultrasound 2000;11: 95–104.
13. Chin CT, Burns PN. Predicting the acoustic response of a microbubble population for contrast imaging in medical ultrasound. Ultrasound Med Biol 2000;26:1293–300.
14. Tiemann K, Becher H, Bimmel D, Schlief R, Nanda NC. Stimulated acoustic emission nonbackscatter contrast effect of microbubbles seen with harmonic power Doppler imaging. Echocardiography 1997;14:65–70.
15. Tiemann K, Pohl C, Schlosser T, Goenechea J, Bruce M, Veltmann C, Kuntz S, Bangard M, Becher H. Stimulated acoustic emission: pseudo-Doppler shifts seen during the destruction of nonmoving microbubbles. Ultrasound Med Biol 2000;26:1161–7.
16. Hope Simpson D, Chin CT, Burns PN. Pulse inversion Doppler: a new method for detecting non-linear echoes from microbubble contrast agents. IEEE Trns Ferroelec Freq Contr 1999;46:372–82.
17. Burns PN, Hope Simpson D, Averkiou MA. Nonlinear imaging. Ultrasound Med Biol 2000;26(Suppl1):19–22.

18. Averkiou M, Powers J, Skyba D, Bruce M, Jensen S. Ultrasound contrast imaging research. Ultrasound Q 2003;19: 27–37.
19. Simpson DH, Burns PN, Averkiou MA. Techniques for perfusion imaging with microbubble contrast agents. IEEE Trans Ultrason Ferroelectr Freq Control 2001;48: 1483–94.
20. Bosniak MA. Difficulties in classifying cystic lesions of the kidney. Urol Radiol 1991;13:91–3.
21. Kim AY, Kim SH, Kim YJ, Lee IH. Contrast-enhanced power Doppler sonography for differentiation of cystic renal lesions: preliminary study. J Ultrasound Med 1999;18:581–8.
22. Jamis-Dow CA, Choyke PL, Jennings SB, et al. Small (< or = 3 cm) renal masses: detection with CT versus US and pathologic correlation. Radiology 1996;198:785–8.
23. Ascenti G, Zimbaro G, Mazziotti S, Gaeta M, Settineri N, Scribano E. Usefulness of power Doppler and contrast enhanced sonography in the differentiation of hyperechoic renal masses. Abdom Imaging 2001;26:654–60.
24. Middleton WD. Doppler US evaluation of renal artery stenosis: past, present and future. Radiology 1992;184: 307–308.
25. Melany ML, Grant EG, Duerinckx AJ, et al. Ability of a phase shift US contrast agent to improve imaging of the main renal arteries. Radiology 1997;205:147–152.
26. Claudon M, Rohban T: Levovist in the diagnosis of renal artery stenosis: results of controlled multicentre study. Radiology 1997;205:242.
27. Calliada F, Bottinelli O, Campani R, et al. Optimisation of colour and spectral Doppler scanning of the renal arteries using a US contrast agent and second harmonic imaging. Radiology 1997;205:241.
28. Lencioni R, Pinto S, Cioni D, et al. Contrast-enhanced Doppler ultrasound of the renal artery stenosis. Echocardiography 1999;16:767–773.
29. Sauvain JL, Bourscheid D, Pierrat V, et al. Duplex Doppler ultrasonography of renal parenchymal arteries: Normal and pathological aspects. Ann Radiol 1991;34:237–247.
30. Cronan JJ, Tublin ME. Role of the resistive index in experimental partial and complete ureteral obstruction. Acad Radiol 1995;2:373–378.
31. Coley BD, Arellano RS, Talner LB, et al. Renal resistive index in experimental partial and complete ureteral obstruction. Acad Radiol 1995;2:373–78.
32. Claudon M, Barnewolt CE, Taylor GA, et al. Renal blood flow in pigs: changes depicted with contrast enhanced harmonic US imaging during acute urinary obstruction. Radiology 1999;212:725–731.
33. Skyba DM, Jayaweea AR, Goodman NC, et al. Quantification of myocardial perfusion with myocardial contrast echocardiography during left atrial injection of contrast: implications for venous injection. Circulation 1994;90:1513–21.
34. Wei K, Jayaweera AR, Firoozan S, et al. Quantification of myocardial blood flow with ultrasound-induced destruction of the microbubbles administered as a constant venous infusion. Circulation 1998;97:473–83.

17 The Transplant Kidney

G.M. Baxter

Introduction

The superficial position of the transplant kidney is particularly advantageous when imaging with ultrasound, and indeed a significant amount of useful information can be gleaned in terms of structure and function using a combination of gray-scale and color Doppler ultrasound. The use of a 4-MHz probe gives ideal resolution of the transplant kidney itself and, with the use of color Doppler, the main transplant renal artery and vein, can normally be followed back to their origins from the external iliac artery and vein, respectively. These qualities make ultrasound well-suited for imaging the patient in the early transplant period, where color Doppler gives an overview of overall renal perfusion and with the use of spectral Doppler can perform serial measurements in an effort to delineate an improving or deteriorating situation. In addition, it can easily detect perirenal collections and is an excellent detector of significant hydronephrosis. Apart from the early period, its main use is in the detection of renal artery stenosis (RAS), although it can clearly detect other more chronic complications such as arteriovenous fistula (AVF), long-term hydronephrosis, etc. (see Chapter 5, Renal Transplantation, for details).

Given the improvements in image quality in the last decade, it is difficult to perceive of situations when the use of a microbubble contrast agent may be useful in the transplant kidney. However, many questions remain unanswered with conventional imaging and, although it is fair to say at present there is no definitive renal transplant application, a number of workers are beginning to take preliminary steps to see if functional imaging can be of clinical use, not just in the native kidney but also within the renal transplant.[1,2,3] The techniques of functional imaging are essentially as described for the native kidney in the earlier part of this chapter. The technique itself depends upon multiple factors and, as this work is very much in its preliminary stages, much regarding this technique remains to be standardized.

The potential applications of these microbubble agents are discussed below.

Hydronephrosis

It is well-recognized that many "normal" transplant kidneys may have some element of hydronephrosis. In the early transplant period approximately 35–40% of kidneys suffer from delayed function and as such it is difficult to know whether these mild hydronephroses are functionally significant or not. It has already been demonstrated in animal studies that by inducing obstructive hydronephrosis and increasing intrarenal pressure, following intravenous injection of a contrast agent the time-intensity curve is altered in those kidneys with severe acute obstruction.[4] Whilst the clinical situation is slightly different in the transplant kidney, this may be one potential application of this technique.

Monitoring In The Early Postoperative Transplant Period

One of the main difficulties in patients with delayed function is not knowing whether this reflects acute tubular necrosis (ATN) or acute rejection. As symptoms are generally absent, the diagnosis is clinically very difficult; in our center we perform routine monitoring with spectral Doppler ultrasound every second day until function begins. Decision-making is based upon the principle that if the Doppler spectral waveforms deteriorate, then this is likely to initiate earlier transplant biopsy. However, should the waveforms remain fairly stable over a period of time, then in general transplant biopsy is delayed. If a diagnosis of acute rejection is made on biopsy, then further monitoring following treatment is also performed to monitor treatment response.

This type of monitoring can be useful clinically but is not perfect and indeed there is some element of interpretative subjectivity involved. In addition to ultrasound, some centers still perform nuclear medicine studies in the early transplant period to help assess vascular function.

It is now possible to give an intravenous injection of microbubble contrast agent and produce a very similar time-intensity arterial curve to that obtained at diethylene triamine pentaacetate (DTPA) renography

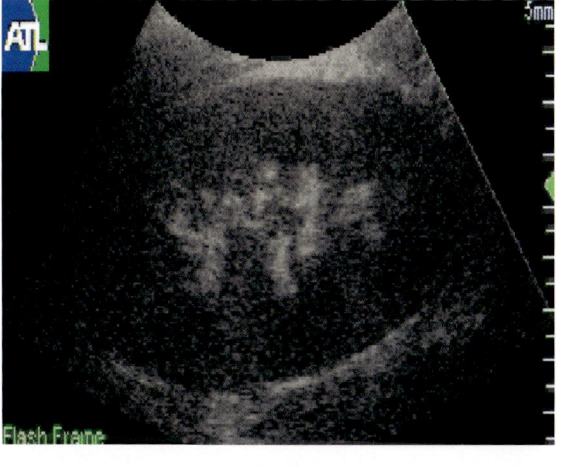 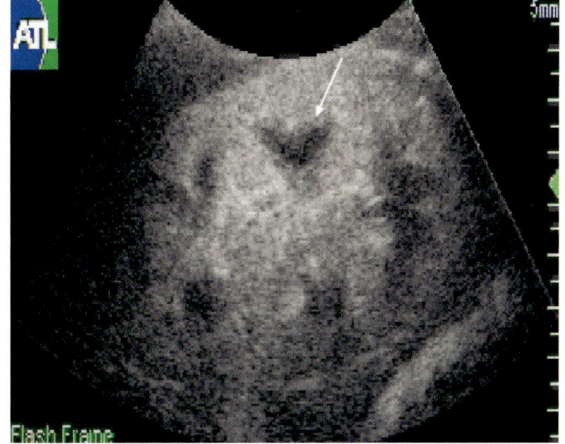
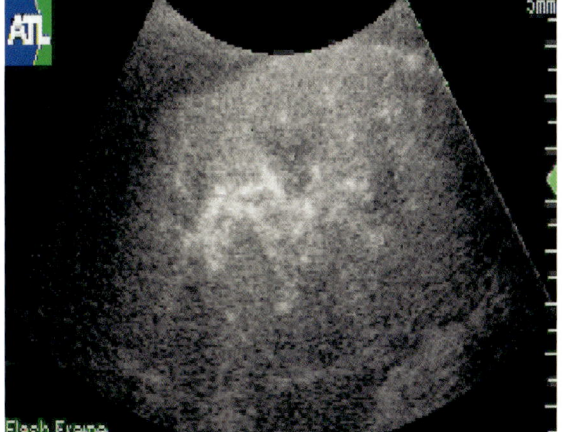 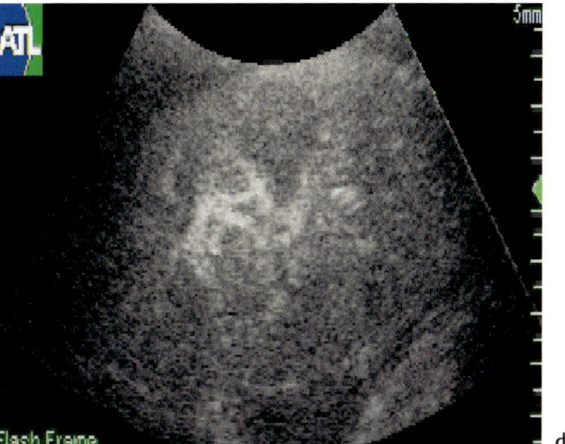

Fig. 17.**1 A series of still images taken from a dynamic study of a transplant kidney following the intravenous injection of the microbubble agent Sonovue.** This study was conducted in the early postoperative phase, as the kidney had delayed function. **a** The baseline scan prior to contrast injection. **b** Shortly after injection, showing good cortical enhancement highlighted against the darker pyramids (arrow); **c,d** Later images which show an even distribution of contrast in both the cortex and pyramids

and essentially show the same information as the isotope study,[5] with the added benefit of the gray-scale anatomical picture and quantitative spectral Doppler measurements. It is too early to say whether this will have any significant effect on prognosis. However, this method is an entirely "nonradioactive" way of producing anatomical and functional information (Figs. 17.**1**, 17.**2**).

It is too early to determine whether there is "hidden information" in the curves that may help differentiate ATN from acute rejection or even that they may contain some prognostic information for the longevity of the transplant. In one study differences in time to peak enhancement values and wash-in and wash-out curves were noted between normal transplant kidneys and those with a parenchymal insult, i.e. ATN or acute rejection. In addition, heterogenous enhancement of cortical contrast was noted in the latter group.[6] Furthermore, it is also possible with this dynamic method to calculate an arterial venous transit time; this again is a topic of clinical research rather than application.

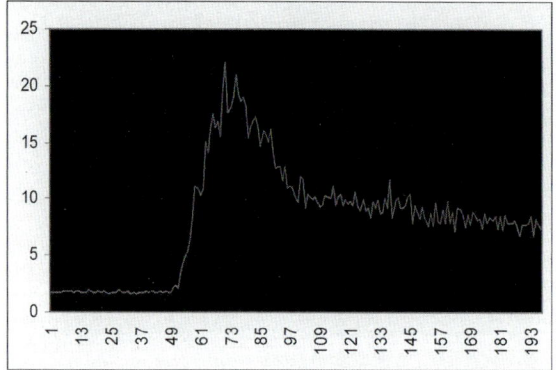
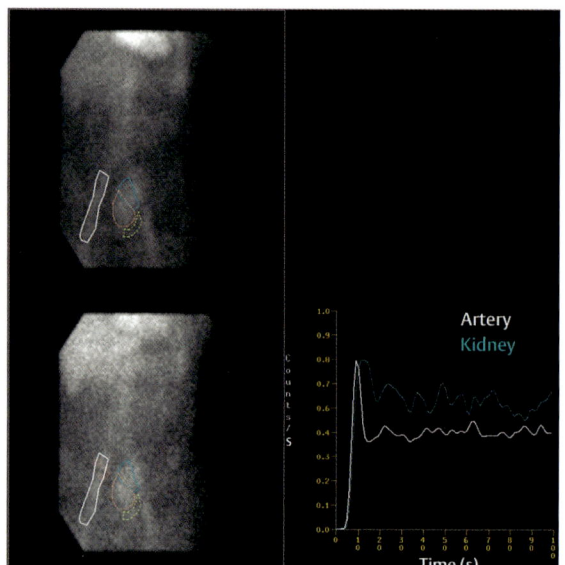

Fig. 17.2 **a** With a region of interest over the renal cortex during dynamic Sonovue injection, a time-intensity curve can be plotted (time is shown along the x-axis and intensity on the y-axis). Various parameters can be measured, including the arrival time from injection, the gradient of the curve, time-to-peak and peak value, and the area under the curve. This curve bears a striking similarity to that of an early DTPA study in the same patient (Fig. 17.2**b**). **b** A DTPA study in the same patient as Figures 17.1 and 17.2**a**, showing normal uptake and handling by the transplant kidney. The gradient of the curve is very similar and much of the information in this study can also be appreciated in the dynamic Sonovue study

Vascular Applications

Vascular Occlusion

The diagnosis of renal artery occlusion is a catastrophic event for any transplant patient. Whilst in the majority the kidney is devoid of intrarenal arterial blood flow, the main renal artery cannot be identified and therefore the clinical diagnosis is not in doubt, on some occasions the finding of renal artery occlusion is unexpected and occasionally small amplitude waveforms are seen within the main renal artery. In this latter situation the injection of a contrast agent will undoubtedly increase confidence and confirm the initial suspicion of transplant artery occlusion.

Furthermore, sometimes multiple renal arteries are transplanted with the kidney and one may suffer damage in the early postoperative period. It is useful to know whether there has been a segmental infarction and, if so, its extent. Although it may seem slightly odd, given the high quality of imaging possible with the transplant, this is in fact a difficult diagnosis to make on conventional color Doppler scanning and indeed a more dynamic analysis following the injection of a microbubble contrast agent is much more revealing in this clinical situation. Indeed microbubble-enhanced ultrasound has been shown to quantify total and regional blood flow when compared with direct flow measurement in dogs (Fig. 17.3).[7]

Renal Artery Stenosis

It has already been shown in the native kidney that the use of microbubble agents does not alter the overall sensitivity or specificity of color Doppler ultrasound in the diagnosis of RAS, but it can rescue failed conventional examinations allowing a greater number of vessels to be interrogated.[8] It has also been shown that intrarenal Doppler spectral waveforms are also improved following contrast injection.[9]

In the transplant kidney, however, the vast majority of transplant artery stenoses can be diagnosed with conventional color Doppler, although in some scenarios, for a number of reasons, for example, patient build, deeply situated iliac vessels, bowel gas, etc., the transplant origin can be difficult to visualize absolutely confidently. In this scenario, injection of a contrast agent may improve on the conventional image and allow precise angle correction for peak systolic velocity (PSV) assessment. The transplant artery is invariably tortuous and as a consequence it is not always possible to see every twist and turn of the vessel; again this can be improved following the injection of a contrast agent (Fig. 17.4).

It is not clear what the role of functional imaging, i.e. time-intensity curves, is in the diagnosis of transplant artery stenosis, although a significant difference in transit time for patients with RAS has been shown.[10] One potential application may be in the follow-up of such patients who are treated with either angioplasty,

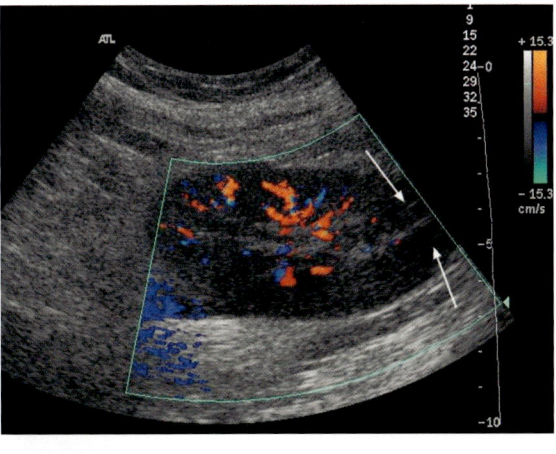
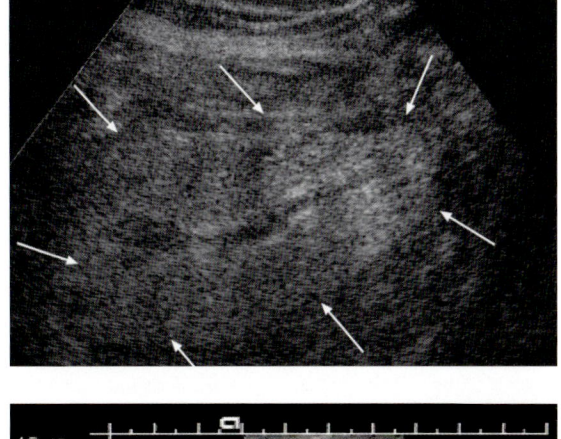
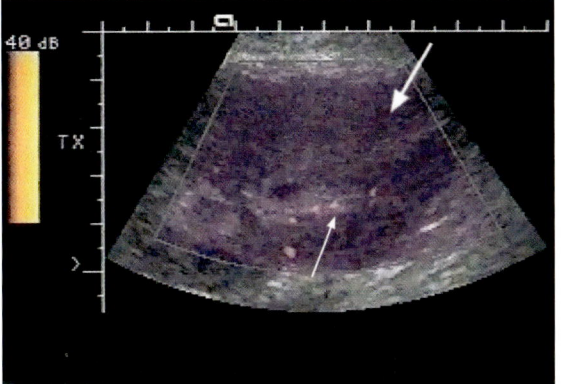
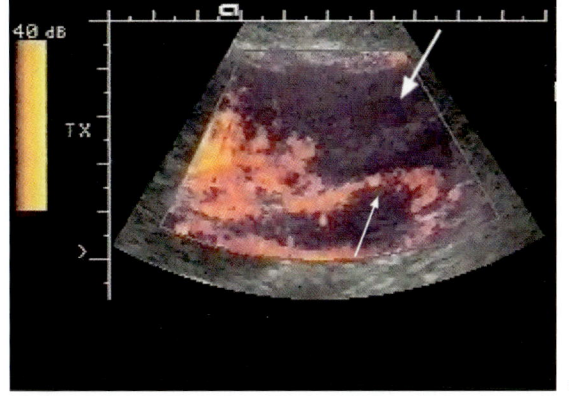

Fig. 17.3 **a** Color Doppler ultrasound of a transplant kidney in the early postoperative period showing a lack of color flow from the lower pole (arrows). It was not clear if this was technical or if the vascular supply to this area was compromised. **b** Following intravenous Sonovue it is clear that the microbubble agent has been evenly distributed to all areas of the transplant kidney (arrows). There is no evidence of focal infarction and the appearances were presumably technical. **c** In another patient a baseline scan shows minimal flow to the lower pole of the transplant kidney (small arrow), but the lack of any significant vessel in this area (big arrow) was suggestive of lower pole infarction. **d** Following intravenous microbubbles it can be seen that the lower pole is devoid of vessels (large arrow) apart from one remaining large lower pole artery (small arrow). The appearances therefore confirmed the suspicion of lower pole infarction

stenting, or both. In such a case, time-intensity curve profiles before and after angioplasty may be helpful, but again this remains an area of research. It is also tempting to postulate that these curves may change following the administration of an angiotensin-converting enzyme (ACE) inhibitor and help differentiate those patients with RAS and those without.

Summary points:
- Microbubble contrast agents have a number of potential uses in the transplant kidney
- Functional studies with microbubbles have demonstrated similar curves to DTPA studies
- Transit studies with microbubbles are possible and may prove helpful in the future
- Elucidation of vascular problems including renal RAS, vessel occlusion, and segmental infarction is easily resolved with microbubble agents
- Microbubbles can help aid the differentiation of tumor and cyst
- Early results are encouraging. However, standardization of the functional techniques are required

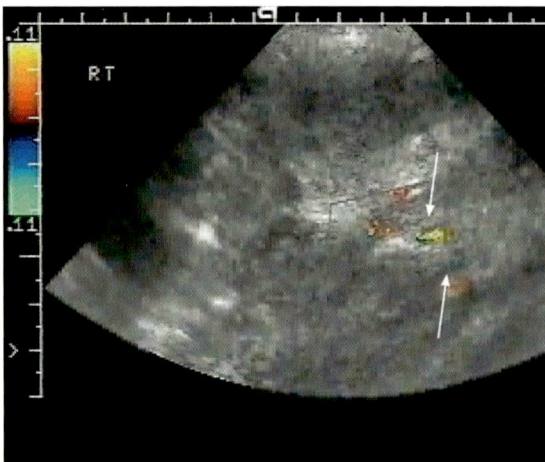

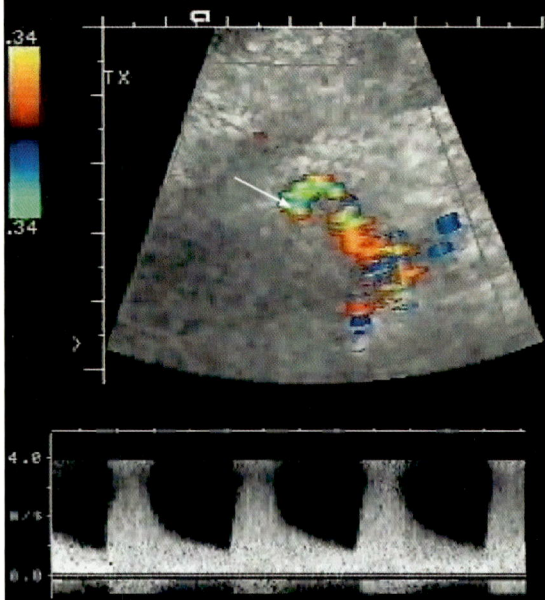

Fig. 17.4 **a** Conventional color Doppler scan of the proximal transplant renal artery close to the origin from the iliac artery. Although a little color flow can be seen (arrows), it is difficult to differentiate the transplant artery from the iliac artery or indeed to plot the course of the transplant artery to allow accurate angle correction for Doppler estimation of the PSV. **b** Following the injection of a microbubble agent, the course of the transplant artery was easily appreciated. An accurate spectral Doppler waveform was measured from the main renal vessel (arrow) and this showed a markedly elevated velocity of 3.5–4.0 ms^{-1} indicative of an RAS

Renal Masses

Transplant kidneys, like native kidneys, may develop either cysts or tumors. With the increased longevity of the transplant kidney, there is a definite but small increase in the incidence of tumors in the transplant population. These may occur at multiple sites and the most frequent tumors are skin-related, i.e. melanoma or lymphoma. The differentiation of a cyst from tumor or elucidation of a "complicated cyst" can be helped with the use of microbubble agents;[11] a difference in cortical enhancement between the normal cortex and tumor has also been demonstrated in rabbits following injection.[12] It is important to remember that complimentary imaging modalities, including computed tomography (CT), also provides a useful role.

Potential Applications

A number of other potential applications can be considered: Is there a relationship between time-intensity curves and the creatinine clearance? Can these curves give an overall prognosis for the kidney or predict chronic rejection? Are such time-intensity curves useful for monitoring drug-related studies? These all remain potential and fruitful areas of clinical research.

In conclusion, microbubble agents are beginning to be utilized in the evaluation of native and transplant kidneys. This work remains at a very embryonic level, most of the initial work with these agents having to date centered on the liver. However, undoubtedly the use of such agents in this area will increase in the future. Although there are no specific applications as yet within the transplant kidney, early use would suggest they may be helpful on occasion in the evaluation of possible transplant artery stenosis, segmental infarction, vessel occlusion, detection of vesicoureteric reflux (VUR),[13] and for helping to differentiate complicated masses.[11] Many questions and areas with regard to these techniques and their standardization are only beginning to be addressed[14] as our knowledge of these agents slowly increase. The future of these agents and their development brings us into a new, exciting area with many potential possibilities, and undoubtedly their use with more defined roles will develop in time.

References

1. Schlosser T, Pohl C, Veltmann C, Lohmaier S, Goenechea J, Ehlgen A, et al. Feasibility of the flash-replenishment concept in renal tissue: which parameters affect the assessment of the contrast replenishment? Ultrasound in Medicine and Biology 2001;27(7):937–944.
2. Cosgrove D, Eckersley R, Blomley M, Harvey C. Quantification of blood flow. Europena Radiology 2001;11(8):1338–1344.
3. Krix M, Kauczor HU, Delorme S. Quantification of tissue perfusion with novel ultrasound methods. Radiology 2003;43(10):823–830.
4. Claudon M, Barnevolt CE, Taylor GA, Dunning PS, Gobet R, Badawy AB. Renal blood flow in pigs: changes depicted with contrast enhanced harmonic US imaging during acute urinary obstruction. Radiology 1999;212:725–731.

5. Hosotani Y, Takahashi N, Kiyomoto H, Ohmori K, Hitomi H, Fujioka H, et al. A new method for evaluation of split renal cortical blood flow with contrast echography. Hypertension Res 2002;25(1):77–83.
6. Lefevre F, Correas JM, Briancon S, Helenon O, Kessler M, Claudon M. Contrast-enhanced sonography of the renal transplant using triggered pulse inversion imaging: preliminary results. Ultrasound in Medicine and Biology 2002;28(3):303–314.
7. Wei K, Le E, Bin JP, Coggins M, Thorpe J, Kaul S. Quantification of renal blood flow with contrast-enhanced ultrasound. Journal of the American College of Cardiology 2001;37(4):1135–1140.
8. Claudon M, Plouin PF, Baxter GM, Rhoban T, Maniez Devos D. Renal arteries in patients at risk of renal artery stenosis: Multicenter evaluation of the echo-enhancer SH U 508A at color and spectral Doppler US. Radiology 2000;214:739–746.
9. Missouris CG, Allen CM, Balen FG, Buckenham T, Lees WR, MacGregor GA. Non-invasive screening for renal artery stenosis with ultrasound contrast enhancement. Journal of Hypertension 1996;14(4):519–524.
10. Bertolotto M, Quaia E, Rimondini A, Lubin E, Pozzi Mucelli R. Current role of color Doppler ultrasound in acute renal failure. Radiology Medicine 2001;102(5–6):340–347.
11. Correas J, Claudon M, Tranquart F, Helenon O. Contrast-enhanced ultrasonography: renal applications. Journal of Radiology 2003;84(12,2):2041–2054.
12. Chomas JE, Pollard RE, Sadlowski AR, Griffey SM, Wisner ER, Ferrara KW. Contrast-enhanced US of microcirculation of superficially implanted tumors in rats. Radiology 2003;229(2):439–436.
13. Kmetec A, Bren AF, Kandus A, Fettich J, Butorovic-Ponokvar J. Contras- enhanced ultrasound voiding cystography as a screening examination for vesicoureteral reflux in the follow-up of renal transplant recipients: a new approach. Nephrology Dialysis Transplantation 2001;16(1):120–123.
14. Lucidarme O, Franchi-Abella S, Correas JM, Bridal SL, Kurtisovski E, Berger G. Blood-flow quantification with contrastenhanced ultrasound: "entrance I the section" phenomenon - phantom and rabbit study. Radiology 2003; 228(2):298–299.

Index

A

Abscess
  prostate gland 142
  renal 34
  testicular 165
Acquired cystic disease of the kidneys (ACDK) 41, 44–45, 217
  hemorrhage 45
  malignant transformation 41, 45
Acquired immune deficiency syndrome (AIDS) 36
Acute cortical necrosis 31
Acute interstitial nephritis 31
Acute renal failure see Renal failure
Acute renal parenchymal disease 10
  see also Parenchymal diseases
Acute tubular necrosis (ATN) 31–32
  renal transplantation and 58, 264–265
Adenocarcinoma 111–112
Adenoma 109
  epididymal 175–176
Adrenal glands
  anatomy 222
  congenital anomalies 222
  cysts 223
  ectopic 222
  fusion 222
  hemorrhage 222
  tumors 223
Adrenal rest cells 164
Agenesis
  adrenal 222
  renal 27, 209
Amyloid 40
Analgesia 72
Aneurysms 38, 105
  AVF complications 51
  pseudoaneurysm 219
Angiography 239
  renal artery stenosis 246
Angiomyolipoma 110, 217
Antibiotic prophylaxis 71
Appendix testis 156, 157, 158–159
  torsion 170–171, 225–226
Arteriovenous fistula (AVF) 38, 83
  following renal transplantation 64–65
  in hemodialysis 48–49
    complications 49–51
    types of 48
  priapism and 187
Arteriovenous malformations 105

Arteritis, giant cell 40
Atrophy
  kidney 26–27
  testis 165
Autonephrectomy 35
Autosomal dominant polycystic kidney disease (ADPKD) 106–108, 215
Autosomal recessive polycystic kidney disease (ARPKD) 106, 215

B

Benign prostatic hyperplasia/hypertrophy (BPH) 93–94, 140–142
Biopsy
  postprostatectomy bed 149
  prostate 148
  renal 78–79
Bladder
  anatomy 130–131
    children 208
  calculi 91, 137
  congenital anomalies 136, 220–221
    exstrophy 220
  diverticula 136–137, 221
  hematoma 137
  interventional ultrasound 140
  neuropathic 221
  postoperative appearances 139–140
  trauma 85, 97, 221
  tumors 92–93, 221
    carcinoma 138–139, 241–242
    see also Bladder cancer treatment
  ultrasound examination 133–134
Bladder cancer treatment 193–195
  metastatic disease 195
  muscle-invasive disease 194–195
  prognosis 194
  superficial disease 194
Bladder-wall abnormalities
  diffuse 137–138
  focal 138–139
Bone scintigraphy 238–239
Brachytherapy, prostate cancer 149, 197

C

Calcification
  bladder-wall 138
  epididymal 171–172
  penile fibrosis 188

  renal cysts 103–104
  testicular macrocalcification 166
Calculi 90–91
  assessment 244–245
  bladder 91, 137
  renal 90–91, 123–124
    children 218
    dialysis and 45
Calyceal diverticula 104
Captopril renography 238
Carcinoma
  penile 98, 189
  prostate 94–95, 144–147
    follow-up 147
    staging 144–147, 242–244
  renal cell (RCC) 96
    children 218
    investigation 201
    staging 240–241
    treatment 201–202
  testicular 159
    embryonal 160–161
  transitional cell (TTC) 112–113, 126
    bladder 138–139, 241–242
    with acquired cystic disease of the kidneys 41, 45
Carcinoma in situ (CIS) 194
Cavernosal herniation 189
Chemotherapy
  bladder cancer 194–195
    with radiotherapy 195
  prostate cancer 198
  renal cell carcinoma 202
  testicular tumors
    germ cell tumors 200–201
    seminoma 200
Children
  adrenal anomalies 222–223
  anatomy 207–208
    bladder 208
    kidney 207
    testis 208
  bladder abnormalities 136, 220–221
  congenital renal anomalies 208–212
    duplication anomalies 209
    hydronephrosis 209–212
    renal agenesis/hypoplasia 209
    renal ectopia 208–209
    renal fusion 208
  cystic renal disease 215–217
    genetic disease 215
    nongenetic disease 216–217
  megacalycosis 212

Children
- megaureters 126, 212
- pelviureteric junction (PUJ) obstruction 91–92, 126, 211
- posterior urethral valve 211–212
- renal calcification 218
- renal transplantation 219
- renal trauma 218
- renal tumors 217–218
  - benign 217
  - malignant 217–218
- testicular anomalies 223–226
- ultrasound imaging 207
- ureteroceles 212
- urinary tract infections 90, 213–214
  - fungal balls 214
  - pyelonephritis 213–214
  - pyonephrosis 214
- vascular anomalies 218–219
- vesicoureteric junction obstruction 211
- vesicoureteric reflux 90, 125–126, 212

Choriocarcinoma 161
Chronic kidney disease (CKD) 3, 31
- causes 11
- consequences 12
- definition 9
- imaging 11–12
- incidence 3
- natural history 8–9
- see also Renal disease

Coagulopathy 71
Collecting system 22–24
- congenital abnormalities 125–126
  - duplex systems 25, 104, 125, 209
  - megaureter 126
  - vesicoureteric reflux 125–126
- obstruction see Obstruction
- retroperitoneal fibrosis 127
- tumors 126–127
- see also Ureters

Computed tomography (CT) 234–236
- bladder carcinoma 242
- calculus disease 244–245
- prostate carcinoma 242
- renal cell carcinoma 240–241
- renal outflow obstruction 246
- renal trauma assessment 248

Congenital adrenal hyperplasia 222
Connective tissue disorders 40
Continuous ambulatory peritoneal dialysis 46–48
Contrast agents see Ultrasound contrast agents
Cortical disorders 30–31
Cross-fused ectopia 208
Cryptorchidism 223
Cyclosporine toxicity 62, 65
Cystectomy 194
Cystic dysplasia
- kidney 108, 216
- testis 224

Cystic malignancy 106

Cystitis 89
- bladder-wall abnormalities 137–138
Cystography 238
Cystourethrography 248
Cysts
- adrenal 223
- epidermoid 161
- epididymal 98, 175
- lymphatic 104–105
- Müllerian 140
- prostate gland 153
  - drainage 149
- renal see Renal cysts

D

Delayed function, following renal transplantation 59–60
Diabetes 39
Dialysis 47–51
- continuous ambulatory peritoneal dialysis 46–48
- hemodialysis 48–49
- peritonitis and 47
- renal calculi and 45
- secondary hyperparathyroidism 45
Diuresis renography 238
Diverticula
- bladder 136–137, 221
- calyceal 104
- renal pelvic 104
Doppler ultrasound
- erectile dysfunction investigation 246
- renal artery stenosis investigation 246
Drainage of perinephric collections 77–78

E

Eagle–Barrett syndrome 221
Echogenicity 19–20
Ectopic adrenal gland 222
Ectopic kidneys 25–26, 208–209
- cross-fused ectopia 208
Ectopic ureters 125
Ejaculatory ducts 133
- developmental anomalies 140
Emphysematous pyelonephritis 34, 89–90, 119
End-stage renal disease (ESRD) 41, 54–55
Epidermoid cyst 161
Epididymis 157, 171–173
- adenomatoid tumor 175–176
- calcification 171–172
- cysts 98, 175
- inflammatory disease 173, 224
- leiomyoma 176
Epididymitis 173
- children 224
- chronic 173
Epididymo-orchitis 98, 173
Erectile dysfunction 99, 182–187

- arterial impotence assessment 184–185
- baseline imaging 182
- false positive venous leak 186–187
- priapism 187
- stimulated color Doppler ultrasound 183
- ultrasound imaging protocol 183
- venogenic impotence assessment 185
Exstrophy, bladder 220

F

Fetal lobulation 24
Fibromuscular dysplasia (FMD) 79
Fibrosis
- penile 188
- retroperitoneal 127
Focal infection 110
Fracture, penile 97, 189
Functional renal imaging 261–262
Fungal infections 36
- fungal balls 214

G

Genital injury 97, 189
Germ cell tumors, testis 160–161, 199
- children 226
- mixed 160
- regressed/burnt-out 161
- seminomatous 160, 200
- treatment 200–201
Giant cell arteritis 40
Glomerular filtration rate (GFR) 5, 8–9
- measurement 237
- urinary volume and 7–8
Glomerulonephritis 30

H

Hematoma 105, 114–115
- bladder 137
- penile 189
Hematuria 92–93
- macroscopic 7
- microscopic 5–6
Hemodialysis 48–49
- arteriovenous fistula complications 49–51
Hemolytic uremic syndrome 41
Hemoperitoneum 48
Hemorrhage
- acquired cystic disease of the kidneys 45
- adrenal 222
- embolization 85
- following renal transplantation 61
- renal cysts 103
Henoch–Schonlein purpura 40
Hepatorenal syndrome 40

Hernia
    cavernosal 189
    inguinal 168
Histocompatibility testing 55
HIV-associated nephropathy (HIVAN) 36
Hormonal therapy, prostatic cancer 198
Horseshoe adrenal gland 222
Horseshoe kidneys 26, 208
Human leukocyte antigen (HLA) matching 55
Hydatid disease 36, 103
Hydrocele 168, 224
Hydronephrosis 91–92, 104, 209–212
    nonobstructive 212–213
        megacalycosis 212
        megaureters 212
        vesicoureteric reflux 212
    obstructive 211–212
        pelviureteric junction obstruction 211
        posterior urethral valve 211–212
        ureteroceles 212
        vesicoureteric junction obstruction 211
    transplant kidney 264
Hyperparathyroidism, secondary 45
Hyperplasia
    benign prostatic (BPH) 93–94, 140–142
    congenital adrenal 222
Hypoplasia
    adrenal 222
    renal 26–27, 209

I

Immunosuppression 56
Immunotherapy, renal cell carcinoma 202
Impotence *see* Erectile dysfunction
Infections 8, 33–36
    focal 110
    renal cyst infection 103
    renal transplantation complications 62, 65
    see also Urinary tract infection (UTI)
Infertility 99
    male 144
Inflammatory disease
    epididymis 173, 224
    ureters 127–128
Inflammatory pseudotumor 110
Informed consent 71
Inguinal hernia 168
Injury *see* Trauma
Intravenous urogram (IVU) 233–234
    bladder carcinoma 241–242
    calculus disease 244–245
    renal outflow obstruction 246
    renal trauma assessment 248

K

Kidney
    anatomy 4, 16–17
        children 207
        relationships 15–16
    ectopic 25–26, 208–209
        cross-fused ectopia 208
    function 4–5
    horseshoe 26, 208
    pelvic 209
    size and volume 18–19
    transplantation *see* Renal transplantation; Transplant kidney
    trauma 96–97
    see also Renal disease; Renal failure

L

Leiomyoma, epididymal 176
Leiomyosarcoma 114
Leukemia
    renal, children 218
    testis 162, 226
Leydig cell tumors 226
Lipoma, extratesticular 175
Liposarcoma 177
Loin pain 7
Lower urinary tract symptoms (LUTS) 93–94, 141–142
Lymphatic cysts 104–105
Lymphoma
    renal 113
        children 218
    testicular 162, 226

M

Macrocalcification, testicular 166
Magnetic resonance (MR) imaging 236
    MR urography 245
    prostate carcinoma 242–244
    renal artery stenosis 246
    renal cell carcinoma 241
Male infertility 144
Medulla disorders 31–33
Medullary cystic disease complex 108, 215
Medullary sponge kidney 32
Megacalycosis 212
Megaureters 126, 212
Mesoblastic nephroma 217
Metastases
    from bladder carcinoma 242
    from renal cell carcinoma 241
    renal 113
    testicular 163
Metastatic disease treatment
    bladder cancer 195
    prostate cancer 198
    renal cell carcinoma 202
Microbubble behavior 254–255
    functional renal imaging 261–262
    see also Ultrasound contrast agents
Microlithiasis, testicular 166, 224
Micturating cystourethrography (MCU) 234
Milk of calcium cysts 104
Müllerian cysts 140
Multicystic dysplastic kidney 108, 216
Multilocular cystic nephroma 105, 216

N

Necrosis
    acute cortical 31
    acute tubular (ATN) 31–32
        renal transplantation and 58, 264–265
    renal papillary 32
Nephrectomy
    partial 202
    radical 201–202
Nephritis, acute interstitial 31
Nephrocalcinosis 32–33
    causes 33
    children 218
    cortical 31
Nephrolithiasis, children 218
Nephroma
    mesoblastic 217
    multilocular cystic 105, 216
Nephrostomy 72–77
    anatomy 73
    complications 77
    dilated system 74
    follow-up 77
    guidance 73
    indications 72–73
    nondilated system 73–74
    primary antegrade ureteric stenting 74–75
    transplant kidneys 76
Neuroblastoma 223
Neuropathic bladder 221
Nonlinear imaging modes 255–256
Nuclear renography 246

O

Obstruction 10–11, 119–123
    acute 119–122
    chronic 122
    following renal transplantation 61
    investigation 246, 260
    pelviureteric junction 91–92, 126, 211
    upper urinary tract 91–92
    vesicoureteric junction 211
Obstructive hydronephrosis *see* Hydronephrosis
Occlusion
    renal artery 38
        transplant kidney 266
    renal vein 39

Oncocytoma 109
Orchitis 165
   epididymo-orchitis 98, 173

P

Pancreas transplant 67
Pancreatitis 48
Parenchymal diseases 29–41
   cortical disorders 30–31
   disorders of the medulla/pyramids 31–33
   renal infections 33–36
   ultrasound examination 29–30
   vascular disorders 36–39
Parenchymal thickness 19
Patient preparation 70, 71–72
Pediatric disorders *see* Children
Pelvic kidney 209
Pelvicalyceal dilatation 119
   without obstruction 123
Pelvicalyceal injuries 84
Pelviureteric junction (PUJ) obstruction 91–92, 126, 211
Penis
   anatomy 181–182
   carcinoma 98, 189
   injury 97, 189
   structural pathology 188–190
      fibrosis 188
      masses 189–190
      tunica albuginea defect 188–189
   urethral ultrasound 190
   see also Erectile dysfunction
Percutaneous nephrostomy (PCN) *see* Nephrostomy
Peritonitis 47
Persistent prostatic utricle 140
Peyronie disease 188
Pheochromocytoma 223
Plain abdominal radiograph 233
Polyarteritis nodosa (PAN) 40
Polycystic kidney disease 106–108
      autosomal dominant (ADPKD) 106–108, 215
      autosomal recessive (ARPKD) 106, 215
Polyorchidism 159
Posterior urethral valve (PUV) 211–212
Postoperative monitoring 264–265
Posttransplant collections 61–62
   drainage 77–78
Power modulation 255
Priapism 85, 187
Prostate
   ablation 149
   abscess 142
      drainage 149
   anatomy 131–132
      prostatic urethra 132
      zonal anatomy 132
      benign prostatic hyperplasia/hypertrophy (BPH) 93–94, 140–142
   biopsy 148
   brachytherapy 149
   carcinoma 94–95, 144–147
      follow-up 147
      staging 144–147, 242–244
      see also Prostate cancer treatment
   cysts 143
      drainage 149
   postoperative bladder appearances 139
   ultrasound examination 134–136
Prostate cancer treatment 195–199
   hormone-refractory disease 198–199
   intracapsular disease 197
   locally advanced disease 197–198
   metastatic disease 198
Prostatectomy, radical 197
Prostatitis 89, 142
Proteinuria 5–6
Prune belly syndrome 221
Pseudoaneurysm 219
Pseudotumor
   fibrous 176
   inflammatory 110
Pulsatility index (PI) 57
Pulse/phase inversion harmonic (PIH) imaging 255
Pyelonephritis 34, 89–90
   children 213
      chronic 214
   emphysematous 34, 89–90, 119
   xanthogranulomatous 35, 214
Pyonephrosis 119, 214
Pyramid disorders 31–33

R

Radiofrequency (RF) ablation 80–82
Radiography, abdominal 233
Radionuclide imaging 236–237
Radiotherapy
   bladder cancer 194–195
      with chemotherapy 195
   prostate cancer 197–198
   renal cell carcinoma 202
   seminoma 200
Reflux nephropathy 214
Rejection, following renal transplantation 59
   acute 65
   chronic 65
Renal arteries
   aneurysms 38
   occlusion 38
      transplant kidney 266
   stenosis (RAS) 12, 36–38
      investigation 246, 259–260
      transplant kidney 266–267
      ultrasound applications 79–80
   ultrasound imaging 21–22
Renal biopsy 78–79
Renal calculi 90–91, 123–124
   dialysis and 45
Renal cell carcinoma (RCC) 96
   children 218
   investigation 201
   staging 240–241
   treatment 201–202
      non-surgical 202
      surgical 201–202
Renal colic 90–91
Renal cysts 95, 102–108, 256
   complicated 103–104
      calcification 103–104
      hemorrhage 103
      infection 103
      septations 103
   congenital cystic renal disease 106–108
      medullary cystic disease complex 108
      multicystic dysplastic kidney 108
      polycystic kidney disease 106–108
      tuberous sclerosis 108
      von Hippel–Lindau disease 108
   simple 102
      children 216
      differential diagnosis 104–106
      multiple 102
   transplant kidney 268
   see also Acquired cystic disease of the kidneys (ACDK)
Renal disease
   end-stage (ESRD) 41, 54–55
   incidence 3
   investigations 9–12
      renal masses 239–240, 256–257
   natural history 8–9
   presentation 5–8
   see also Chronic kidney disease (CKD); Renal failure; *Specific diseases*
Renal duplication 209
Renal failure 6–7
   acute (ARF) 7
      acute renal parenchymal disease 10
      investigations 9–11
      postrenal 10
      prerenal 9–10
   chronic (CRF) 7, 44–51
      dialysis 46–51
      diseases associated with native kidneys 44–46
Renal function 4–5
Renal fusion 208
Renal imaging
   dynamic 237–238
   static 237
Renal length 16
Renal mass investigation 239–240, 256–257
   transplant kidney 268
Renal outflow obstruction *see* Obstruction
Renal papillary necrosis 32
Renal pelvic diverticula 104
Renal pelvic tumors 112–113
Renal sinus 22–24
   splitting 23, 25, 119

Renal transplantation 54–67
  children 219
  combined renal and pancreas transplant 67
  complications 58–67
    early 58–62
    late 62–67
    long-term 67
  contraindications 55
  donor supply 55
  histocompatibility testing 55
  history 54
  immunosuppression 56
  postoperative monitoring 264–265
  preoperative management 55
  surgery 55–56
  see also Transplant kidney
Renal veins
  occlusion 39
  thrombosis 38–39
    children 218–219
  ultrasound imaging 22
Renography
  captopril 238
  diuresis 238
  nuclear 246
Resistive index (RI) 57
  obstruction diagnosis 121–122
Rete testis 158
Retroperitoneal fibrosis 127
Rhabdomyosarcoma 177, 221, 226

S

Sarcoma 114
Schistosomiasis 36, 139
Sclerosing peritonitis 47
Screening, targeted 8
Scrotal sac
  abnormalities 98, 153
    edema 177
    inflammatory disease, children 224
  vasculature 153–154
Sedation 72
Segmental testicular infarction 164
Seminal vesicles 133
  developmental anomalies 140
  drainage 149
Seminoma 160, 200
  treatment 200
Septa of Bertin 25
Septated cysts 103
Shrunken kidneys, bilateral 12
Sickle cell disease 40
Sperm granuloma 175
Spermatic cord 168
  spontaneous detorsion 170
  torsion 168–170
    children 224–225
    testicular appendage 170–171, 225–226
Spermatocele 175
Splenogonadal fusion 163–164

Staghorn calculi 124
Stauffer syndrome 96
Steal syndrome 50
Stenosis see Renal arteries
Stenting, ureteric 74–75
Systemic lupus erythematosus (SLE) 40

T

Tacrolimus toxicity 62, 65
Teratoma 161
Testicular prosthesis 166
Testicular rupture 167
Testicular tumors 98, 159–164
  children 226
  germ cell tumors 160–161, 199, 226
  investigation 244
  nongerm cell tumors 162–164
  staging system 200
  treatment 199–201
Testis 155–156
  abscess 165
  anatomy 153–154
    children 208
  atrophy 165
  congenital anomalies 223–224
  macrocalcification 166
  microlithiasis 166, 224
  normal variants 157–159
    appendix testis 156, 157, 158–159
    polyorchidism 159
    rete testis 158
    transmediastinal artery 157
    two-tone testis 158
  orchitis 165
  postoperative appearance 166
  segmental infarction 164
  torsion 98, 168–170
    children 224–225
    congenital 223–224
    spontaneous detorsion 170
    testicular appendage 170–171, 225–226
  trauma 97, 167, 226
  tumors see Testicular tumors
  ultrasound examination 155
Thrombosis
  arteriovenous fistula complications 49–50
  following renal transplantation 60–61
    arterial 60
    venous 60–61
  renal vein 38–39
    children 218–219
Transitional cell carcinomas (TTCs) 112–113, 126
  bladder 138–139, 241–242
    staging 242
Transmediastinal artery 157
Transplant artery stenosis 63–64
Transplant kidney 264
  hydronephrosis 264
  imaging 56–57

  postoperative monitoring 264–265
  renal artery stenosis 266–267
  renal masses 268
  vascular occlusion 266
Transplantation see Renal transplantation
Transrectal ultrasound (TRUS) 134–135
  benign prostatic hyperplasia 94, 141–142
  interventional 148–149, 197
  male infertility assessment 144
  prostate carcinoma 94–95, 144–147
  prostatitis 142
Transurethral resection of the prostate (TURP) 94
Trauma
  bladder 85, 97, 221
  genital 97, 189
  investigation 246–248
  pelvicalyceal 84
  renal 82–83, 96–97, 114–115
    children 218
    classification 114, 115
  testis 97, 167, 226
  ureters 84–85, 97
  vascular injuries 83–84
Tuberculosis 35
Tuberous sclerosis 108, 215
Tunica albuginea defect 188–189
Two-tone testis 158

U

Ultrasound contrast agents 253–254
  applications in transplant kidney 264–268
    postoperative monitoring 264–265
    potential applications 268
    renal masses 26
    vascular applications 266–267
  clinical applications 256–262
    acute urinary obstruction 260
    focal renal lesions 256–258
    functional renal imaging 261–262
    renal artery stenosis 259–260
  microbubble behavior 254–255
  nonlinear imaging modes 255–256
Ultrasound imaging 12, 17–27
  bladder 133–134
    interventional 140
  children 207
  congenital variants 25–27
  erectile dysfunction 183
  normal variants 24–25
  parenchymal diseases 29–30
  parenchymal thickness 19
  prostate gland 134–136
  renal collecting system 22–24
  renal echogenicity 19–20
  renal size 18–19
  renal vasculature 21–22
  technique 17–18
  testis 155

Ultrasound imaging
    transplant kidney 56–57
    urethra 190
Ultrasound-guided procedures 70–71
    drainage of perinephric collections 77–78
    nephrostomy 72–77
    radiofrequency ablation 80–82
    renal artery stenosis 79–80
    renal biopsy 78–79
    trauma and emergencies 82–85
        bladder injuries 85
        pelvicalyceal injuries 84
        priapism 85
        renal tract trauma 82–83
        renal vascular injuries 83–84
        ureteric injuries 84–85
Urachal anomalies 220
Ureteric colic 90
Ureteric jets 122
Ureteric stenting 74–75
Ureteroceles 125, 212
Ureteroneocystostomy 85
Ureters
    duplex 25, 209
    ectopic 125
    inflammatory disorders 127–128
    injuries 84–85, 97
    megaureters 126, 212
    tumors 126–127

Urethral gland, posterior (PUV) 211–212
Urethral ultrasound 190
Urethritis 89
Urinary bladder see Bladder
Urinary calculus disease 90–91
Urinary leak, following renal transplantation 61
Urinary tract infection (UTI) 89–90
    children 90, 213–214
    complicated 89
    following renal transplantation 65
    recurrent 8
    uncomplicated 89–90
    see also Infections
Urinary tract obstruction see Obstruction
Urine discoloration 8
Urine volume 7–8
Urodynamics 246

V

Varicocele 171
Vascular disorders 36–39
    children 218–219
    injuries 83–84
    see also Renal arteries
Vasectomy 171
Venous hypertension 50–51

Venous thrombosis
    following renal transplantation 60–61
    renal vein 38–39
        children 218–219
Vesicoureteric junction (VUJ) obstruction 211
Vesicoureteric reflux (VUR) 90, 125–126, 212
Volume measurements 18–19
Von Hippel-Lindau disease 108

W

Wegener granulomatosis 40
Wilms tumor 217
Woolfian duct anomalies 140

X

Xanthogranulomatous pyelonephritis 35, 214

Y

Yolk sac tumor 161

Radiology

www.thieme.com

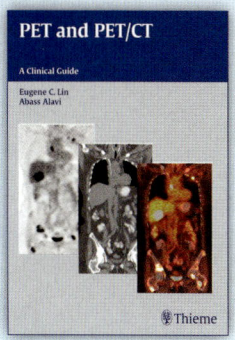

PET and PET/CT
A Clinical Guide
E. C. Lin, M.D.
A. Alavi, M.D.

© 2006, 200 pp., 227 illus.
softcover
ISBN-10: 3-13-141731-5
ISBN-13: 978-3-13-141731-2
€ 59.95

Presenting both oncological and nononcological applications, this book covers the full range of scenarios the clinician is likely to encounter in the professional setting. With a special focus on PET/CT correlation and FDG oncological imaging, this text addresses the important role of PET/CT in managing patients with brain neoplasms; thyroid cancer; breast cancer; gastric cancer; lymphoma; melanoma; pancreatic cancer; gynecological neoplasms; urological neoplasms; musculoskeletal neoplasms, and more. Each chapter in the Oncological Applications section of the text focuses on a particular disease, allowing the reader to quickly access the information relevant to managing a specific clinical situation. Thorough review of the existing scientific literature and pointers on how to interpret and report images provide readers with the tools to sharpen their assessment and decision-making skills.

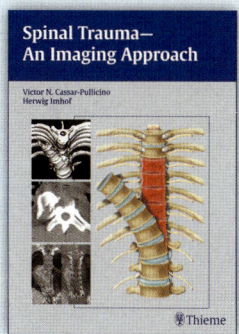

Spinal Trauma:
An Imaging Approach
V. N. Cassar-Pullicino, M.D.
H. Imhof, M.D.

© 2006, 224 pp., 250 illus.
hardcover
ISBN-10: 3-13-137471-3
ISBN-13: 978-3-13-137471-4
€ 119.95

The diagnosis of trauma to the spine-where the slightest oversight may have catastrophic results-requires a thorough grasp of the spectrum of resultant pathology as well as the imaging modalities used in making an accurate diagnosis.
In Spinal Trauma, the internationally renowned team of experts provides a comprehensive, cutting-edge exposition of the current vital role of imaging in the diagnosis and treatment of injuries to the axial skeleton. Beginning with a valuable clinical perspective of spinal trauma, the book offers the reader a unique overview of the biomechanics underlying the beautifully illustrated pathology of cervical trauma.

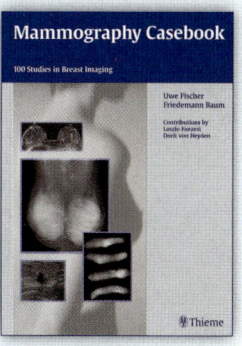

Mammography Casebook
U. Fischer, M.D.

© 2006, 360 pp., 1715 illus.
hardcover
ISBN-10: 3-13-140351-9
ISBN-13: 978-3-13-140351-3
€ 129.95

Mammography Casebook presents 100 case studies in breast imaging. In a unique step-by-step layout, the imaging presented is of superb quality and clarity and includes the full range of digital and conventional mammograms, ultrasound, panoramic ultrasound, color-coded Doppler sonography, and contrast-enhanced MR mammography. In the second part of each case the findings are analyzed and categorized according to BI-RADS criteria and standard terminology; differential diagnoses are considered and the correlation with the eventual histological results is examined. Where relevant, further procedures such as core biopsy and specimen radiography are shown in additional image sequences.
Finally, the unique lesson of each case is succinctly and memorably summarized. Both the experienced mammographer and the beginner in breast imaging will treasure this book as it extends their knowledge, confidence and diagnostic technique.

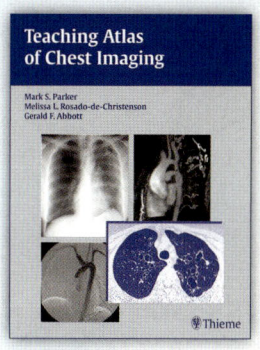

Teaching Atlas
of Chest Imaging
M. S. Parker, M.D.
M. L. R. De Christenson, M.D.
G. F. Abbott, M.D.

© 2006, 800 pp., 1064 illus.
hardcover
ISBN-10: 3-13-139021-2
ISBN-13: 978-3-13-139021-9
€ 129.95

With this book, you will learn to interpret chest images and recognize the imaging findings, generate an appropriate differential diagnosis, and understand the underlying disease process.
The atlas begins with a review of normal thoracic radiography, CT, and MR anatomy, and goes on to present cases on a wide range of congenital, traumatic, and acquired thoracic conditions. Each case is supported by a discussion of etiology, pathology, imaging findings, treatment, and prognosis in a concise, bullet format to give you a complete clinical overview of each disorder. Images demonstrate normal and pathologic findings, and complementary scans demonstrate additional imaging manifestations of disease entities.
A must for residents, fellows, and general radiologists, as well as thoracic radiologists, pulmonary physicians, and thoracic surgeons who have to read chest images.

Easy ways to order

Online: www.thieme.com
E-mail: custserv@thieme.de
Fax: +49 711 8931 410

Thieme International
P.O.Box 30 11 20
70451 Stuttgart
Germany

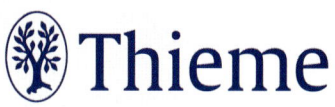

```
RC      Ultrasound of the
874       urogenital system.
.U47
2006
```

35010000521557

$129.95

DATE			

SOUTH UNIVERSITY
709 MALL BLVD.
SAVANNAH, GA 31406

BAKER & TAYLOR